Ultimate Review for the Neurology Boards

Ultimate Review for the Neurology Boards

Third Edition

EDITORS

Alexander D. Rae-Grant, MD

Staff, Mellen Center for Multiple Sclerosis
Director, Center for Continuing Education
Jane and Lee Seidman Chair for Advanced Neurological Education
Cleveland Clinic
Cleveland, Ohio

Seby John, MD

Cerebrovascular Center
Neurological Institute
Cleveland Clinic
Cleveland, Ohio

John A. Morren, MD/MBBS(Hons)

Clinical Assistant Professor of Medicine (Neurology)
Cleveland Clinic Lerner College of Medicine of Case Western Reserve University
Staff, Neuromuscular Center
Neurological Institute
Cleveland Clinic
Cleveland, Ohio

Hubert H. Fernandez, MD

Professor of Medicine (Neurology)
Cleveland Clinic Lerner College of Medicine
James and Constance Brown Endowed Chair in Movement Disorders
Center for Neurological Restoration
Cleveland Clinic
Cleveland, Ohio

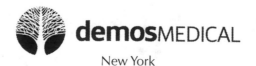

demosMEDICAL

New York

Visit our website at www.demosmedical.com

ISBN: 9781620700815
e-book ISBN: 9781617052590

Acquisitions Editor: Beth Barry
Compositor: S4Carlisle

Library of Congress Cataloging-in-Publication Data

Names: Fernandez, Hubert H., author. | Rae-Grant, Alexander, author. | John,
  Seby, author. | Morren, John Anthony, author.
Title: Ultimate review for the neurology boards / Alexander D. Rae-Grant,
  Seby John, John A. Morren, Hubert H. Fernandez.
Description: Third edition. | New York : Springer Publishing Company, [2016]
  | Hubert H. Fernandez's name appears first in the previous edition. |
  Includes bibliographical references and index.
Identifiers: LCCN 2016003524| ISBN 9781620700815 | ISBN 9781617052590 (e-book)
Subjects: | MESH: Nervous System Diseases | Neurology | Specialty Boards | Outlines
Classification: LCC RC343.6 | NLM WL 18.2 | DDC 616.80076—dc23 LC record available at
http://lccn.loc.gov/2016003524

Special discounts on bulk quantities of Demos Medical Publishing books are available to corporations, professional associations, pharmaceutical companies, health care organizations, and other qualifying groups. For details, please contact:

For details, please contact:
Special Sales Department
Demos Medical Publishing
11 West 42nd Street, 15th Floor, New York, NY 10036
Phone: 800-532-8663 or 212-683-0072; Fax: 212-941-7842
E-mail: specialsales@demosmedical.com

Printed in the United States of America by McNaughton & Gunn.
16 17 18 19 20 / 5 4 3 2 1

Contents

Contributors   *vii*
Preface   *ix*
Acknowledgments   *xi*

INTRODUCTION: PREPARING FOR YOUR BOARDS

I. How to Use This Book   *xiii*

II. Preparing for Your Board Examination   *xiv*

BASIC NEUROSCIENCES

1. Neurochemistry/Pharmacology   *1*

2. Neurogenetics   *23*

3. Neurohistology, Embryology, and Developmental Disorders   *51*

4. Clinical Neuroanatomy   *61*

CLINICAL NEUROLOGY

5. Stroke   *115*

6. Head Trauma   *139*

7. Neurocritical Care   *147*

8. Dementia   *167*

9. Headache Syndromes   *179*

10. Neuromuscular Disorders   *185*

11. Epilepsy and Related Disorders   *249*

12. Movement Disorders   *301*

13. Demyelinating Disorders   *327*

14. Infections of the Nervous System   *337*

15. Neurotoxicology and Nutritional Disorders   *375*

16. Sleep and Sleep Disorders   *391*

NEUROPHYSIOLOGY

17.   Nerve Conduction Studies (NCS) and Electromyography (EMG)   *401*

18.   Electroencephalography (EEG)   *415*

19.   Evoked Potentials   *429*

20.   Sleep Neurology   *449*

PEDIATRIC NEUROLOGY

21.   Pediatric Neurology   *461*

SUBSPECIALTIES

22.   Neurourology   *493*

23.   Neuro-ophthalmology   *499*

24.   Neuro-otology   *525*

25.   Neurorehabilitation   *531*

26.   Neuroendocrinology   *535*

27.   Neuro-oncology and Transplant Neurology   *541*

28.   Adult Psychiatry   *561*

29.   Child Psychiatry   *595*

30.   Neurobehavior and Neuropsychology   *607*

50 PRACTICE QUESTIONS WITH ANSWERS

Practice Questions and Answers   *621*

Index   *639*

Contributors

Russell Cerejo, MD
Fellow, Cerebrovascular Fellow
Neurological Institute
Cleveland Clinic
Cleveland, Ohio
Chapter 5: Stroke

Marisa Clifton, MD
Fellow, Female Pelvic Medicine and Reconstructive
    Surgery
Glickman Urological Institute
Cleveland Clinic
Cleveland, Ohio
Chapter 22: Neurourology

Mita Deoras, MD
Fellow, Sleep Disorders Center
Neurological Institute
Cleveland Clinic
Cleveland, Ohio
Chapter 16: Sleep and Sleep Disorders

Rachel Donaldson, DO
Fellow, Neuromuscular Center
Neurological Institute
Cleveland Clinic
Cleveland, Ohio
*Chapter 3: Neurohistology, Embryology, and
    Developmental Disorders*

Richard Drake, PhD
Director of Anatomy, Professor of Surgery
Lerner College of Medicine
Cleveland Clinic
Cleveland, Ohio
Chapter 4: Clinical Neuroanatomy

Camilo Garcia, MD
Epilepsy Center
Neurological Institute
Cleveland Clinic Florida
Weston, Florida
Chapter 18: Electroencephalography (EEG)

Joao Gomes, MD
Attending, Vascular Neurology and Neurocritical Care
Summa Health
Akron, Ohio
Chapter 7: Neurocritical Care

Pravin George, DO
Fellow, Neurosciences Critical Care Unit
Johns Hopkins University
Baltimore, Maryland
Chapter 6: Head Trauma
Chapter 7: Neurocritical Care

Gary Hsich, MD
Center for Pediatric Neurology
Department of Neurology
Neurological Institute
Cleveland Clinic
Cleveland, Ohio
Chapter 21: Pediatric Neurology

Ahmed Itrat, MD
Fellow, Cerebrovascular Center
Neurological Institute
Cleveland Clinic
Cleveland, Ohio
Chapter 27: Neuro-oncology and Transplant Neurology

M. Cecilia Lansang, MD
Associate Professor of Medicine, Cleveland Clinic Lerner
    College of Medicine
Department of Endocrinology
Cleveland Clinic
Cleveland, Ohio
Chapter 26: Neuroendocrinology

Lisa Lystad, MD
Division of Neuro-ophthalmology
Cole Eye Institute
Cleveland Clinic
Cleveland, Ohio
Chapter 23: Neuro-ophthalmology

Jennifer M. McBride, PhD
Director of Histology, Associate Professor of
    Surgery
Lerner College of Medicine
Cleveland Clinic
Cleveland, Ohio
Chapter 4: Clinical Neuroanatomy

Jhanvi Menon, MD
Fellow, Neuromuscular Center
Neurological Institute
Cleveland Clinic
Cleveland, Ohio
*Chapter 15: Neurotoxicology and Nutritional
    Disorders*

Lileth Mondok, MD
Center for Pediatric Neurology
Department of Neurology
Neurological Institute
Cleveland Clinic
Cleveland, Ohio
Chapter 21: Pediatric Neurology

Courtenay K. Moore, MD
Associate Professor of Surgery, Cleveland Clinic Lerner
    College of Medicine
Fellowship Director, Female Pelvic Medicine and
    Reconstructive Surgery
Glickman Urological Institute
Cleveland Clinic
Cleveland, Ohio
Chapter 22: Neurourology

John A. Morren, MD/MBBS(Hons)
Clinical Assistant Professor of Medicine
    (Neurology)
Cleveland Clinic Lerner College of Medicine of Case
    Western Reserve University
Staff, Neuromuscular Center
Neurological Institute
Cleveland Clinic
Cleveland, Ohio
*Chapter 17: Nerve Conduction Studies (NCS) and
    Electromyography (EMG)*
Chapter 19: Evoked Potentials
Chapter 20: Sleep Neurology
Chapter 10: Neuromuscular Disorders

Oluwadamilola (Lara) Ojo, MD
Fellow, Center for Neurological Restoration
Neurological Institute
Cleveland Clinic
Cleveland, Ohio
Chapter 12: Movement Disorders

Shnehal Patel, MD, MPH
Fellow, Center for Neurological Restoration
Neurological Institute
Cleveland Clinic
Cleveland, Ohio
Chapter 25: Neurorehabilitation
Chapter 30: Neurobehavior and Neuropsychology

Gregory Pontone, MD
Assistant Professor
Department of Psychiatry and Behavioral Sciences
Johns Hopkins University School of Medicine
Baltimore, Maryland
Chapter 28: Adult Psychiatry
Chapter 29: Child Psychiatry

Alexander D. Rae-Grant, MD
Staff, Mellen Center for Multiple Sclerosis
Director, Center for Continuing Education
Jane and Lee Seidman Chair for Advanced Neurological
    Education
Cleveland Clinic
Cleveland, Ohio
Chapter 8: Dementia
Chapter 11: Epilepsy and Related Disorders
Chapter 13: Demyelinating Disorders

Ian Rossman, MD, PhD
Fellow, Neuroimmunology; Pediatric Neurologist
Mellen Center for Multiple Sclerosis; Center for Pediatric
    Neuroscience
Neurological Institute
Cleveland Clinic
Cleveland, Ohio
Chapter 2: Neurogenetics

Aasef Shaik, MD, PhD
Fellow, Center for Neurological Restoration
Neurological Institute
Cleveland Clinic
Cleveland, Ohio
Chapter 1: Neurochemistry/Pharmacology
Chapter 24: Neuro-otology

Lakshmi Shankar, MD
Fellow, Cerebrovascular Center
Neurological Institute
Cleveland Clinic
Cleveland, Ohio
Chapter 14: Infections of the Nervous System

Qingshan Teng, MD, MS
Fellow, Neuromuscular Center
Neurological Institute
Cleveland Clinic
Cleveland, Ohio
Chapter 9: Headache Syndromes

Preface

Ultimate Review for the Neurology Boards, Third Edition, continues the tradition of providing a brief but comprehensive source for study or simply review. The authors and editors have tried hard to include the most up-to-date material while keeping the verbiage to a minimum. We have followed a point form outline style where possible, also including tables and lists where long paragraphs would be problematic. A brief Cheat Sheet at the end of most chapters provides a simple quick study section for key facts or potential "board question" information, often those tricky eponyms that we all learn and rapidly forget. We have included some suggested readings for those who want to dive deeper into a review, but have not exhaustively referenced the chapters for the sake of space and clarity. Finally, there are 50 all-new questions with answers and explanations at the end of the book for self-assessment.

The editors hope this text will provide a useful tool to students of neurology at multiple levels, and will help in review for whatever neurological examination looms in the future for the reader.

Alexander D. Rae-Grant
Seby John
John A. Morren
Hubert H. Fernandez

Acknowledgments

The editors would like to acknowledge the support of Christine Moore, our editorial assistant, who valiantly assisted in organizing authors, managing editors, modifying manuscripts, and generally making the entire contraption function.

Thanks go to our authors, who carefully reviewed and updated the chapters to reflect recent changes in understanding of disease and approaches to treatment within the bounds of the *Ultimate* review format.

We would like to acknowledge the support of the leadership of the Neurological Institute at the Cleveland Clinic for encouraging our authors and editors to contribute to clinical pedagogy.

We would also like to thank our editor, Beth Barry, at Demos for her assistance and support during the editing of this third edition of *Ultimate Review for the Neurology Boards.*

The editors would also like to thank their loving wives (Mary Bruce, Ritika, Divya, and Cecilia) and their wonderful children (Michael, Tucker, George, Sasha, Jordan, and Annella Marie) for their unconditional support and understanding during this process.

Alexander D. Rae-Grant
Seby John
John A. Morren
Hubert H. Fernandez

INTRODUCTION

Preparing for Your Boards

I. How to Use This Book

Neurology covers a broad spectrum of disease processes and complex neuroanatomy, neurophysiology, and neuropathology. Moreover, your certification examination will also include psychiatry and other neurologic subspecialties such as neuro-ophthalmology, neuro-otology, and neuroendocrinology, to name a few. Covering all of the possible topics for these boards is not only impossible, it is impractical. Although this book is entitled *Ultimate Review for the Neurology Boards*, it is not intended to be your single source of study material in preparing for your examination. Rather, it presumes that throughout your residency training, or at the very least, several months before your board examination date, you will have already read primary references and textbooks (and, therefore, carry a considerable fund of knowledge) on the specific broad categories of neurology. Because you cannot possibly retain all the information you have assimilated, we offer this book as a convenient way of tying it all together. The point-form information will help you recall specific facts, associations, and clues that may help with answering questions correctly.

Ultimate Review for the Neurology Boards contains detailed chapters on subjects included on the neurology board examination.

For maximal retention within the shortest amount of time, we have used an expanded outline format in this manual.

The main headings and subtopics are in **bold**. A few phrases or a short paragraph is spent on subtopics that we think are of particular importance. Crucial or essential data within the outlines are *italicized* or in **bold**. Thus, we present three levels of learning in each chapter. We suggest that you first read the entire chapter, including the brief sentences on each subtopic. After the first reading, you should go back a second time, focusing only on the headings and subtopics in **bold** and the *italicized* words within the outline. If you need to go back a third time to test yourself, or, alternatively, if you feel you already have a solid fund of knowledge on a certain topic, you can just concentrate on the backbone outline in **bold** to make sure you have, indeed, retained everything.

Whenever appropriate, illustrations are liberally sprinkled throughout the text to tap into your "visual memory." Quick pearls (such as mnemonics to remember long lists and confusing terminology, tables to organize a complex body of information) and high-yield topics are preceded with this symbol "**NB:**" (for *nota bene,* Latin for "note well"), to make sure you do not miss them. We have added a few suggested readings where pertinent to help you extend your learning both for the exams and for your education.

Some chapters overlap. For example, some diseases discussed in the chapter on pediatric neurology and the chapter on neurogenetics can also be found in the individual chapters of the Clinical Neurology section. This overlap is intended to maximize memory retention through repetition.

We have included 50 questions at the end of the book to help you practice for the tests. One of the best preparation methods for taking exams is practicing the exam situation over and over. We hope these questions will give you a chance to try out your hand at answering questions.

Good luck, and we hope you pass your boards in one attempt!

II. Preparing for Your Board Examination

Although most residents initially feel that after a busy residency training it is better to "take a break" and postpone their certification examination, we believe that, in general, it is best to take your examination right after residency, when "active" and "passive" learning are at their peak. There will never be "a perfect time" (or "enough time") to review for your boards. The board examination is a present-day reality that you will need to prepare for whether you are exhausted, in private practice, expecting your first child, renovating your newly purchased 80-year-old house, or burning candles in your research laboratory. You just need to squeeze in the time to study. Luckily, all the others taking these tests are in the same boat, so you are not alone!

Here are a few pointers to help you prepare for the board examination. All or some of them may be applicable to you:

A. Board preparation starts from day 1 of your residency training. Although most residency programs are clinically oriented and have a case-based structure of learning, here are some suggestions as to how you can create an "active" learning process out of your clinical training, rather than just passively learning from your patients and being content with acquiring clinical skills.

1. Imagine you are on your sixth month of a boring ward rotation carrying eight patients on your service. The following table contains the diagnoses of your patients in the neurology ward and the reading initiative we recommend. The point here is to use your patient caseload to suggest topic areas for review. Our experience is that case-based learning "sticks" better than starting on page one of any textbook.

PATIENT	DIAGNOSIS	READING INITIATIVE
1	Thalamic lacunar stroke	Master the anatomy of the thalamus.
2	Embolic stroke	Become familiar with the literature on the use of heparin versus aspirin.
3	Guillain-Barré syndrome	Master the differential diagnosis of axonal versus demyelinating polyneuropathy.
4	Amyotrophic lateral sclerosis	Master the differential diagnosis of motor neuron diseases.
5	25-year-old with stroke, unclear etiology	Master the data on stroke risk factors.
6	Seizure breakthrough for overnight observation	Know all the mechanisms of action of antiepileptic agents.
7	Hemorrhagic stroke	Know and be able to differentiate the MRI picture of a hyperacute, acute, subacute, and chronic bleed.
8	Glioblastoma	Know the pathology of all glial tumors.

2. Always carry a small notebook that fits in your coat pocket so you can write down all the questions and observations that may arise in the course of your day. If possible, do not sleep without answering those questions. Likewise, jot down all the new information you have learned. Read through these notes one more time before you call it a night.

3. Follow your grand rounds schedule. Read the topic(s) beforehand. This will help you in two ways: (a) the talk itself will serve as reinforcement because you already read about it; and (b) you can ask more intelligent questions that will, at the very least, impress your colleagues and mentors, if not make you learn and appreciate neurology even more.

4. For the driven resident: have a monthly schedule of books or book chapters to read. Maximize your reading on your light or elective rotations. On the average, a "good" resident reads 25 to 50 pages per day (from journals, notes, books, etc.). If you read more than 50 pages per day, you are driven and will be rewarded with an almost effortless board review period. If you read less than 10 pages per day, or, even worse, are an occasional reader, you are relying on passive learning and will need to make up a lot of lost time (and knowledge) during your board review.

B. Take your Residency In-Service Training Examination (RITE)/in-service examination seriously. If possible, prepare for it weeks in advance. People who do well every year are the ones who pass their written board examination on the first attempt.

C. Know all board examination requirements several months before you finish your residency training. Know all the deadlines. READ THE INSTRUCTIONS CAREFULLY! Check the name on your identification and the name on your admission slip to make sure they are identical. Contact the American Board of Psychiatry and Neurology (ABPN) if they are not. Ideally, you should be distracted as little as possible when your examination date approaches.

D. Start your formal board review midway (that is, January 2) of your senior year. Make a general, realistic schedule. Do not make it too ambitious or too detailed. Otherwise, you will find yourself frustrated and always catching up to your schedule. As we mentioned, there will never be a perfect time to study for your boards—you need to create your own time. Consider working with a study group, which will provide peer support and pressure to continue studying.

E. In general, start with topics you know the most about (and, therefore, are least likely to forget), such as clinical neurology, and end with topics you know the least about (and, thus, are more likely to forget in a short amount of time), such as neurogenetics, metabolic disorders, neuroanatomy, neurochemistry, and so forth.

F. Use your book allowance wisely. Read and underline books during residency that fit your taste and that you are likely to use for your board review. Underlined books are less overwhelming, provide a sense of security that you have already been through the material (even if you have forgotten its contents), make review time more efficient, and significantly reinforce learning and retention.

G. End your formal review at least 2 weeks before the date of your written boards. Earmark 1 week for the psychiatry portion (do not forget to read on child psychiatry topics) and 1 week for recapping high-yield topics, reviewing questions and answers, looking at radiology and pathology pictures, and reading the answers to past RITE/in-service examinations (they do repeat!).

H. Arrive at your examination site city at least 24 hours before the exam. You do not want to realize on the day of your examination that your hotel reservation was inadvertently misplaced or that your flight was canceled because of a snow storm. Make sure your cell phone is fully charged and that you have your driver's license with you. DO AS MUCH AS YOU CAN BEFOREHAND SO YOU DON'T HAVE TO WORRY ABOUT DETAILS.

I. You might consider bringing ear plugs, an extra sweater, and a reliable watch. When one of us took our boards in the basement of a hospital, there was a general announcement through the public-address system every 30 minutes. We have heard different stories: the heater was not working, a dog convention was going on in the next room, and so forth. **It is best to be prepared.**

J. If this is the second or third time you are taking the boards, consider the benefits of a small study group or having a study partner. You will be amazed that two or three people assigned the same topic to read will emphasize different items. It could very well be that you are underlining the wrong words and need someone to give you a different perspective. At the very least, a study group will keep you on pace with your schedule.

Basic Neurosciences

CHAPTER 1

Neurochemistry/Pharmacology

I. Neurotransmitters (NTs) and Receptors

A. Miscellaneous

1. *Three major categories of NTs*
   a. **Amino acids**
      i. *Glutamate*
      ii. *γ-Aminobutyric acid (GABA)*
      iii. *Aspartic acid*
      iv. *Glycine*
   b. **Peptides**
      i. *Vasopressin*
      ii. *Somatostatin*
      iii. *Neurotensin*
   c. **Monoamines**
      i. *Norepinephrine (NE)*
      ii. *Dopamine (DA)*
      iii. *Serotonin (5-hydroxytryptamine [5-HT])*
      iv. *Acetylcholine (ACh)*
2. Monoamine NTs are nearly always (with a few exceptions) inhibitory.
3. *ACh is the major NT in the peripheral nervous system (the only other peripheral NT being NE).*
4. *Major NTs of the brain are glutamate and GABA.*
5. Peptides perform specialized functions in the hypothalamus and other regions.

A. **Miscellaneous** (*cont'd*)

   6. *Peripheral nervous system has only two NTs:*

     a. ACh

     b. NE

   7. *Excitatory NTs*

     a. Glutamate

     b. Aspartate

     c. Cystic acid

     d. Homocystic acid

   8. *Inhibitory NTs*

     a. GABA

     b. Glycine

     c. Taurine

     d. β-Alanine

   9. *Excitatory/inhibitory pairs*

     a. Glutamate (+): GABA (−) in the brain

     b. Aspartate (+): glycine (−) in the ventral spinal cord

B. **ACh**

   1. Miscellaneous

     a. First NT discovered

     b. The major NT in the peripheral nervous system

       i. *Provides direct innervation of skeletal muscles*

       ii. *Provides innervation of smooth muscles of the parasympathetic nervous system*

     c. Major locations of ACh

       i. *Autonomic ganglia*

       ii. *Parasympathetic postganglionic synapses*

       iii. *Neuromuscular junction (NMJ)*

       iv. *Renshaw cells of spinal cord*

     d. Roles of ACh

       i. *Thermal receptors*

       ii. *Chemoreceptors*

       iii. *Taste*

       iv. *Pain perception (possibly)*

     e. Primarily (but not always) an *excitatory* NT

     f. Main effect of ACh on pyramidal cells is via muscarinic receptor-mediated depletion of K^+ currents, which results in hyperexcitability

     g. Most dietary choline comes from phosphatidyl choline found in the membranes of plants and animals.

     h. Phosphatidyl choline is converted to choline, which is then transported across the blood-brain barrier.

     i. Acetylcoenzyme A and choline are independently synthesized in the neuronal cell body and independently transported along the axon to the synapse in which they are conjugated into Ach.

   2. Synthesis: *Rate limiting: supply of choline*

   3. Release

    a. Voltage-gated calcium channel is open as the action potential (AP) reaches the terminal button of the presynaptic neuron, producing an influx of calcium ions that allows exocytosis of presynaptic vesicles containing ACh into the synaptic cleft.

    b. The activation of postsynaptic ACh receptors results in an influx of Na^+ into the cell and an efflux of K^+, which depolarizes the postsynaptic neuron, propagating a new AP.

4. Receptors

    a. Muscarinic receptors

        i. *Subtypes*

            (A) *M1, 3, 5: activate phosphatidyl inositide hydroxylase*

            (B) *M2, 4: inhibit adenyl cyclase*

        ii. *Agonists*

            (A) Bethanecol

            (B) Carbachol

            (C) Pilocarpine

            (D) Methacholine

            (E) Muscarine (from *Amanita* mushroom)

        iii. *Antagonists*

            (A) Atropine

            (B) Scopolamine

            (C) Trihexyphenidyl

    b. Nicotinic receptors

        i. *Antagonists (nondepolarizing)*

            (A) Tubocurarine

            (B) Atracurium

            (C) α-Neurotoxin of sea snakes

            (D) Procainamide

            (E) Aminoglycoside antibiotics

        ii. *Antagonists (depolarizing)*

            (A) Succinylcholine

        iii. *Receptor inactivation*

            (A) Myasthenia gravis

        iv. *Receptor deficiency*

            (A) Congenital myasthenia gravis

        v. *ACh release augmentation*

            (A) Black widow spider latrotoxin

        vi. *ACh release blockade*

            (A) Botulism

            (B) Lambert-Eaton syndrome

            (C) Tick paralysis

            (D) β-Neurotoxin of sea snakes

    c. Specific locations of muscarinic and nicotinic receptors

        i. Both nicotinic and muscarinic

            (A) *Central nervous system (CNS) (muscarinic > nicotinic receptor concentrations)*

      i. Both nicotinic and muscarinic (*cont'd*)

        (B) *All sympathetic and parasympathetic preganglionic synapses*

      ii. *Muscarinic only*

        (A) *All postganglionic parasympathetic terminals*

        (B) *Postganglionic sympathetic sweat glands*

      iii. *Nicotinic only*

        (A) *NMJ*

        (B) *Adrenal medulla*

      iv. In brain: muscarinic $>$ nicotinic

5. Vesicle transport

    a. SNARE proteins:

      i. Mediate docking of synaptic vesicles with the presynaptic membrane

      ii. Targets of the bacterial neurotoxins responsible for botulism and tetanus

    b. SNAP-25:

      i. Synaptosomal-associated protein 25 (SNAP-25) accounts for the membrane fusion (bringing the synaptic vesicle and plasma membranes together).

      ii. Botulinum toxins A, C, and E cleave SNAP-25, leading to muscle paralysis as intended in clinically induced botulism.

6. Inactivation

    a. Metabolism

      i. Within synaptic cleft by acetylcholinesterase

      ii. Acetylcholinesterase found at nerve endings is anchored to the plasma membrane through a glycolipid.

7. *Cholinergic agonists*

AGONISTS	SOURCE	MODE OF ACTION
Nicotine	Alkaloid prevalent in the tobacco plant	Activates nicotinic class of ACh receptors, locks the channel open
Muscarine	Alkaloid produced by *Amanita muscaria* mushrooms	Activates muscarinic class of ACh receptors
α-Latrotoxin	Protein produced by the black widow spider	Induces massive ACh release, possibly by acting as a Ca^{2+} ionophore

8. *Cholinergic antagonists*

ANTAGONISTS	SOURCE	MODE OF ACTION
Atropine/ scopolamine	Alkaloid produced by the deadly nightshade, *Atropa belladonna*	Blocks ACh actions only at muscarinic receptors
Botulinum toxin	Eight proteins produced by *Clostridium botulinum*	Inhibits the release of ACh
β-Bungarotoxin	Protein produced by *Bungarus* genus of snakes	Prevents ACh receptor channel opening
d-Tubocurarine	Active ingredient of curare	Prevents ACh receptor channel opening at motor end plate

9. *Specific agonist/antagonist action*

    a. *Presynaptic NMJ release blockade*

        i. Botulinum toxin: block presynaptic vesicle mobility (see Sections 5.a and b)

        ii. Lambert-Eaton syndrome: block presynaptic Ca^{2+} channels

        iii. Sea snake venom

    b. *Postsynaptic NMJ receptor blockade*

        i. Myasthenia gravis: ACh receptor antibody

        ii. Succinylcholine: depolarizing blockade

        iii. Curare: nondepolarizing blockade

        iv. α-Bungarotoxin: irreversible ACh receptor blockade

10. *Anticholinesterases*

    a. *Reversible*

        i. Neostigmine

        ii. Pyridostigmine

        iii. Physostigmine

        iv. Donepezil, galantamine, rivastigmine, tacrine

    b. *Irreversible*

        i. With irreversible anticholinesterases, receptors can be regenerated with pralidoxime (peripherally) and atropine (centrally).

        ii. Agents

            (A) Organophosphates

            (B) Carbamates

            (C) Nerve gas

11. *Conditions/medications that increase ACh concentration*

    a. Acetylcholinesterase inhibitors

        i. Pyridostigmine

        ii. Physostigmine

        iii. Edrophonium

        iv. Donepezil, galantamine, rivastigmine, tacrine

        v. Organophosphates

        vi. Black widow venom

        vii. β-Bungarotoxin

    b. Enhances of neurotransmission

        i. Pyridostigmine

        ii. 3,4-diaminopyridine

C. Catecholamines

1. Miscellaneous

    a. *Principal catecholamines*

        i. *NE*

        ii. *Epinephrine*

        iii. *DA*

    b. Synthesis

    c. Tyrosine (TYR) transported to catecholamine-secreting neurons in which it is converted into DA, NE, and epinephrine

1. Miscellaneous (*cont'd*)

   d. Direct innervation of the sympathetic nervous system (except for sweat glands) due to NE

   e. *β-Noradrenergic receptors inhibit feeding, whereas α receptors stimulate feeding.*

2. **DA**

   a. Miscellaneous

      i. 3 to 4 times more dopaminergic cells in the CNS than adrenergic cells

      ii. DA made in the substantia nigra: *neurons in the pars compacta of the substantia nigra account for 80% of DA in the brain; neuromelanin is a DA polymer that makes the substantia nigra appear dark.*

      iii. Highest concentration of DA: striatum (caudate and putamen)—although made in the substantia nigra, is transported to the striatum from the substantia nigra in vesicles

      iv. Two primary DA-receptor types found in striatum: D1 (stimulatory) and D2 (inhibitory)

      v. D2 receptors are found predominantly on dopaminergic neurons functioning primarily as autoreceptors to inhibit DA synthesis and release.

      vi. *Four main dopaminergic tracts*

         (A) The *nigrostriatal tract* accounts for most of the brain's DA.

         (B) The *tuberoinfundibular tract* controls release of prolactin via D2 receptors.

         (C) *The mesolimbic tract*

         (D) *The mesocortical tract*

      vii. Parkinson's disease develops when striatal DA is depleted by $>$80% ($<$20% of original concentration remaining)

	SCHIZOPHRENIA	PARKINSON'S DISEASE	HUNTINGTON'S DISEASE
DA transporter	Normal	Decreased (midbrain DA also decreased)	—
D1 receptor	Normal	Increased	Decreased
D2 receptor	Increased in caudate and putamen	Increased	Decreased
Linkage between D1 and D2	Decreased	Normal with treatment	Decreased

   b. *Synthesis*

      i. *Rate-limiting step: TYR hydroxylase conversion to L-dopa*

      ii. DA is feedback inhibitor

      iii. TYR

         (A) Not an essential amino acid because it can be synthesized in the liver from phenylalanine

         (B) Cannot be synthesized in the brain

         (C) Must enter the brain by the large neutral amino acid transporter, which transports TYR, phenylalanine, tryptophan, methionine, and the branch-chained amino acids

      iv. L-TYR converted to L-dopa within the brain

      v. DA is synthesized in the cytoplasm.

c. Receptors

   i. The receptor that determines whether the transmitter is excitatory or inhibitory

   ii. *D1 receptor (subtypes D1 and D5)*

     (A) *Postsynaptic receptors*

       (1) *Excitatory*

       (2) *Stimulates cyclic adenosine monophosphate (cAMP)*

     (B) D1 receptor: ↑ adenylate cyclase

     (C) D1-receptor activation is required for full postsynaptic expression of D2 effects

   iii. *D2 receptor (subtypes D2, D3, and D4)*

     (A) *Presynaptic receptor: inhibitory (high affinity)*

     (B) *Postsynaptic receptor*

       (1) *Inhibitory (low affinity)*

       (2) *Genetic polymorphisms exist for the D4 receptor that may provide basis for genetic-based schizophrenia*

   iv. *Tardive dyskinesia may be due to supersensitivity of DA receptors that have been chronically clocked (i.e., psychotropic agents)*

   v. Tuberoinfundibular DA system: regulated by prolactin

d. Inactivation

   i. Reuptake

     (A) Presynaptic intraneuronal monoamine oxidase (MAO) converts DA → 3,4-dihydroxyphenylacetic acid (DOPAC)

     (B) Extraneuronal MAO and catechol-O-methyltransferase convert DA → homovanillic acid; CNS DA metabolite: homovanillic acid

3. **NE**

a. Miscellaneous

   i. Neuropeptide Y: co-localized with NE in sympathetic nerve terminals, innervating blood vessels

   ii. *Most concentrated in CNS within locus ceruleus of the pons followed by lateral tegmental area*

   iii. Electrical stimulation of the locus ceruleus produces arousal.

   iv. Benzodiazepines decrease firing in the locus ceruleus, which reduces release of NE to rest of brain, causing relaxation and sedation.

   v. *Antidepressant effect of MAO inhibitors (MAOIs) is more related to NE than to DA.*

b. Synthesis

   i. *Rate-limiting step*

     (A) *TYR hydroxylase*

     (B) NE is feedback inhibitor.

   ii. NE is synthesized in the storage vesicles.

   iii. TYR hydroxylase is inhibited by α-methyl-p-TYR.

c. Release and vesicle storage

   i. Calcium influx with depolarization

   ii. Amphetamines increase release.

      c. Release and vesicle storage (*cont'd*)

         iii. Inhibition of transport

            (A) Reserpine

            (B) Tetrabenazine

         iv. NE is displaced from vesicles by:

            (A) Amphetamine

            (B) Ephedrine

    d. *Receptors*

       i. *α-1*

          (A) *Postsynaptic*

          (B) *Most sensitive to epinephrine*

          (C) *Blocked by prazosin and clonidine*

       ii. *α-2*

          (A) *Presynaptic*

          (B) *Inhibits adenyl cyclase via G-protein effects*

          (C) *Inhibited by yohimbine and clonidine*

    e. Inactivation

       i. Metabolism

          (A) Catechol-O-methyltransferase in synaptic cleft

          (B) Reuptake

             (1) Primary mode of NE termination

             (2) *Reuptake inhibited by:*

                (a) Cocaine

                (b) Tricyclic antidepressants (TCAs) (desipramine)

                (c) Tetracyclic antidepressant (maprotiline)

                (d) Selective serotonin reuptake inhibitors (SSRIs)

  f. Other medication effects

       i. *Lithium*

          (A) *Decreases NE release*

          (B) *Increases NE reuptake*

4. Epinephrine

  a. Miscellaneous

       i. *Epinephrine is found with NE in:*

          (A) *Lateral tegmental system*

          (B) *Dorsal medulla*

          (C) *Dorsal motor nucleus*

          (D) *Locus ceruleus*

  b. Synthesis: epinephrine synthesis occurs only in adrenal medulla via phenylethanolamine N-methyltransferase.

5. Medications

  a. *Catecholamine agonists/antagonists*

       i. *Neuroleptics*

          (A) *Based on D2- and D4-receptor antagonism in the mesolimbic and mesocortical pathways*

          (B) *Antagonism of nigrostriatal pathways produces extrapyramidal side effects.*

          (C) Antagonism in the chemoreceptor trigger zone produces antiemetic effect.

(D) *Older neuroleptics mainly block D2 receptor but can block multiple DA receptors.*

(E) D2 affinity correlates to efficacy.

(F) *Clozapine*

    (1) *Neuroleptic that is more selective for the D1 and D4 receptors; also binds to:* 5-HT$_2$ *receptor,* α_1-*adrenergic receptor, muscarinic receptor, histamine (histamine$_1$) receptor*

    (2) DA neurons in ventral tegmentum develop depolarization inactivation, but neurons in the substantia nigra do not have this effect (i.e., minimal parkinsonism).

  ii. *Amphetamines*

    (A) *Increase release of DA and NE centrally and peripherally*

    (B) *Decrease reuptake of DA*

  iii. *MAOIs: decrease metabolism of DA*

  iv. *Cocaine: blocks reuptake of DA and NE*

  v. *TCAs: block reuptake of DA*

  vi. *Reserpine and tetrabenazine: prevent vesicle storage of DA, epinephrine, and 5-HT, both centrally and peripherally*

  vii. *Selegiline and rasagiline: MAO$_B$ inhibitor, increasing DA stores*

D. 5-HT

  1. Miscellaneous

    a. An *indolamine*

    b. Most prominent effects on cardiovascular system, with additional effects in the respiratory system and the intestines

    c. *Vasoconstriction is a classic response to the administration of 5-HT.*

    d. Only 1% to 2% of 5-HT in the body is in the brain; widely distributed in platelets, mast cells, etc.; greatest concentration of 5-HT (90%) is found in the enterochromaffin cells of the gastrointestinal tract.

    e. *High concentration in CNS found in:*

      i. *Raphe nuclei that project to the limbic system*

      ii. *Pons/upper brainstem*

      iii. *Area postrema*

      iv. *Caudal locus ceruleus*

      v. *Interpeduncular nucleus*

      vi. *Facial (cranial nerve VII) nucleus*

    f. *Raphe nuclei*

      i. *5-HT neurons are located in the CNS.*

      ii. Projects caudally mainly to the medulla and spinal cord for the regulation of pain

      iii. Projects rostrally to the limbic structures and the cerebral cortex

      iv. Stimulation produces similar effects as lysergic acid diethylamine (LSD)

    g. *5-HT and NE regulate arousal.*

    h. *Low 5-HT associated with anxiety and impulsive behavior*

      i. *5-HT syndrome*

      ii. *SSRI + MAOI*

      iii. *Clinical: restlessness, tremor, myoclonus, hyperreflexia, diarrhea, diaphoresis, confusion, and possible death*

h. *Low 5-HT associated with anxiety and impulsive behavior (cont'd)*

  iv. *Must wait 2 to 3 weeks after stopping MAOI before initiating SSRI*

  v. *Must wait 5 weeks after stopping SSRI before initiating MAOI*

2. *Synthesis*

  a. *Rate-limiting step: tryptophan hydroxylase*

  b. *5-HT in the brain is independently synthesized from tryptophan transported across the blood-brain barrier.*

3. Receptors

RECEPTOR	LINKED TO/ASSOCIATIONS	AGONIST	ANTAGONIST
$5\text{-}HT_{1a}$	G-protein → inhibit adenyl cyclase	Buspirone	None
$5\text{-}HT_{1b/1d}$, both act as autoreceptors	G-protein → inhibit adenyl cyclase	Sumatriptan ($5\text{-}HT_{1d}$)	None
$5\text{-}HT_{1C}$	G-protein → increase DAG and IP_3	LSD α-Methyl-5-HT	Ritanserin Pizotifen Clozapine
$5\text{-}HT_2$	G-protein → increase DAG and IP_3	LSD α-Methyl-5-HT	Ritanserin Pizotifen Clozapine
$5\text{-}HT_3$	Ion channel	2-α-5-HT	Metoclopramide Ondansetron (potent) Cocaine (weak)

Abbreviation: DAG: dimeric acidic glycoprotein.

  a. Most receptors are coupled to G proteins that affect the activities of adenylate cyclase or phospholipase C.

  b. *5-HT₁ receptor function*

    i. *Thermoregulation*

    ii. *Sexual behavior*

    iii. *Hypotension*

  c. *5-HT₂ receptor function*

    i. *Vascular contraction*

    ii. *Platelet aggregation*

  d. *5-HT₃ receptor function: ion channels*

4. Inactivation

  a. Metabolism

  b. Reuptake

    i. Primary mode of inactivation

    ii. Mechanism similar to NE

  c. 5-HT also converted to melatonin (only in pineal gland)

5. Agonists/antagonists

  a. Storage

    i. Disrupted by reserpine and tetrabenazine

      (A) *Reserpine (an extract of the Rauwolfia plant) prevents the transport of all the monoamines and ACh into storage vesicles in the presynaptic membrane, allowing MAO metabolism to occur.*

   b. Release

      i. *Increased release of 5-HT*

        (A) *Amphetamine*

        (B) *Fenfluramine*

      ii. *Increased release and blocked reuptake of 5-HT*

        (A) *Clomipramine*

        (B) *Amitriptyline*

   c. Reuptake

      i. *Blocked by:*

        (A) *TCAs: inhibit NE and 5-HT reuptake by presynaptic nerve terminals*

        (B) *SSRIs (fluoxetine, sertraline): selectively prevent the reuptake of 5-HT*

        (C) *Clomipramine: although a TCA, it is an SSRI.*

   d. LSD

      i. Acts most strongly on the $5\text{-}HT_2$ receptors (and some effect on NE receptors)

      ii. Small doses potentiate 5-HT activity.

      iii. High doses inhibit 5-HT activity, leading to psychedelic action.

   e. *5-HT agonists*

      i. *Sumatriptan: potent $5\text{-}HT_2$ agonist*

      ii. *Methysergide*

      iii. *Cyproheptadine*

   f. *5-HT antagonist: clozapine*

E. Glutamate

  1. Miscellaneous

    a. *Excitatory* NT

    b. Glutamate is NT of corticostriate fibers.

    c. *Most common NT in the brain*

    d. *High concentration in dorsal spinal cord and dentate nucleus*

    e. Aspartic acid and glutamate have the capacity for neuronal damage via excitotoxicity

  2. *Receptors*

    a. *N-methyl-D-aspartate*

      i. Only known receptor that is regulated both by a ligand (glutamate) and by voltage

      ii. *Mainly activate Ca^{2+} channels*

      iii. *N-methyl-D-aspartate receptor locations*

        (A) *Cortex*

        (B) *Hippocampal neurons, particularly the CA1 region*

        (C) *Amygdala*

        (D) *Basal ganglia*

      iv. *Five binding sites alter channel opening*

        (A) *Glutamate (increase)*

        (B) *Glycine (increase)*

        (C) *Polyamine (increase): binds the hallucinogenic substance phencyclidine*

          iv. *Five binding sites alter channel opening* (*cont'd*)

              (D) *Magnesium (decrease)*

              (E) *Zinc (decrease)*

         v. *Glycine binding is required for activation.*

         vi. *Voltage-dependent blockers*

              (A) *Phencyclidine*

              (B) *Ketamine*

              (C) *Magnesium*

        vii. *Voltage-independent blocker: zinc*

       viii. Associated with long-term potentiation and long-term depression, which are integral for learning and memory

    b. *AMPA*

       i. Mainly activate *sodium channel*

      ii. Major source of excitatory postsynaptic potentials (EPSPs)

     iii. Receptor affinity: AMPA > glutamate > kainate

      iv. *GluR3 receptor: implicated in Rasmussen's encephalitis*

    c. *Kainate*

       i. Receptor affinity: kainate > glutamate > AMP

      ii. No specific antagonists

     iii. Derived commercially from seaweed

    d. 1-amino-1,3-cyclopentone dicarboxylic acid (ACPD): G-coupled formation of IP_3

    e. L-AP4

       i. G-coupled formation of AMP

      ii. Inhibitory autoreceptor

  3. Inactivation

  4. Other

    a. *Caffeine:* increases alertness and possibly produces anxiety by blocking adenosine receptors that normally inhibit glutamate release

    b. *Mercury poisoning:* damage to astrocytes prevents resorption of glutamate, resulting in excitotoxicity.

    c. *Lamotrigine* inhibits release of excitatory NTs glutamate and aspartate.

F. **GABA**

  1. Miscellaneous

    a. *Inhibitory NT: inhibitor of presynaptic transmission in the CNS and retina*

    b. *30% to 40% of all synapses (second only to glutamate as a major brain NT)*

    c. *Most highly concentrated in the basal ganglia (with projections to the thalamus); also concentrated in the hypothalamus, periaqueductal gray, and hippocampus*

  2. Synthesis: *glutamate decarboxylase decreased in striatum of Huntington's disease*

  3. *Receptors*

    a. *Connected to a chloride ion channel, allowing chloride to enter the cell and increasing the threshold for depolarization*

    b. *GABA-A*

       i. Fast inhibitory postsynaptic potentials (IPSPs)

      ii. Increase chloride conductance

     iii. Five binding sites

         (A) *Benzodiazepine: increases chloride conductance of presynaptic neurons*

        (B) *Barbiturate: prolongs duration of chloride channel opening*

        (C) Steroid site

        (D) Picrotoxin site

        (E) GABA site

     iv. CNS locations

        (A) *Cerebellum: highest concentration in granule cell layer*

        (B) *Cortex*

        (C) *Hippocampus*

        (D) *Basal ganglia*

     v. GABA-A receptor binds

        (A) GABA

        (B) Benzodiazepine

        (C) β-Carbolines

        (D) Picrotoxin-like convulsant drugs: noncompetitive antagonist

        (E) Bicuculline: competitive antagonist

        (F) Barbiturates

  c. *GABA-B*

     i. *Slow IPSPs*

     ii. *Increased K^+ conductance via K^+ channels*

     iii. *Coupled to G-protein that uses adenyl cyclase as a second messenger*

     iv. *Agonist: baclofen*

     v. *Antagonist: phaclofen*

     vi. CNS locations

        (A) Cerebellum

        (B) Cord

4. Inactivation

  a. Reuptake

  b. Enzyme metabolism

5. Agonists/antagonists

  a. *Inhibitors of GABA transaminase*

     i. *Valproic acid*

     ii. *Vigabatrin*

6. Other

  a. *Benzodiazepines*

     i. Increase the frequency of chloride channel opening

     ii. Enhance the effect of GABA on GABA-A receptors

  b. *Caffeine:* neutralizes the effects of benzodiazepines by inhibiting GABA release

  c. *Barbiturates:* prolong the duration of opening

G. MAO

1. Miscellaneous

  a. *Antidepressant effect of MAOIs is more related to NE than DA.*

  b. MAO$_A$

     i. *MAO$_A$ inhibitors have proven to be better antidepressants because MAO$_A$ metabolizes NE and 5-HT; therefore, inhibition increases NE and 5-HT levels.*

    b. MAO$_A$ (*cont'd*)

        ii. *MAO$_A$-inhibiting drugs given for depression have critically elevated blood pressure in patients eating tyramine-containing foods (e.g., cheese).*

    c. *MAO$_B$*

        i. Alcohol also selectively inhibits MAO$_B$.

        ii. MAO$_B$ is the most common form in the striatum.

        iii. *MAO$_B$ metabolizes the neurotoxin 1-methyl-4-phenyl-1,2,3,6-tetrahydropyridine (MPTP).*

        iv. *Selegiline, rasagiline: specific MAO$_B$ inhibitor*

    d. Mitochondrial MAO degrades intraneuronal DA, NE, and 5-HT that is not protected within storage vesicles.

    e. **Hypertensive crisis**

        i. *MAO in the gastrointestinal system usually prevents entrance of large amounts of ingested tyramine (or other pressor amines).*

        ii. If MAOI is used, then ingested tyramine can be absorbed and produce sympathetic response.

        iii. Clinical: sudden occipital or temporoparietal headache, sweating, fever, stiff neck, photophobia (can be mistaken for meningitis)

        iv. *Foods to avoid with MAOIs*

            (A) *Aged cheese*

            (B) *Smoked or pickled meats, fish, or poultry*

            (C) *Caviar*

            (D) *Non-fresh meat*

            (E) *Liver*

            (F) *Nondistilled alcohol*

            (G) *Broad beans (fava, Italian green, Chinese pea pods)*

            (H) *Banana peel*

            (I) *Sausage*

            (J) *Corned beef*

            (K) *Sauerkraut*

        v. *Medications/drugs to avoid with MAOIs*

            (A) *Amphetamines*

            (B) *Cocaine*

            (C) *Anorectics/dietary agents*

            (D) *Catecholamines*

            (E) *Sympathomimetic precursors (DA, levodopa)*

            (F) *Sympathomimetic (ephedrine, phenylephrine, phenylpropanolamine, pseudoephedrine)*

            (G) *Meperidine*

        vi. Treatment of hypertensive crisis: *phentolamine, 5 mg intravenously, or nifedipine, 10 mg sublingually*

  2. Location

    a. Outer surface of presynaptic mitochondria

    b. Postsynaptic cell membrane

  3. Inhibitors

    a. *MAO$_A$: clorgyline*

    b. MAO$_B$: selegiline, pargyline, rasagiline

    c. Nonspecific MAOIs: phenelzine, isocarboxazid, tranylcypromine

H. Glycine

1. Miscellaneous

    a. Inhibitory NT of cord for inhibitory interneurons (Renshaw cells), which inhibit anterior motor neurons of the spinal cord

    b. Glycine binds to a receptor that makes the postsynaptic membrane more permeable to Cl$^-$ ion, which hyperpolarizes the membrane, making it less likely to depolarize (inhibitory NT).

    c. Opposite function of aspartate in the spinal cord

    d. Anoxia results in loss of inhibitory neurons and decreased glycine.

2. Synthesis

3. Inactivation: deactivated in the synapse by active transport back into the presynaptic membrane

4. Agonists/antagonists

    a. Antagonist

        i. *Strychnine*

            (A) *Antagonist*

            (B) *Noncompetitively blocks glycine > GABA receptors by inhibiting opening of the chloride channel, which subsequently results in hyperexcitability*

        ii. *Tetanus toxin: blocks release of glycine and GABA*

    b. Agonist: glycine > β-alanine > taurine >> alanine/serine

I. Aspartate

1. Miscellaneous

    a. Primarily localized to the ventral spinal cord

    b. Opens an ion channel

    c. Excitatory NT, which increases the likelihood of depolarization in the postsynaptic membrane

    d. Opposite function of glycine in the spinal cord

    e. Aspartate (+) and glycine (−) form an excitatory/inhibitory pair in the ventral spinal cord.

    f. Nonessential amino acid found particularly in sugar

2. Inactivation: reabsorption into the presynaptic membrane

J. Histamine

1. Miscellaneous

    a. Histamine acts as an NT and is found *in mast cells (but histamine of mast cells is not an NT).*

    b. Highest concentration within hypothalamus

2. Synthesis

3. Receptors

    a. Histamine$_1$ receptor

    b. Histamine$_2$ receptor

    c. Histamine$_3$ receptor: functions in autoregulation

J. **Histamine** (*cont'd*)

    4. Agonists/antagonists

        a. Histamine$_1$-receptor antagonists

           i. Diphenhydramine

           ii. Chlorpheniramine

           iii. Promethazine

        b. Histamine$_2$-receptor antagonists: cimetidine

        c. α-Fluoromethylhistidine: selective inhibitor of histamine decarboxylase

K. **Neuropeptides**

    1. Miscellaneous

        a. Most common NTs in the hypothalamus

        b. Very potent compared to other NTs

        c. May modulate postsynaptic effects of NTs by prolonging effect via second messengers

        d. Neuropeptides coexist with other NTs

NT	NEUROPEPTIDE
GABA	Somatostatin
	Cholecystokinin
Ach	Vasoinhibitory peptide (VIP)
	Substance P
NE	Somatostatin
	Enkephalin
	Neuropeptide Y
DA	Cholecystokinin
	Neurotensin
Epinephrine	Neuropeptide Y
	Neurotensin
5-HT	Substance P
	Enkephalin
Vasopressin	Cholecystokinin
	Dynorphin
Oxytocin	Enkephalin

    2. Synthesis: ribosomal synthesis

    3. Inactivation: extracellular action is terminated via hydrolysis by proteases and diffusion; not inactivated by reuptake.

    4. Subtypes

        a. Enkephalins

           i. *Enkephalin receptor*

               (A) Opiates and enkephalins bind to the receptor.

               (B) Highest concentration found in the sensory system, limbic system, hypothalamic region, amygdala, and periaqueductal gray

               (C) Located on presynaptic synapses

           ii. *Opiates and enkephalins inhibit the firing of locus ceruleus neurons.*

L. **Opioids**

1. *Receptors*

	μ RECEPTOR	δ RECEPTOR	κ RECEPTOR
Agonist	β endorphin[a]	Leu-enkephalin[a]	Dynorphins[a]
	Morphine	Met-enkephalin	
Antagonist	Naloxone	Naloxone (weak)	Naloxone (very weak)
	Naltrexone		
Function	Analgesia	Cardiac affects	Salt and water resorption
			Analgesia

[a]Most potent.

a. κ Receptor differs from μ and δ receptors because it cannot reverse morphine withdrawal.

M. **Substance P**

1. Release
    a. Ca^{2+} dependent
    b. Inhibited by morphine
2. Agonists/antagonists
    a. *Capsaicin: depletes substance P (analgesic effect)*

N. *Quick reference for NTs*

NT	SYNTHESIZED FROM	SITE OF SYNTHESIS
ACh	Choline	CNS, parasympathetic nerves
5-HT	Tryptophan	CNS, chromaffin cells of gut, enteric cells
GABA	Glutamate	CNS
Glutamate	—	CNS
Aspartate	—	CNS
Glycine	—	Spinal cord
Histamine	Histidine	Hypothalamus
Adenosine	ATP	CNS, peripheral nerves
Adenosine triphosphate	—	Sympathetic, sensory, and enteric nerves
Nitric oxide	Arginine	CNS, gastrointestinal

O. *Other*

1. Quisqualate-type receptor is coupled to phospholipase C.
2. CNS sites of high neurochemical concentrations
    a. NE: locus ceruleus
    b. 5-HT: median and dorsal raphe
    c. DA: substantia nigra
    d. GABA: cerebellum
    e. Cholinergic: substantia innominata and nucleus basalis of Meynert
    f. Histamine: hypothalamus

O. *Other* (*cont'd*)

    3. Calmodulin: prominent calcium-binding protein in the CNS

    4. Ascending pathways mediating arousal

II. Neurochemistry

A. **Electrolyte concentrations**

ION	INTRACELLULAR CONCENTRATION (mEq/L)	EXTRACELLULAR CONCENTRATION (mEq/L)
Na^+	15	140
K^+	135	4
Ca^{2+}	2×10^{-4}	4
Mg^{2+}	40	2
Cl^-	4	120
HCO_3^-	10	24

B. **Basic neurophysiology**

    1. *Action potential (AP)*

        a. Definition: a self-propagating regenerative change in membrane potential

        b. An AP only develops if the depolarization reaches the threshold determined by the voltage-dependent properties of the sodium channels; sodium channels are also time dependent, staying open for only a limited period.

        c. *Ion fluxes and membrane potentials*

            i. Most of the charge movement in biological tissue is attributed to passive properties of the membrane or changes in ion conductance.

            ii. Important cations: K^+, Na^+, Ca^{2+}

            iii. Important anions: Cl^-, proteins

        d. *Three phases*

            i. *Resting membrane potential*

                (A) *Potential* $= -70\,mV$

                (B) Due to difference in permeability of ions and sodium-potassium pump forcing K^+ in and Na^+ out

                (C) Resting membrane potential based on outward K^+ current through passive leakage channels

                (D) If resting membrane potential is diminished and threshold is surpassed and the AP is generated

            ii. *Depolarization*

                (A) *Potential* $= +40\,mV$

                (B) Dependent on sodium permeability

                    (1) Voltage-gated opening of sodium channels

                        (*a*) Sodium permeability increases as membrane potential decreases from the resting membrane potential (–70 mV) toward 0.

                        (*b*) When the membrane potential reaches approximately –55 mV, sodium channels open dramatically.

(c) The transient increase in sodium permeability allows results in membrane potential of +40 mV.

(d) Voltage-dependent potassium channels will also open in conjunction with sodium channels.

iii. *Repolarization:* closure of voltage-gated sodium channels reestablishes potassium as the determining ion of the membrane potential.

e. Myelinated are faster than unmyelinated nerves

i. *Myelin decreases membrane capacitance and conductance and the time constant.*

ii. Increases the space constant of the segment of axon between the nodes of Ranvier

iii. Velocity is proportional to axon radius.

2. *Neuromuscular junction (NMJ)*

a. Presynaptic components

i. Motor neuron

ii. Axon

iii. Terminal bouton

(A) *Synaptic vesicles: contain 5,000 to 10,000 molecules (1 quanta) of ACh*

(B) *Release based on voltage-gated calcium channels*

b. Synaptic cleft: 200 to 500 μm

c. Postsynaptic components

i. Motor end plate

ii. ACh receptors

iii. Voltage-gated sodium channels

3. Synaptic transmission

a. *AP is based on sodium inward current and potassium outward current through voltage-dependent channels.*

b. *When AP reaches presynaptic region, it causes release of NT.*

c. NTs bind to postsynaptic receptors, opening postsynaptic membrane channels.

d. Depending on the ionic currents flowing through the transmitter (ligand)-operated channels, two types of postsynaptic potentials are generated.

i. *EPSPs*

(A) Occur when sodium inward current prevails

(B) Increase the probability that AP will be propagated

ii. *IPSPs*

(A) Occur when potassium outward current or chloride inward current prevails

(B) Cause hyperpolarization of the postsynaptic membrane, making it more difficult to reach the threshold potential

e. Summation

i. EPSPs and IPSPs interact to determine whether AP is propagated postsynaptically.

ii. *Temporal summation: EPSPs/IPSPs sequentially summate at a monosynaptic site.*

iii. *Spatial summation: EPSPs/IPSPs simultaneously evoke an end-plate potential polysynaptically.*

3. Synaptic transmission (*cont'd*)

    f. Depolarization of the nerve terminal results in opening of all ionic channels, including those for calcium; calcium entry causes release of NT from the pre-synaptic terminal, which binds to postsynaptic receptor sites.

    g. Chemical transmission is the main mode of neuronal communication and can be excitatory or inhibitory (if postsynaptic binding opens sodium channels and/or calcium channels → EPSP; if it opens potassium channels and/or Cl channels → IPSP); most common excitatory NT is glutamate; common inhibitory NTs are GABA and glycine.

C. *Membrane channel dysfunction*

1. *Sodium channel*

    a. Sodium channel inhibitors

        i. Tetrodotoxin (puffer fish)

        ii. Saxitoxin (dinoflagellate, shellfish)

    b. Sodium channel potentiators

        i. Batrachotoxin (arrow poisoning)

        ii. Grayanotoxin (Amazon amphibians)

    c. Sodium channel closure inhibitors

        i. Scorpion toxin

        ii. Sea anemone toxin

    d. Mutational disorders

        i. Failure of sodium channel to inactivate

        ii. Disorders

            (A) *Hyperkalemic periodic paralysis*

            (B) *Paramyotonia congenita*

2. *Potassium channel*

    a. Antagonists

        i. Tetraethyl ammonium chloride: voltage-gated potassium channels

        ii. 4-Aminopyridine: antagonizes fast voltage-gated potassium channels

    b. Mutational disorders: hypokalemic periodic paralysis

3. *Calcium channel disorders*

    a. Absence seizures: thalamic calcium channels

    b. Hypokalemic periodic paralysis

CHEAT SHEET

1. Postganglionic sympathetic neurons to sweat glands use ACh as NT.
2. Botulinum toxin works on SNAP-25 protein to exert its pharmacological effect.
3. Two types of dopamine receptors: D1 stimulatory and D2 inhibitory
4. Parkinson's disease is manifestation of striatal dopamine depletion.
5. *Locus ceruleus* stores NE and epinephrine.
6. Syndrome associated with NMDA-receptor antibody: paraneoplastic phenomenon of ovarian cancer, leads to dystonia, opsoclonus, myoclonus, psychosis, epilepsy.

(continued)

7. Antibodies targeting glutamate decarboxylase represent the autoimmune form of stiff-person syndrome, downbeat nystagmus, slow saccades, opsoclonus.

8. Avoid tyramine-containing food products, which interact with MAOI. Cottage cheese, ricotta, and cream cheese do *not* interact with MAOI.

9. 3,4 diaminopyridines may be used in the treatment of Lambert-Eaton myasthenic syndrome.

10. Calcium channel blockers worsen weakness in myasthenia gravis patients.

11. Paraneoplastic syndromes: anti-Yo—pancerebellar degeneration, directed at cytoplasm of Purkinje cells; anti-Tr, anti-Hu also associated with cerebellar degeneration.

12. Entacapone, tolcapone—COMT inhibitors, prolong action of dopamine by inhibiting metabolism, reduction of "wearing off" in Parkinson's disease patients

13. Memantine—moderate affinity, noncompetitive, NMDA receptor antagonist, inhibits excessive Ca^{2+} influx induced by chronic overstimulation of receptor

14. Patients with inborn errors of metabolism such as mitochondrial disease or urea cycle defect are more prone to valproate induced liver toxicity.

15. Pyridoxine-dependent seizures: Diminished gamma amino decarboxylase enzyme activity; the enzyme needs vitamin B_6 as cofactor to break down glutamic acid to GABA. Absence of cofactor results in increased glutamic acid levels and subsequently seizures.

16. Clopidogrel: irreversible blockade of ADP receptor on platelet membrane, receptor involved in platelet aggregation, blocks activation of glycoprotein 2b/3b pathway

17. Dipyridamole: inhibits uptake of adenosine into platelets, increases concentration of adenosine → acts on A2 receptor ⇢ stimulates adenylate cyclase to increase cAMP levels → inhibits platelet aggregation

18. Aspirin: irreversible inactivation of COX enzyme (required for production of thromboxane) → blocks production of thromboxane A2 in platelets → inhibits aggregation

19. Triptans: selectively active two 5-HT1 sub-types—1B and 1D. 1B receptor located in cranial blood vessels and trigeminal nerve terminals. Mechanism: binding → vasoconstriction → modulation of neuropeptide release. 5-HT receptor (serotonin): seven subtypes, involved in various disorders—anxiety, depression, schizophrenia, migraine.

20. Serotonin syndrome: excessive serotonin agonism in CNS and PNS. Triad: neuromuscular hyperactivity, autonomic hyperactivity, altered mental status. Causes: SSRI, SNRI, MAOI, triptans, opioids, lithium, illicit drugs. NMS: caused by antipsychotics; similar symptoms as serotonin syndrome.

(continued)

21. Hyperkalemic periodic paralysis: AD, episodic weakness, attacks 1 to 4 hours, generalized, triggered by rest after exercise, electrical myotonia, ictal elevated K levels, caused by mutation of Na channel SCN4A, symptomatic management, avoid triggers, thiazide diuretics

22. Hypokalemic periodic paralysis: decreased K levels, AD, mutation of Ca channel CACNA1S, attacks hours to days, induced by exercise, large meals, and ETOH

23. Grapefruit juice inhibits CYP3A4, increases levels of carbamazepine.

24. Calcitonin gene related peptide (GCRP): release is associated with migraine HA; blocking receptor stops migraine.

Suggested Readings

Brunton, L, Chabner, B, Knollman B. *Goodman and Gilman's the Pharmacological Basis of Therapeutics.* New York, NY: McGraw Hill;2010.

Kandel, ER, Schwartz, JH, Jessell, TM, Siegelbaum, SA, Hudspeth, AJ. *Principles of Neural Science.* 5th ed. New York, NY: McGraw-Hill;2012.

CHAPTER 2

Neurogenetics

I. The Central Dogma of Genetics

A. Deoxyribonucleic acid (DNA)

1. DNA is the molecular blueprint.
2. The *genome* refers to a species' entire collection of DNA:
   a. Human genome: 3 billion nucleotide bases subdivided into 23 paired chromosomes
   b. Chromosomes 1 through 22 are *autosomal chromosomes*; X and Y are *sex chromosomes*.
      i. Females are 46, XX; Males are 46, XY.

B. Genes

1. The human genome contains approximately 20,000 genes.
2. Genes specify amino acid sequences of proteins.
3. Approximately 1.5% of the human genome consists of protein-coding regions.
4. Noncoding sequences have structural or regulatory functions.
5. Gene structure:
   a. *Promoters:* sequences of DNA upstream from the start codon
      i. Binding sites for transcriptional machinery
      ii. Transcription factors can activate or repress transcription at this site.
   b. *Exons:* sequences of DNA that code for specific amino acid sequences
      i. *Codons:* groups of three nucleotides (*trinucleotides*) that code for particular amino acids
      ii. Start and stop codons are trinucleotides recognized by transcriptional complexes at the beginning and the terminus of the exon, respectively.
   c. *Introns:* intervening DNA sequences between exons that are not expressed in the final amino acid sequence
6. Copies of the same gene are called *alleles*.
7. Noncoding regions: help regulate gene expression
   a. Distal promoters, enhancers, silencers, insulators, five-prime untranslated region (5' UTR), and the three-prime untranslated region (3' UTR)
   b. Intergenic noncoding regions: important for chromosomal structure and replication
      i. Examples: the centromere and telomere

C. Transcription: DNA is transcribed into *heteronuclear ribonucleic acid (RNA)* containing both introns and exons (and UTRs).

1. Splicing: heteronuclear RNA is *spliced*, or edited, at specific sequences known as *splice sites.*
   a. Introns are excised and adjacent exons are fused together.
   b. Splicing yields *messenger RNA (mRNA).*

1. Splicing (*cont'd*)

    c. Splice-site variants: allow a single gene to produce more than one mRNA, yielding similar proteins with different biological functions

D. **Translation**: mRNA is translated into a protein on cytoplasmic ribosomes.

1. *Transfer RNA (tRNA):*

    a. Binds to one specific amino acid

    b. Contains a trinucleotide *anticodon* that binds a specific mRNA codon

    c. tRNA links together specific amino acids and mRNA, allowing amino acids to bind together (i.e., be translated) into the primary sequence of the protein.

    d. Posttranslational modifications: Linear amino acid strands will be further processed, folded, and shuttled to the protein's functional site.

        i. Many posttranslational modifications, such as *glycosylation,* occur in the Golgi or cytosol, are enzyme-mediated, and require chaperone proteins.

        ii. Modifications are typically covalent additions of functional groups such as glycosylation, phosphorylation, methylation, ubiquitination, nitrosylation, acetylation, lipidation, or removal of regulatory subunits.

E. **Mutations:** changes in the genome that affect the production of proteins. There are myriad causes of mutations with varying effects. The following are common types of mutations, arranged by size from smallest to largest:

MUTATION	MUTATION TYPE	LEADS TO
Point mutation: Single-nucleotide base change	Silent	Same amino acid, results in a normally functioning protein
	Neutral	Similar amino acid substitution, results in a normally or almost normally functioning protein
	Missense	Amino acid substitution and potentially abnormal protein
	Nonsense	Results in a premature stop codon, resulting in an abnormal or no protein
Insertions or deletions	Frame shift	Disrupts the "reading frame," so the three-nucleotide codons are out of sequence; results in abnormal or no protein
	In-frame mutation	Insertion/deletion resulting in a sequence divisible by 3; may cause abnormal or no protein
	Chromosomal deletion	Interstitial loss of DNA affecting all genes in that region; may result in fusion gene formation; effects depend on location and size of the deletion
	Chromosomal duplication	Duplication of a part or whole chromosome; effects depend on the location and size of the duplication

(continued)

MUTATION	MUTATION TYPE	LEADS TO
	Chromosomal translocation	An exchange of part of one chromosome with another nonhomologous chromosome; effects depend on the location, size, and whether associated deletions or duplications are present; fusion genes may form
	Chromosomal inversion	A portion of a chromosome becomes reversed within the chromosome; effects depend on the location, size, and whether associated deletions or duplications are present; fusion genes may form
Splice-site mutation	Any of the above mutations that disrupt recognition of a splice site during mRNA processing	Improper inclusion of intronic RNA or exclusion of exonic RNA in the mRNA, resulting in an abnormal or no protein
Gene fusion	Production of a single mRNA from two typically separate genes	Chimera protein that may or may not have loss or gain of function
Dynamic mutations	Trinucleotide repeat expansion	Increasing number of trinucleotide repeats, typically glutamate codons, resulting in larger mRNAs; increased risk of genetic disease with larger trinucleotide repeats. *Genetic anticipation* refers to earlier disease expression in subsequent generations, and is a common consequence of trinucleotide repeat expansion.

1. **Mitochondrial DNA (mtDNA):**

   a. Mitochondria have their own DNA separate from the chromosomal DNA.

   b. mtDNA has approximately 16,500 nucleotide bases and codes for 37 proteins (including 22 tRNAs).

      i. mtDNA mutations: point mutations, deletions, duplications, or insertions in mtDNA

      ii. Can result in abnormal proteins, many of which are critical for mitochondrial function

      iii. Note: there are over 1,000 chromosomal genes encoding mitochondrial proteins, and mutations affecting these genes can result in mitochondrial dysfunction and disease.

F. **Effects of mutations**

   1. **Gene dosage effects:**

      a. **Haploinsufficiency:** loss of a gene copy resulting in less protein production than is required by a cell for normal function. Some cancers result from haploinsufficiency of a tumor suppressor gene.

F. **Effects of mutations** (*cont'd*)

2. **Loss of function:** mutations that disrupt protein structure, binding sites, functional domains, or loci of posttranslational modifications. These proteins may be less functional or nonfunctional, may not localize properly within the cell, or may be degraded by a cell more quickly than the normal protein. Loss of function mutations are common in many recessive neurologic diseases.

3. **Gain of function:** a mutation resulting in increased activity, increased half-life, or the creation of a new and abnormal function that disrupts other functions in the cell. Gain of function mutations in the *SCN9A* gene have been implicated in some patients with idiopathic small fiber neuropathy.

4. **Dominant negative:** a mutation in one copy of a gene may result in an abnormal protein that disrupts the function of the normal protein made by the nonmutated copy of the gene. Dominant negative mutations in the *ClC-1* gene give rise to both dominant and recessive forms of the channelopathy myotonia congenita.

5. **Lethal mutations:** these are not compatible with life and often result in spontaneous abortion, intrauterine fetal demise, or death in the neonatal period.

G. **Nonmutational DNA variants**

VARIANT	SIZE OF VARIANT	CHARACTERISTICS
Single-nucleotide polymorphism (SNP)	Single base change, typically in noncoding regions	Common occurrences, ~1% or more frequent in a population
		Typically binary (e.g., A or T)
		~1 million SNPs across the human genome
		SNP allele frequencies vary across ethnicities
		May be linked with disease or phenotype
		SNPs can alter transcriptional regulation
Copy-number variation (CNV)	Vary from 1,000 nucleotides (1 kilobase or Kb) to > 1,000 Kb (megabase, or Mb)	A deletion or duplication of a region of a gene
		~13% of the human genome consists of CNVs
		Stable and heritable from parents to offspring
		CNV gains are more common than losses
		May be responsible for phenotypic variation, increased or decreased susceptibility to diseases
Variants of unknown significance (VUS)	Variable	These are genetic changes that may be as small as single base substitutions or large copy-number variants. These VUSs have yet to be characterized, and their effects are not known. Some VUSs occur in coding regions of genes known to be associated with disease and are likely pathogenic. Others may be found in both unaffected parents and their affected offspring, and are less likely to be deleterious.

H. Patterns of inheritance

1. *Autosomal dominant (AD):* inheritance or de novo mutation of **one** allele is sufficient to produce disease; *50% of offspring of an affected individual will receive the disease allele and therefore have the disease.*

   Penetrance: The degree of phenotypic expression of a mutation. For AD-inherited diseases this can be variable even within a family, with some members minimally affected while others with the same mutation will be severely affected. When all carriers are affected, this is 100% penetrance.

   The absence of a family history does NOT preclude an autosomal dominant disease because variable penetrance, questions of paternity, and de novo mutation can all result in an affected offspring.

2. *Autosomal recessive (AR):* two mutated alleles must be present for the disease to manifest. If both parents are each unaffected carriers of an AR mutation, on average 25% of their offspring will have two normal copies of the gene (noncarriers), 50% will be unaffected carriers with a single copy of the mutated gene, and *25% of the offspring will inherit both mutated alleles and be affected.* Typically, carriers are asymptomatic.

3. *X-linked recessive:* Gene mutations on the X chromosome can be inherited by both male and female offspring.

   a. Males only have one X chromosome (from their mother); therefore in X-linked recessive diseases, a male receiving a mutated allele will manifest the disease, and a female offspring will not.

   b. An unaffected carrier female has a 50% chance of transmitting an X-linked recessive disease to her sons.

   c. Males with X-linked diseases CANNOT transmit the disease to male offspring, although 100% of their female offspring will receive the disease-causing allele and be asymptomatic carriers.

   d. If a male with an X-linked recessive disease and an unaffected female carrier have children:

      i. 50% of their male offspring will be expected to inherit the disease (from their mother)

      ii. 50% of their female offspring will be unaffected carriers (from either mother or father)

      iii. 50% of their female offspring will also inherit the disease (one copy from each parent)

4. *X-linked dominant:* these mutations are often so deleterious that survival of the offspring is contingent on having at least one normal functioning copy of the gene.

   a. Because males only have one X chromosome, these mutations are typically lethal in male fetuses and likely result in spontaneous abortion, although rarely male patients are found with X-linked dominant diseases.

   b. Because females contain two X chromosomes, they can survive with the disease-causing mutation.

   c. The degree of severity of X-linked dominant diseases varies between individuals due to X-inactivation, a process by which one copy of a female's two X chromosomes is transcriptionally silenced. Rett syndrome, caused by a mutation in the *MECP2* gene, is an example of an X-linked dominant disease.

5. *Genomic imprinting:* DNA and histone methylation allow transcriptional silencing of individual genes, as well as regions of chromosomes. Genomic imprinting is the regulation of gene expression depending on the parental origin of the gene. In

5. *Genomic imprinting* (*cont'd*)

paternal imprinting, genes inherited from the father are silenced through methylation, and only those from the mother are expressed. Maternal imprinting is the opposite.

   a. *Prader-Willi:* **Paternally inherited** mutation (maternal imprinting). You can remember this because both Prader and paternal start with P.

   b. *Angelman's:* **Maternally inherited** mutation (paternal imprinting). You can remember this because there is an M in Angelman's.

6. *Mitochondrial: at fertilization, the ovum contributes all of the mitochondria,* and the sperm contributes none. *Thus, mitochondrial inheritance is exclusively maternal,* and ALL her offspring are at risk of manifesting a mitochondrially inherited mutation.

   a. Heteroplasmy: within individual cells there exist thousands of copies of mtDNA, some of which may be mutated, and others normal. This is called heteroplasmy.

      i. The degree of heteroplasmy correlates with disease severity, with a critical level of heteroplasmy above which symptoms are more likely to manifest.

      ii. Patients with mitochondrial disease tend to accumulate heteroplasmy throughout their lives. Thus, patients with high levels of heteroplasmy at birth are at increased risk of earlier-onset disease.

II. Genetic Testing

A. Cytogenetic analyses

   1. **Karyotyping:**

      a. **Method:** chromosomes from cells in metaphase are examined by microscope.

      b. **Resolution:** very large chromosomal abnormalities, approximately 5 Mb, and breakpoint resolution from 5 to15 Mb

      c. **Utility:** to determine genetic sex; validate a diploid state (having two copies of all autosomal chromosomes); rule out monoploidy (one set of chromosomes) or polyploidy (more than two copies of all chromosomes); rule out monosomy (loss of one chromosome) or polysomy (greater than two copies of a chromosome); detect inversions, translocations, ring chromosomes, and isochromosomes (a chromosome with either two long or two short arms, rather than one of each)

      d. **Clinical example:** to confirm Turner syndrome (monosomy X) or Down syndrome (trisomy 21).

   2. **Fluorescent in situ hybridization (FISH):**

      a. **Method:** fluorescently labeled probes detect the presence or absence of specific DNA sequences on chromosomes. Unlike karyotyping, FISH can be performed on frozen or fixed tissue.

      b. **Resolution:** 1 to 5 Mb, depending on technique

      c. **Utility:** detection of chromosomal rearrangements, deletions, and duplications; confirmatory test for abnormal karyotype.

      d. **Clinical example:** detection of specific chromosomal abnormalities associated with tumors, such as fusion genes; to confirm diagnosis of velocardiofacial (also known as DiGeorge) syndrome, the most common microdeletion syndrome, caused by deletion of 22q11.2

   3. **Comparative genomic hybridization (CGH):**

      a. **Method:** similar technology to FISH. CGH compares copy numbers of chromosomal regions between two biological samples by labeling each sample a different color, and identifying a relative abundance or absence of a signal, to indicate a chromosomal duplication or deletion, respectively.

b. **Resolution:** resolution is about 5 Mb; array-based CGH allows high-throughput genome-wide analysis of copy-number changes at a resolution of 5 to 10 Kb.

c. **Utility:** to identify deletions, duplications, or unbalanced translocations

d. **Clinical example:** to detect patterns of chromosomal aberrations in solid tumors; disease-causing deletions such as 5p deletions in cri-du-chat syndrome

B. Genotyping

1. **Microarray:** automated, chip-based platforms allowing the simultaneous analysis of multiple genes, polymorphisms, or gene expression levels

    a. **Whole-genome chromosomal microarrays and SNP arrays:**

       i. Method: CGH (as described earlier). This is the standard-of-care, cost-effective screening test to detect microdeletions and duplications.

       ii. Resolution: 5 Kb.

       iii. Utility: Cost-effective screening test

       iv. SNP arrays detect deletions/duplications, but also detect individual SNP alleles across the genome to identify regions of lost heterozygosity (see Section II.B.1.b, Loss of heterozygosity).

       v. Where available, SNP arrays should be ordered instead of chromosomal microarrays.

    b. **Loss of heterozygosity:**

       i. There should be relative heterozygosity of SNP alleles between maternally inherited and paternally inherited chromosomes.

          (A) In consanguineous families, maternally and paternally inherited SNPs may be more homozygous than expected from unrelated parents.

          (B) Increased SNP homozygosity is synonymous with a "loss of heterozygosity."

          (C) Recessive disease-causing alleles are more common in consanguineous families; thus regions with a high degree of lost heterozygosity are more likely to contain deleterious recessive mutations than are areas of preserved heterozygosity.

          (D) Similarly, uniparental disomy (two copies of a single chromosome inherited from the same parent) will result in lost heterozygosity; uniparental disomy can result in imprinting-related and autosomal recessive diseases.

          (E) Utility: SNP arrays can indicate *regions of interest* in which *deleterious mutations* are more likely to be found, and help guide further genetic testing.

2. **Single-gene sequencing:**

    a. Next Generation (or NextGen) sequencing has improved the accuracy and speed of gene sequencing at the individual nucleotide level.

       i. **Method:** multiplex ligation-dependent probe amplification (MLPA) is one of the many methods, and is extremely efficient and precise, and has a lower cost.

       ii. **Resolution:** a single nucleotide base. HOWEVER, gene sequencing will not detect deletions or duplications.

          (A) NOTE: some labs will reflex to a deletion/duplication analysis if sequencing fails to detect a mutation, but clinicians may need to request this additional analysis.

       iii. **Utility:** mutation analysis, copy-number variant detection, deletion/duplication analysis, and SNP detection

a. Next Generation (*cont'd*)

iv. **Caution:** Single-gene sequencing remains high cost, and unless serving as a confirmatory test, phenotypic gene panels or whole-exome sequencing are likely better testing strategies.

3. **Gene panels:** simultaneous sequencing of multiple genes associated with a particular phenotype

a. **Method:** most panels incorporate NextGen sequencing to detect point mutations as well as deletion/duplication analyses.

b. **Resolution:** single-nucleotide point mutations, copy-number variants, and microdeletions/duplications

c. **Utility:** gene panels allow sequencing of large numbers of genes for a fraction of the cost of sequencing even a couple of individual genes.

i. **Disadvantages:** gene panels include genes that may not be relevant to a patient's case; may detect VUSs in more than one gene that cause confusion and trepidation for patients and their families; turnaround time for many gene panels may take months.

ii. **Advantages:** cost savings; gene panels are frequently updated to include new genes; therefore, many companies will re-run patient samples for free if the initial analysis failed to identify a mutation.

d. **Clinical example:** epilepsy panels (neonatal, infant-onset, etc.), X-linked intellectual disability panel, hereditary polyneuropathy panels, and so forth.

4. **Mitochondrial DNA sequencing:** NextGen sequencing of the mtDNA can be obtained commercially when there is a high index of suspicion for a mitochondrial disease. Many companies include mtDNA sequencing as part of their whole-exome sequencing.

5. **Whole-exome sequencing (WES):** the entirety of the protein-coding regions of the genome, or the *exome*, makes up only about 1.5% of human DNA, but contains approximately 85% of the disease-causing mutations.

a. **Method:** high-throughput DNA sequencing to simultaneously and accurately sequence the roughly 180,000 exons in the human exome, and mtDNA in its entirety

i. WES analyses include samples from parents and the affected child to exclude as pathogenic any VUSs found in unaffected parents; sequencing of parent–child triads increases diagnostic yield in many cases.

ii. Often phenotypic information is used to more closely probe genes known to be associated with certain diseases/phenotypes.

b. **Resolution:** single-nucleotide bases

i. Limitations: inability to detect mutations and pathogenic copy-number variants in noncoding and structural DNA; its lack of deletion/duplication detection and nonuniform coverage of the exome may contribute to both false positives and false negatives.

c. **Utility:** although expensive, WES is the most cost-efficient and broad-based clinical genetic test available. Recommended for patients with complex phenotypes, particularly if previous gene testing has been uninformative. Turnaround time may take 6 months, although focused, emergency sequencing/interpretation is available for critical cases.

d. **Clinical/ethical considerations:** WES interpretation is extremely complex and should be carried out by genetic counselors and medical geneticists. Ethical issues abound, including the reporting of potentially actionable mutations in a patient or his or her parents not associated with the clinical phenotype in question (e.g., Huntington's mutation in an asymptomatic parent).

6. **Whole-genome sequencing (WGS):** at the time of this writing, WGS remains largely experimental and rarely used clinically. Unlike WES, WGS sequences the entire coding and noncoding genome, almost 3 billion base pairs. This is an expensive and very time-consuming technology, and has the potential for even greater ethical challenges than WES.

III. Oncogenes and Chromosomal Aberrations in Central Nervous System (CNS) Tumors:

Proto-oncogenes are normal genes that exist in the genome and regulate or support important cellular functions related to mitosis, homeostasis, and apoptosis. When mutated, these genes (oncogenes) have the potential to promote tumor formation through either loss or gain of function, resulting in uncontrolled cell proliferation, growth, or prolonged survival.

TUMOR OR SYNDROME	COMMON MUTATION	CHARACTERISTICS
Low-grade astrocytoma	Gain of Ch 7	
Anaplastic astrocytoma	Gain Ch 7, 19, 20; Loss Ch 10, 22, X/Y	
Low grade oligo-dendrogliomas/oligoastrogliomas	Loss of heterozygosity of 1p and 19q	Pathognomonic diagnostic feature
Glioblastoma multiforme	Loss of Ch 10	80% of cases
	Gain of Ch 7 Loss Ch 22, Ch 17 (*p53* tumor suppressor genes) Loss Ch 9 (*CDKN2*) Amplification of epidermal growth factor receptor (*EGFR* on 7p)	
Retinoblastoma	*RB1* on Ch 13q14	60% are sporadic, require two mutations, typically only affect one eye, not heritable
		40% inherited as germline mutation; need second mutation in retinal cells to develop retinoblastoma; have increased risk of other cancers, including pinealoblastoma, osteosarcoma, and aggressive melanoma
Familial isolated pituitary adenoma	*AIP* on Ch 11q13.3	20% of familial cases of isolated pituitary adenoma; due to AD mutation with incomplete penetrance
	MEN1 on Ch 11q13	Associated with multiple endocrine neoplasia
Ependymoma	Monosomy of Ch 22, deletions or translocations of Ch 22q	

(continued)

TUMOR OR SYNDROME	COMMON MUTATION	CHARACTERISTICS
Li-Fraumeni cancer susceptibility syndrome	*p53* mutation (distal Ch 17p)	Increased incidence of early breast cancer, childhood sarcomas, and brain tumors; 50% likelihood of cancer diagnosis by age 30

The following tables provide a reference for genetic diseases important to neurology. The most important/high-yield genetic variants appear in **BOLD.**

IV. Dementia

DISEASE	INHERITANCE	CHROMOSOME	GENE/PROTEIN
Alzheimer's	AD	**21q21.3**	***APP*/Amyloid precursor protein**
Alzheimer's	AD	**14q24.3**	***PSEN1*/Presenilin-1**
Alzheimer's	AD	1	***PSEN2*/Presenilin-2**
Alzheimer's	**Risk factor only**	19q	***APOE4*/Apolipoprotein E4**
Familial prion disorders	AD	**20p**	***PRNP*/Prion protein**

Creutzfeldt-Jakob (fCJD)
 	
Gerstmann-Sträussler syndrome (GSS)
 	
Fatal familial insomnia (FFI)
	Insertional mutations in *PRNP*:
	  2–7 Octapeptide repeats → fCJD
	  8–9 Octapeptide repeats → GSS
	
	Disease-modifying alleles:
	Codon 129, Methionine or Valine
	  Met/Met: Earlier onset, shorter disease course
	Codon 178 Aspartate/Asparagine heterozygotes AND:
	  Methionine at Codon 129 → FFI phenotype
	  Valine at Codon 129 → fCJD		

Fragile X	AD	**Xq27.3**	***FMR1*/Fragile X mental retardation protein (FMRP)**
Cerebral amyloid angiopathy	AD	**20**	***APP*/Amyloid precursor protein**
	AD	20q11.21	*CST3*/Cystatin-C
	AD	13q14.3	*ITM2B*/ Integral membrane protein 2B

V. Movement Disorders

A. Parkinson's disease/parkinsonism

LOCUS/DISEASE	CHROMOSOME	GENE/PROTEIN	INHERITANCE	DISEASE
PARK1	**4q21**	***SNCA*/α Synuclein**	AD	EOPD
PARK2	6q25.2-27	*PARK2*/Parkin	AR	EOPD

(continued)

LOCUS/DISEASE	CHROMOSOME	GENE/PROTEIN	INHERITANCE	DISEASE
PARK3	2p13	NOTE: *SPR*/sepiapterin reductase localizes to this region	AD	Classic PD
PARK4	4q22.1	*SNCA*/α Synuclein triplications and duplications	AD	EOPD
PARK5	4p14	*UCHL1*/Ubiquitin carboxy-terminal hydrolase L1	AD	Classic PD
PARK6	1p36	*PINK1*/Serine/threonine-protein kinase PINK1	AR	EOPD
PARK7	1p36.23	*PARK7*/Protein DJ-1	AR	EOPD
PARK8	12q12	*LRRK-2*/Leucine-rich repeat kinase 2	AD	Classic PD
PARK9	1q36.13	*ATP13A2*/Probable cation-transporting ATPase 13A2	AR	Atypical PD
PARK10	1p32	SNP-associations with *EIF2B3* (1p34.1) and *USP24* (1p32.3)	?	Classic PD
PARK11	2q37.1	*GIGYF2*/GRB10-Interacting GYF Protein 2	AD	Late-onset PD
PARK12	Xq21-q25	*TAF1*/Transcription initiation factor TFIID subunit 1	X-linked	Classic PD
PARK 13	2p13.1	*HTRA2*/HTRA serine peptidase 2 (unconfirmed)	AD or risk factor	Classic PD
PARK14	22q13.1	*PLA2G6*/Phospholipase A2, group VI	AR	EODPD
PARK15	22q12-q13	*FBXO7*/F-box only protein 7	AR	EOPPS
PARK16	1q32	Risk factor/gene unkown	?	Classic PD
PARK17	16q11.2	*VPS35*/Vacuolar protein sorting-associated protein 35	AD	Classic PD
PARK18	3q27.1	*EIF4G1*/Eukaryotic translation initiation factor 4 gamma, 1	AD	Classic PD
Frontotemporal dementia with parkinsonism-17	**17q21.1**	***MAPT*/Microtubule-associated protein Tau**	**AD**	**FTD**
Familial multisystem degeneration with parkinsonism	mtDNA11778	Mitochondrial mutation	Maternally transmitted	

Abbreviations: EODPD, early-onset dystonia-parkinsonism; EOPD, early-onset PD; EOPPS, early-onset parkinsonian pyramidal syndrome; FTD, frontotemporal dementia; PD, Parkinson's disease.

B. Trinucleotide-repeat diseases

DISEASE	INHERITANCE	REPEATS	CHROMOSOME	PROTEIN
Huntington's	AD	**CAG**	**4p16**	**Huntingtin**
Fragile X	AD	**CGG**	**Xq27.3**	**FMR-1**
Myotonic dystrophy	AD	**CTG**	**19**	**Myotonin**
Spinocerebellar ataxia type 1 (SCA 1)	AD	CAG	6p23	Ataxin-1
SCA 2	AD	CAG	12q24	Ataxin-2
SCA 3 (Machado-Joseph)	AD	CAG	14q32	Ataxin-3
SCA 6	AD	CAG	19p13	Voltage-dependent calcium channel
SCA 7	AD	CAG	13p12	Ataxin-7
SCA 12	AD	CAG	5q31-33	Regulatory subunit of protein phosphatase (PP2A)
SCA 17	AD	CAG	6q27	TATA-binding protein
Spinobulbar muscular atrophy (Kennedy's)	**X-linked recessive**	**CAG**	**Xq12**	**Androgen receptor**
Dentatorubropal-lidoluysian atrophy	AD	CAG	12p13	Atrophin-1
Friedreich's ataxia	**AR**	**GAA**	**9q13-21.1**	**Frataxin**

Abbreviations: A, Adenine; C, Cytosine; G, Guanine; T, Thymine.

The majority of trinucleotide repeats are CAG repeats. Here are mnemonics to help remember the non-CAG repeats:

DISEASE	TRINUCLEOTIDE REPEAT	MNEMONIC
Fragile X	CGG	"**C**hild (with) **G**iant **G**onads"
Myotonic dystrophy	CTG	"**C**ontinues **T**o **G**rasp"
Friedreich's ataxia	GAA	"**G**erman (name) **A**taxi**A**"

C. Dystonia

DYSTONIA TYPE	GENE	INHERITANCE	CHROMOSOME	GENE/MUTATION
Early-onset generalized torsion dystonia	**DYT 1**	**AD**	**9q34**	***TOR1A*/Torsin A GAG deletion**
AR torsion dystonia	DYT 2	AR	1p35.1	*HPCA*/Hippocalcin
X-linked dystonia parkinsonism	DYT 3	X-linked	Xq13.1	*TAF1*-unconfirmed
Non-DYT1 torsion dystonia	DYT 4	AD	19p13.3	*TUBB4A*/Tubulin beta 4A

(continued)

DYSTONIA TYPE	GENE	INHERITANCE	CHROMOSOME	GENE/MUTATION
Dopa-responsive dystonia and parkinsonism (Segawa syndrome)	**DYT 5a**	**AD**	**14q22.2**	***GCH1*/GTP cyclohydrolase I** **NOTE: Identical to DYT14**
Segawa syndrome—recessive	DYT 5b	AR	11p15.5	*TH*/Tyrosine hydroxylase
Segawa syndrome—recessive	NA	AR	2p13.2	*SPR*/Sepiapterin reductase
Adolescent and early-adult torsion dystonia of mixed phenotype	DYT 6	AD	8p11.21	*THAP1*/THAP domain-containing protein 1
Adult-onset focal dystonia	DYT 7	AD	18p	Unknown
Paroxysmal nonkinesiogenic dyskinesia	DYT 8	AD	2q35	*PNKD*/Myofibrillogenesis regulator 1
Paroxysmal choreoathetosis with episodic ataxia and spasticity	DYT 9	AD	1p34.2	SLC2A1 = GLUT1/Facilitated glucose transporter 1 NOTE: Same as DYT18, and GLUT1 deficiency syndrome (De Vivo syndrome)
Paroxysmal kinesiogenic dyskinesia	DYT 10	AD	16p11.2	*PRRT2*/Proline-rich transmembrane protein 2
Myoclonus dystonia	**DYT 11**	**AD**	**7q21.3**	***SGCE*/ε-sarcoglycan**
Rapid-onset dystonia parkinsonism	DYT 12	AD	19q13.2	*ATP1A3*/ATPase Na+/K+ transporting, alpha-3 Same gene as alternating hemiplegia of childhood-2
Early- and late-onset cervical cranial dystonia	DYT 13	AD	1p36.32-p36.13	Unknown
Adult-onset cranial-cervical dystonia	DYT 25	AD	18p11	*GNAL*/Guanine nucleotide-binding protein, alpha-activating activity polypeptide, olfactory type

D. AR ataxias with known gene loci

DISEASE	CHROMOSOME	GENE
Friedreich's ataxia	**9q21.11**	**FXN/Frataxin**
Ataxia telangiectasia	11q22.3	*ATM*/Ataxia-telangiectasia mutated gene
Ataxia with isolated vitamin E deficiency	8q12.3	*TTPA*/alpha-tocopherol transporter protein
AR ataxia of Charlevoix-Saguenay	13q12.12	*SACS*/Sacsin
Ataxia with oculomotor apraxia	**9p21.1**	**APTX/Aprataxin**
Spinocerebellar ataxia, AR 1 (previously, Ataxia, neuropathy, high α-fetoprotein)	9q34.1	*SETX*/Senataxin
Infantile onset olivopontocerebellar atrophy	10q24.31	C10orf2
Ataxia, deafness, optic atrophy	6p21-23	Unknown
Unverricht-Lundborg	**21q22.3**	**CSTB/Cystatin B**

E. AD ataxias

DISEASE	CHROMOSOME	GENE	MUTATION
SCA 1	6p22.3	*ATXN1*	CAG expansion
SCA 2	12q24.12	*ATXN2*	CAG expansion
SCA 3/Machado-Joseph disease	14q32.12	**ATXN3**	CAG expansion
SCA 4	16q22.1	—	—
SCA 5	11q13.2	*SPTBN2*	—
SCA 6	19p13.2	*CACNA1*	CAG expansion
SCA 7	3p14.1	*ATXN7*	CAG expansion
SCA 8	13q21.33	*ATXN8OS*	CTG/CAG expansion
SCA 10	22q13.31	*ATXN10*	ATTCT expansion
SCA 11	15q15.2	*TTBK2*	—
SCA 12	5q32	*PPP2R2B*	CAG expansion
SCA 13	19q13.33	*KCNC3*	—
SCA 14	19q13.42	*PRKCG*	—
SCA 15	3p26.1	*ITPR1*	Also causes SCA29
SCA 17	6p27	*TBP*	CAG or CAA expansion
Dentatorubropallidoluysian atrophy	12p13.31	*ATN1*	CAG expansion
Episodic ataxia 1	12p13.32	**KCNA1**	—
Episodic ataxia 2	19p13.2	**CACNA 1**	—

VI. Neuromuscular Disorders

DISEASE	GENE	CHROMOSOME
Familial amyotrophic lateral sclerosis (FALS) FTD/ALS ALS6 ALS10	**SOD1 (20% FALS)** C9orf72 (20-30% FALS) *FUS/TLS* (~4% FALS) *TARDBP* (1-4% FALS)	**21q22.11** 9p21.2 16p11.2 1p36.2
ALS2, juvenile onset	ALS2	2q33.1
Charcot-Marie-Tooth 1A	**PMP22 (Duplication)**	**17p12**
Charcot-Marie-Tooth 1B	MPZ	1q23.3
Hereditary neuropathy with liability to pressure palsy/Tomaculous neuropathy	**PMP22 (Deletion/ Mutation)**	**17p12**
Charcot-Marie-Tooth 2A2 (most common form of CMT2, ~20%)	—*MFN2*	1p36.22
Charcot-Marie-Tooth 3 (Dejerine-Sottas disease)	—Multiple genes impli- cated, most commonly: **PMP22** *MPZ* *EGR2* *PRX*	17p12 1q23.3 10q21.3 19q13.2
Charcot-Marie-Tooth X1	**GJB1/Cx32**	**Xq13.1**
Familial amyloidotic peripheral neuropathy	*TTR*	18q12.1
Familial dysautonomia (Riley Day syndrome)	*IKBKAP*	9q31.3
Duchenne's and Becker's muscular dystrophy	**DMD/Dystrophin**	**Xp21.2-p21.1**
Myotonic dystrophy type 1	**DMPK (>50 CTG repeats)**	**19q13.32**
Myotonic dystrophy type 2	*ZNF9* (CCTG repeat)	3q21.3
Nemaline myopathy (AD)	Multiple genes, most commonly: *NEB* (~50%) *ACTA1* (15–25%) *TPM3* (2–3%)	2q23.3 1q42.13 1q21.3
Central core myopathy Minicore myopathy with external ophthalmoplegia Malignant hyperthermia susceptibility	*RYR1*/Ryanodine receptor	19q13.2
Myotubular/Centronuclear myopathy	*MTM1*	Xq28
Ullrich's congenital muscular dystrophy (AD/AR)	**COL6A3** **COL6A1** **COL6A2**	**2q37.3** **21q22.3** **21q22.3**
Bethlem myopathy (allelic AD, milder phenotype of Ullrich's)	**COL6A3** **COL6A1** **COL6A2**	**2q37.3** **21q22.3** **21q22.3**

(continued)

DISEASE	GENE	CHROMOSOME
Congenital muscular dystrophy type 1 (merosin deficient)	*LAMA2*	6q22.33
Walker-Warburg congenital muscular dystrophy type A1 (dystroglycanopathy)	**POMT1**	**9q34.13**
Congenital muscular dystrophy type A2 (dystroglycanopathy)	**POMT2**	**14q24.3**
Muscle-brain-eye congenital muscular dystrophy type A3 (dystroglycanopathy)	**POMGNT1**	**1p34.1**
Fukuyama congenital muscular dystrophy (dystroglycanopathy)	**FKTN/FUKUTIN**	**9q31.2**
Congenital muscular dystrophy type A5 (with or without intellectual disability) (dystroglycanopathy)	*FKRP/FUKUTIN-*related protein	19q13.32
Severe childhood muscular dystrophy (limb-girdle MD, type 2D, AR)	**SGCA**	17q21.33
Spinal muscular atrophy (SMA) 1 (Werdnig-Hoffman) SMA II, infantile chronic SMAIII, juvenile onset (Wohlfart-Kugelberg-Welander) SMAIV, adult onset	**SMN1** SMA-phenotype modifier genes: *SMN2* *NAIP* *GTF2H1/BTF2*	**5q13.2** 5q13.2 5q13.2 5q13.2
Spinobulbar muscular atrophy (Kennedy's)	**AR/Androgen receptor**	**Xq21.312**
Fascioscapulohumeral dystrophy (FSHD) type 1	D4Z4 microsatellite repeat contraction (1–10 repeats only; normal 11–150 repeats)	4q35
FSHD type 2	Digenic inheritance: Mutation *SMCHD1* Permissive allele 4A161 in *DUX4*	18q11.32 4q35
Limb-girdle muscular dystrophies (LGMD), type 1 (AD) LGMD1A (myotilinopathy) LGMD1B LGMD1C (caveolinopathy):	Multiple genes/subtypes *MYOT* *LMNA* *CAV3*	5q31.2 1q22 3p25.3
LGMD, type 2 (AR) LGMD2A (calpainopathy) LGMD2B (dysferlinopathy) Sarcoglycanopathies: LGMD2C LGMD2D LGMD2E LGMD2F	Multiple genes/subtypes *CAPN3* *DYSF* *SGCG* *SGCA* *SGCB* *SGCD*	15q15.1 2p13.2 13q12.12 17q21.33 4q12 5q33.2-33.3
Emery-Dreifuss muscular dystrophy	**EMD**	**Xq28**

(continued)

DISEASE	GENE	CHROMOSOME
Distal myopathy type 1 (Laing)	*MYH7*	14q11.2
Kearns-Sayre syndrome	—	**mtDNA deletion (1–10 Kb)**
(Chronic) Progressive external ophthalmoplegia (PEA), AD	Autosomal and mitochondrial mutations/ deletions	
	MT-TL1	mtDNA
PEA1, AD	*POLG*	15q26.1
PEA2, AD	*ANTI*	4q35.1
PEA3	*C10ORF2/TWINKLE*	10q24
PEA4	*POLG2*	17q23.3
PEA5	*RRM2B*	8q23
PEA6, AD	*DNA2*	10q21.3
Myoclonic epilepsy with ragged red fibers (MERFF)	*MTTK* *MTTL1* *MTTH* *MTTS1* *MTTS2* *MTTF* *MTND5*	mtDNA
Mitochondrial encephalomyopathy with lactic acidosis and stroke-like episodes (MELAS)	**Most common:** ***MTTL1* c.3243A-G** Others: *MTTQ* *MTTH* *MTTK* *MTTC* *MTTS1* *MTND1* *MTND5* *MTND6* *MTTS2*	mtDNA
Sodium channelopathies: Hyperkalemic periodic paralysis Paramyotonia congenital Hypokalemic periodic paralysis 2	***SCN4A***	**17q22.3**
Calcium channelopathy: Hypokalemic periodic paralysis	*CACNA1S/CACNL1A3*	1q32.1
Chloride channelopathy AD myotonia congenita (Thomsen's) AR myotonia congenital (Becker)	***CLCN1*** ***CLCN1***	**7q34** **7q34**
McArdle's disease (glycogen storage disease V, myophosphorylase deficiency)	*PYGM*	11q13.1
acute intermittent porphyria	*HMBS*	11q23.3

(continued)

DISEASE	GENE	CHROMOSOME

Hereditary spastic paraplegia (HSP)
   AD
   AR
   X-linked
Maternal (mitochondrial)
	~56 HSP loci and 41 HSP-related genes	See "Hereditary Spastic Paraplegia Overview" on the GeneReview's website: http://www.ncbi.nlm.nih.gov/books/NBK1509/

Hyperekplexia (startle)	*GLRA1*	5q33.1
Congenital myasthenic syndromes (multiple genes identified, all code for neuromuscular junction proteins)	Most common: *CHRNE* (50%) *RAPSN* (15%–20%) *COLQ* (10%–15%) *DOK7* (10%–15%) *CHAT* (4%–5%) *GFPT1* (2%)	17p13.2 11p11.2 3p25.1 4p16.3 10q11.23 2p13.3

VII. Stroke/Narcolepsy/Seizures

DISEASE	GENE	CHROMOSOME
Cerebral autosomal dominant arteriopathy with subcortical infarcts and leukoencephalopathy (CADASIL)	**NOTCH3**	**19p13.12**
Cerebral autosomal recessive arteriopathy with subcortical infarcts and leukoencephalopathy (CARASIL)	*HTRA1*	10q26.13
Homocystinuria (cystathionine beta-synthase deficiency)	*CBS*	21q22.3
Cystatin 3/cerebral amyloid angiopathy	*CST3*	20p11.21
Mitochondrial encephalomyopathy with lactic acidosis and stroke-like episodes (MELAS)	Most common: *MTTL1* c.3243A-G Others: *MTTQ* *MTTH* *MTTK* *MTTC* *MTTS1* *MTND1* *MTND5* *MTND6* *MTTS2*	mtDNA

(continued)

DISEASE	GENE	CHROMOSOME
Familial cerebral cavernous malformations		
Type 1	*CCM1/KRIT1*	**7q21.2**
Type 2	*CCM2*	7p13
Type 3	*CCM3/PDCD10*	3q26.1
Narcolepsy 1	*HCRT*	**17.q21.2**
Benign familial neonatal seizures (BFNS)		
BFNS1	*KCNQ2*	**20q13.33**
BFNS2	*KCNQ2*	**8q24.22**
BFNS3	*SCN2A*	**2q24.3**
Dravet's (formerly "severe myoclonic epilepsy of infancy")	*SCN1A* Potential modifier: *SCN9A*	**2q24.3** 2q24.3
Generalized epilepsy with febrile seizures plus (GEFS+), Types 1-9	Multiple loci/ genes,	
Type 1	*SCN1B*	**19q13.12**
Type 2	*SCN1A*	**2q21.3**
Type 3	*GABRG2*	5q34
GLUT1 deficiency (DeVivo syndrome)	*SLC2A1*	**1p34.2**
Juvenile myoclonic epilepsy	*EFHC1*	6p12.2
Myoclonic epilepsy (Unverricht-Lundborg)	*CSTB*	21q22.3
Lafora body disease	*NHLRC1* *EPM2A*	6p22.3 6p24.3

VIII. Genetic Syndromes Associated With Brain Tumors (From Kesari and Wen 2004)

SYNDROME	INHERITANCE	GENE PROTEIN CHROMOSOME	ASSOCIATED TUMORS
Neurofibromatosis type 1 (von Recklinghausen syndrome)	AD	*NF1* **neurofibromin** **17q11.2**	Schwannomas, astrocytomas, optic nerve gliomas, meningiomas, neurofibromas, neurofibrosarcomas
Neurofibromatosis type 2	AD	*NF2* **merlin** **22q12.2**	Bilateral vestibular schwannomas, astrocytomas, multiple meningiomas, ependymomas

(continued)

SYNDROME	INHERITANCE	GENE PROTEIN CHROMOSOME			ASSOCIATED TUMORS
von Hippel-Lindau disease	AD	**VHL** **VHL** **3p25.3**			Hemangioblastomas, paragangliomas, pancreatic cysts, retinal angiomas, renal cell carcinomas, pheochromocytomas
Li-Fraumeni syndrome	AD	*TP53* p53 17p13.1			Gliomas, sarcomas, osteosarcomas, breast cancer, leukemias
Mismatch repair cancer syndrome (Turcot's syndrome)	AD	*APC* (adenomatous polyposis coli) 5q22.2			Gliomas, medulloblastomas, adenomatous colon polyps, adenocarcinoma
Basal cell nevus (Gorlin's syndrome)	AD	*PTCH1* Patched1 9q22.32	*PTCH2* Patched2 1p34.1	*SUFU* Suppressor of Fused 10q24.32	Basal cell carcinoma, medulloblastomas

IX. Channelopathies With Neurologic Manifestations (Excluding Seizure Disorders Listed in Part VII)

DISEASE	GENE	ION CHANNEL
Hyperkalemic periodic paralysis	**SCN4A**	Sodium channel
Paramyotonia congenita	**SCN4A**	Sodium channel
Potassium-aggravated myotonia	*SCN4A*	Sodium channel
Hypokalemic periodic paralysis type 2	*SCN4A*	Sodium channel
Erythromelalgia	*SCN9A*	Sodium channel
Paroxysmal extreme pain disorder	*SCN9A*	Sodium channel
Congenital insensitivity to pain disorder	*SCN9A*	Sodium channel
Myotonia congenita	**CLCN1**	Chloride channel
Hypokalemic periodic paralysis type 1	**CACNA1S/ CACNL1A3**	Calcium channel
Episodic ataxia type 2 (with nystagmus)	**CACNA1A**	Calcium channel
Familial hemiplegic migraine	**CACNA1A** **ATP1A2** **SCN1A**	Calcium channel Na$^+$/K$^+$ ATPase Sodium channel
SCA 6	*CACNA1A*	Calcium channel

(continued)

DISEASE	GENE	ION CHANNEL
Timothy syndrome	*CACNA1C*	Calcium channel
Episodic ataxia type 1 (with myokymia)	**KCNA1**	Potassium channel
Neuromyotonia	*KCNA1*	Potassium channel
Andersen-Tawil syndrome	*KCNJ2*	Potassium channel
Jervell Lange Nielsen syndrome	*KCNQ1* (90%) *KCNE1* (10%)	Potassium channel
Nonsyndromic dominant progressive deafness	*KCNQ4*	Potassium channel
Alternating hemiplegia of childhood	**ATP1A3**	Na$^+$/K$^+$ ATPase
Hereditary hyperekplexia	*GLRA1*	Glycine receptor

X. Pediatric Neurology

A. Phakomatoses

DISEASE	PROTEIN	CHROMOSOME
Neurofibromatosis 1	**Neurofibromin**	**17q11.2**
Neurofibromatosis 2	**Merlin**	**22q11-13.1**
Legius syndrome	SPRED1	15q14
von Hippel-Lindau	**VHL**	**3p25.3**
Tuberous sclerosis	**TSC1 (hamartin)** **TSC2 (tuberin)**	**9q34.13** **16p13.3**
Ataxia telangiectasia	ATM	11q22.3
Sturge-Weber	GNAQ	9q21.2
Klippel-Trenaunay-Weber	—	8q22.3
Incontinentia pigmenti	IKBKG (Nemo)	Xq28

B. Lysosomal storage diseases

DISEASE	INHERITANCE	ENZYME DEFICIENCY (GENE)	CHROMOSOME
Neuronal ceroid lipofuscinosis			
CLN10/CTSD (Congenital)	AR	Cathepsin D (*CTSD*)	11p15.5
CLN1 (Classic Infantile)	AR	**Palmitoyl-protein thiesterase-1 (PPT1)**	**1p34.2**
CLN2 (Late Infantile)	AR	**Tripeptidyl-peptidase 1 (TTP1)**	**11q15.4**
CLN3 (Atypical Juvenile)	AR	**Battenin (CLN3)**	**16p11.2**
CLN6 (Adult)	AR	CLN Protein 6 (*CLN6*)	15q23
CLN13 (Adult)	AR	Cathepsin F (*CTSF*)	11q13.2

(continued)

B. Lysosomal storage diseases (*cont'd*)

DISEASE	INHERITANCE	ENZYME DEFICIENCY (GENE)	CHROMOSOME
Mucopolysaccharidoses (MPS)			
MPS1 Hurler, Scheie, and Hurler-Scheie	AR	**α-L-iduronidase (*IDUA*)**	4p16.3
MPS2 Hunter	**X-linked recessive**	**Iduronate sulfatase (*IDS*)**	**Xq28**
MPS3A Sanfilippo A	AR	Heparan sulfamidase (*SGSH*)	17q25.3
MPS3B Sanfilippo B	AR	N-acetylglucosamini-dase (*NAGLU*)	17q21.2
MPS3C Sanfilippo C	AR	Heparan-α-glucos-aminide N-acetyltrans-ferase (*HGSNAT*)	8p11.21
MPS3D Sanfilippo D	AR	N-acetylglucosamine 6-sulfatase (*GNS*)	12q14.3
MPS4A Morquio A	AR	Galactose-6-sulfate sul-fatase (*GALNS*)	16q24.3
MPS4B Morquio B	AR	β-galactosidase (*GLB1*)	3p22.3
MPS6 Maroteaux–Lamy syndrome	AR	N-acetylgalac-tosamine-4-sulfatase (*ARSB*)	5q14.1
MPS7 Sly	AR	β-glucuronidase (*GUSB*)	7q11.21
MPS9 Natowicz	AR	Hyaluronidase (*HYAL1*)	3p21.31
Sphingolipidoses			
Gangliosidoses			
GM1 Gangliosidosis	AR	β-galactosidase 1 (*GLB1*)	3p22.3
GM2 Gangliosidosis			
Sandhoff	**AR**	**Hexosaminidase A Hexosaminidase B (*HEXB*)**	5q13.3
Tay-Sachs	**AR**	**Hexosaminidase A (*HEXA*)**	15 q23
GM2 AB Variant	AR	GM2 Activator protein (*GM2A*)	5q33.1
Glycolipidoses			
Fabry's	**X-linked recessive**	**α-galactosidase A (*GLA*)**	**Xq22.1**
Niemann-Pick type A Niemann-Pick type B	**AR**	**Acid sphingomyelinase (*SMPD1*)**	11p15.4
Niemann-Pick type C1	AR	Niemann-Pick C1 choles-terol transporter (*NPC1*)	18q11.2

(continued)

DISEASE	INHERITANCE	ENZYME DEFICIENCY (GENE)	CHROMOSOME
Niemann-Pick type C1	AR	Niemann-Pick C2 cholesterol transporter (*NPC2*)	14q24.3
Krabbe's	**AR**	**Galactocerebrosidase (*GALC*)**	**14q31.3**
Metachromatic leukodystrophy	**AR**	**Arylsulfatase A (*ARSA*)**	**22q13.33**
Glucocerebrosidosis			
Gaucher's	AR	β-glucocerebrosidase (*GBA*)	1q22
Mucolipidoses			
Sialidosis type I and II	AR	Neuraminidase 1 (*NEU1*)	6p21.33
Mucoliposis II alpha/beta (I-cell disease)	AR	N-acetylglucosamine-1-phosphotransferase (*GNPTAB*)	12q23.2
Glycogen storage disease (GSD)			
Pompe's (GSD type II)	**AR**	**α-1,4 glycosidase (acid maltase) (*GAA*)**	**17q25.3**
Danon disease (GSD type IIb)	**X-linked recessive**	**Lysosome-associated membrane protein-2 (*LAMP2*)**	**Xq24**
McArdle's (GSD type V)	AR; rarely AD	Myophosphorylase (*PYGM*)	11q13.1
Lactate dehydrogenase deficiency (GSD XI)	AR	Lactate dehydrogenase A (*LDHA*) Lactate dehydrogenase B (*LDHB*)	11p15.1 12q12.1
Other lysosomal storage diseases			
Cystinosis	AR	Cystinosin (*CTNS*)	17p13.2
Fucosidosis	AR	α-L-fucosidase (*FUCA1*)	1p36.11

C. Other inborn errors of metabolism

DISEASE	INHERITANCE	ENZYME DEFICIENCY (GENE)	CHROMOSOME
Amino Acidopathies			
Phenylketonuria	AR	phenylalanine hydroxylase (*PAH*)	12q23.2

Maple syrup urine disease
    Type Ia
    Type Ib
    Type II
	AR	Branched-chain alpha-keto acid dehydrogenase complex:
		E1 alpha subunit (*BCKDHA*)
		Beta polypeptide (*BCKDHB*)
		Dihydrolipoyl transacylase (*DBT*)
			19q13.2
			6q14
			1p21.2

(continued)

C. Other inborn errors of metabolism (*cont'd*)

DISEASE	INHERITANCE	ENZYME DEFICIENCY (GENE)	CHROMOSOME
Aspartylglucosaminuria	AR	Aspartylglucosaminidase (*AGA*)	4q34.3
Methylmalonic aciduria	AR	Methylmalonyl-CoA mutase (MUT)	6p12.3
Homocystinuria	AR	Cystathionine beta-synthase (CBS)	21q22.3
Tyrosinemia	AR	Fumarylacetoacetate hydrolase (FAH)	15q25.1
Hartnup	AR	Solute carrier family 6 member 19 (*SLC6A19*)	5p15.33
Nonketotic hyper-glycinemia (glycine encephalopathy)	AR	Three glycine cleavage proteins: P (*GLDC*) T (*GCST*) H (*GCSH*)	9p24.1 3p21.31 16q23.2
Glutaric academia I	AR	glutaryl-CoA dehydrogenase (*GCDH*)	19p13.2
Fatty Acid Oxidation			
Carnitine transport defect	AR	Organic cation transporter 2 (*SLC22A5*)	5q31.1
Carnitine palmitoyltrans-ferase deficiency 1A	AR	Carnitine palmitoyltransferase deficiency 1A (*CPT1A*)	11q13.3
Carnitine palmitoyl-transferase deficiency 2	AR	carnitine palmitoyltransferase II (*CPT2*)	1p32.3
Very long-chain acyl-coenzyme A dehy-drogenase deficiency (VLCAD deficiency)	AR	(*ACADVL*)	17p13.1
Long-chain 3-hydroxyacyl-coenzyme A dehy-drogenase deficiency (LCHAD deficiency)	AR	(*HADHA*)	2p23.3
Medium-chain acyl-coenzyme A dehy-drogenase deficiency (MCAD deficiency)	AR	(*ACADM*)	1p31.1
Short-chain acyl-coenzyme A dehy-drogenase deficiency (SCAD deficiency)	AR	(*ACADS*)	12q24.31
Trifunctional protein deficiency	AR	Mitochondrial trifunctional protein subunit alpha or beta (*HADHA/HADHB*)	2p23.3

(continued)

DISEASE	INHERITANCE	ENZYME DEFICIENCY (GENE)	CHROMOSOME
Peroxisomal Biogenesis Disorders			
PBD-Zellweger spectrum		Multiple pexin genes: PEX1, PEX2, PEX3, PEX5, PEX6, PEX12, PEX14, PEX26	
Infantile refsum	AR	*PEX1*	7q21.2
Neonatal adrenoleu-kodystrophy	AR	*PEX1*	7q21.2
Zellweger syndrome	AR	*PEX1*	7q21.2
Rhizomelic chondro-dysplasia punctata	AR	Peroxisomal type 2 targeting signal receptor (*PEX7*)	6q23.3
Urea Cycle Disorders			
Argininosuccinic aciduria	AR	Argininosuccinate lyase (*ASL*)	7q11.21
N-Acetylglutamate synthase deficiency	AR	(*NAGS*)	17q21.31
Ornithine transcarba-mylase deficiency	**X-linked recessive**	**Ornithine Transcarbamylase (OTC)**	**Xp21.1**
Carbamoyl phosphate synthetase I deficiency	AR	(*CPS1*)	2q34
Citrullinemia	AR	Argininosuccinate synthetase (*ASS1*)	9q34.11
Argininemia	AR	Arginase (*ARG1*)	6q23.2

D. Other metabolic/genetic disorders

DISEASE	INHERITANCE	PROTEIN (GENE)	CHROMOSOME
Wilson's disease (hepatolen-ticular degeneration)	**AR**	**Cu(2+)-transporting ATPase, beta polypeptide (ATP7B)**	**13p14.3**
Menke's	X-linked recessive	Cu(2+)-transporting AT-Pase, alpha polypeptide (*ATP7A*)	Xq21.1
Pantothenate kinase-associated neurode-generation (PKAN); Neurodegeneration with brain iron accumulation	**AR**	**Pantothenate kinase-2 (PANK2)**	**20p13**
Lesch-Nyhan	**X-linked recessive**	**Hypoxanthine-guanine-phosphoribosyl transferase (HPRT1)**	**Xq26**
Galactosemia 1	AR	Galactose-1-phosphate uridyl transferase (*GALT*)	9p13

(continued)

D. Other metabolic/genetic disorders (*cont'd*)

DISEASE	INHERITANCE	PROTEIN (GENE)	CHROMOSOME
Pyruvate dehydrogenase deficiency	X-linked recessive	E1-alpha (*PDHA1O*)	Xp22.12
Pyruvate carboxylase deficiency (Leigh's)	AR	Pyruvate carboxylase (*PC*)	11q13.2
Abetalipoproteinemia (Bassen-Kornzweig)	AR	Microsomal triglyceride transfer protein (*MTTP*)	4q23
Familial hypobetalipoproteinemia	AR	Apolipoprotein B (*APOB*)	2p24.1
Kallmann's anosmia-hypogonadism	**X-linked recessive**	**Anosmin (*KAL1*)**	**Xp22.31**
Ataxia/sideroblastic anemia	X-linked recessive	ATP-binding cassette transporter 7 (*ABCB7*)	Xq13.3
Aicardi syndrome	**X-linked dominant**	**(*AIC*)**	**Xp22**
Rett syndrome	**X-linked dominant**	**Methyl-CpG-binding protein 2 (*MECP2*)**	**Xq28**
CDKL5	**X-linked dominant**	**Cyclin dependent kinase-like 5 (*CDKL5*)**	**Xp22.13**
Neuronal Migration Disorders			
Lissencephaly (LIS)			
LIS1, classic (Miller-Dieker)	**AR**	**LIS1(*PAFAH1B1*)**	**17p13.3**
Cobblestone	AR	Congenital muscular dystrophies (see previous discussion)	
LIS2 (Norman-Roberts syndrome)	AR	Reelin (*RELN*)	7q22.1
LIS3	AR	Alpha-1-tubulin (*TUBA1A*)	12q13.12
LISX1	**X-linked dominant**	**Doublcortin (*DBX*)**	**Xq23**
LISX2	X-linked recessive	Aristaless-related homeobox protein (*ARX*)	Xp21.3
Holoprosencephaly 3	AD	Sonic Hedgehog (*SHH*)	7q36.3
Schizencephaly	?	(*SIX3*) (*SHH*) (*EMX2*)	2p21 7q36.3 10q26.11

E. Leukodystrophies

DISEASE	INHERITANCE	PROTEIN (GENE)	CHROMOSOME
Alexander disease	**AD**	**Glial fibrillary acid protein (*GFAP*)**	**17q21.31**
Pelizaeus-Merzbacher	**X-linked recessive**	**Proteolipoprotein 1 (*PLP*)**	**Xq22.2**

(continued)

DISEASE	INHERITANCE	PROTEIN (GENE)	CHROMOSOME
Adrenoleukodystrophy Adrenomyeloneuropathy	**X-linked recessive**	**ATPase-binding cassette transporter (ABCD1)**	**Xq28**
Cerebrotendinous xanthomatosis	AR	Sterol 27-hydroxylase (CYP27A1)	2q35
Canavan disease	**AR**	**Aspartoacylase (ASPA)**	**17p13.2**
Leukoencephalopathy with vanishing white matter	AR	Mutations in the translation initiation factor EIF-2B: EIF2B1 EIF2B2 EIF2B3 EIF2B4 EIF2B5	12q24.31 14q24.3 1p34.1 2p23.3 3q27.1
Refsum (classic adult) Peroxisome biogenesis disorder 9B (phenotype identical to refsum)	AR AR	phytanoyl-CoA hydroxylase (PHYH) Peroxin-7 (PEX7)	10p13 6q23.3
Krabbe's	**AR**	**Galactocerebrosidase (GALC)**	**14q31.3**
Metachromatic leukodystrophy	**AR**	**Arylsulfatase A (ARSA)**	**22q13.33**

F. Other mitochondrial disorders (not included in earlier discussion)

Complex I	Nicotinamide adenine dinucleotide-coenzyme Q reductase	Congenital lactic acidosis, hypotonia, seizures, and apnea Exercise intolerance and myalgia Kearns-Sayre syndrome Mitochondrial encephalomyopathy with lactic acidosis and stroke-like episodes Progressive infantile poliodystrophy Subacute necrotizing encephalomyelopathy (Leigh disease)
Complex II	Succinate-coenzyme Q reductase	Encephalomyopathy
Complex III	Coenzyme QH_2-cytochrome-c reductase	Cardiomyopathy Kearns-Sayre syndrome Myopathy and exercise intolerance with or without progressive external ophthalmoplegia
Complex IV	Cytochrome-c oxidase	Fatal neonatal hypotonia Menke's syndrome Myoclonic epilepsy with ragged red fibers Progressive infantile poliodystrophy Subacute necrotizing encephalomyelopathy (Leigh disease)

(continued)

F. **Other mitochondrial disorders (not included in earlier discussion)** (*cont'd*)

Complex V	Adenosine triphos-phate synthase	Congenital myopathy Neuropathy, retinopathy, ataxia, and dementia Retinitis pigmentosa, ataxia, neuropathy, and dementia
Leber hereditary optic atrophy	18 allelic variants listed in Online Mendelian Inheritance in Man	Degeneration of retinal ganglion cells Acute to subacute bilateral vision loss Males are affected younger than females Male predominance (3-8:1 M:F, depending on mutation)
Neuropathy, ataxia, retinitis pigmentosa syndrome (NARP)	subunit 6 of mitochondrial H(+)-ATPase (*MTATP6*)	Developmental delay, retinitis pigmentosa, dementia, seizures, ataxia, proximal neurogenic muscle weakness, sensory neuropathy, hearing loss, cardiac conduction defects

Suggested Readings

Gene Reviews: http://www.ncbi.nlm.nih.gov/books/NBK1116/

Gene Test Registry: http://www.ncbi.nlm.nih.gov/gtr/

Kesari S, Wen PY. Neurooncolgy. In: Samuels M, ed. Manual of Neurologic Therapuetics, 7th edition. Philadelphia: PA, Lippincott Williams & Wilkins;2004. pp115-178.

Online Mendelian Inheritance in Man: http://www.omim.org/

CHAPTER 3

Neurohistology, Embryology, and Developmental Disorders

I. Neurohistology

A. **Neurons:** classified by the number of processes

1. *Pseudounipolar:* located in the spinal dorsal root ganglia and sensory ganglia of the cranial nerves V, VII, IX, X

2. *Bipolar:* found in the cochlear and vestibular ganglia of cranial nerve VIII, in the olfactory nerve, and in the retina

3. *Multipolar:* the largest population of nerve cells in the nervous system; includes the motor neurons, neurons of the autonomic nervous system, interneurons, pyramidal cells of the cerebral cortex, and Purkinje cells of the cerebellar cortex

B. **Nissl substance:** consists of rosettes of polysomes and rough endoplasmic reticulum; therefore, it has a role in protein synthesis; found in the nerve cell body (perikaryon) and dendrites and not in the axon hillock or axon

C. **Axonal transport:** mediates the intracellular distribution of secretory proteins, organelles, and cytoskeletal elements; inhibited by colchicine, which depolarizes microtubules

1. *Fast anterograde axonal transport:* responsible for transporting all newly synthesized membrane organelles (vesicles) and precursors of neurotransmitters; occurs at *a rate of 200 to 400 mm per day;* mediated by neurotubules and kinesin; neurotubule dependent

2. *Slow anterograde transport:* responsible for transporting fibrillar cytoskeletal and protoplasmic elements; occurs at a rate of 1 to 5 mm per day

3. *Fast retrograde transport:* returns used materials from the axon terminal to the cell body for degradation and recycling at a rate of 100 to 200 mm per day; transports nerve growth factor, neurotropic viruses, and toxins (e.g., herpes simplex, rabies, poliovirus, and tetanus toxin); mediated by neurotubules and dynein

D. **Wallerian degeneration:** anterograde degeneration characterized by the disappearance of axons and myelin sheaths and the secondary proliferation of Schwann cells; occurs in the central nervous system (CNS) and peripheral nervous system (PNS)

E. **Chromatolysis:** the result of retrograde degeneration in the neurons of the CNS and PNS; there is loss of Nissl substance after axotomy

> **NB:** Axonal sprout grows at the rate of 3 mm per day in the PNS.

F. **Glial cells:** nonneural cells of the nervous system

   1. *Macroglia:* consists of astrocytes and oligodendrocytes

       a. *Astrocytes:* project foot processes that envelop the basement membrane of capillaries, neurons, and synapses; form the external and internal glial-limiting membranes of the CNS; play a role in the metabolism of certain neurotransmitters (e.g., γ-aminobutyric acid, serotonin, glutamate); buffer the potassium concentration of the extracellular space; form glial scars in damaged areas of the brain; contain glial fibrillary acidic protein, a marker for astrocytes; contain glutamine synthetase

       b. *Oligodendrocytes:* myelin-forming cells of the CNS; *one oligodendrocyte can myelinate up to 30 axons.*

   2. *Microglia:* arise from monocytes and function as the scavenger cells (phagocytes) of the CNS

   3. *Ependymal cells:* ciliated cells that line the central canal and ventricles of the brain; also line the luminal surface of the choroid plexus; produce the cerebrospinal fluid

   4. *Tanycytes:* modified ependymal cells that contract capillaries and neurons; mediate cellular transport between the ventricles and the neuropil; project to hypothalamic nuclei that regulate the release of gonadotropic hormone from the adenohypophysis

   5. *Schwann cells:* derived from the neural crest; myelin-forming cells of the PNS; *one Schwann cell can myelinate only one internode;* separated from each other by the nodes of Ranvier.

G. **Blood–brain barrier:** consists of the tight junctions of nonfenestrated endothelial cells; some authorities include the astrocytic foot processes; although the *blood-cerebrospinal fluid barrier* consists of the tight junctions between the cuboidal epithelial cells of the choroid plexus, it is permeable to some circulating peptides (e.g., insulin) and plasma proteins (e.g., prealbumin).

> **NB:** Areas of the brain that contain no blood-brain barrier include the subfornical organ, area postrema, and neurohypophysis.

H. **Classification of nerve fibers**

FIBER	DIAMETER (μM)	CONDUCTION VELOCITY (M/SEC)	FUNCTION
Sensory axons			
Ia (A)	12–20	70–120	Proprioception, muscle spindles
Ib (A)	12–20	70–120	Proprioception, Golgi tendon organs
II (A)	5–12	30–70	Touch, pressure, and vibration
III (A)	2–5	12–30	Touch, pressure, fast pain, and temperature

(continued)

FIBER	DIAMETER (μM)	CONDUCTION VELOCITY (M/SEC)	FUNCTION
IV (C)	0.5–1.0	0.5–2.0	Slow pain and temperature (unmyelinated fibers)
Motor axons			
α(A) (alpha)	12–20	15–120	Innervate the extrafusal muscle fibers
γ(A) (gamma)	2–10	10–45	Innervate the intrafusal muscle fibers
Preganglionic autonomic fibers (B)	<3	3–15	Myelinated preganglionic autonomic fibers
Postganglionic autonomic fibers (C)	1	2	Unmyelinated postganglionic autonomic fibers

I. **Cutaneous receptors**

1. *Free nerve endings:* nociceptors (pain) and thermoreceptors (cold and heat)
2. *Encapsulated endings:* touch receptors (Meissner's corpuscles) and pressure and vibration receptors (Pacinian corpuscles)
3. *Merkel disks:* unencapsulated light-touch receptors

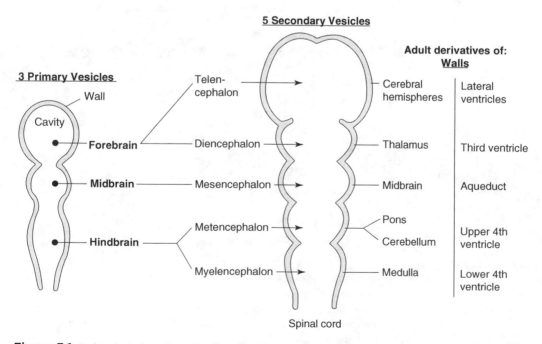

Figure 3.1 Embryologic derivatives of walls and cavities.

II. Embryology

A. **NB: Ectoderm is the main embryonal layer forming the nervous system.**

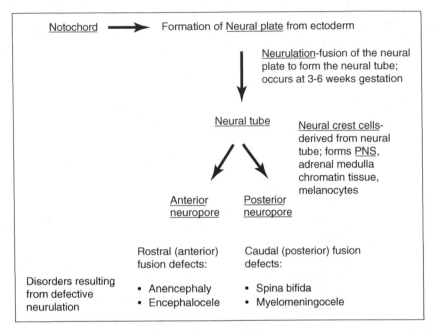

Figure 3.2 Neural tube formation.

B. **Segmentation of neural tube**

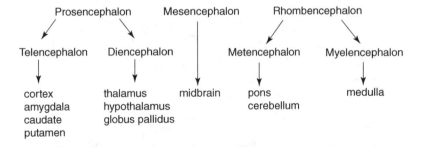

> **NB:** Telencephalon produces the cerebral hemispheres and striatum except for the globus pallidus, which is from the diencephalon.

C. **Sulcus limitans:** marks boundary between basal and alar plates

   1. *Alar plate* forms: posterior horn, gray matter, cerebellum, inferior olive, quadrigeminal plate, red nucleus, sensory brainstem nuclei

   2. *Basal plate* forms: anterior horn, gray matter, motor nuclei of the cranial nerves

D. **Cells derived from neural crest:** *chromaffin cells, preganglionic sympathetic neurons, dorsal root ganglia cells, skin melanocytes, adrenal medulla, cranial nerve sensory ganglia, autonomic ganglia, cells of pia/arachnoid, Schwann cells, odontoblasts* (which elaborate predentin)

> **NB:** The olfactory epithelium is from the ectoderm.

E. **Neural tube formation**

1. Closure of neural tube: *begins at the region of 4th somite* and proceeds in cranial and caudal directions; fusion begins on day 22

2. *Anterior neuropore: closes on day 25*

3. *Posterior neuropore: closes on day 27*

> **NB:** α-Fetoprotein is found in the amniotic fluid and maternal serum; it is an indicator of neural tube defects (e.g., spina bifida, anencephaly); it is reduced in mothers of fetuses with Down syndrome.

F. **Secondary neurulation** (caudal neural tube formation): forms on days 28 to 32; forms the sacral/coccygeal segments, filum terminale, ventriculus terminalis

G. **Neuronal proliferation:** radial glia—earliest glia in embryonic CNS, provide guidance for neuron migration from ventricular region to cortex, may be *precursors to astrocytes/oligodendrocytes* but persist as Bergmann glia in mature cerebellum (which are special cerebellar cells whose processes extend to the pial surface)

1. *Phase 1:* between 2 and 4 months; neuronal proliferation and generation of radial glia

2. *Phase 2:* between 5 and 12 months; mostly glial multiplication

H. **Neuronal migration:** radial cells send foot processes from the ventricular surface to the pial surface, forming a limiting membrane at the pial surface; proliferate units of the ventricular zone migrate via the radial glia scaffolding to become the neuronal cell columns; the later migrating cells take a more superficial position (inside-out pattern). Types:

1. *Radial:* primary mechanism for formation of the cortex and deep nuclei, cerebellar Purkinje cells, and cerebellar nuclei

2. *Tangential:* originates in the germinal zones of the rhombic lip and migrate to form the external and internal granular layers

> **NB:** All six layers of cerebral cortex are present at 27 weeks gestation (layer 1 is the most superficial):
>
> 1. Molecular layer
> 2. External granular layer
> 3. External pyramidal layer
> 4. Internal granular layer
> 5. Internal pyramidal layer
> 6. Multiform layer

I. **Myelination:** begins in the *4th month of gestation*

1. *PNS:* myelinates before CNS; motor fibers myelinate before sensory; myelination in the PNS is accomplished by the *Schwann cells.*

2. *CNS:* sensory areas myelinate before motor, association cortices myelinate last; *most rapid myelination is between birth and age 2 years;* myelination in the cerebral association cortex continues into the 3rd decade; myelination in the CNS is accomplished *by oligodendrocytes* (which are not found in the retina).

I. Myelination (*cont'd*)

> **NB:** The lateral corticospinal tract does not fully myelinate until age 2 years (correlating to development of motor skills); the earliest structures to be myelinated at 14 weeks include medial longitudinal fasciculus/dorsal roots/cranial nerves (except II, VIII, and sensory V); myelination continues until age 12 years.

J. **Positional changes in the spinal cord**

1. *Newborn:* the conus medullaris *ends at L3.*

2. *Adult:* the conus medullaris *ends at L1.*

K. **Optic nerve and chiasma:** derived from the diencephalon; the optic nerve fibers occupy the choroid fissure; failure of this fissure to close results in coloboma iridis.

L. **Pituitary gland:** derived from two embryologic substrata

1. *Adenohypophysis:* **derived from the ectodermal diverticulum of the primitive mouth cavity (stomodeum), which is also called *Rathke pouch;* remnants of Rathke pouch may give rise to a craniopharyngioma.**

2. *Neurohypophysis:* **develops from a ventral evagination of the hypothalamus (neuroectoderm of the neural tube)**

III. Developmental Disorders

A. **Disorders of primary neurulation**

1. **Anencephaly:** *meroanencephaly; failure of anterior neuropore closure* (less than day 24); as a result, the brain does not develop; frequency: 1:1,000; risk in subsequent pregnancies is 5% to 7%; 75% are stillborn; absence of both cerebral hemispheres and variable portions of the brainstem

    a. *Holoacrania:* up to the foramen magnum

    b. *Meroacrania:* slightly higher than the foramen magnum

2. **Encephalocele:** restricted to anterior neuropore defects; herniation of neural tissues into midline skull defects; 75% are occipital, 50% have hydrocephalus.

3. **Spina bifida:** results from failure of the posterior neuropore to form; the defect usually occurs in the *sacrolumbar region.*

    a. *Spina bifida occulta:* skin-covered defect; rarely associated with a neurologic deficit; frequency: 10%; associated with diastematomyelia, lipomeningocele, tethered cord, filum terminale, intraspinal dermoid, epidermoid cyst

    b. *Spina bifida aperta:* associated with a neurologic deficit in 90%; 85% with spinal dysraphism

        i. **Meningocele:** herniation of cerebrospinal fluid–filled sac without neural elements

        ii. **Myelomeningocele:** herniated neural elements covered by meningeal sac; 80% are lumbar; 90% have hydrocephalus if lumbar is involved; symptoms include motor, sensory, and sphincter dysfunction.

        iii. **Myeloschisis:** neural elements at surface completely uncovered; associated with malformed skull base; most babies stillborn

        iv. **Myelocystocele:** herniation of meninges and cord with dilated central canal

4. **Arnold-Chiari malformation**

    a. Chiari I: typical characteristics include:

      i. Kinked cervical cord

      ii. Brainstem elongation

      iii. Cerebellar tonsillar dysmorphic tissue displaced downward (radiologically, cerebellar tonsils are > 5 mm below foramen magnum)

      iv. Beaked mesencephalic tectum

      v. Atretic aqueduct

      vi. Small cerebellum with small posterior fossa and large foramen magnum

    b. Chiari II: similar to Chiari I *plus lumbar spinal fusion defect;* almost 100% with myelomeningocele; 96% with cortex malformation (heterotopia, polymicrogyria); with hydrocephalus (due to 4th ventricle obstruction); with tectum deformity; frequency: 1:1,000

    c. Chiari III: Chiari II *plus occipital encephalocele or myelocerebellomeningocele* (due to cervical spina bifida with cerebellum herniating through the foramen magnum); with downbeat nystagmus or periodic alternating nystagmus, cranial nerve dysfunction, altered respiratory control, abnormal extraocular movements

    d. Chiari IV: with cerebellar hypoplasia

5. **Meckel's syndrome:** associated with *maternal hyperthermia/fever on days 20 to 26; characterized by encephalocele, microcephaly, micro-ophthalmia, cleft lip, polydactyly, polycystic kidneys, ambiguous genitalia*

> **NB:** Chromosomal abnormalities associated with neural tube defects: trisomy 13 and 18; other causes of neural tube defects: teratogens (thalidomide, valproate, phenytoin), single mutant gene (Meckel's syndrome), multifactorial

B. **Disorders of secondary neurulation:** occult dysraphic states; 100% have abnormal conus and filum; 90% with vertebral abnormalities; 80% have overlying dermal lesions (dimple, hair tuft, lipoma, hemangioma), although with an intact dermal layer over lesions; 4% have siblings with a disorder of primary neurulation.

1. **Caudal regression syndrome:** 20% infants of diabetic mothers; characterized by dysraphic sacrum and coccyx with atrophic muscle and bone; symptoms: delayed sphincter control and walking, back and leg pain, scoliosis, pes cavus, leg asymmetry

2. **Myelocystocele:** cystic central canal

3. **Diastematomyelia:** bifid cord

4. **Meningocele: rare;** no associated hydrocephalus

5. **Lipomeningocele**

6. **Subcutaneous lipomas/teratoma**

7. **Dermal sinus**

C. **Disorders of porencephalic development**

1. **Aprosencephaly:** absent telencephalon and diencephalon

2. **Atelencephaly:** absent telencephalon (diencephalon present); characterized by intact skull and skin, cyclopia with absent eyes, abnormal limbs, and abnormal genitalia

C. **Disorders of porencephalic development** (*cont'd*)

3. **Holoprosencephaly:** single-lobed cerebrum and only one ventricle; 100% associated with anosmia; facial defects include *ethmocephaly* (hypertelorism with proboscis between eyes), *cebocephaly* (single nostril), *cyclopia* (single eye with or without proboscis), *cleft lip;* associated with hypoplastic optic nerves; corpus callosum may be absent; associated chromosomal abnormality: *trisomy 13 (Patau syndrome)* or ring 13; also the most severe manifestation of **fetal alcohol syndrome** (i.e., the most common cause of mental retardation and is associated *with microcephaly and congenital heart disease*); 2% are infants of diabetic mothers; 6% recurrence rate.

   a. *Alobar:* characterized by facial anomalies, hypotelorism, microphthalmia, micrognathia

   b. *Semilobar:* facial anomalies are less severe and less common; septum pellucidum and corpus callosum are absent; the falx and interhemispheric fissure are partially developed posteriorly.

   c. *Lobar:* shallow, incomplete interhemispheric fissure anteriorly; septum pellucidum is absent; facial anomalies are uncommon.

4. **Agenesis of corpus callosum:** associated with:

   a. *Holoprosencephaly*

   b. *Absent septum pellucidum*

   c. *Schizencephaly and other migrational disorders*

   d. *Chiari type 2*

   e. *Septo-optic dysplasia:* absent or hypoplastic septum pellucidum, hypoplastic optic nerves, schizencephaly in approximately 50% but normal-sized ventricles, pituitary axis dysfunction (50% with diabetes insipidus)

   f. **Aicardi syndrome:** *X-linked dominant* condition with agenesis of the corpus callosum, neuronal migrational defects and chorioretinal lacunes

   g. **Dandy-Walker malformation:** failure of foramen of Magendie development; cystic dilation of 4th ventricle and cerebellar vermis agenesis with enlarged posterior fossa; elevation of the inion; agenesis of the corpus callosum; 70% with migrational disorders; associated with cardiac abnormalities and urinary tract infections; frequency: 1:25,000; may result from riboflavin inhibitors, posterior fossa trauma, or viral infection

D. **Disorders of proliferation**

1. **Microcephaly:** decreased size of proliferative units; head circumference less than 2 standard deviations below the mean

2. **Radial microbrain:** decreased number of proliferative units

3. **Megalencephaly:** well-formed but large brain; weight of brain greater than 2 standard deviations above the mean

4. **Hemimegalencephaly: enlargement of one cerebral hemisphere; often associated with seizures and hemiparesis**

E. **Neuronal migrational disorders**

> **NB:** Schizencephaly involves clefts <u>lined with cortex</u> that span from the pail surface to the ventricles. With porencephaly, the cerebrospinal fluid (CSF)-filled space usually results from infarction and is not a consequence of malformation during cortical development.

   1. **Schizencephaly:** clefts between ventricles and subarachnoid space lined with gray matter; no gliosis; associated with heterotopias in the cleft wall

   2. **Lissencephaly:** few or no gyri (smooth surface)

     a. **Miller-Dieker syndrome:** lissencephaly, 90% with *chromosome 17 deletion, LIS1 gene;* characterized by microcephaly, seizures, hypotonia, craniofacial defects (micrognathia), cardiac defects, genital abnormalities

     b. X-linked lissencephaly: DCX gene mutation, encodes doublecortin protein

     c. Cobblestone lissencephaly (type II): typically autosomal recessive, reduced amount of gyri and sulci, giving appearance of cobblestones; indistinguishable cortical layers; associated with Walker-Warburg syndrome, muscle-eye-brain disease, and Fukuyama muscular dystrophy

   3. **Pachygyria:** few broad, thick gyri

   4. **Polymicrogyria:** too many small gyri (like a wrinkled chestnut); seen in Zellweger syndrome (cerebrohepatorenal syndrome): autosomal recessive peroxisomal disorder linked to *chromosome 13,* characterized by increased very long chain fatty acids in blood, polymicrogyria, heterotopias, seizures, hepatomegaly, renal cysts

   5. **Heterotopias:** rests of neurons in the white matter secondary to arrested radial migration; associated with seizures; may be periventricular, laminar (in the deep white matter) or band-like (between the cortex and the ventricular surface)

     a. Periventricular nodular heterotopia: arrested neuronal migration at subventricular area, FLNa gene mutations, chromosome X; commonly associated with epilepsy

F. **Disorders of myelination**

   1. Aminoaciduria/organic acidurias

     a. Ketotic hyperglycinemia

     b. Nonketotic hyperglycinemia

     c. Phenylketonuria

     d. Maple syrup urine disease

     e. Homocystinuria

   2. Hypothyroidism

   3. Malnutrition

   4. Periventricular leukomalacia

   5. Prematurity

G. **Congenital hydrocephalus:** frequency: 1:1,000; common etiologies are:

   1. Aqueductal stenosis: 33%

   2. Chiari types 2 and 3: 28%

   3. Communicating hydrocephalus: 22%

   4. Dandy-Walker malformation: 7%

   5. Others: tumors, vein of Galen, X-linked aqueductal stenosis

> **NB:** The most common cause of congenital hydrocephalus is aqueductal stenosis.

H. **Walker-Warburg syndrome:** associated with congenital muscular dystrophy, cerebellar malformation, retinal malformation, and macrocephaly

I. **Hydranencephaly:** results from bilateral hemisphere infarction secondary to occlusion of the carotid arteries; hemispheres are replaced with hugely dilated ventricles

CHEAT SHEET

Chiari II	Most with myelomeningocele and hydrocephalus
Aicardi syndrome	X-linked, agenesis corpus callosum, neuronal migration defects
Dandy-Walker syndrome	Dilation of 4th ventricle, cerebellar vermis agenesis, agenesis of corpus callosum
Miller-Dieker syndrome	Lissencephaly, most chromosome 17 deletion
Walker-Warburg syndrome	Congenital muscular dystrophy, cerebellar malformation, retinal malformation, macrocephaly

Suggested Readings

Moore, KL, Persaud, TVN, Torchia, MG. *The Developing Human: Clinically Oriented Embryology.* Philadelphia, PA: Elsevier;2016.

Prayder, D, Brugger, PC, Nemec, U, et al. Cerebral malformations. *Fetal MRI.*2011:287–308.

Prayson, R A. *Neuropathology.* Philadelphia, PA: Elsevier Churchill-Livingstone;2005.

CHAPTER 4

Clinical Neuroanatomy

I. Skull, Cerebrovascular Supply, and Venous Drainage

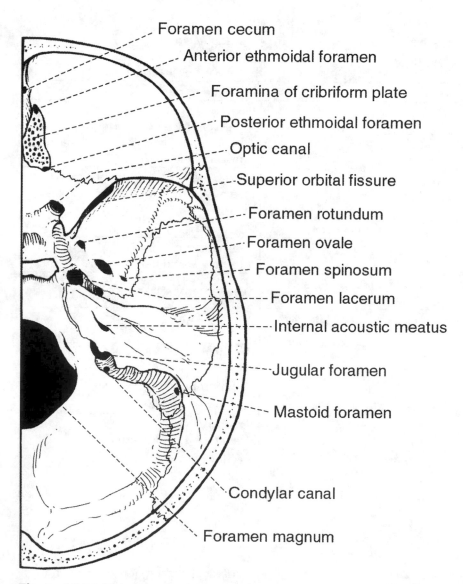

Foramen cecum
Anterior ethmoidal foramen
Foramina of cribriform plate
Posterior ethmoidal foramen
Optic canal
Superior orbital fissure
Foramen rotundum
Foramen ovale
Foramen spinosum
Foramen lacerum
Internal acoustic meatus
Jugular foramen
Mastoid foramen
Condylar canal
Foramen magnum

Figure 4.1 Basal view of the skull highlighting the foramina.

A. Foramina of the skull

FORAMEN	STRUCTURES
Foramen cecum	Vein to superior sagittal sinus
Anterior ethmoidal foramen	Anterior ethmoidal artery, vein, and nerve
Foramina of cribriform plate	Olfactory nerve bundles
Posterior ethmoidal foramen	Posterior ethmoidal artery, vein, and nerve
Optic canal	CN II Ophthalmic artery
Superior orbital fissure	CN III CN IV Ophthalmic nerve CN VI Superior ophthalmic vein
Foramen rotundum	Maxillary nerve
Foramen ovale	Mandibular nerve Accessory meningeal artery Lesser petrosal nerve (occasionally) Emissary veins
Foramen spinosum	Middle meningeal artery and vein Meningeal branch of the mandibular nerve
Foramen of Vesalius (inconstant)	Small emissary vein
Foramen lacerum	Internal carotid artery Internal carotid nerve plexus
Hiatus of canal of lesser petrosal nerve	Lesser petrosal nerve
Hiatus of canal of greater petrosal nerve	Greater petrosal nerve
Internal acoustic meatus	CN VII CN VIII Labyrinthine artery
Vestibular aqueduct	Endolymphatic duct
Mastoid foramen	Emissary vein Branch of occipital artery
Jugular foramen	Inferior petrosal sinus CN IX CN X CN XI Sigmoid sinus Posterior meningeal artery
Condylar canal (inconstant)	Emissary vein Meningeal branch of the ascending pharyngeal artery

(continued)

FORAMEN	STRUCTURES
Hypoglossal canal	CN XII
Foramen magnum	Medulla oblongata Meninges Vertebral arteries Spinal roots of CN XI

B. **Arterial supply**

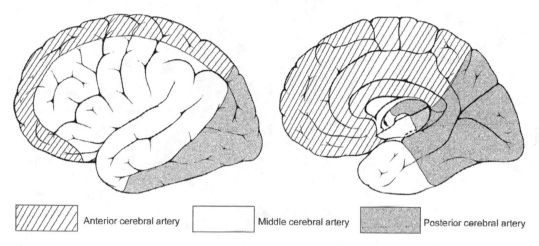

Anterior cerebral artery   Middle cerebral artery   Posterior cerebral artery

Figure 4.2 Sagittal view and section of the brain showing the major arterial supplies.

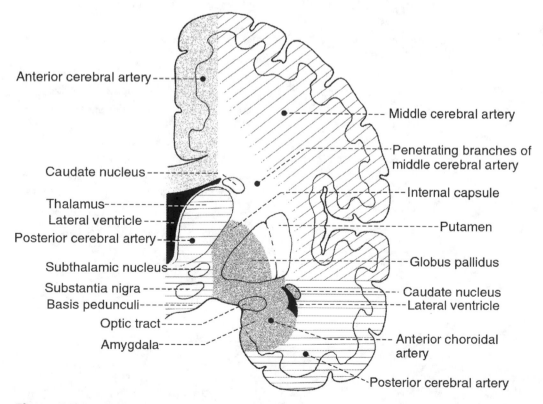

Figure 4.3 Coronal section of the brain at the level of the internal capsule and thalamus showing the arterial supply.

C. **Venous drainage**

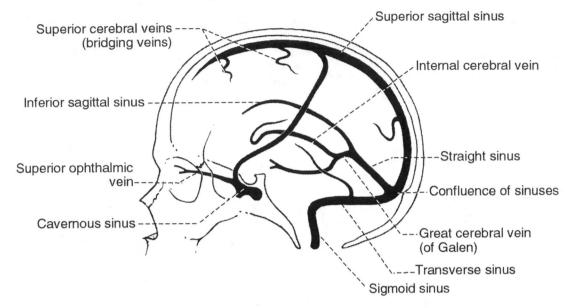

Superior cerebral veins
(bridging veins)

Superior sagittal sinus

Internal cerebral vein

Inferior sagittal sinus

Superior ophthalmic
vein

Straight sinus

Confluence of sinuses

Cavernous sinus

Great cerebral vein
(of Galen)

Transverse sinus

Sigmoid sinus

Figure 4.4 The venous system.

II. Cerebral Cortex: Thin gray covering of both hemispheres of the brain; two types: neocortex (90%) and allocortex (10%); motor cortex is the thickest (4.5 mm) and visual cortex is the thinnest (1.5 mm).

A. **Layers of the neocortex: layers II and IV are mainly afferent; layers V and VI are mainly efferent.**

1. *Layer I:* molecular layer

2. *Layer II:* external granular layer

3. *Layer III:* external pyramidal layer; gives rise to association and commissural fibers

4. *Layer IV:* internal granular layer; receives thalamocortical fibers from the thalamic nuclei of the ventral tier and also input from the lateral geniculate body

5. *Layer V:* internal pyramidal layer; gives rise to corticobulbar, corticospinal, and corticostriatal fibers; contains giant pyramidal cells of Betz (found only in the motor cortex)

6. *Layer VI:* multiform layer; major source of corticothalamic fibers; gives rise to projection, commissural, and association fibers

B. Functional areas

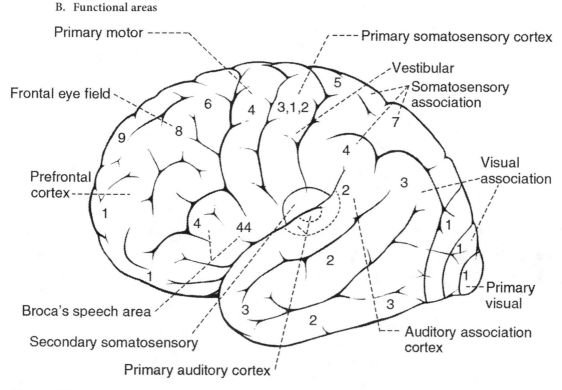

Figure 4.5 Gross lateral view of the brain illustrating the functional (Brodmann's) areas.

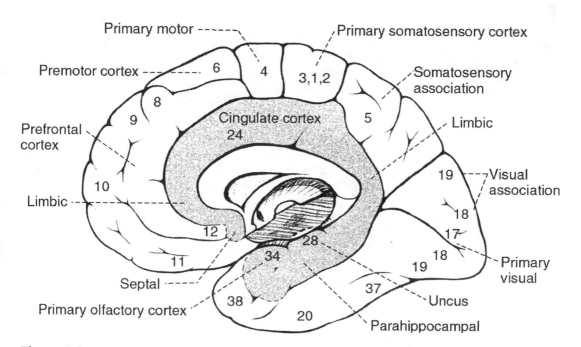

Figure 4.6 Medial surface of the brain hemisphere highlighting the functional (Brodmann's) areas.

1. *Frontal lobe*
   a. *Motor cortex (Brodmann's area 4) and premotor cortex (Brodmann's area 6):* destruction causes contralateral spastic paresis.
   b. *Frontal eye field (Brodmann's area 8):* destruction causes deviation of the eyes to the ipsilateral side.
   c. *Broca's speech area (Brodmann's areas 44 and 45):* located in the posterior part of the inferior frontal gyrus in the dominant hemisphere; destruction results in expressive, nonfluent aphasia.
   d. *Prefrontal cortex (Brodmann's areas 9–12, 46, 47):* destruction of the anterior two-thirds results in deficits in concentration, orientation, abstracting ability, judgment, and problem-solving ability; destruction of the orbital (frontal) lobe results in inappropriate social behavior.

> **NB:** Medial frontal cortex lesions may result in akinetic mutism, whereas orbitofrontal cortex lesions may result in impulsive and antisocial behavior. Left dorsolateral frontal lesions may produce depression.

2. *Parietal lobe*
   a. *Sensory cortex (Brodmann's areas 3, 1, 2):* destruction results in contralateral hemihypesthesia and astereognosis.
   b. *Superior parietal lobule (Brodmann's areas 5 and 7):* destruction results in contralateral astereognosis and sensory neglect.

> **NB:** Asomatognosia is a form of neglect in which patients deny ownership of their limbs (also described as lack of awareness of the condition of all or part of one's body). It frequently accompanies anosognosia (an inability or refusal to recognize a defect or disorder that is clinically evident). The lesion is located in the nondominant supramarginal gyrus (and/or angular gyrus).

   c. **Inferior parietal lobule of the dominant hemisphere: damage results in Gerstmann's syndrome: (1) right-left disorientation, (2) finger agnosia, (3) dysgraphia (+/- dyslexia), (4) dyscalculia,** possibly contralateral hemianopia, or lower quadrantanopia as well.
   d. *Inferior parietal lobule of the nondominant hemisphere:* destruction results in topographic memory loss, anosognosia, construction apraxia, dressing apraxia, contralateral sensory neglect, contralateral hemianopia, or lower quadrantanopia.
3. *Temporal lobe*
   a. *Primary auditory cortex (Brodmann's areas 41 and 42):* unilateral destruction results in slight hearing loss; bilateral loss results in cortical deafness.

b. *Wernicke's speech area in the dominant area (Brodmann's area 22):* found in the posterior part of the superior temporal gyrus; destruction results in receptive, fluent aphasia.

c. *Olfactory bulb, tract, and primary cortex (Brodmann's area 34):* destruction results in ipsilateral anosmia; irritative lesion of the uncus results in olfactory and gustatory hallucinations.

d. *Hippocampal cortex (archicortex):* bilateral lesions result in the inability to consolidate short-term memory into long-term memory.

e. **Anterior temporal lobe (including amygdaloid nucleus):** bilateral damage results in Klüver-Bucy syndrome—visual agnosia, hyperphagia, docility, hypersexuality.

f. **Inferomedial occipitotemporal cortex:** bilateral lesions result in the inability to recognize once-familiar faces (prosopagnosia).

4. *Occipital lobe*

a. Bilateral lesions: cortical blindness

> **NB:** Individuals with Anton's syndrome have cortical blindness, often with denial or unawareness of the blindness.

b. *Unilateral lesions:* contralateral hemianopia or quadrantanopia

5. *Corpus callosum*

a. *Anterior corpus callosum lesions:* may result in akinetic mutism or tactile anomia

b. *Posterior corpus callosum (splenium) lesion:* may result in alexia without agraphia

> **NB:** Left posterior cerebral artery syndrome presents alexia without agraphia (often also have right homonymous hemianopia and achromatopsia and/or color anomia). The lesion is in the splenium of the corpus callosum.

> **NB:** Surface dyslexia is characterized by impairment in linking the visual form system with the phonological output lexicon. Patients are therefore unable to access the visual word images to link to proper pronunciation and will need to rely on "print-to-sound conversion" and have difficulty reading words that do not sound the way they are spelled (e.g., words such as *yacht* and *thought* pronounced as spelled).

c. *Split-brain syndrome:* a disconnection syndrome that results from transection of the corpus callosum (e.g., in a patient with alexia in the left visual field, the verbal symbols seen on the right visual cortex have no access to the language centers of the left hemisphere)

III. Spinal Cord: An elongated, cylindrical mass of nerve tissue occupying the upper two-thirds of the adult spinal canal within the vertebral column; normally 42 to 45 cm long; *conus medullaris:* the conical distal end of the spinal cord; *filum terminale:* extends from the tip of the conus and attaches to the distal dural sac; it consists of pia and glial fibers and often contains a vein.

A. Segments and divisions: divided into 30 segments—8 cervical, 12 thoracic, 5 lumbar, 5 sacral, and a few small coccygeal segments; cross sections show a deep anterior median fissure (commonly contains a fold of pia and blood vessels; its floor is the anterior/ventral white commissure) and a shallow posterior median sulcus; the dorsal nerve roots are attached to the spinal cord along the posterolateral sulcus; the ventral nerve roots exit the spinal cord in the anterolateral sulcus.

B. Gray matter

1. *Columns:* a cross section of the spinal cord shows an H-shaped internal mass of gray matter surrounded by white matter; made up of two symmetric portions joined across the midline by a transverse connection (commissure) of gray matter that contains the minute central canal or its remnants.

a. *Ventral (anterior) gray column:* contains the cells of origin of the fibers of the ventral roots

b. *Intermediolateral gray column:* position of the gray matter between the dorsal and ventral gray columns; a prominent lateral triangular projection in the thoracic and upper lumbar regions but not in the midsacral regions; contains the preganglionic cells of the sympathetic division of the autonomic nervous system

c. *The dorsal gray column:* reaches almost to the posterolateral sulcus; Lissauer's tract: dorsolateral fasciculus, compact bundle of small fibers as part of the pain pathway

2. *Laminas:* a cross section of the gray matter shows a number of laminas (layer of nerve cells), termed *Rexed laminas* after the neuroanatomist who described them.

a. *Lamina I:* thin marginal layer, contains neurons that respond to noxious stimuli and send axons to the contralateral spinothalamic tract.

b. *Lamina II:* substantia gelatinosa; small neurons, some respond to noxious stimuli; substance P is the neuropeptide involved in pathways mediating sensitivity to pain, which is found in high concentration in laminae I and II.

c. *Laminae III and IV:* nucleus proprius; main input is from fibers that convey position and light-touch sense.

d. *Lamina V:* this layer contains cells that respond to both noxious and visceral afferent stimuli.

e. *Lamina VI:* the deepest layer of the dorsal horn and contains neurons that respond to the mechanical signals from joints and skin.

f. *Lamina VII:* a large zone that contains the cells of the dorsal nucleus of Clarke medially, as well as a large portion of the ventral gray column; Clarke's column contains cells that give rise to the posterior cerebellar tract; also contains the intermediolateral nucleus.

g. *Laminae VIII and IX:* represent motor neuron groups in the medial and lateral portions of the ventral gray column; the medial portion contains the lower motor neurons (LMNs) that innervate the axial musculature; the lateral motor neuron column contains LMNs for the distal muscles of the arm and leg; in general, motor neurons for flexor muscles are located more centrally, whereas motor neurons for extensor muscles are located more peripherally.

h. *Lamina X:* represents the small neurons around the central canal or its remnants.

C. **White matter**

1. *Columns:* each lateral half of the spinal cord has white columns (funiculi)—dorsal (posterior), lateral, ventral (anterior); the dorsal column lies between the posterior median sulcus and the posterolateral sulcus (in the cervical region, it is divided into fasciculus gracilis and fasciculus cuneatus); the lateral column lies between the posterolateral sulcus and the anterolateral sulcus; the ventral column lies between the anterolateral sulcus and the anterior median fissure.

2. *Tracts*

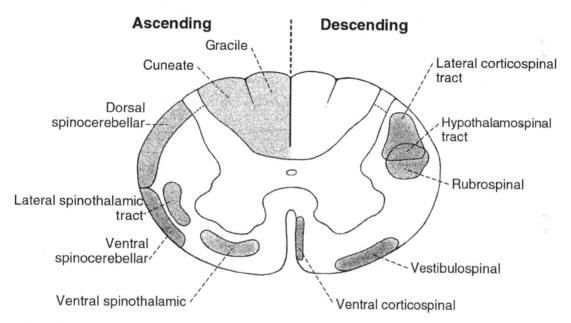

Figure 4.7 Cross section of the spinal cord highlighting the major ascending and descending tracts.

a. *Descending tracts in the spinal cord*

TRACT	ORIGIN	TERMINATION	LOCATION	FUNCTION
Pyramidal/ corticospinal	Motor and premotor cortex	Contralateral anterior horn cells (**after crossing the pyramidal decussation at the medulla**)	Lateral column	Fine motor function (distal musculature)

(continued)

a. Descending tracts in the spinal cord (cont'd)

TRACT	ORIGIN	TERMINATION	LOCATION	FUNCTION
Anterior (ventral) corticospinal	Motor and premotor cortex	**Descends uncrossed in the spinal cord then later decussates via anterior white commissure to** the contralateral anterior horn neurons (interneurons and LMNs)	Anterior column	Gross and postural motor function (proximal and axial)
Lateral vestibulospinal	Lateral vestibular nucleus	Descend uncrossed to the anterior horn interneurons and motor neurons (for extensors)	Ventral column	Postural reflexes
Medial vestibulospinal	Medial vestibular nucleus	Descends crossed and uncrossed to the anterior horn interneurons and motor neurons	Ventral column	Postural reflexes
Rubrospinal	Red nucleus	Immediately crosses and terminates in contralateral ventral horn interneurons	Lateral column	Motor function
Medial reticulospinal	Pontine reticular formation	Descends uncrossed fibers to the ventral horn	Ventral column	Motor function (excitation of flexor and proximal trunk and axial motor neurons)
Lateral reticulospinal	Medullary reticular formation	Descends crossed and uncrossed to most of the ventral horn and the basal portion of the dorsal horn	Lateral column	Modulation of sensory transmission and spinal reflexes; excitation and inhibition of axial (neck and back) motor neurons
Descending autonomic	Hypothalamus, brainstem	Poorly defined fiber system projecting to the preganglionic autonomic fibers	Lateral columns	Modulation of autonomic functions
Tectospinal	Superior colliculus of the midbrain	Contralateral ventral horn interneurons	Ventral column	Reflex head turning
Medial longitudinal fasciculus (MLF)	Vestibular nuclei	Only up to the cervical gray	Ventral column	Coordination of head and eye movements

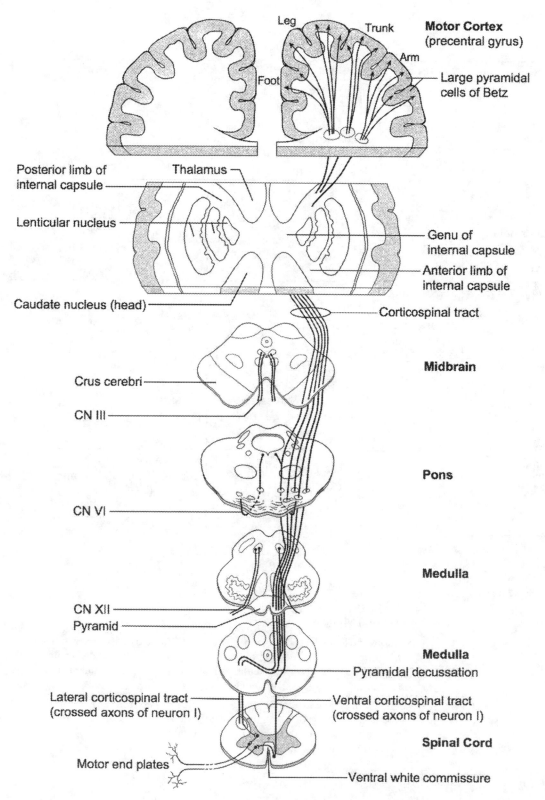

Figure 4.8 The route of the lateral corticospinal tract in the spinal cord from the motor and premotor cortex down to the contralateral anterior horn cells after crossing the pyramidal decussation at the medulla.

2. *Tracts* (cont'd)

    b. *Ascending tracts of the spinal cord*

TRACT	ORIGIN	TERMINATION	LOCATION	FUNCTION
Dorsal column system	Skin, joints, tendons	Dorsal column nuclei; 2nd-order neurons project to the contralateral thalamus (crossing at the lemniscal decussation in medulla)	Dorsal column	(Conscious) proprioception, fine-touch, two-point discrimination
Spinothalamic	Skin	Dorsal horn; 2nd-order neurons project to the contralateral thalamus (cross in the spinal cord close to the level of entry)	Ventrolateral column	Sharp pain, temperature, crude touch
Dorsal spinocerebellar	Muscle spindles, Golgi tendon organs, touch and pressure receptors	Cerebellar paleocortex (via ipsilateral inferior cerebellar peduncle)	Lateral column	(Unconscious) proprioception-stereognosis
Ventral spinocerebellar	Muscle spindles, Golgi tendon organs, touch and pressure receptors	Cerebellar paleocortex (via contralateral and some ipsilateral superior cerebellar peduncle)	Lateral column	(Unconscious) proprioception-stereognosis
Spinoreticular	Deep somatic structures	Ipsilateral reticular formation of the brainstem	Polysynaptic, diffuse in the ventrolateral column	Deep and chronic pain

> **NB:** The dorsal and ventral spinocerebellar tracts are the most lateral tracts in the spinal cord and are most likely to be affected first from an extrinsic lateral insult.

D. **Spinal cord syndromes**

    1. **Small central lesion (e.g., syringomyelia):** affects the decussating fibers of the spinothalamic tract from both sides without affecting other ascending or descending fibers, **producing dissociated sensory abnormalities with loss of pain and temperature sensibility in appropriate dermatomes but with preserved vibration and position sense.**

    2. *Large central lesion:* in addition to the pain and temperature pathways, portions of the adjacent tracts, gray matter, or both, are affected, producing LMN weakness in the segments involved, together with upper motor neuron (UMN) dysfunction, and occasionally with joint position and vibration sense loss below the lesion.

> **NB:** Central cord syndrome at the cervical levels may produce LMN findings in the upper extremities, UMN findings in the lower extremities, and a disturbance of pain and temperature sensation noticeable in the upper extremities.

3. *Dorsal column lesion* (e.g., *tabes dorsalis*): proprioception and vibratory sensation are involved, with other functions remaining normal.

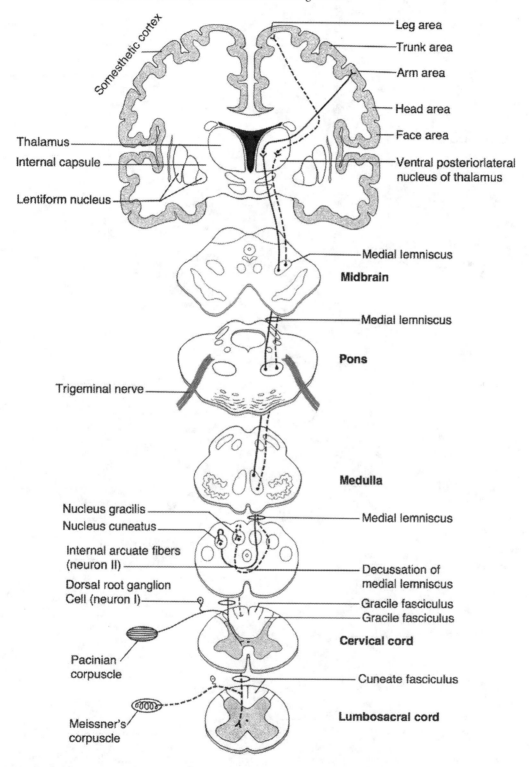

Figure 4.9 The route of the **dorsal column system** from the dorsal column nuclei to the **contralateral thalamus** to its termination in the sensory cortex.

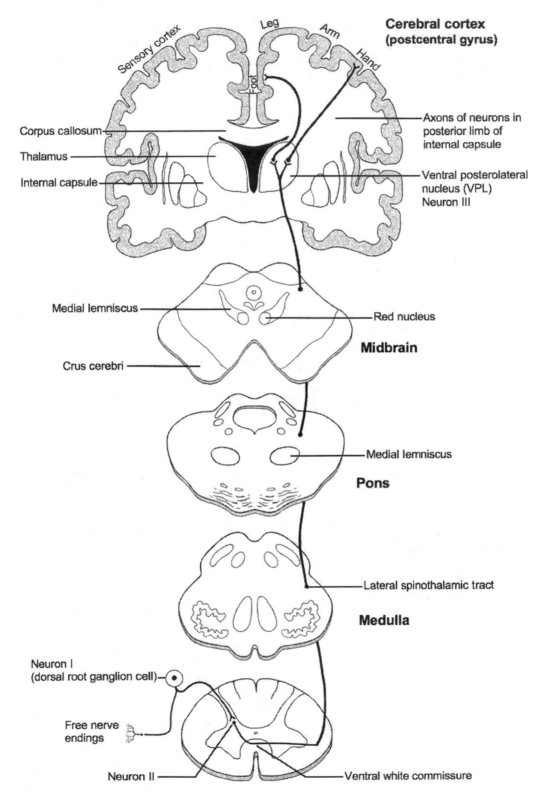

Figure 4.10 The route of the **lateral spinothalamic tract** from the nucleus in the dorsal horn through the **contralateral** thalamus to its termination in the sensory cortex.

> **NB:** Examples of conditions presenting findings from dorsal column lesions include latent *Treponema pallidum* infection and vitamin B$_{12}$ deficiency

4. Brown-Sequard syndrome: hemisection of the spinal cord as a result of bullet or stab wound, syrinx, tumor, hematomyelia, and so forth; signs:

   a. Ipsilateral LMN paralysis in the segment of the lesion (damage of the LMNs)

   b. Ipsilateral UMN paralysis below the level of the lesion (due to damage of the corticospinal tract)

   c. Ipsilateral cutaneous anesthesia in the segment of the lesion (damage of yet uncrossed afferent fibers)

   d. Ipsilateral loss of proprioceptive, vibratory, and two-point discrimination sense below the level of the lesions (damage of dorsal columns)

   e. Contralateral loss of pain and temperature sense below the lesion (damage of spinothalamic tracts that have already crossed)

5. *Subacute combined degeneration of the spinal cord: deficiency of vitamin B$_{12}$ (cyanocobalamin) results in degeneration of dorsal and lateral columns;* loss of position sense, two-point discrimination, and vibratory sensation; ataxic gait (damage to the spinocerebellar tracts), muscle weakness, hyperactive reflexes, spasticity of the extremities, and positive Babinski sign.

6. Spinal shock: acute transection of or severe injury to the spinal cord from sudden loss of stimulation from higher levels or from overdose of spinal anesthetic; all body segments below the level of the injury become paralyzed and have no sensation; all reflexes (including autonomic) are suppressed; usually transient; may disappear in 3 to 6 weeks followed by a period of increased UMN signs.

> **NB:** Autonomic dysreflexia may occur in patients with lesions at T5, T6, and above. Symptoms include diaphoresis, hypertension, tachycardia, and others. If not treated promptly, death may result.

7. Combined UMN and LMN disease (e.g., amyotrophic lateral sclerosis): damage to the corticospinal tracts with pyramidal (UMN) signs and by damage to the anterior horn cells to produce LMN signs; no sensory deficits

> **NB:** About 5%–10% of ALS is familial. Mutations in the *C9orf72* gene are responsible for 30%–40% of familial ALS in Europe and the U.S. Superoxide dismutase (*SOD1*) gene mutations cause 15%–20% of familial ALS, and *TARDBP* and *FUS* gene mutations each account for ~5% of cases.

8. Ventral spinal artery occlusion: causes infarction of the anterior two-thirds of the spinal cord but spares dorsal columns and horns; damage to the following structures: lateral corticospinal tracts (bilateral spastic paresis with pyramidal signs below the lesion), lateral spinothalamic tracts (bilateral loss of pain and temperature sensation below the lesion), hypothalamospinal tract (at T2 and above, results in bilateral Horner's syndrome), ventral (anterior) horns (results in bilateral flaccid paralysis of the innervated muscles), corticospinal tracts to the sacral parasympathetic centers at S2 through S4 (results in bilateral damage and loss of voluntary bladder and bowel control).

D. **Spinal cord syndromes** (*cont'd*)

9. Cauda equina syndrome: for spinal roots L3 through coccygeal; results usually from a nerve root tumor (also ependymomas, dermoid tumor, or from a lipomas of the terminal cord); clinical: severe radicular unilateral pain; sensory distribution in unilateral saddle-shaped area; unilateral muscle atrophy; absent quadriceps (L3–L4) and ankle jerks (S1); incontinence and sexual functions are not marked (initially, at least); onset is often gradual.

10. Conus medullaris syndrome: for segments S3 through coccygeal; usually results from an intramedullary tumor, such as ependymomas; clinical: pain usually bilateral but not severe, sensory distribution in bilateral saddle-shaped area, muscle changes are not marked, quadriceps reflexes are normal (ankle jerk may be affected), incontinence and sexual functions are severely impaired, onset is often sudden and bilateral.

> **NB:** The collateral blood supply at the T5 through T7 level of the spinal cord (SC) is relatively tenuous, making this "watershed" area most susceptible to ischemia.

IV. Peripheral Nerves

A. **Brachial plexus: originates from the anterior rami of spinal nerves C5 through T1; variations are common.**

1. *Certain muscles of the shoulder girdle innervated by nerves* that **originate *proximal to the formation of the brachial plexus;*** these muscles are important to evaluate clinically and by nerve conduction study/electromyography (EMG) when trying to determine if the lesion is at the level of the plexus or roots.

    a. **Serratus anterior:** innervated by the long thoracic nerve (C5–C7)

    b. **Rhomboids:** innervated by the dorsal scapular nerve (C5)

2. *Trunks of the brachial plexus*

    a. *Upper trunk:* C5, C6; branches include:

        i. **Suprascapular nerve:** innervates the supraspinatus and infraspinatus muscles

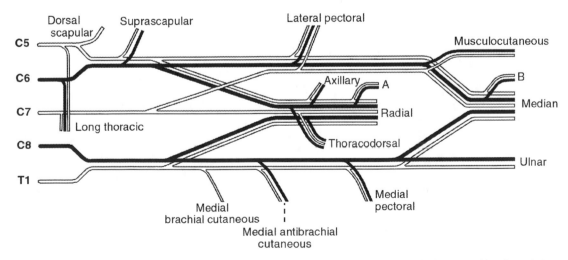

Figure 4.11 Schematic diagram of the brachial plexus. A, branch to extensor carpi radialis longus and brachioradialis; B, branch to flexor carpi radialis and pronator teres.

> **NB:** The suprascapular nerve is susceptible to compression in the suprascapular notch.

ii. **Nerve to the subclavius muscle:** innervates the subclavius

b. *Middle trunk:* C7

c. *Lower trunk:* C8, T1

3. *Cords of the brachial plexus*

a. *Lateral cord:* formed by the anterior divisions of the upper and middle trunks (C5–C7); branches include

i. *Part of the median nerve:* supplies pronator teres, flexor carpi radialis

> **NB:** The sensory supply to the median nerve derives from the lateral cord.

ii. *Musculocutaneous nerve:* supplies the biceps, brachialis, and coracobrachialis

iii. *Lateral antebrachial cutaneous nerve (continuation of the musculocutaneous nerve):* skin of the lateral forearm

iv. *Branch to the pectoral nerve:* supplies the pectoralis major

b. *Medial cord:* formed by the anterior division of the lower trunk (C8, T1)

i. *Part of the median nerve:* supplies the flexor digitorum superficialis, one-half of the flexor digitorum profundus, pronator quadratus, flexor pollicis longus, and 1st and 2nd lumbricals, abductor pollicis brevis, opponens pollicis, and one-half of flexor pollicis brevis (superficial head)

> **NB:** Martin-Gruber anastomosis occurs in 15% to 30% of the population, consisting of a communicating branch from the median nerve to the ulnar nerve in the forearm to supply the first dorsal interosseous, and/or adductor pollicis, and/or abductor digiti minimi.

ii. *Ulnar nerve:* supplies one-half of the flexor digitorum profundus, flexor carpi ulnaris, 3rd and 4th lumbricals, interossei, adductor pollicis, abductor digiti minimi, opponens digiti minimi, and one-half flexor pollicis brevis (deep head)

iii. *Medial cutaneous nerve:* supplies the skin to the medial arm

iv. *Medial antebrachial cutaneous nerve:* supplies the skin to the medial forearm

> **NB:** This nerve is a branch of the medial cord and would be expected to be injured in neurogenic thoracic outlet syndrome, and would be spared in an ulnar nerve mononeuropathy at the elbow.

v. *Medial pectoral nerve:* supplies the pectoralis major and minor muscles

A. **Brachial plexus** (*cont'd*)

 c. *Posterior cord:* formed by the posterior division of the upper, middle, and lower trunks (C5–T1); branches include:

  i. *Upper and lower subscapular nerves:* supplies the subscapularis and teres major

  ii. *Thoracodorsal nerve:* supplies latissimus dorsi

  iii. *Axillary nerve:* supplies the deltoid and teres major

  iv. *Radial nerve:* supplies the triceps, brachioradialis, extensor carpi radialis longus, extensor carpi radialis brevis, anconeus, supinator, extensor digitorum communis, extensor carpi ulnaris, abductor pollicis longus, extensor pollicis longus, extensor pollicis brevis, and extensor indicis proprius muscles

  v. *Posterior antebrachial cutaneous nerve*

 4. *Anatomic lesions of the brachial plexus*

> **NB:** Lesions in the brachial plexus will spare the paraspinal muscles at the corresponding levels.

 a. *Trunk lesions*

  i. *Upper trunk lesion:* **Erb-Duchenne paralysis**; nerves involved: *suprascapular nerve* (paralysis of the shoulder adductors/external rotators), C5, C6 portions of the *lateral cord and posterior cord* (paralysis of forearm flexors, elbow flexors, external rotators of the forearm), *lateral antebrachial cutaneous nerve;* clinical presentation: arm is adducted, internally rotated and extended *(porter tip position)* with sparing of the intrinsics, absent biceps/brachioradialis reflexes, absent sensation over the lateral forearm

  ii. *Lower trunk lesions:* **Klumpke's paralysis**—involves the C8, T1 portion of the *medial cord; paralysis of the finger flexors and intrinsics; paresis of triceps and extensor digitorum communis* (C8, T1 portion of the posterior cord); the arm is mildly flexed at the elbow and wrist, with a *"useless" hand;* may be accompanied by Horner's syndrome

  iii. *Middle trunk lesions:* rarely in isolation

 b. *Cord lesions*

  i. *Lateral cord:* weakness in the elbow and wrist flexors; sensory loss over the lateral forearm

  ii. *Medial cord:* weakness in the hand intrinsics and partial weakness in long finger flexors; sensory loss over medial forearm

  iii. *Posterior cord:* weakness in shoulder abduction and elbow/wrist/finger extensors; sensory loss over posterior aspect of the arm and hand

> **NB:** Idiopathic brachial plexopathy (Parsonage Turner syndrome)—most common among young, healthy males; 25% preceded by a viral syndrome; symptoms include **pain (severe at onset)**, weakness, paresthesias; elevated cerebrospinal fluid protein in 10%; two-thirds begin to improve by 1 month and two-thirds recover by 1 year.

 5. *Muscles innervated by the brachial plexus*

MUSCLE	NERVE	SPINAL SEGMENT	ACTION/TEST
Trapezius	Spinal accessory	C3, C4	Have the patient elevate shoulder against resistance.
Rhomboids	Dorsal scapular	C5	With the patient's hand behind the back, order to press against you while you press on the palm.
Serratus anterior	Long thoracic	C5–C7	Have the patient push against a wall.
Pectoralis major	Lateral and medial pectoral	C6–C8	Have the patient adduct the upper arm against resistance.
Supraspinatus	Suprascapular	C5, C6	With the arm close to the body, have the patient abduct the upper arm against resistance.
Infraspinatus	Suprascapular	C5, C6	Have the patient externally rotate the upper arm at the shoulder against resistance.
NB: Latissimus dorsi	Thoracodorsal	C6–C8	With the upper arm up at shoulder level, have the patient adduct against resistance.
Teres major	Subscapular	C5–C7	Have the patient adduct the elevated upper arm against resistance.
Biceps	Musculocutaneous	C5, C6	Have the patient flex supinated forearm against resistance.
Deltoid	Axillary	C5, C6	Have the patient abduct the upper arm against resistance while elevated to the level of the shoulder.
Triceps	Radial	C6–C8	Have the patient extend the forearm at the elbow against resistance.
Brachioradialis	Radial	C5, C6	Have the patient flex the forearm against resistance with the forearm midway between pronation and supination.
Extensor carpi radialis	Radial	C5, C6	Have the patient extend and abduct the hand at the wrist against resistance.
Supinator	Radial	C6, C7	Have the patient supinate the forearm against resistance with the forearm extended at the elbow.
Extensor carpi ulnaris	Posterior interosseous	C7, C8	Have the patient extend and adduct the hand at the wrist against resistance.
Extensor digitorum	Posterior interosseous	C7, C8	Have the patient maintain extension of fingers at the metacarpophalangeal joints against resistance.
Abductor pollicis longus	Posterior interosseous	C7, C8	Have the patient abduct the thumb at the carpometacarpal joint in a plane at right angles to the palm.
Extensor pollicis longus	Posterior interosseous	C7, C8	Have the patient extend the thumb at the interphalangeal joint against resistance.

(continued)

5. *Muscles innervated by the brachial plexus (cont'd)*

MUSCLE	NERVE	SPINAL SEGMENT	ACTION/TEST
Extensor pollicis brevis	Posterior interosseous	C7, C8	Have the patient extend the thumb at the metacarpophalangeal joint against resistance.
Pronator teres	Median	C6, C7	Have the patient pronate the forearm against resistance.
Flexor carpi radialis	Median	C6, C7	Have the patient flex the hand at the wrist against resistance.
Flexor digitorum superficialis	Median	C7–T1	Have the patient flex the finger at the proximal interphalangeal joint against resistance.
Flexor digitorum profundus I, II	Anterior interosseous	C7–T1	Have the patient flex the distal phalanx of the index finger against resistance.
Flexor pollicis longus	Anterior interosseous	C7–T1	Have the patient flex the distal phalanx of the thumb against resistance.
Abductor pollicis brevis	Median	T1>C8	Have the patient abduct the thumb at right angles to the palm against resistance.
Opponens pollicis	Median	C8, T1	Have the patient touch the base of the little finger with the thumb against resistance.
1st lumbrical-interosseous	Median and ulnar	C8, T1	Have the patient extend the finger at the proximal interphalangeal joint against resistance.
Flexor carpi ulnaris	Ulnar	C7–T1	Have the patient flex and adduct the hand at the wrist against resistance.
Flexor digitorum profundus III, IV	Ulnar	C7–T1	Have the patient flex the distal interphalangeal joint against resistance.
Adductor digiti minimi	Ulnar	C8, T1	Have the patient adduct the little finger against resistance.
Flexor digiti minimi	Ulnar	C8, T1	Have the patient flex the little finger at the metacarpophalangeal joint against resistance.
1st dorsal interosseous	Ulnar	C8, T1	Have the patient abduct the index finger against resistance.
2nd palmar interosseous	Ulnar	C8, T1	Have the patient adduct the index finger against resistance.
Adductor pollicis	Ulnar	C8, T1	Have the patient adduct the thumb at right angles to the palm against resistance.

B. **Median nerve: derived from the lateral cord (C5, C6) and medial cord (C8, T1) of the brachial plexus; passes between the two heads of the pronator teres muscle**

1. *Innervates: pronator teres, flexor carpi radialis, flexor digitorum superficialis, and palmaris longus muscles*

2. *Anterior interosseous innervation—flexor digitorum profundus (the radial half, i.e., the lateral two out of the four tendons), flexor pollicis longus, pronator quadratus*

3. *Branches to palmar cutaneous nerve*, which supplies the skin of the proximal median palm; arises at the lower part of the forearm; travels superficial to the flexor retinaculum; therefore, this portion of the median nerve **usually remains spared in carpal tunnel syndrome.**

   The median nerve passes **through** the carpal tunnel to innervate the abductor pollicis brevis, opponens pollicis, one-half of flexor pollicis brevis (superficial head), skin of the distal median palm and 1st through 3rd digits, and one-half of the 4th digit.

4. *Clinical syndromes*

   a. **Carpal tunnel syndrome:** *symptoms:* pain, tingling, or burning in thumb, 1st two fingers, most prominent at night, aggravated by activities involving repetitive wrist action; *clinical findings:* thenar muscle weakness, sensory deficit, *Phalen's sign, Tinel's sign* (to percussion at wrist flexor crease); *EMG/nerve conduction study (NCS):* relative slowing of the conduction between the palm and wrist as compared to the adjacent ulnar nerve may be the most sensitive method of detecting carpal tunnel syndrome, the motor conduction and compound motor action potential amplitude are normal in the majority, unless severe disease.

> **NB:** The median sensory nerve action potential is the most sensitive study for the detection of carpal tunnel syndrome. Motor studies are recorded over the abductor pollicis brevis.

   b. **Anterior interosseous nerve syndrome:** *symptoms:* spontaneous onset or associated with vigorous exercise, pain over proximal flexor surface of the forearm but can be painless, weakness is a common complaint; *clinical:* tenderness over proximal flexor surface of the forearm, weakness of the flexor pollicis longus is most common, no weakness of the thenar muscles, no sensory deficit; *etiology:* accessory head of the flexor pollicis longus, fibrous origin or tendinous origin of the flexor digitorum superficialis to the long finger; *EMG:* abnormalities in the flexor pollicis longus, 1st and 2nd flexor digitorum profundus, and pronator quadratus sparing all other muscles, especially thenar groups

> **NB:** Approximately one-half of the cases of Martin-Gruber anastomosis arise from the anterior interosseous nerve.

   c. **Pronator syndrome:** *symptoms:* pain in the flexor muscles of the proximal forearm, paresthesias of the hand, symptoms worse with forceful pronation, weakness of grip is not a common complaint; *clinical:* tenderness over pronator teres, Tinel's sign over site of entrapment, weakness is often slight, sensory deficit over the cutaneous distribution of the median nerve including the thenar eminence; *etiology:* hypertrophy of the pronator teres, fibrous band from the ulnar head of the pronator teres to the "sublimis bridge," ligament from medial epicondyle to the radius; *EMG/NCS:* **sparing of the pronator teres**, abnormalities of other median innervated forearm muscles plus the thenar muscles, slowing of the conduction through proximal forearm distal latencies

4. *Clinical syndromes (cont'd)*

d. **Humeral supracondylar spur syndrome (ligament of Struthers):** presents clinically like a pronator syndrome; aggravated by forearm supination and elbow extension, which may obliterate the radial pulse, the spur may be palpable, EMG abnormalities of all median nerve–innervated muscles, including pronator teres; supracondylar conduction abnormalities may be demonstrated

C. **Ulnar nerve: derived directly from the lower trunk and medial cord (C8, T1) of the brachial plexus; in the midarm, it becomes superficial and reaches the groove behind the median epicondyle; it passes between the two heads of the flexor carpi ulnaris (cubital tunnel); runs down the medial forearm, innervating the flexor carpi ulnaris and the ulnar half of the flexor digitorum profundus.**

1. Before entry into the Guyon's canal, gives off two small branches: *dorsal cutaneous* (supplies the dorsal ulnar aspect of the hand) and *palmar cutaneous* (supplies the skin of the ulnar palm)

2. *Within Guyon's canal,* gives off two branches: *superficial branch* to the skin over the distal ulnar palm and 5th digit and one-half of 4th digit, and *deep branch* to innervate adductor digiti minimi, opponens digiti minimi, flexor digitorum minimi, 3rd and 4th lumbricals, all interossei, one-half flexor pollicis brevis (deep head), adductor pollicis

> **NB:** The ulnar nerve does not supply sensory innervation proximal to the wrist.

3. *Clinical syndromes*

a. *Compression at the elbow:* site of compression: adjacent to posterior aspect of medial epicondyle of the humerus is most common (due to trauma), *cubital tunnel syndrome* (due to entrapment between the two heads of the flexor carpi ulnaris), *arcade of Struthers syndrome* (due to entrapment as the nerve passes through the medial intermuscular septum); *clinical:* gradual onset of pain along the ulnar side of the forearm and/or hand, numbness in the ring and little fingers, atrophy and weakness of ulnar innervated intrinsic hand muscles, weakness of 4th and 5th flexor digitorum profundus, flexor carpi ulnaris is seldom weak (except entrapment at the arcade of Struthers), hypesthesia and hypalgesia over cutaneous distribution of the ulnar nerve in most cases, nerve in the ulnar groove may enlarge and sublux/dislocate; *EMG/NCS:* abnormally large motor unit potentials with decreased recruitment is common, positive waves and fibrillation also seen frequently (if injury active/ongoing), findings are much more prominent in the hand than the forearm (except in the Arcade of Struthers syndrome), conduction delay is the earliest finding.

b. **Distal ulnar nerve compression syndrome:** *symptoms:* gradual or sudden onset, aching pain along the ulnar side of hand, sensory symptoms may be absent in type 2; *etiology:* fibrous scaring after fracture or soft tissue injury, ganglion, hemorrhage (hemophilia), lipoma, other tumors, ulnar artery disease

i. *Type 1:* atrophy and weakness of all ulnar innervated intrinsic muscles of the hand, sensory loss in the ulnar cutaneous distribution sparing the dorsum of the hand; EMG/NCS: confined to the ulnar innervated intrinsic muscles, motor conduction delay from wrist to hypothenar muscles, sensory conduction delay from the digit to the wrist

ii. *Type 2:* atrophy and weakness of all ulnar innervated intrinsic muscles or all but the hypothenar group, no sensory deficit; EMG/NCS: may spare hypothenar muscles on EMG, may have no conduction delay to hypothenar muscles, conduction delay to the 1st dorsal interosseous, no conduction delay from the digit to the wrist

iii. *Type 3:* sensory loss in the ulnar cutaneous distribution sparing the dorsum of the hand, no motor deficit; EMG/NCS: no EMG abnormality (except possibly palmaris brevis), no conduction delay of hypothenar muscles or 1st dorsal interosseous, with sensory conduction delay from digit to wrist

D. **Radial nerve: derived from the posterior cord (C5–C8) of the brachial plexus; courses down on medial side of the humerus; winds obliquely around the humerus in the spiral groove and branches to triceps; passes between the head of the triceps, passes into the forearm and branches to brachioradialis, the extensor carpi radialis brevis, and longus muscles**

1. Divides into

   a. *Deep radial nerve:* deep motor branch, major terminal portion of the nerve, passes through the supinator muscle (via arcade of Frohse) and becomes the *posterior interosseous nerve, which* innervates extensor groups of forearm and wrist

   b. *Superficial radial nerve:* superficial sensory branch

2. **Posterior interosseous syndrome:** *symptoms:* usually painless, progression most often gradual, begins with a fingerdrop and then progresses from one finger to another, incomplete wristdrop develops later; *clinical:* no weakness proximal to elbow, weakness of muscles of the extensor surface of forearm (except brachioradialis, extensor carpi radialis, and supinator), no sensory deficit; etiology: tumors (usually lipomas), bursitis or synovitis, chronic trauma; *EMG/NCS:* EMG sparing brachioradialis, extensor carpi radialis, and supinator, delayed latency from elbow to extensor indicis

E. **Musculocutaneous nerve: derived from the lateral cord (C5–C7) of the brachial plexus; pierces coracobrachialis then passes between biceps and brachialis and supplies these muscles; continues as the lateral cutaneous nerve of the forearm**

1. **Coracobrachialis syndrome:** *symptoms:* painless weakness of elbow flexion, onset related to strenuous exercise or associated with general anesthesia, recovery is spontaneous and usually complete; *clinical:* weakness is limited to the biceps and brachialis, sensory deficit in the distribution of the lateral cutaneous nerve; *EMG/NCS:* abnormalities noted in biceps and brachialis, but **coracobrachialis spared;** conduction block can be detected proximal to axilla.

F. **Lumbar plexus: produced by the union of the ventral rami of the 1st three lumbar nerves and the greater part of the 4th, with contribution from the subcostal nerve; lies anterior to the vertebral transverse processes, embedded in the posterior part of the psoas major**

1. *1st lumbar nerve:* receives fibers from the subcostal nerve and divides into:

   a. *Upper branch:* splits into iliohypogastric and ilioinguinal (supplying the skin over the root of the penis, adjoining part of the femoral triangle, and upper part of the scrotum) nerves

   b. *Lower branch:* joins a twig from the 2nd lumbar nerve and becomes the *genitofemoral nerve* (divides further into genital—supplying the cremaster muscle and the skin of the scrotum, and femoral—supplying the skin over the upper part of the femoral triangle, branches); all three nerve branches run parallel to the lower intercostal nerves and supply the transverse and oblique abdominal muscles

2. Large part of the *2nd lumbar* and the entire *3rd* (and the offshoot from the 4th lumbar nerve): split into *ventral (anterior) division* and *dorsal (posterior) division,* which unite to constitute:

   a. Femoral nerve

   b. Obturator nerve

3. The lower part of the ventral ramus of the 4th lumbar joins the ventral ramus of the 5th to form the *lumbosacral trunk.*

G. Sacral plexus: formed by the lumbosacral trunk and the ventral rami of the 1st three sacral nerves and the upper part of the 4th sacral ramus; a flattened band that gives rise to many branches before its largest part passes below the piriformis muscle to form the sciatic nerve

> **NB:** The sciatic nerve is divided into the common fibular (peroneal) division and tibial division.

H. Coccygeal plexus: the lower part of the ventral ramus of the 4th and 5th sacral nerves and the coccygeal nerves form the small coccygeal plexus; it consists of two loops on the pelvic surface of the coccygeus and levator ani muscles; anococcygeal nerve: supplies the skin between the anus and coccyx

I. Muscles innervated by the lumbar plexus

MUSCLES	NERVE	SPINAL SEGMENT	ACTION/TEST
Iliopsoas	Femoral, L1–L3 spinal nerve branches	L1–L3	Have the patient flex the thigh against resistance with the leg flexed at the knee and hip.
Quadriceps femoris	Femoral	L2–L4	Have the patient extend the leg against resistance with the limb flexed at the hip and knee.
Adductors	Obturator	L2–L4	Have the patient adduct the limb against resistance while lying on back with leg extended at the knee.
Gluteus medius and minimus	Superior gluteal	L4–S1	Have the patient lie on his back and internally rotate the thigh against resistance with the limb flexed at the hip and knee; or, while the leg is extended, have the patient abduct the limb against resistance.
Gluteus maximus	Inferior gluteal	L5–S2	While the patient lies on his back with the leg extended at the knee, extend the limb at the hip against resistance; or while the patient lies on his face, have him elevate the leg against resistance.
Hamstring: semitendinosus, semimembranosus, biceps	Sciatic	L5–S2	While the patient lies on his back with the limb flexed at the hip and knee, have him flex the leg at the knee against resistance.
Gastrocnemius	Tibial	S1, S2	With the leg extended, have the patient plantar flex the foot against resistance.
Soleus	Tibial	S1, S2	With the limb flexed at the hip and knee, have the patient flex the foot against resistance.
Tibialis posterior	Tibial	L4, L5	Have the patient invert the foot against resistance.

(continued)

MUSCLES	NERVE	SPINAL SEGMENT	ACTION/TEST
Flexor digitorum longus; flexor hallucis longus	Tibial	L5-S2	Have the patient flex the toes against resistance.
Small muscles of the foot	Medial and lateral plantar	S1, S2	Have the patient cup the sole of the foot.
Tibialis anterior	Deep fibular (peroneal)	L4, L5	Have the patient dorsiflex the foot against resistance.
Extensor digitorum longus	Deep fibular (peroneal)	L5, S1	Have the patient dorsiflex the toes against resistance.
Extensor hallucis longus	Deep fibular (peroneal)	L5, S1	Have the patient dorsiflex the distal phalanx of the big toe against resistance.
Extensor digitorum brevis	Deep fibular (peroneal)	L5, S1	Have the patient dorsiflex the proximal phalanges of the toes against resistance.
Peroneus longus and brevis	Superficial fibular (peroneal)	L5, S1	Have the patient evert the foot against resistance.

> **NB:** The short head of the biceps femoris is the only muscle supplied by the peroneal division of the sciatic nerve proximal to the knee.

J. **Clinical syndromes of nerves in the lower limb**

1. *Lateral femoral cutaneous nerve:* arises from the lumbar plexus by fusion of the dorsal division of the ventral rami of L2 and L3; **meralgia paresthetica:** burning, numbness, tingling sensation over the anterolateral thigh; usually most intense in the distal half of the thigh, aggravated by standing, walking, relieved by sitting; etiology: intrapelvic—diverticulitis, uterine fibroid; extrapelvic at the anterior superior iliac spine—pressure by belts, girdles, backpacks; stretch by obesity, pregnancy, physical maneuvers (e.g., getting on bicycle)

2. *Femoral nerve:* arises from the lumbar plexus within the psoas muscle, formed by the posterior division of the ventral rami of L2 through L4

   a. *Intrapelvic compression:* symptoms: pain in the inguinal region partially relieved by flexion and external rotation of the hip, dysesthesia over the anterior thigh and anteromedial leg; clinical: weakness of hip flexion and knee extension, impaired quadriceps reflex, sensory deficit in the cutaneous distribution of the femoral nerve, pain with hip extension; etiology: iliacus hematoma, tumor, extension of disease from the hip joint

> **NB:** Psoas abscess may cause compression of the lumbar plexus, as can hematoma in hemophiliac patients.

   b. *Compression in the inguinal region:* symptoms: similar to intrapelvic compression; clinical: same as intrapelvic compression except that there is no weakness of hip flexion; etiology: femoral lymphadenopathy, lithotomy position

3. *Saphenous nerve:* compression at the knee symptoms: history of prolonged external compression over the anteromedial aspect of the knee, numbness limited to the cutaneous distribution of the saphenous nerve; clinical: *no weakness or reflex changes;* etiology: horseback riding, pressure during sleep

> **NB:** Saphenous neuropathy causes exquisite pain in the distribution of the saphenous nerve.

J. **Clinical syndromes of nerves in the lower limb** (*cont'd*)

4. *Obturator nerve:* symptoms: pain in the groin and along the medial aspect of the thigh, numb patch over the medial aspect of the thigh, worse with adduction and extension of the hip; clinical: *weakness of hip adduction,* impaired adductor reflex, patch of numbness over the medial aspect of the thigh; etiology: high retroperitoneal hemorrhage, surgical procedures (intra- and extrapelvic), tumor

5. *Superior gluteal nerve:* symptoms: pain in the upper gluteal region, limping gait; clinical: no sensory deficit or reflex changes, weakness of gluteus medius and tensor fascia lata; etiology: involvement at the sciatic notch (in conjunction with the sciatic nerve), posttraumatic entrapment

6. *Inferior gluteal nerve:* symptoms: pain in the posterior gluteal region, limping gait; clinical: no sensory or reflex changes, weakness of gluteus maximus; etiology: involvement at the sciatic notch, neoplasm

7. *Sciatic nerve:* originates from the ventral rami of L4 through S3, leaves the pelvis through the sciatic notch; two trunks: *lateral trunk (forms the common fibular [peronea] nerve) and medial trunk (forms the tibial nerve)*

    a. *Intrapelvic involvement:* symptoms: pain in the posterior aspect of the thigh and leg, extending into the foot, numbness/paresthesia may be present along the sciatic cutaneous distribution, nocturnal pain prominent in tumor patients, may be associated with low back pain; etiology: tumors, intrapelvic surgical procedures, piriformis syndrome.

    b. *Compromise at the notch:* symptoms: similar to intrapelvic involvement; clinical: findings predominate in the fibular (peroneal) division, may present as a fibular (peroneal) nerve injury, glutei and hamstrings may or may not be involved; etiology: injection palsy, compression during coma, tumor.

    c. *Focal involvement in the thigh:* symptoms: similar to intrapelvic and sciatic thigh lesions; etiology: tumors, entrapment by the myofascial band

8. *Common fibular (peroneal) nerve:* continuation of the lateral trunk of the sciatic nerve; separates from the sciatic nerve in the upper popliteal fossa, passes behind the fibular head, pierces the superficial head of fibularis (peroneus) longus muscle to reach the anterior compartment of the leg; *divides into: superficial and deep branch;*

    The sciatic nerve gives rise to two sensory nerves in the popliteal fossa: sural nerve and superficial fibular (peroneal) nerve.

    a. **Crossed-leg palsy:** involves the *common fibular (peroneal) nerve* at the head of the fibula, or occasionally the deep or superficial branches individually near their origin; symptoms: footdrop, unstable ankle, paresthesias over anterolateral leg and dorsum of the foot; clinical: weakness of dorsiflexors and evertors of the foot, sensory deficit over the anterolateral leg and dorsum of the foot; etiology; external pressure over the head of the fibula (crossed legs, bed positioning, etc.), internal pressure (squatting), predisposing factors—rapid weight change, especially loss

> **NB:** An L5 lesion will also involve the invertors of the foot (namely, the tibial-innervated tibialis posterior muscle).

b. **Anterior compartment syndrome:** clinical: tenderness to palpation over the anterior compartment, pain with passive plantar flexion of the foot and flexion of the toes, weakness of the anterior compartment muscles (tibialis anterior, extensor hallucis longus, extensor digitorum longus), sensory deficit over the cutaneous distribution of the deep fibular (peroneal) nerve; etiology: increased anterior compartment pressure due to bleeding, increased capillary permeability (trauma, postischemia), increased capillary pressure (exercise, venous obstruction)

> **NB:** An area of sensory loss between the big and the 2nd toe is the typical distribution for a deep peroneal mononeuropathy.

c. **Lateral compartment syndrome:** symptoms are the same as for the anterior compartment syndrome except that the pain is localized over the lateral aspect of the leg; pain with passive inversion of the foot, weakness of the fibularis muscles (peronei), sensory deficit over the cutaneous distribution of the superficial fibular (peroneal) nerve.

d. **Anterior tarsal tunnel syndrome:** symptoms: pain in the ankle and dorsum of the foot, dysesthesia in the distribution of the deep fibular (peroneal) nerve, nocturnal exacerbation, walking provides partial relief; clinical: weakness of extensor digitorum brevis only, no reflex changes, hypesthesia in the cutaneous distribution of the deep fibular (peroneal) nerve; etiology: edema, swelling due to ankle injuries, tight boots.

> **NB:** An accessory deep fibular (peroneal) nerve may exist and innervate the extensor digitorum brevis, passing behind the lateral malleolus. It will manifest in NCS as a smaller compound motor action potential with stimulation of the deep fibular (peroneal) nerve in the ankle (at routine site) when compared to stimulation at the knee.

9. *Tibial nerve:* continuation of the medial trunk of the sciatic nerve; from the ventral rami of L5 through S2; innervates the posterior calf muscles; *branches into medial plantar nerve and lateral plantar nerve*

a. **Deep posterior compartment syndrome:** tenderness over the distal posteromedial leg; pain with passive foot dorsiflexion and toe extension; weakness of plantar flexion, inversion of the foot and flexion of the toes; plantar hypesthesia

b. **Tarsal tunnel syndrome:** symptoms: burning pain and paresthesias in toes and soles of the foot, aggravated by ambulation, nocturnal exacerbations; clinical: tenderness to palpation over the flexor retinaculum, sensory deficit over the distribution of the tibial nerve; etiology: compression within the flexor retinaculum at the ankle

10. *Digital nerve:* **Morton's neuroma**—metatarsal pain and pain in the toes, *typically the 3rd and 4th,* numbness in one or two toes; clinical: hypesthesia of apposing surfaces of two toes, palpation of the nerve across the deep transverse metatarsal ligament with passive hyperextension of the toes causes acute tenderness; etiology: fixed hyperextended M-P joint secondary to trauma or rheumatoid arthritis, high-heeled shoes, work-related stooping, interphalangeal fracture, barefoot running on a hard surface, shortened heel cord

V. Spinal Reflexes and Muscle Tone

A. Monosynaptic reflex response: mediated by two neurons, one afferent and one efferent (e.g., deep tendon reflexes); polysynaptic reflex response: involves several neurons, termed interneurons or internuncial cells, in addition to afferent and efferent neurons

B. Muscle spindles: receptor organs that provide the afferent component of many spinal stretch responses; encapsulated structures, 3 to 4 mm in length; consist of 2 to 12 thin muscle fibers of modified striated muscle; because they are enclosed in a fusiform spindle, they are termed intrafusal muscle fibers (to contrast them with large extrafusal fibers); they are connected to the muscle's tendons in parallel with the extrafusal fibers; the sensory function of the intrafusal fibers is to inform the nervous system of the length and rate of change in length of the extrafusal fibers. Types of spindles:

1. *Nuclear bag fiber:* longer, larger fiber containing large nuclei closely packed in a central bag

2. *Nuclear chain fiber:* shorter, thinner, and contains a single row of central nuclei

3. *Bag$_2$:* intermediate in structure between bag and chain fibers

> **NB:** Both bag and chain fibers are innervated by γ motor neurons, which terminate in two types of endings—plates (occur chiefly on nuclear bag fibers) and trails (occur mostly on nuclear chain fibers, but found on bag fibers as well); muscle spindles are supplied by group 1a and group 2 nerve fibers.

C. Motor neurons: muscle contraction in response to a stimulus involves activation of the α, β, and γ motor neurons of lamina IX

1. α *Motor neurons: largest of the anterior horn cells;* may be stimulated monosynaptically by group 1a primary and 2 secondary afferents, corticospinal tract fibers, lateral vestibulospinal tract fibers, reticulospinal and raphe spinal tract fibers; however, the vast majority are stimulated through interneurons in the spinal cord gray matter; they *activate the large extrafusal skeletal muscle fibers and interneurons in the ventral horn* (*Renshaw cells*, which are capable of inhibiting α motor neurons, producing a negative feedback response).

2. γ *Motor neurons: fusimotor neurons; innervate the intrafusal muscle fibers only, thus do not produce extrafusal muscle contraction;* smaller, not excited monosynaptically by segmental inputs, not involved in inhibitory feedback by Renshaw cells; discharge spontaneously at high frequencies

   a. *Dynamic* γ *motor neurons:* affects the afferent responses to phasic stretch more than static stretch; terminate in plate endings on nuclear bag fibers

   b. *Static* γ *motor neurons:* increase spindle response to static stretch; terminate in trail endings on bag and chain fibers

3. β *Motor neurons:* have axons intermediate in diameter between α and β motor neurons; *innervate extrafusal and intrafusal muscle fibers*

D. Stretch reflex: the basic neural mechanism for maintaining tone in muscles (e.g., tapping the patellar tendon stretches the extrafusal fibers of the quadriceps femoris group); because the intrafusal fibers are arranged in parallel with the extrafusal fibers, the muscle spindles will also be stretched, which then stimulates the sensory nerve endings in spindles (particularly group 1a); group 1a monosynaptically stimulates the α motor neurons that supply the quadriceps muscle and polysynaptically inhibits the antagonist muscle group (the hamstring muscles); thus, the quadriceps suddenly contract and the hamstring relaxes, causing the leg to extend the knee.

E. Golgi tendon organs: encapsulated structures attached in series with the large, collagenous fibers of tendons at the insertions of muscles and along the fascial covering of muscles; *group 1b afferents terminate* in small bundles within the capsule; when muscle contraction occurs, shortening of the contractile part of the muscle results in lengthening of the noncontractile region where the tendon organs are located, resulting in vigorous firing of the Golgi tendon organs; their afferents project to the spinal cord, where they polysynaptically inhibit the α motor neurons innervating the agonist muscle and facilitate motor neurons of the antagonist muscle; central action of the Golgi tendon organs is responsible for the "clasp knife" phenomenon in spasticity.

VI. Basal Ganglia and Cerebellum

A. **Basal ganglia:** function is to control and regulate activities of the motor and premotor cortical areas so that voluntary movements can be performed smoothly; consists of five subcortical nuclei

1. *Caudate:* **derived from the telencephalon;** three parts: head, body, and tail (ending near the amygdala); along with the putamen, is the major input nuclei of the basal ganglia (i.e., receives most of the input from the cerebral cortex); **caudate + putamen = striatum;** major neurotransmitter: GABA (inhibitory)

> **NB:** The recurrent artery of Heubner, a branch of the anterior cerebral artery, supplies the anteromedial part of the head of the caudate nucleus, adjacent parts of the internal capsule and putamen, and parts of the septal nuclei.

2. *Putamen:* **derived from the telencephalon;** means "shell"; **putamen + globus pallidus = lentiform nucleus**

3. *Globus pallidus:* **derived from the diencephalon;** histologically resembles substantia nigra pars reticulata (SNr) and, along with it, serves as the major output nuclei of the basal ganglia; two divisions: globus pallidus interna (GPi) and externa (GPe); neurotransmitter: major GABA (inhibitory)

> **NB:** The caudate and the putamen serve as the primary input nuclei for the basal ganglia, whereas the **globus pallidus, which projects to the ventral anterior nucleus of the thalamus, is the primary output nucleus.**

4. *Substantia nigra:* **derived from the diencephalon;** means "black substance"; lies in the midbrain and composed of two zones: SNr (pale, GABA-ergic) and substantia nigra pars compacta ([SNc] dark, composed of dopaminergic neurons)

5. *Subthalamic nucleus:* **derived from the diencephalon;** involved in the **indirect pathway;** major neurotransmitter: *glutamate (excitatory)*

> **NB:** The subthalamic nucleus receives inhibitory input from the external part of the globus pallidus and sends excitatory input to the GPi.

A. **Basal ganglia** (*cont'd*)

    6. *Basal ganglia connections*

        a. *Direct pathway*

            i. In the *normal state*, dopamine (DA) levels are relatively constant; this produces an output (neurotransmitter release/GABA) from the striatum that is inhibitory in nature (and can be thought of as braking signal to the GPi and SNr); these two populations of neurons (GPi and SNr) also produce an output to the thalamus that is also inhibitory (GABA); so, in effect, the greater the inhibitory signal is to the GPi and SNr, the smaller the inhibitory signal is to the thalamus (braking the brake); the output from the thalamus (to the motor areas of the brain) is excitatory (so by increasing the braking signal from the striatum to the GPi and SNr, the braking signal to the thalamus is diminished and the excitatory output from the thalamus is increased).

           ii. *With Parkinson's disease (PD)*, there is a progressive loss of the DA cells (in the SNc); with the diminished DA signal, the output from the striatum (remember, it is inhibitory or a brake signal) is diminished, and in turn will release the GPi and SNr from inhibition, allowing a larger inhibitory or braking signal to be sent to the thalamus (so by unbraking a brake, the thalamus sends a smaller excitatory signal, which is consistent with the bradykinesia seen in PD).

> NB: GABA is inhibitory, and glutamate is excitatory.

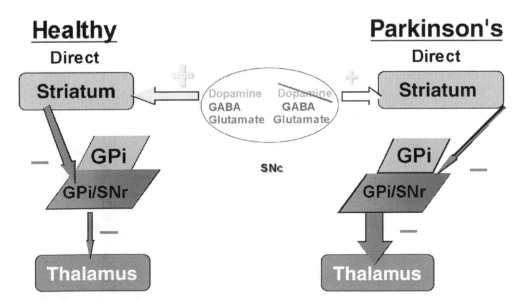

Figure 4.12 Schematic diagram of the direct pathway of the basal ganglia.

b. *Indirect pathway:* DA stimulates the DA receptors in the striatum (as discussed for the *direct pathway*); this courses through a series of inhibitory and excitatory nuclei (**GPe, subthalamic nucleus,** GPi/SNr) and results in the **final inhibitory signal to the thalamus;** *output of the globus pallidus = GABA (inhibitory), subthalamic nucleus = glutamate (excitatory).*

> **NB:** The GPe is part of the indirect pathway (not the direct pathway!) that projects inhibitory fibers to the subthalamic nucleus.

B. **Cerebellum: three primary functions: maintenance of posture, maintenance of muscle tone, and coordination of voluntary motor activity**

1. *Cerebellar peduncles*

   a. *Superior cerebellar peduncle:* brachium conjunctivum

      i. *Afferent tract:* ventral spinocerebellar portion of the rostral spinocerebellar tract, and trigeminocerebellar projections

      ii. *Efferent tract:* **dentatothalamic tract—terminates in the ventral lateral nucleus of the thalamus; also rubral** and reticular projections arise from the dentate and interposed nuclei

> **NB:** Lesion in this tract results in palatal tremor.

   b. *Middle cerebellar peduncle:* brachium pontis

      i. Afferent tract: pontocerebellar fibers—crossed fibers from the pontine nuclei that project to the neocerebellum

   c. *Inferior cerebellar peduncle:* restiform body–afferent tracts

      i. Dorsal spinocerebellar

      ii. Cuneocerebellar

      iii. **Olivocerebellar (from the contralateral olivary nucleus)**

      iv. Others: fibers from the vestibular nerve and nuclei, reticulocerebellar fibers, some fibers from the rostral spinocerebellar

2. *Cerebellar cortex, neurons, and fibers*

   a. *Cortex:* has three layers

      i. *Molecular layer:* outer layer underlying the pia; contains stellate cells, basket cells, and dendritic arbor of the Purkinje cells

      ii. *Purkinje cell layer:* lies between the molecular and granule cell layers

      iii. *Granule layer:* inner layer overlying the white matter; contains granule cells, Golgi cells, and **cerebellar glomeruli (which consist of a mossy fiber rosette, granule cell dendrites, and a Golgi cell axon)**

   b. *Neurons and fibers of the cerebellum*

      i. *Purkinje cells:* convey the *only output* from the cerebellar cortex; **project inhibitory output (γ-aminobutyric acid [GABA]) to the cerebellar and vestibular nuclei;** excited by parallel and climbing fibers and inhibited by GABA-ergic basket and stellate cells

      ii. *Granule cells: excite (by way of glutamate)* **Purkinje, basket, stellate, and Golgi cells** through parallel fibers; **excited by mossy fibers and inhibited by Golgi cells**

      iii. *Parallel fibers:* axons of granule cells; extend into the molecular layer

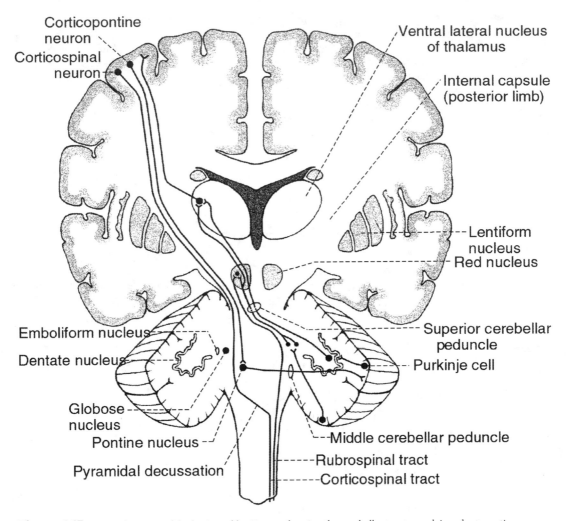

Figure 4.13 Coronal section of the brain and brainstem showing the cerebellar tracts, nuclei, and connections.

b. *Neurons and fibers of the cerebellum (cont'd)*

iv. *Mossy fibers:* the afferent excitatory fibers of the spinocerebellar, pontocerebellar, and vestibulocerebellar tracts; terminate as mossy fiber rosettes on granule cell dendrites; excite granule cells

v. *Climbing fibers:* the *afferent excitatory (by way of aspartate)* fibers of the olivocerebellar tract; arise from the contralateral inferior olivary nucleus and terminate on neurons of the cerebellar nuclei and dendrites of Purkinje cells

> **NB:** The major cerebellar pathway: Purkinje cells of the cerebellar cortex project to the dentate nucleus (also emboliform, globose, and fastigial nuclei); dentate nucleus gives rise to the dentatothalamic tract, which projects (through the superior cerebellar peduncle) **to the contralateral ventral lateral thalamus**, which projects to the ipsilateral primary motor cortex (Brodmann's area 4), which projects ipsilaterally as the corticopontine tract to the pons; the pontine nuclei then project as the pontocerebellar tract (through the middle cerebellar peduncle) to the contralateral cerebellar cortex, where they terminate as mossy fibers.

VII. Brainstem, Cranial Nerves (CNs), and Special Sensory Systems:
The brainstem includes the medulla, pons, and midbrain; extends from the pyramidal decussation to the posterior commissure; receives blood supply from the vertebrobasilar system; contains CNs III–XII, except the spinal part of XI.

A. Brainstem surface anatomy and blood supply

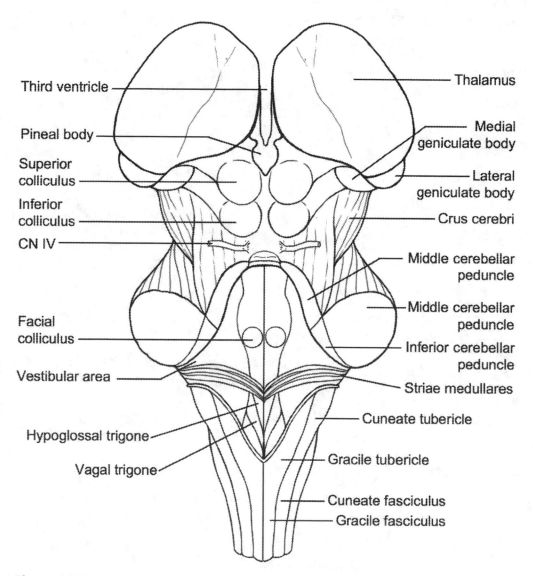

Figure 4.14(A) Dorsal view of the brainstem.

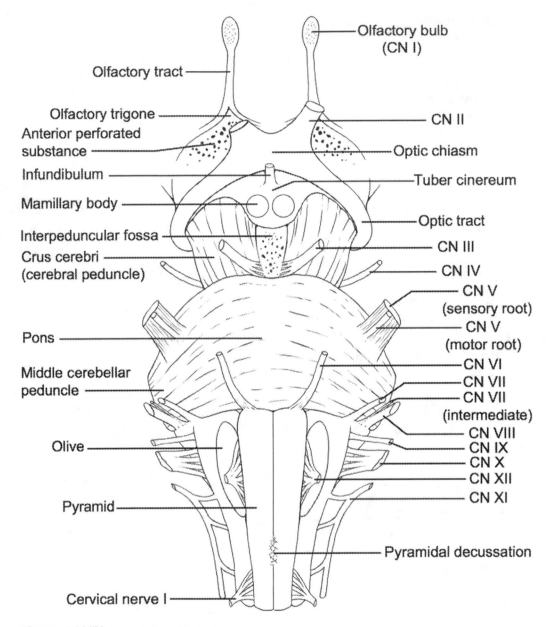

Figure 4.14(B) Ventral view of the brainstem.

B. Functional components of the CNs

1. *General afferent fibers:* have their cells of origin in the cranial and spinal dorsal root ganglia

   a. *General somatic afferent (GSA) fibers:* carry exteroceptive (pain, temperature, and touch) and proprioceptive impulses from sensory endings in the *body wall, tendons, and joints*

   b. *General visceral afferent (GVA) fibers:* carry sensory impulses from the *visceral structures* (hollow organs and glands) within the thoracic, abdominal, and pelvic cavities

2. *Special afferent fibers:* found only in certain CNs
   a. *Special somatic afferent (SSA)* nerves: carry sensory impulses from the special sense organs in the *eye and ear* (vision, hearing, and equilibrium)
   b. *Special visceral afferent (SVA)* fibers: carry information from the *olfactory and gustatory receptors;* designated as visceral because of the functional association with the digestive tract
3. *General efferent fibers:* arise in cells in the spinal cord, brainstem, and autonomic ganglia; innervate all musculature of the body except the branchiomeric muscles
   a. *General somatic efferent (GSE)* fibers: convey motor impulses to *somatic skeletal muscles;* in the head, the somatic musculature is that of the tongue and the extraocular muscles.
   b. *General visceral efferent (GVE)* fibers: autonomic axons that innervate *smooth and cardiac muscle fibers and regulate glandular secretion;* sympathetic or parasympathetic
4. *Special visceral efferent fibers (SVE):* innervate the skeletal musculature of *branchiomeric origin;* striated muscles of the jaw, facial expression, pharynx, and larynx; they are not part of the autonomic nervous system.

CN	GENERAL AFFERENT	SPECIAL AFFERENT	GENERAL EFFERENT	SPECIAL EFFERENT
I		*SVA:* olfactory nerve; consists of unmyelinated axons of bipolar neurons		
II		*SSA:* optic nerve; not a true nerve, rather an evaginated fiber tract of the diencephalon		
III			*GSE:* oculomotor nucleus—innervates ipsilateral inferior rectus, inferior oblique, medial rectus, contralateral superior rectus, and bilateral levators (most medial subnuclei) *GVE:* Edinger-Westphal nucleus—constricts the pupil and participates in light accommodation reflex	
IV			*GSE:* trochlear nucleus—innervates the superior oblique of the contralateral eye	

(continued)

CN	GENERAL AFFERENT	SPECIAL AFFERENT	GENERAL EFFERENT	SPECIAL EFFERENT
V	GSA: trigeminal ganglion—sensory innervation of the face, dura of the anterior and middle cranial fossae; mesen-cephalic nucleus—proprioceptive fibers from the muscles of masti-cation and muscles innervated by the mandibular nerve			SVE: motor nucleus of V—innervates muscles of mastication
VI			GSE: abducens nu-cleus—innervates the lateral rectus	
VII	GSA: geniculate ganglion—conveys pain and tempera-ture from the exter-nal auditory meatus and skin of the ear region GVA: genicu-late ganglion—innervates the soft palate and adjacent pharynx	SVA: geniculate ganglion—innervates taste buds of the anterior two-thirds of the tongue by way of the chorda tympani and lingual nerves; terminates in the nucleus solitaries	GVE: superior sal-ivatory nucleus—preganglionic parasympathetic neurons that inner-vate the lacrimal, submandibular, sublingual glands	SVE: facial nucleus—loops around the abducens nucleus, exits the brainstem, and enters the internal auditory meatus, traverses facial canal and ex-its through the sty-lomastoid foramen; innervates muscles of facial expression, stylohyoid muscle, posterior belly of digastric and stape-dius muscle
VIII		SSA: spiral ganglion—bipolar cells receive stimuli from hair cells in cochlear duct and terminate in dorsal and ventral cochlear nuclei; vestibular ganglion—bipolar cells receive stimuli from hair cells in the maculae and cristae and terminate in four vestibular nuclei		

(continued)

CN	GENERAL AFFERENT	SPECIAL AFFERENT	GENERAL EFFERENT	SPECIAL EFFERENT
IX	*GSA:* superior ganglion of IX—conveys pain and temperature from the external auditory meatus of the ear	*SVA:* inferior ganglion—carries gustatory sensation from the posterior third of the tongue	*GVE:* inferior salivatory nucleus—preganglionic parasympathetic fibers that innervate the parotid gland	*SVE:* nucleus ambiguus of the medulla—innervates the stylopharyngeus muscle
	GVA: inferior petrosal ganglion—carries general sensory input from posterior 3rd of the tongue, upper pharynx, tonsils, tympanic cavity, auditory tube and terminate in nucleus solitarius; also innervates the carotid sinus (baroreceptors) and carotid body (chemoreceptors)			
X	*GSA:* superior (jugular) ganglion—conveys pain and temperature from the skin in the ear region and terminates in the spinal nucleus of V *GVA:* inferior (nodose) ganglion—conveys general sensations from the pharynx, larynx, thoracic and abdominal viscera and terminates in nucleus solitarius	*SVA:* inferior ganglion—receives gustatory sensation from epiglottal taste buds and ends in the nucleus solitarius	*GVE:* dorsal motor nucleus of X—preganglionic parasympathetic fibers, innervates the viscera of the neck and thoracic (heart) and abdominal cavities as far as the left colic flexure	*SVE:* nucleus ambiguus—provides efferent limb of the gag reflex; innervates the pharyngeal arch muscles of larynx, pharynx, striated muscles of the upper esophagus, uvula, levator palatini, and palatoglossus muscles

(continued)

CN	GENERAL AFFERENT	SPECIAL AFFERENT	GENERAL EFFERENT	SPECIAL EFFERENT
XI				*SVE:* cranial division—arises from the nucleus ambiguus and innervates the intrinsic muscles of the larynx; exits through the jugular foramen; spinal division—ventral horn of C1–C6 and innervates sternocleidomastoid and trapezius
XII			*GSE:* hypoglossal nucleus—mediates tongue movement, exits skull through the hypoglossal canal	

C. Trigeminal system: provides sensory innervation to the face, oral cavity, and supratentorial dura (general somatic afferent [GSA] fibers); also innervates the muscles of mastication (special visceral efferent [SVE] fibers)

> **NB:** A lesion in the facial nerve will not affect the muscles of mastication.

1. *Trigeminal ganglion: semilunar or gasserian;* contains pseudounipolar ganglion cells; three divisions:
   a. *Ophthalmic nerve (V1):* lies in the wall of the cavernous sinus; enters *through the superior orbital fissure;* also mediates the afferent limb of the corneal reflex
   b. *Maxillary nerve (V2):* lies in the wall of the cavernous sinus; exits the skull *through the foramen rotundum*
   c. *Mandibular nerve (V3):* exits the skull *through the foramen ovale*

> **NB:** V3 does not go through the cavernous sinus. It will be spared in a cavernous sinus thrombosis.

   d. *Motor (SVE) component of CN V:* accompanies the mandibular nerve *through the foramen ovale;* innervates the muscles of mastication, mylohyoid, anterior belly of digastric, tensors tympani, and veli palatini; innervates the muscles of the jaw, the lateral and medial pterygoids
2. *Trigeminothalamic pathways*
   a. *Ventral trigeminothalamic tract:* mediates pain and temperature sensation from the face and oral cavity

   i. *First-order neurons:* located in the *trigeminal ganglion;* gives rise to axons that descend in the spinal trigeminal tract and synapse with second-order neurons in the spinal trigeminal nucleus

   ii. *Second-order neurons:* located in the *spinal trigeminal nucleus;* gives rise to the decussating axons that terminate in the contralateral ventral postero-medial (VPM) nucleus of the thalamus

   iii. *Third-order neurons:* located in the *VPM nucleus* of the thalamus; project through the posterior limb of the internal capsule to the face area of the somatosensory cortex (Brodmann's areas 3, 1, 2)

  b. *Dorsal trigeminothalamic tract:* mediates tactile discrimination and pressure sensation from the face and oral cavity; receives input from Meissner's and Pacini's corpuscles

   i. *First-order neurons:* located in the *trigeminal ganglion;* synapse in the principal sensory nucleus of CN V

   ii. *Second-order neurons:* located in the *principal sensory nucleus of CN V;* project to the ipsilateral VPM nucleus of the thalamus

   iii. *Third-order neurons:* located in the *VPM nucleus* of the thalamus; project through the posterior limb of the internal capsule to Brodmann's areas 3, 1, 2

 3. *Trigeminal reflexes*

  a. *Corneal reflex:* consensual disynaptic reflex

  b. *Jaw-jerk reflex:* monosynaptic myotatic reflex

  c. *Tearing (lacrimal) reflex*

  d. *Oculocardiac reflex:* pressure of the globe results in bradycardia

 4. *Cavernous sinus:* contains the following structures—*internal carotid artery (siphon), CN III, IV, V1, V2, and VI, postganglionic sympathetic fibers* (en route to the orbit)

D. Auditory system: an exteroceptive special somatic afferent (SSA) system that can detect sound frequencies from 20 to 20,000 Hz; derived from the otic vesicle, which is a derivative of the otic placode, a thickening of the surface ectoderm

 1. *Auditory pathway:*

  a. *Hair cells of the organ of Corti:* innervated by the peripheral processes of bipolar cells of the spiral ganglion; stimulated by vibrations of the basilar membrane

   i. *Inner hair cells:* chief sensory elements; synapse with the dendrites of my-elinated neurons whose axons comprise 90% of the cochlear nerve

   ii. *Outer hair cells:* synapse with the dendrites of unmyelinated neurons whose axons comprise 10% of the cochlear nerve; they reduce the threshold of the inner hair cells.

  b. *Bipolar cells of the spiral (cochlear) ganglion:* project peripherally to the hair cells of the organ of Corti; project centrally as the cochlear nerve to the cochlear nuclei

  c. *Cochlear nerve (CN VIII):* extends from the spiral ganglion to the cerebellopontine angle, where it enters the brainstem

  d. *Cochlear nuclei:* receive input from the cochlear nerve and project to the contralateral superior olivary nucleus and lateral lemniscus

  e. *Superior olivary nucleus:* projects to the lateral lemniscus; plays a role in sound localization; **NB: the trapezoid body, located in the pons, contains decussating fibers from the ventral cochlear nuclei.**

  f. *Lateral lemniscus:* receives input from the contralateral cochlear nuclei and superior olivary nuclei

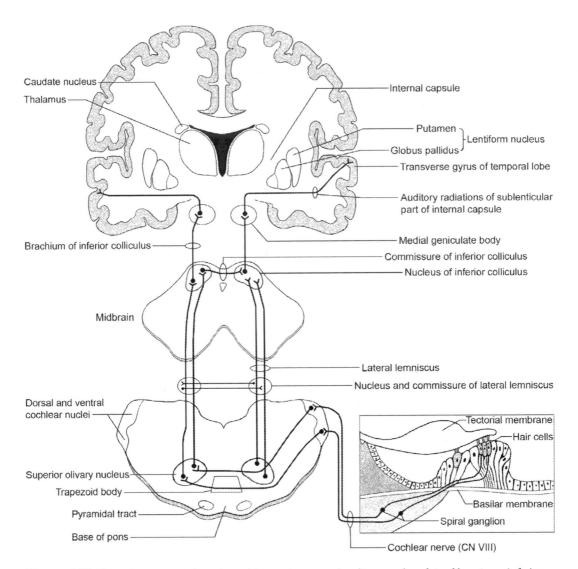

Figure 4.15 The auditory system from the cochlear nucleus, **superior** olivary nucleus, **lateral** lemniscus, **inferior** colliculus, and **medial** geniculate body to the primary auditory cortex.

1. *Auditory pathway (cont'd)*

    g. *Nucleus of the inferior colliculus:* receives input from the lateral lemniscus and projects through the brachium of the inferior colliculus to the medial geniculate body

    h. *Medial geniculate body:* projects through the internal capsule as the auditory radiation to **the primary auditory cortex (transverse temporal gyri of Heschl-Brodmann's areas 41, 42)**

2. *Tuning fork tests*

    a. *Weber's test:* place a vibrating tuning fork on the vertex of the skull; the patient should hear equally on both sides.

        i. Unilateral conduction deafness: hears the vibration more loudly in the affected ear

        ii. Unilateral partial nerve deafness: hears the vibration more loudly in the normal ear

b. *Rinne test:* compares air and bone conduction; place a vibrating tuning fork on the mastoid until the vibration is no longer heard, then hold the tuning fork in front of the ear; the patient should hear the vibration in air after bone conduction is gone.

    i. *Unilateral conduction deafness:* patient does not hear the vibration in air after bone conduction is gone.

    ii. *Unilateral partial nerve deafness:* patient hears the vibration in the air after bone conduction is gone.

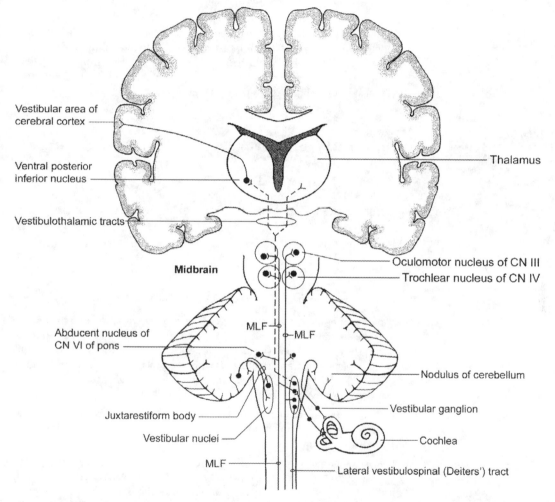

Figure 4.16 The vestibular system from the semicircular ducts, utricle, and saccule and cerebellar projections to the vestibular nuclei to its various projections to the cerebellum, CN III, CN IV, CN VI, spinal cord, and ventral posteroinferior and posterolateral nuclei of the thalamus.

E. **Vestibular system: also derived from the otic vesicle; maintains posture and equilibrium and coordinates head and eye movements**

1. The *labyrinth*

    a. *Three semicircular ducts (superior, lateral, and posterior)* lie within the three semicircular canals; ducts *respond to angular acceleration and deceleration* of the head; contain hair cells in the crista ampullaris; hair cells respond to endolymph flow.

1. The *labyrinth* (*cont'd*)

   b. *Utricle and saccule:* respond to the position of the head with respect to *linear acceleration and pull of gravity;* also contain hair cells whose cilia are embedded in the otolithic membrane

2. *Vestibular pathways*

   a. *Hair cells of the semicircular ducts, saccule, and utricle are innervated by the peripheral processes of bipolar cells* of the vestibular ganglion.

   b. *Vestibular ganglion:* located on the fundus of the internal auditory meatus; project their central processes as the vestibular nerve to the vestibular nuclei and to the flocculonodular lobe of the cerebellum

   c. *Vestibular nuclei:* receive input from semicircular ducts, saccule, utricle, flocculonodular lobe of the cerebellum; project to flocculonodular lobe of the cerebellum, CN III, CN IV, CN VI (through MLF), spinal cord (through the lateral vestibule spinal tract), and ventral posteroinferior and posterolateral nuclei of the thalamus (which project to the postcentral gyrus)

 NB: Cold-water irrigation of the external auditory meatus (stimulation of the horizontal ducts) results in nystagmus to the opposite side; in unconscious patients, no nystagmus is observed; with intact brainstem, deviation of the eyes to the side of the cold irrigation is seen; with bilateral MLF transection, deviation of the abducting eye to the side of the cold irrigation is observed; with lower brainstem damage to the vestibular nuclei, no deviation of the eyes is seen.

F. **Visual system: served by the optic nerve (SSA nerve)**

   1. *Visual pathway:* human retina contains *two types of photoreceptors: rods (mediate light perception, provide low visual acuity, used chiefly in nocturnal vision, contain rhodopsin pigment) and cones (mediate color vision, provide high visual acuity, contain iodopsin pigment);* the *fovea centralis* within the macula is a specialized region in the retina adapted for high *visual acuity and contains only cones;* the pathway includes the following structures:

      a. *Ganglion cells* of the retina: form the optic nerve (CN II); project from the **nasal hemiretina to the contralateral lateral geniculate body and from the temporal hemiretina to the ipsilateral geniculate body**

      b. *Optic nerve:* projects from the lamina cribrosa of the scleral canal, through the optic canal, to the optic chiasm; transection causes ipsilateral blindness, with no direct pupillary light reflex; **NB: a section of the optic nerve at the optic chiasm transects all fibers from the ipsilateral retina as well as fibers from the contralateral inferior nasal quadrant that loop into the optic nerve (fibers of von Willebrand's knee)—a lesion, therefore, causes ipsilateral blindness plus contralateral upper temporal quadrant defect (junction scotoma).**

      c. *Optic chiasm:* contains the decussating fibers from the two nasal hemiretinas and noncrossing fibers from the two temporal hemiretinas and projects to the suprachiasmatic nucleus of the hypothalamus; **midsagittal transection or pressure (e.g., pituitary tumor) causes bitemporal hemianopia;** bilateral lateral compression (e.g., calcified internal carotid artery) causes binasal hemianopia.

      d. *Optic tract:* contains fibers from the ipsilateral temporal hemiretina and contralateral nasal hemiretina; projects to the ipsilateral lateral geniculate body, pretectal nuclei, and superior colliculus; transection causes hemianopia.

e. *Lateral geniculate body:* Six-layer nucleus; *layers 1, 4, and 6 receive crossed fibers; layers 2, 3, and 5 receive uncrossed fibers;* projects through the geniculocalcarine tract to layer IV of Brodmann's area 17.

f. *Geniculocalcarine tract (optic radiation):* projects through two divisions to the visual cortex

    i. *Upper division:* projects to the upper bank of the calcarine sulcus, the *cuneus;* contains input from the superior retinal quadrants, representing inferior visual field quadrants; transection causes contralateral lower quadrantanopia; lesions that involve both cunei *cause a lower altitudinal hemianopia (altitudinopia).*

    ii. *Lower division:* loops from the lateral geniculate body anteriorly **(Meyer's loop),** then posteriorly, to terminate in the lower bank of the calcarine sulcus, the *lingual gyrus;* contains input from the inferior retinal quadrants representing the superior visual field quadrants; **transection causes contralateral upper quadrantanopia ("pie in the sky");** transection of both lingual gyri *causes an upper altitudinal hemianopia.*

g. **Visual cortex (Brodmann's area 17) is located on the banks of the calcarine fissure:** cuneus (upper bank) and lingual gyrus (lower bank); **lesions cause contralateral hemianopia with macular sparing.**

2. *Pupillary light reflex pathway:* has an *afferent limb (CN II)* and *efferent limb (CN III);* the ganglion cells of the retina project bilaterally to the pretectal nuclei, **which projects crossed and uncrossed fibers to the** *Edinger-Westphal nucleus,* **which gives rise to the preganglionic parasympathetic fibers;** these fibers exit the midbrain with CN III and **synapse with postganglionic parasympathetic neurons of the ciliary ganglion,** which innervates the sphincter muscle of the iris.

3. *Pupillary dilatation pathway:* mediated by the *sympathetic division* of the autonomic nervous system; interruption at any level causes *Horner's syndrome* (miosis, hemifacial anhidrosis, ptosis +/− enophthalmos); includes the following structures: hypothalamic neurons of the paraventricular nucleus project directly to the ciliospinal center (T1–T2) of the intermediolateral cell column of the spinal cord, which projects preganglionic sympathetic fibers through the sympathetic trunk to the superior cervical ganglion, which projects postganglionic sympathetic fibers through the perivascular plexus of the carotid system to the dilator muscle of the iris

> **NB:** The pupil in Horner's syndrome is reactive to light.

a. **Argyll-Robertson pupil:** pupillary light-near dissociation—the absence of a miotic reaction to light, both direct and consensual, with the preservation of a miotic reaction to near stimulus (accommodation-convergence); occurs in syphilis and diabetes

> **NB:** This pupil is typically small, irregular, and fixed to light.

b. Relative afferent pupillary defect (RAPD, **Marcus Gunn Pupil**): results from lesion of the optic nerve, the afferent limb of the pupillary light reflex; diagnosis can be made with the **swinging flashlight test.**

> **NB:** When the affected eye is stimulated, the reaction is slower and incomplete, and it may start dilating while still illuminated.

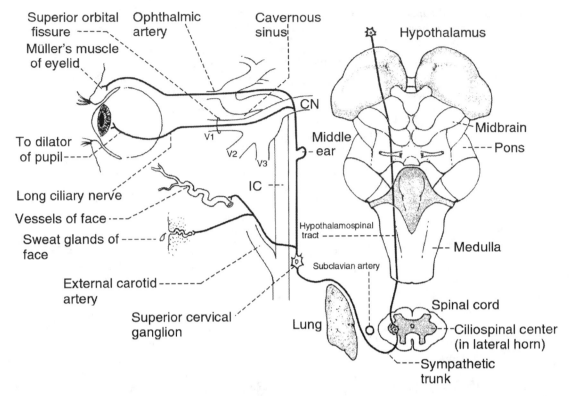

Figure 4.17 The course of the oculosympathetic pathway, where any interruption of this pathway results in Horner's syndrome. Hypothalamic fibers project to the ipsilateral ciliospinal center of the intermediolateral cell column at T1, which then projects preganglionic sympathetic fibers to the superior cervical ganglion. The superior cervical ganglion projects postganglionic sympathetic fibers through the tympanic cavity, cavernous sinus, and superior orbital fissure. CN, cranial nerve; IC, internal carotid.

3. *Pupillary dilatation pathway* (*cont'd*)

   c. **Adie's pupil**: a large tonic pupil that reacts slowly to light but may show a more definite response to accommodation (light-near dissociation); frequently seen in females with absent knee or ankle jerks and impaired sweating

> **NB:** Adie's pupil is caused by degeneration of the nerve cells in the ciliary ganglion.

4. *Near reflex and accommodation pathway:* the cortical visual pathway projects from the primary visual cortex (Brodmann's area 17) to the visual association cortex (Brodmann's area 19), which projects through the corticotectal tract to the superior colliculus and pretectal nucleus, which project to the oculomotor complex of the midbrain; the oculomotor complex includes the following structures:

   a. *Rostral-Edinger-Westphal nucleus:* mediates pupillary constriction through the ciliary ganglion

   b. *Caudal-Edinger-Westphal nucleus:* mediates contraction of the ciliary muscle to increase the refractive power of the lens

   c. *Medial rectus subnucleus of CN III:* mediates convergence

5. *Cortical and subcortical centers for ocular motility*

   a. *Frontal eye field:* located on the posterior part of the middle frontal gyrus (Brodmann's area 8); regulates voluntary (saccadic) eye movements; stimulation causes contralateral deviation of the eyes (i.e., away from the lesion), and destruction causes transient ipsilateral conjugate deviation of the eyes (i.e., toward the lesion).

> **NB:** This means that in a patient with a vascular lesion, the eyes deviate to the side of the lesion, whereas a patient seizing has deviation of the eyes opposite to the lesion.

   b. *Occipital eye fields:* located in Brodmann's areas 18 and 19; controls involuntary (smooth) pursuit and tracking movements; stimulation causes contralateral conjugate deviation of the eyes.

   c. *Subcortical center for lateral gaze:* located in the abducens nucleus of the pons ([?]paramedian pontine reticular formation)

      i. **MLF syndrome or internuclear ophthalmoplegia:** damage to the MLF between the abducens and oculomotor nuclei causes medial rectus palsy in the adducting eye on the attempted lateral conjugate gaze and monocular horizontal nystagmus in the abducting eye (convergence is normal).

      ii. **One-and-a-half syndrome:** bilateral lesions of the MLF and unilateral lesion of the abducens nucleus; on attempted lateral gaze, the only muscle that functions is the intact lateral rectus.

   d. **Subcortical center for vertical gaze:** located in the midbrain at the level of the posterior commissure; called the ***rostral interstitial nucleus*** of the MLF; associated with **Parinaud syndrome** *(paralysis of upward gaze and convergence)*

> **NB:** Parinaud syndrome can result from a pineal gland tumor.

VIII. Thalamus, Hypothalamus, and Basal Ganglia

A. **Thalamus: the largest division of the diencephalon; divided into three unequal parts by the internal medullary lamina; the centromedian nucleus and other intralaminar nuclei are enclosed within the internal medullary lamina in the center of the thalamus.**

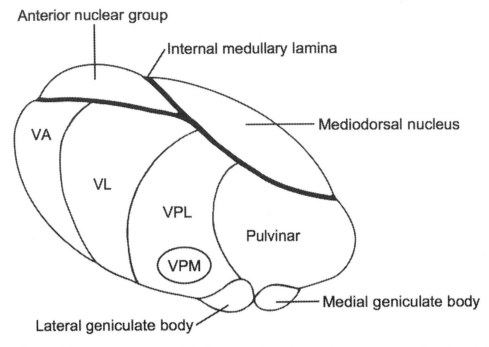

Figure 4.18 Schematic diagram of the thalamus and its various nuclei. VA, ventral anterior; VL, ventral lateral; VPL, ventroposterolateral; VPM, ventroposteromedial.

1. **NB:** *Major thalamic nuclei and their connections*

NUCLEI	INPUT	PROJECTION
Anterior	Mamillary nucleus of the hypothalamus	Cingulate gyrus
Dorsomedial	Prefrontal cortex (parvocellular part)	Prefrontal cortex (parvocellular)
	Amygdala, substantia nigra, orbital portion of the frontal lobe (magnocellular)	Many interconnections with other thalamic nuclei
Centromedian	Globus pallidus	Striatum (caudate and putamen) and to the entire neocortex
Pulvinar	Connects reciprocally with large association areas of the parietal, temporal, and occipital lobes; receives input from the superior colliculus, retina, cerebellum, and other thalamic nuclei	Connects reciprocally with large association areas of the parietal, temporal, and occipital lobes
Ventral tier		
Ventral anterior	Globus pallidus and substantia nigra	Prefrontal, orbital, and premotor cortex
NB: Ventral lateral	Cerebellum, globus pallidus, substantia nigra	Motor and supplementary motor cortex
Ventral posterior		

(continued)

NUCLEI	INPUT	PROJECTION
Ventroposterolateral	Spinothalamic tracts and medial lemniscus	Sensory cortex
Ventroposteromedial	Trigeminothalamic tracts, nucleus soli-tarius (via central tegmental tract)	Sensory cortex
Metathalamus		
Lateral geniculate body	Retinal input (via optic tract)	Visual cortex
Medial geniculate body	Auditory input (brachium of the inferior colliculus)	Primary auditory cortex
Reticular nucleus	Excitatory collateral input from corti-cothalamic and thalamocortical fibers	Inhibitory fibers to the thalamic nuclei

> **NB:** The dorsomedial nucleus is the most implicated in the amnestic confabulation in Korsakoff's syndrome because it receives input from limbic structures and projects diffusely to the frontal cortex.

> **NB:** Sleep spindles are generated in the reticular nucleus of the thalamus.

> **NB:** Pulvinar is associated with visual attention.

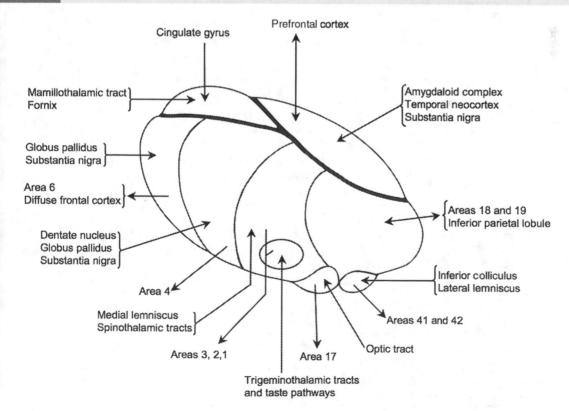

Figure 4.19 The projections of the major thalamic nuclei.

> **NB:** **Lesions in the anterior group are more likely to manifest with amnesia, confabulation, anomia, and preserved visual function.** Lesions in the paramedian area can manifest with decreased consciousness followed by vertical gaze paresis, disinhibition, and occasionally amnesia.

A. **Thalamus** (*cont'd*)

   2. *Blood supply:* Three arteries:

     a. Posterior communicating artery

     b. Posterior cerebral artery

     c. **Anterior choroidal artery (to the lateral geniculate body)**

   3. *Epithalamus:* the most dorsal division of the diencephalon

     a. *Pineal body:* the dorsal diverticulum of the diencephalon; cone-shaped structure that overlies the tectum; no neurons are present.

     b. *Habenular nuclei:* located in the dorsal margin of the base of the pineal body; afferent fibers (via habenulopeduncular tract and stria medullaris): from septal area, lateral hypothalamus, brainstem, interpeduncular nuclei, raphe nuclei, ventral tegmental area; efferent fibers (via habenulopeduncular tract) terminate in the interpeduncular nucleus.

     c. *Habenular commissure:* consists of stria medullaris fibers crossing over to the contralateral habenular nuclei

     d. *Posterior commissure:* located ventral to the base of the pineal body; carries decussating fibers of superior colliculi and pretectum (visual reflex fibers)

B. **Hypothalamus: subserves three systems: autonomic, endocrine, and limbic**

   1. *Hypothalamic nuclei and their functions*

NUCLEUS	FUNCTION
Medial preoptic	Regulates the release of gonadotropic hormones from the adenohypophysis; contains sexually dimorphic nucleus, which depends on testosterone levels for development
Suprachiasmatic	Receives direct input from the retina; role in regulation of circadian rhythms
Anterior	Role in temperature regulation; stimulates the parasympathetic nervous system; destruction results in hyperthermia
Paraventricular	Synthesizes the antidiuretic hormone, oxytocin, and corticotropin-releasing hormone; regulates water conservation; destruction results in diabetes insipidus
Supraoptic	Synthesizes antidiuretic hormone and oxytocin
Dorsomedial	In animals, savage behavior results when this nucleus is stimulated
Ventromedial	Satiety center; when stimulated, inhibits the urge to eat; destruction results in hyperphagia
Arcuate (infundibular)	Gives rise to tuberohypophysial tract; contains neurons that produce dopamine ([DA] i.e., prolactin-inhibiting factor)

(continued)

NUCLEUS	FUNCTION
Mamillary	Receives input from the hippocampal formation through the postcommissural fornix; projects to the anterior nucleus of the thalamus through the mamillothalamic tract; associated with Wernicke's encephalopathy and alcoholism
Posterior hypothalamic	Role in heat conservation and production of heat; lesions result in poikilothermia (inability to thermoregulate)
Lateral hypothalamic	Induces eating when stimulated; lesions cause anorexia and starvation

> **NB:** The paraventricular nucleus provides the bulk of the direct innervation of the preganglionic sympathetic neurons.

> **NB:** The **posterior lateral hypothalamus contains the hypocretin/orexin neurons that have a function in preventing abrupt transitions from wakefulness to sleep**. They project to cholinergic and mono-aminergic neurons in brainstem and ventrolateral preoptic neurons. Narcolepsy results from impaired activity of these neurons.

2. *Circuit of Papez: hippocampal formation—to the mamillary body (and septal area) through the fornix—to the anterior thalamic nucleus (through the mamillothalamic tract)—to the cingulate gyrus (passing through the anterior limb of the internal capsule)—to the entorhinal cortex (through the cingulum)—back to the hippocampal formation (through the perforant pathway)*

> **NB:** During transcallosal surgery to remove a colloid cyst in the third ventricle, the fornix can be damaged, which interrupts Papez's circuit and results in loss of the ability to form new memories.

> **NB:** *Akinetic mutism* may result from lesions in the anterior cingulate gyrus or a disconnection of the limbic connections projecting from the anterior cingulate through subcortical circuits.

3. *Other limbic connections*
   a. *Stria terminalis:* from the amygdala, follows curvature to the tail of the caudate nucleus to the septal nuclei and anterior hypothalamus
   b. *Stria medullaris:* from septal nuclei and anterior hypothalamus to habenular nucleus
   c. *Mamillotegmental tract:* mamillary bodies to raphe nuclei of the midbrain reticular formation
   d. *Medial forebrain bundle:* septal area and amygdala to the raphe nuclei of the midbrain reticular formation

IX. Limbic System

A. Limbic structures

MAIN STRUCTURES	COMPONENTS
Limbic cortex	Parahippocampal gyrus, cingulate gyrus, medial orbitofrontal cortex, temporal pole, anterior insula
Hippocampal formation	Dentate gyrus, hippocampus, subiculum
Amygdala	
Olfactory cortex	
Diencephalon	Hypothalamus, thalamus (anterior & dorsomedial nuclei), habenula
Basal ganglia	Ventral striatum, ventral pallidum
Basal forebrain	
Septal nuclei	
Brainstem	

B. Limbic pathways

1. *Circuit of Papez*: subiculum—fornix—mammillary body—mammillothalamic tract—anterior nucleus of thalamus—anterior limb of internal capsule—cingulate gyrus—cingulum—entorhinal cortex—perforant pathway—subiculum and hippocampus

2. *Olfactory projections*: primary olfactory cortex includes piriform cortex and peri-amygdaloid cortex.

3. *Hippocampal formation projections*: for consolidation of long-term memory

   a. Alvear pathway: axonal projections from entorhinal cortex to CA1 and CA3

   b. Perforant pathway: axonal projections from entorhinal cortex through subiculum to dentate gyrus

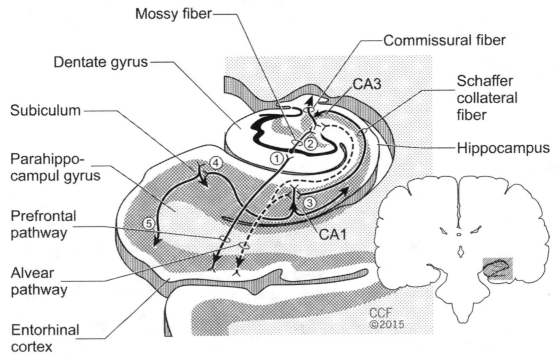

Figure 4.20 Hippocampal formation projections. Reprinted with permission, Cleveland Clinic Center for Medical Art & Photography © 2015. All Rights Reserved.

4. *Amygdala*

   a. *Nuclei*

      i. Corticomedial: near basal forebrain; sends axonal projects to olfactory areas and hypothalamus

      ii. Basolateral: multiple axonal projections to assorted cortical areas, basal forebrain, and medial thalamus

      iii. Central: sends axonals; projects to the hypothalamus and brainstem

   b. *Connections of the amygdala*

      i. Uncinate fasciculus: anterior projection to medial orbitofrontal and cingulate cortices

      ii. Ventral amygdalofugal pathway: anteriorly to forebrain and brainstem structures

      iii. Stria terminalis: along wall of lateral ventricle to hypothalamus and septal area

5. Medial forebrain bundle: to hypothalamus and brainstem

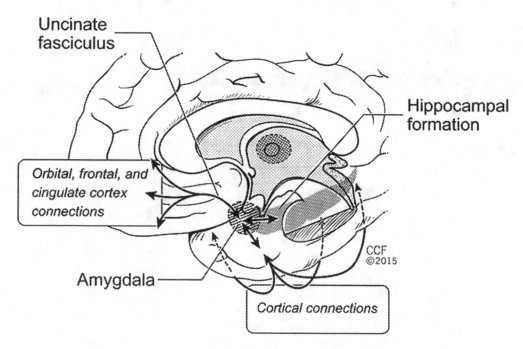

Figure 4.21(A) Connections of the amygdala. Reprinted with permission, Cleveland Clinic Center for Medical Art & Photography © 2015. All Rights Reserved.

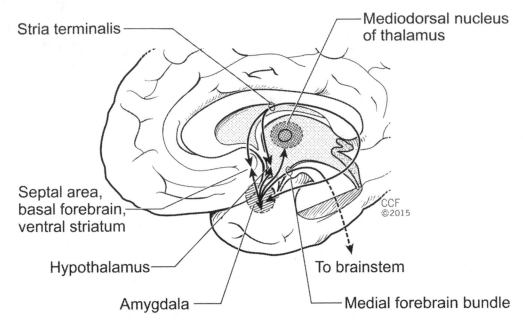

Stria terminalis

Mediodorsal nucleus of thalamus

Septal area, basal forebrain, ventral striatum

Hypothalamus

Amygdala

To brainstem

Medial forebrain bundle

CCF ©2015

Figure 4.21(B) Connections of the amygdala. Reprinted with permission, Cleveland Clinic Center for Medical Art & Photography © 2015. All Rights Reserved.

CHEAT SHEET

Contents of Foramen Ovale:
MALE
M = Mandibular nerve
A = Accessory meningeal artery
L = Lesser petrosal nerve
E = Emissary veins

Anton's syndrome	Cortical blindness with visual anosognosia, bilateral occipital lesions
Gerstmann's syndrome	Inferior parietal lobule (dominant hemisphere); (1) right-left disorientation, (2) finger agnosia, (3) dysgraphia (+/– dyslexia), (4) dyscalculia
Tabes dorsalis	Dorsal column lesion with syphilis, proprioception, and vibration involved
Brown-Sequard syndrome	Hemicord; ipsi LMN at segment, UMN below, ipsi dorsal column, contra spinothalamic
Erb-Duchenne paralysis	C5-6, porter tip position
Klumpke's paralysis	C8-T1, useless hand and Horner's syndrome
Meralgia paresthetica	Lateral femoral cutaneous nerve entrapment, burning anterolateral thigh

(continued)

CHEAT SHEET (continued)

Edinger-Westphal nucleus	Pupilloconstrictor fibers pupils
Horner's syndrome	Miosis, hemifacial anhidrosis, ptosis +/– enophthalmos
Argyll-Robertson pupil	Pupillary light-near dissociation
Marcus Gunn pupil	Relative afferent pupillary defect
Adie's pupil	Large tonic pupil reacting slowly to light, more to accommodation

Suggested Readings

Blumenfeld, H. *Neuroanatomy Through Clinical Cases*. Sunderland, MA: Sinauer Associates;2011.

Purves, D. *Neuroscience*. Sunderland, MA: Sinauer;2008.

"The Brain From Top to Bottom: http://thebrain.mcgill.ca/avance.php

CHAPTER 5

Stroke

I. Definitions

A. **Ischemic stroke:** an episode of neurological dysfunction caused by focal cerebral, spinal, or retinal infarction (clinical syndrome)

B. **Central nervous system (CNS) infarction:** brain, spinal cord, or retinal cell death attributable to ischemia, based on:

   1. Pathological, imaging, or other objective evidence of cerebral, spinal cord, or retinal focal ischemic injury in a defined vascular distribution; or

   2. Clinical evidence of cerebral, spinal cord, or retinal focal ischemic injury based on symptoms persisting ≥24 hours or until death, and other etiologies excluded

C. **Transient ischemic attack (TIA):** a transient episode of neurological dysfunction caused by focal brain, spinal cord, or retinal ischemia without acute infarction

> **NB:** Up to one-third of patients with symptoms lasting less than 24 hours are found to have an infarction..

II. Epidemiology

A. **Stroke incidence:** in the United States, *≈795,000 people experience new or recurrent strokes* per year, with 130,000 deaths per year.

B. **Stroke prevalence:** measures the total number of cases, new and old, at a particular time in a defined population; in the United States, stroke *prevalence is 3,000,000.*

C. Stroke is the *fifth most common* cause of death in the United States, and leading cause of long-term disability.

D. Between 1990 and 2010 the global stroke mortality has decreased.

III. Frequency of Strokes

TYPE		
Ischemic	87%	
Large-vessel disease		20%
Cardioembolism		30%
Small-vessel disease		20%
Other		3%
Unknown		27%
Hemorrhage		
Subarachnoid hemorrhage (SAH)	3%	
Intracerebral hemorrhage (ICH)	10%	

IV. Pathophysiology

A. Cerebral blood flow (CBF)

Normal	50 cc/100 g/min
Change in electrophysiologic activity	20 cc/100 g/min
Irreversible ischemia	10 cc/100 g/min

B. When blood supply is interrupted for 30 seconds, brain metabolism is altered: *1 minute, neuronal function ceases; 5 minutes,* a chain of events that results in cerebral *infarction ensues;* evolution of an infarct: local vasodilatation → stasis of the blood column with segmentation of red cells; edema → necrosis of brain tissue.

   1. *Coagulation necrosis:* the infarcted area is pale and swollen—blurred border between gray and white matter at *6 to 24 hours; "red neuron"* (neuronal shrinkage and eosinophilia); astrocytes and oligodendrocytes; microglial cells disintegrate and give rise to somewhat granular appearance of the background; polymorphonucleocytes surround vessels; red cell extravasation; edematous swelling (may occur in 3–4 days).

   2. *Liquefaction (or absorption):* represents removal of debris by macrophages *72 to 96 hours later;* glitter cells—lipid-laden macrophages; sharpened demarcation between normal and infarcted tissue; tissue becomes mushy; there is hypertrophy (12–36 hours), then hyperplasia (48 hours to months) of astrocytes; macrophages clear debris at 1 cc/month.

V. Risk Factors

A. Nonmodifiable risk factors

   1. *Age: strongest determinant of stroke;* incidence rises exponentially with age >65 years.

   2. Sex: *male*

   3. Race: in the United States, *African American* followed by *Hispanic* and *Caucasian* (extracranial > intracranial disease); Asian population has a higher incidence of intracranial stenosis.

B. Modifiable risk factors

   1. *Hypertension:* there is a fourfold increased risk of stroke with duration and severity of blood pressure (BP), especially among African Americans. It increases the risk by accelerating the progression of atherosclerosis and predisposing to small-vessel

disease. Target blood pressure should be systolic BP <140/90. Choice of agent depends on comorbid conditions.

2. *Cardiac disease:* atrial fibrillation; valvular heart disease; myocardial infarction (MI), coronary artery disease (CAD), cardiomyopathy,

   a. *Chronic nonvalvular atrial fibrillation stroke risk: 5% per year*

   b. *Valvular atrial fibrillation: 17-times-higher stroke risk*

   c. Risk stratification is done using CHA$_2$DS$_2$ VASc score.

CHA$_2$DS$_2$ VASc	
Congestive heart failure—1 point	1 point
Hypertension—1 point	1 point
Age 65–74 y—1 point	1 point
≥75 y—2 points	2 points
Diabetes mellitus—1 point	1 point
Stroke/TIA—2 points	2 points
Vascular disease (e.g., peripheral artery disease, myocardial infarction, aortic plaque)	1 point
Female sex	1 point
Levels of risk for thromboembolic stroke Low risk = 0 points (antiplatelets) Moderate risk = 1 point (anticoagulation) High risk = ≥2 points (anticoagulation)	

   d. Cardiomyopathy: stroke risk reduction for low-ejection fraction can be achieved with either anticoagulation or antiplatelets depending on the individual case.

3. *Diabetes mellitus type 2: carries a 1.8 to 6.0 relative stroke risk*

   a. *Treatment: glycemic control with hemoglobin A1C <7 and hypertension control with angiotensin-converting enzyme (ACE) inhibitors or angiotensin receptor blockers*

4. *Blood lipids:* relative stroke risk is 1.5. Treatment includes HMG-CoA reductase inhibitor with high doses for atherosclerotic disease.

5. *Cigarette smoking:* 1.9 increased risk for stroke; cessation reduces risk by 50% in 1 year and to baseline by 5 years.

6. *Alcohol:* a *J-shaped* relationship shows increased risk with moderate to heavy alcohol consumption (>14 oz of alcohol per month).

7. *Asymptomatic carotid artery disease:* >70% stenosis; risk is ~2% per year. Medical management with aspirin and HMG-CoA reductase inhibitor is recommended. Carotid endarterectomy (CEA) can be considered if perioperative risk is <3%.

8. Symptomatic carotid artery disease: >70% to 99% stenosis; risk of stroke is ~24.5% in 2 years. Greater benefit is obtained when CEA is performed within 2 weeks from stroke or TIA, if perioperative risk rate <6%. The 5-year absolute risk reduction with CEA for symptomatic carotid stenosis or >70% is 16. Benefit of CEA is lower in women, although patients who present with retinal ischemic symptoms have lower recurrent stroke risk as compared with hemispheric symptoms. Carotid artery stenting should be considered in patients who cannot undergo CEA. In patients with symptomatic carotid stenosis of 50% to 69%, the 5-year absolute risk reduction rate is 4.6%.

9. Symptomatic intracranial stenosis: if stroke or TIA (within 30 days) attributable to severe stenosis (70%–99%), the addition of clopidogrel 75 mg/d to aspirin 325 mg

B. **Modifiable risk factors** (*cont'd*)

for 90 days along with maintenance of systolic BP below 140 mmHg and high-intensity HMG-Co-A reductase might be reasonable. Warfarin-Aspirin Symptomatic Intracranial Disease (WASID) trial showed no benefit of anticoagulation compared with antiplatelets for symptomatic intracranial stenosis. Stenting vs. Aggressive Medical Management for Preventing Recurrent Stroke in Intracranial Stenosis (SAMMPRIS) and Vitesse Intracranial Stent Study for Ischemic Stroke Therapy (VISSIT) trial showed no benefit of intracranial stenting compared with aggressive medical management.

10. Most atherosclerosis occur in major cerebral arteries proximally at branching points:

   a. *Bifurcation of common carotid artery into external carotid artery and internal carotid artery (ICA)—62%*

   b. *Origin of middle cerebral artery (MCA)—10%*

   c. *Origin of anterior cerebral artery (ACA)—1%*

   d. *Origin of vertebral artery—15%*

   e. *Others—11%*

C. **Potential risk factors**

   1. *Physical inactivity*

   2. *Oral contraceptives: increased risk of cerebral venous thrombosis if concurrent hypercoagulable genetic condition; risk of ischemic stroke may be increased if patients have migraines.*

   3. *Drug abuse*

      a. Cocaine: risk of ischemic stroke may be up to 7 times higher; mechanism includes vasospasm and vasculitis.

      b. Opioids: septic emboli from intravenous drug abuse

   4. *Coagulopathy*

      a. Lupus anticoagulant

      b. Heparin-induced thrombocytopenia

   5. Others

      a. *Heredity*

      b. *Aortic arch plaques*

      c. *Migraine*

      d. *Obstructive sleep apnea*

VI. Clinical Stroke Syndromes

A. **Common carotid:** *anatomy:* **the right common carotid artery arises from the brachiocephalic (innominate) artery, and the left common carotid directly from the aortic arch; the common carotids ascend to approximately the C4 level (just below the angle of the jaw) then divide into external and internal branches.**

   1. Internal carotid artery (ICA): anatomy: there are seven segments of the ICA:

      a. C1: cervical segment—branches: none

      b. C2: petrous segment—branches: vidian, caroticotympanic

      c. C3: lacerum segment—branches: none

      d. C4: cavernous segment—branches: meinigohypophyseal, inferolateral trunk, capsular

      e. C5: clinoid segment—branches: none

      f. C6: ophthalmic segment—branches: ophthalmic, superior hypophyseal

      g. C7: communicating segment—branches: posterior communicating, anterior choroidal

    i. *Two mechanisms:* embolus from an unstable plaque in ICA goes to distal vessel *(artery-to-artery embolism)* or occlusion (or severe stenosis) of carotid artery leads to hypoperfusion in the distal vasculature *(also known as watershed or border-zone ischemia).*

    ii. *MCA/posterior cerebral artery (PCA) border zone:* affects temporo-occipital portion of distal MCA territory; produces quadrant/hemianopic field defect, transcortical aphasia, or hemi-inattention (depending on hemisphere).

    iii. *MCA/ACA border zone:* affects superficial frontal and parietal parasagittal cortical area; produces *proximal* $>>$ *distal sensory motor deficit* in the contralateral upper extremities; variable lower extremity involvement, sparing face and hand.

    iv. ICA nourishes optic nerve and retina: transient painless monocular blindness (amaurosis fugax) occurs in symptomatic carotid occlusion; stenosis, ulcerations, dissections of ICA may be a source of fibrin platelet emboli or may cause reduction of blood flow.

2. External carotid artery (ECA) branches and significance

    a. Superior thyroid artery

    b. Ascending pharyngeal artery—neuromeningeal branch supplies the dura and lower cranial nerves

    c. Lingual artery

    d. Facial artery—via the angular artery, anastomoses with branches of the ophthalmic artery

    e. Occipital artery—anastomoses with segmental branches of the vertebral artery

    f. Posterior temporal artery

    g. Superficial temporal artery

    Internal maxillary artery—a major branch, the middle meningeal artery enters the skull via the foramen spinosum; is a common cause of epidural hematoma.

B. **Middle cerebral artery (MCA):** *anatomy:* **four segments: M1—main MCA trunk with deep penetrating vessels and lenticulostriate arteries, M2—in the Sylvian fissure where the two divisions arise, M3—cortical branches, M4—over the cortical surface**

1. *Territory* encompasses:

    a. Cortex and white matter of the *inferior parts of frontal lobe,* including areas four and six, centers for lateral gaze, Broca's area

    b. Cortex and white matter of *parietal lobe,* including sensory cortex and *angular and supramarginal*

    c. *Superior parts of the temporal lobe* and insula, including Wernicke's area

    d. Penetrating branches: *putamen, outer globus pallidus, posterior limb of internal capsule, body of caudate, corona radiata*

2. *Stem occlusion:* blocking deep penetrating and superficial cortical branches— *contralateral hemiplegia* (face, arm, and leg), *hemianesthesia, homonymous hemianopia,* deviation of head and eyes toward side of the lesion; left hemisphere lesions—*global aphasia;* right hemisphere—*anosognosia and amorphosynthesis*

3. *Superior division:* supplies rolandic and prerolandic areas—dense sensorimotor of face and arm $>>$ leg; ipsilateral deviation of head and eye; brachiofacial paralysis, no impairment of consciousness; left-sided lesions—initial global aphasia, then predominantly motor

    a. *Ascending frontal branch:* initial mutism and mild comprehension defect, then slightly dysfluent, agrammatic speech with normal comprehension

    b. *Rolandic branches:* sensorimotor paresis with severe dysarthria but little aphasia

    c. *Cortical-subcortical branch:* brachial monoplegia

    d. *Ascending parietal:* no sensorimotor defect, only a conduction aphasia

B. **Middle cerebral artery (MCA)** (*cont'd*)

4. *Inferior division:* left sided—*Wernicke's* aphasia; right sided—*left visual neglect;* superior *quadrantanopia* or homonymous hemianopia; agitated confusional state from temporal lobe damage

5. Other cortical syndromes

    a. Dominant parietal lobe: *Gerstmann syndrome*—finger agnosia, acalculia, right-left confusion, alexia (supramarginal gyrus), alexia with agraphia (angular gyrus), ideational apraxia

    b. Nondominant parietal lobe: anosognosia, autoprosopagnosia, neglect, constructional apraxia, dressing apraxia

    c. Bilateral anterior poles of the temporal lobes: *Klüver-Bucy* syndrome; docility, hyper-oral, hypersexual, hypomobile, hypermetamorphosis, visual agnosia

> **NB:** In addition to prosopagnosia (deficit in facial recognition), other *nondominant* hemisphere deficits include auditory agnosia (deficit in recognition of sounds), autotopagnosia (inability to localize stimuli on the affected side), and phonagnosia (inability to recognize familiar voices). Pure word deafness (inability to recognize spoken language) is a *dominant* hemisphere deficit!

    d. Aphasias

TYPE	COMPREHENSION	FLUENCY	REPETITION	NAMING
Broca	Normal	Impaired	Impaired	Impaired
Wernicke	Impaired	Normal	Impaired	Impaired
Conduction	Normal	Normal	Impaired	Normal/impaired
Transcortical motor	Normal	Impaired	Normal	Impaired
Transcortical sensory	Impaired	Normal	Normal	Impaired
Mixed transcortical	Impaired	Impaired	Normal	Impaired
Global	Impaired	Impaired	Impaired	Impaired

C. **Anterior cerebral artery (ACA): supplies anterior three-fourths of the medial surface of cerebral hemisphere, including medial-orbital surface of frontal lobe, strip of lateral surface of cerebrum along the superior border, anterior four-fifths of corpus callosum, deep branches supplying anterior limb of internal capsule, inferior part of caudate, anterior globus pallidus**

1. *Stem occlusion:* proximal to the anterior communicating artery, usually well tolerated; if both arteries arise from one ACA, paraplegia, abulia, motor aphasia, frontal lobe personality changes; distal to the anterior communicating artery—sensorimotor defect of contralateral foot $>>$ shoulder and arm; motor in foot and leg $>>$ thigh; sensory is more of discriminative modalities and is mild or absent; head and eyes deviated ipsilaterally, urinary incontinence, contralateral grasp reflex, paratonic rigidity (gegenhalten); left sided—may have alien hand.

2. *Branch occlusions:* fragments of the total syndrome (usually spastic weakness and cortical sensory loss of foot or leg); occlusion of Heubner's artery: may give rise to transcorticomotor aphasia

3. *Penetrating branches:* transient hemiparesis, dysarthria, abulia or agitation; left side—stuttering and language difficulty; right side—visuospatial neglect; bilateral caudate—syndrome of inattentiveness, abulia, forgetfulness, sometimes agitation and psychosis

D. **Anterior choroidal artery: long narrow artery from ICA just above the posterior communicating artery; supplies internal globus pallidus, posterior limb of internal capsule, contiguous structures such as the optic tract; choroid plexus of lateral**

ventricles; clinical: contralateral hemiplegia, hemihypesthesia, homonymous hemianopsia; cognitive function is spared; no uniform syndrome

E. **Posterior cerebral artery (PCA): in 70%, both PCAs originate from the bifurcation
of the basilar artery; in 20% to 25%, one of the PCAs comes from the ICA in the remainder, both PCAs from ICA. (Fetal origin of the PCA: posterior communicating
artery diameter is large and the ipsilateral P1 segment is hypoplastic.)**

1. *Anatomy*

   a. *Interpeduncular branches/mesencephalic artery:* supply red nucleus, substantia
   nigra, medial cerebral peduncles, medial longitudinal fasciculi, medial lemnisci

   b. *Thalamoperforate/paramedian thalamic arteries:* inferior, medial, and anterior thalami

   c. *Thalamogeniculate branches:* geniculate body, posterior thalamus

   d. *Medial branches:* lateral cerebral peduncles, lateral tegmentum, corpora quad-
   rigemina, pineal gland

   e. *Posterior choroidal:* posterosuperior thalamus, choroid plexus, posterior hypothalamus, psalterium (decussation of fornices)

   f. *Cortical branches:* inferomedial temporal lobe, medial occipital, including lin-
   gula, cuneus, precuneus, and visual areas 17, 18, and 19

2. *Syndromes*

   a. Anterior and proximal syndromes, involves interpeduncular, thalamic perforant, thalamogeniculate branches

      i. *Thalamic syndrome of Dejerine and Roussy:* infarction of sensory relay nu-
      clei (due to occlusion of thalamogeniculate)—deep and cutaneous sen-
      sory loss contralateral, with transient hemiparesis; after an interval, pain,
      paresthesia, hyperpathia of affected parts; distortion of taste, athetotic pos-
      turing of hand; depression

      ii. *Central midbrain and subthalamic syndromes:* due to occlusion of interpe-
      duncular branches; oculomotor palsy with contralateral hemiplegia *(We-
      ber syndrome),* palsies of vertical gaze, stupor, coma, movement disorders
      (usually contralateral ataxic tremor)

      iii. *Anteromedial-inferior thalamic syndromes:* occlusion of thalamoperforate
      branches; hemiballismus, hemichoreoathetosis; deep sensory loss, hemi-
      ataxia, tremor; occlusion of dominant dorsomedial nucleus gives rise to
      Korsakoff syndrome

   b. *Cortical syndromes*

      i. Occlusion of branches to temporal and occipital lobes: homonymous
      hemianopsia; macular and central vision may be spared owing to collat-
      eralization of occipital pole from distal branches of MCA (or ACA); visual
      hallucination in blind parts *(Cogan)* or metamorphopsia, palinopsia

      ii. Dominant hemisphere: alexia, anomia (most severe for colors and visually
      presented material—may describe their function and use them but not
      name them), visual agnosia, occasional memory impairment

   c. Bilateral cortical syndromes: result of successive infarctions from embolus or
   thrombus of upper basilar artery

      i. *Cortical blindness:* blindness with unformed visual hallucinations; pupillary re-
      flexes preserved, optic discs normal; patient may be unaware *(Anton syndrome)*

      ii. If confined to occipital poles, may have homonymous central scotomas

      iii. *Balint's syndrome:* from bilateral occipital-parietal border zones

         (A) Oculomotor apraxia

         (B) Optic ataxia (failure to grasp objects under visual guidance)

         (C) Asimultanagnosia

  c. Bilateral cortical syndromes (*cont'd*)

   iv. Bilateral inferomedial temporal lobes: *Korsakoff amnestic state*

   v. Bilateral mesial-temporal-occipital lesions: prosopagnosia

F. Vertebral artery

1. *Anatomy:* chief arteries of the medulla; supplies lower three-fourths of pyramid, medial lemniscus, all of lateral medullary region, restiform body, posterior-inferior part of cerebellar hemisphere; long extracranial course and passes through transverse processes of C6 through C2 before entering the cranial cavity—may be subject to trauma, spondylotic compression.

2. *Syndromes*

 a. *Lateral medullary syndrome/Wallenberg syndrome:* vestibular nuclei (nystagmus, oscillopsia, vertigo, nausea, vomiting); spinothalamic tract (contralateral impairment of pain and thermal sense over one-half the body); descending sympathetic tract (ipsilateral Horner's—ptosis, miosis, anhidrosis); cranial nerves (CNs) IX and X (hoarseness, dysphagia, ipsilateral paralysis of palate and vocal cord, diminished gag); otolithic nucleus (vertical diplopia and illusion of tilting of vision); olivocerebellar and/or spinocerebellar fibers/restiform body (ipsilateral ataxia of limbs, falling to ipsilateral side); nucleus and tractus solitarius (loss of taste); descending tract and nucleus of V (pain, burning, impaired sensation on ipsilateral one-half of face; rarely nucleus cuneatus and gracilis (ipsilateral numbness of limbs); most likely due to occlusion of vertebral artery or posterior-inferior cerebellar artery.

 b. Opalski syndrome: considered a variant of lateral medullary syndrome with ipsilateral hemiplegia, likely due to caudal extension of the infarct due to involvement of perforator branches arising from the distal vertebral artery.

 c. *Medial medullary syndrome:* involves medullary pyramid (contralateral paralysis of arm and leg); medial lemniscus (contralateral impaired tactile and proprioceptive sense over one-half the body); CN XII (ipsilateral paralysis and, later, hemiatrophy of the tongue).

 d. Hemimedullary infarction (Babinski–Nageotte syndrome): occlusion of the ipsilateral vertebral artery proximal to the posterior-inferior cerebellar artery and its anterior spinal artery causes medial medullary syndrome and lateral medullary syndrome simultaneously.

 e. *Posterior medullary region:* ipsilateral cerebellar ataxia and, rarely, hiccups.

 f. *Avellis syndrome:* tegmentum of medulla: CN X, spinothalamic tract (paralysis of soft palate and vocal cord and contralateral hemianesthesia).

 g. *Jackson syndrome:* tegmentum of medulla: CN X, XII, corticospinal tract (Avellis syndrome plus ipsilateral tongue paralysis).

G. Basilar artery

1. *Branches*

 a. Paramedian

 b. Short circumferential (supplying lateral two-thirds of pons and middle and superior cerebellar peduncles)

 c. Long circumferential (anterior-inferior cerebellar artery and superior cerebellar artery)

 d. Paramedian (interpeduncular) at the bifurcation of the basilar artery supplying subthalamic and high midbrain

2. *Syndromes*

 a. *Basilar artery syndrome:* bilateral corticobulbar and corticospinal tracts (paralysis/weakness of all extremities plus all bulbar musculature); ocular nerves, medial longitudinal fasciculus, vestibular apparatus (diplopia, paralysis of conjugate gaze, internuclear ophthalmoplegia, horizontal and/or vertical nystagmus); visual cortex (blindness; visual field defects); cerebellar peduncles and hemispheres (bilateral cerebellar ataxia); tegmentum of midbrain/thalami (coma); medial lemniscus-spinothalamic tracts (may be strikingly intact, syringomyelic, reverse, or involve all modalities)

b. *Medial inferior pontine syndrome* (occlusion of paramedian branch of basilar artery): paramedian pontine reticular formation (paralysis of conjugate gaze to the side of lesion but preservation of convergence); vestibular nuclei (nystagmus); middle cerebral peduncle (ipsilateral ataxia of limbs and gait); CN VI (ipsilateral diplopia on lateral gaze), corticobulbar and corticospinal tract (contralateral paresis of face, arm, and leg); medial lemniscus (contralateral tactile dysfunction and proprioceptive sense over one-half the body)

c. *Lateral inferior pontine syndrome* (occlusion of anterior-inferior cerebellar artery): CN VIII (horizontal and vertical nystagmus, vertigo, nausea, oscillopsia, deafness, and tinnitus); CN VII (ipsilateral facial paralysis); paramedian pontine reticular formation (paralysis of conjugate gaze to side of lesion); middle cerebellar peduncles and cerebellar hemisphere (ipsilateral ataxia); main sensory nucleus and descending tract of V (ipsilateral impairment of sensation over face); spinothalamic tract (contralateral impairment of pain and thermal sense over one-half the body)

d. *Millard-Gubler syndrome* (base of pons): CN VI and VII and corticospinal tract (facial and abducens palsy plus contralateral hemiplegia)

e. *Medial midpontine syndrome* (paramedian branch of midbasilar artery): middle cerebellar peduncle (ipsilateral ataxia of limbs and gait); corticobulbar and corticospinal tracts (contralateral paralysis of face, arm, and leg; deviation of eyes); medial lemniscus (variable—usually pure motor)

f. *Lateral midpontine syndrome* (short circumferential artery): middle cerebellar peduncle (ipsilateral ataxia); motor nucleus of V (ipsilateral paralysis of masticatory muscles); sensory nucleus of V (ipsilateral sensory facial impairment)

g. *Medial superior pontine syndrome* (paramedian branches of upper basilar artery): superior and middle cerebellar peduncle (ipsilateral cerebellar ataxia); medial longitudinal fasciculus (ipsilateral internuclear ophthalmoplegia); central tegmental bundle (rhythmic myoclonus of palate, pharynx, vocal cords, etc.); corticobulbar and corticospinal tracts (contralateral paralysis of face, arm, and leg); medial lemniscus (rarely with sensory impairment)

h. *Lateral superior pontine syndrome (syndrome of superior cerebellar artery):* middle and superior cerebellar peduncles, dentate nucleus (ipsilateral ataxia, falling to side of lesion); vestibular nuclei (dizziness, nausea, horizontal nystagmus); descending sympathetic fibers (ipsilateral Horner's); spinothalamic tract (contralateral impairment of pain and temperature sense of face, limb, trunk); medial lemniscus—lateral portion (contralateral impaired touch, vibration, position sense of leg >> arm); other—ipsilateral paresis of conjugate gaze, skew deviation

i. Base of midbrain *(Weber syndrome):* CN III (ipsilateral oculomotor palsy) plus corticospinal tract (crossed hemiplegia)

j. Tegmentum of midbrain *(Claude syndrome):* CN III, red nucleus, and brachium conjunctivum (contralateral cerebellar ataxia and tremor)

k. *Benedikt syndrome:* CN III, red nucleus, plus corticospinal tract

l. *Nothnagel syndrome:* CN III (unilateral or bilateral); superior cerebellar peduncles (ocular palsies, paralysis of gaze, cerebellar ataxia); usually caused by a tumor

m. *Parinaud syndrome:* dorsal midbrain—supranuclear mechanism for upward gaze and other structures in periaqueductal gray (paralysis of upward gaze and accommodation, fixed pupils)

VII. TIA

A. Etiology: causes for TIA are the same as those for ischemic stroke. Management of TIA mainly includes risk stratification and identifying a treatable cause.

B. Presentation and subsequent stroke risk: presenting symptoms are often similar to ischemic stroke symptoms but usually last for a few minutes. Estimated risk of stroke 2 days after TIA is around 4%, and in the next 90 days is around 9%. The Age, Blood pressure, Clinical presentation, Duration of symptoms, Diabetes (ABCD2) score can be used to stratify the stroke risk after a TIA. (See accompanying table.)

C. Management: monitor patients for 24 hours for symptom recurrence. Brain MRI to evaluate for acute ischemic stroke or for old stroke burden, arterial imaging, and cardiac evaluation including rhythm monitoring and echocardiogram. Patients should be started on aspirin unless there is indication for anticoagulation. Clopidogrel in High-risk patients with Acute Nondisabling Cerebrovascular Events (CHANCE) study showed benefit of dual antiplatelet therapy (aspirin + clopidogrel) for 21 days, after a TIA or mild ischemic stroke.

ABCD2 Score for TIA Risk Stratification (Score 0–7)				
Age	>60			1 point
Blood pressure	>140 mmHg systolic or >90 mmHg diastolic			1 point
Clinical presentation	Unilateral weakness			2 points
	Any speech impairment without unilateral weakness			1 point
Duration of symptoms	<10 minutes			0 point
	10-59 minutes			1 point
	≥60 minutes			2 points
Diabetes	Positive history			1 point
90-day stroke risk				
Very low = 0-1 points	Low = 2-3 points	Moderate = 4-5 points	High = 6-7 points	
1.7%	3.3%	9.8%	17.8%	

VIII. Lacunar Stroke: These are usually <15 mm in diameter and occur due to occlusions of penetrating small-end arteries of the anterior or posterior circulation.

A. Pathology: lipohylinosis, or atherosclerosis, underlies small-vessel occlusion related to hypertension primarily, but diabetes and hyperlipidemia might play a role.

B. Syndromes and locations

1. *Pure motor* hemiparesis: internal capsule, adjacent corona radiata, paramedian pons, or medullary pyramid

2. *Pure sensory* stroke: ventral posterior thalamus

3. *Sensory-motor stroke*: thalamus, corona radiata

4. *Clumsy-hand dysarthria*: anterior limb of the internal capsule, genu, or pons

5. *Ataxia hemiparesis*: pons, internal, capsule, deep grey nuclei, cerebellum

IX. Acute Stroke Therapy

A. **Supportive care and treatment:** all stroke patients regardless of the type must be first stabilized with regard to airway, breathing, and circulation (ABCs). Once the patient is stabilized, efforts should be made to identify the exact time the patient was last seen well. *Keep in mind that symptom onset may be reported when the patient was found, which is different from when patient was last seen normal.* Evaluation should also rule out any potential stroke mimics. The National Institute of Health Stroke Scale (NIHSS) performed at the bedside will help establish the severity of the stroke. A noncontrast CT scan of the head must be performed to rule out hemorrhagic stroke.

B. **Thrombolysis therapy:** Once a hemorrhagic stroke is ruled out with a CT scan, all efforts should be made to establish reperfusion for ischemic stroke.

   1. **Intravenous:** The National Institute of Neurological Disorders and Stroke (NINDS) Tissue Plasminogen Activator (tPA) trial established the efficacy of intravenous (IV) tPA for patients presenting within 3 hours from symptom onset. Compared with the placebo group, patients treated with tPA had a 16% absolute increase in favorable outcomes at 3 months. IV tPA is approved by the U.S. Food and Drug Administration (FDA) for ischemic stroke presenting within 3 hours from last known normal. No consent is required for this time window. See the accompanying table for inclusion/exclusion criteria and testing recommended prior to initiation of IV tPA. For patients presenting after 3 hours but before 4.5 hours, the European Cooperative Acute Stroke Study (ECASS) III was the first study to show a statistical benefit for IV tPA use with a slightly higher intracranial hemorrhage rate. The American Heart Association and American Stroke Association recommend the use of IV tPA for patients (see inclusion/exclusion criteria in the following table) presenting between 3 and 4.5 hours from last known normal; however, this is not FDA approved.

   2. Orolingual angioedema that can occur due to IV tPA varies from a rate of 1.3% to 5.1% and is usually mild, transient, and contralateral to the ischemic hemisphere. Increased risk of angioedema is associated with ACE inhibitor use. Treatment includes close monitoring, intravenous ranitidine, diphenhydramine, and methylprednisolone.

TESTING PRIOR TO IV T-PA ADMINISTRATION FOR ACUTE ISCHEMIC STROKE
Noncontrast brain CT or brain MRI
Blood glucose
Oxygen saturation
Serum electrolytes/renal function tests*
Complete blood count, including platelet count*
Markers of cardiac ischemia*
Prothrombin time/INR*
Activated partial thromboplastin time*
ECG*

Abbreviations: ECG, electrocardiogram; ECT, ecarin clotting time; INR, international normalized ratio; TT, thrombin time.

*Although it is desirable to know the results of these tests before giving intravenous recombinant tissue-type plasminogen activator, fibrinolytic therapy should not be delayed while awaiting the results unless

(1) there is clinical suspicion of a bleeding abnormality or thrombocytopenia,

(2) the patient has received heparin or warfarin, or

(3) the patient has received other anticoagulants (direct thrombin inhibitors or direct factor Xa inhibitors).

B. **Thrombolysis therapy** (*cont'd*)

INCLUSION AND EXCLUSION CRITERIA FOR IV TPA UNDER 3 HOURS

Inclusion criteria
- Diagnosis of ischemic stroke causing measurable neurological deficit
- Onset of symptoms <3 hours before beginning treatment
- Age ≥18 years

Exclusion criteria
- Significant head trauma or prior stroke in previous 3 months
- Symptoms suggest subarachnoid hemorrhage
- Arterial puncture at noncompressible site in previous 7 days
- History of previous intracranial hemorrhage
- Intracranial neoplasm, arteriovenous malformation, or aneurysm
- Recent intracranial or intraspinal surgery
- Elevated blood pressure (systolic >185 mmHg or diastolic >110 mmHg)
- Active internal bleeding

Acute bleeding diathesis, including but not limited to:
- Platelet count <100,000/mm
- Heparin received within 48 hours, resulting in abnormally elevated aPTT greater than the upper limit of normal
- Current use of anticoagulant with INR >1.7 or PT >15 seconds
- Current use of direct thrombin inhibitors or direct factor Xa inhibitors with elevated sensitive laboratory tests (such as aPTT, INR, platelet count, and ECT; TT; or appropriate factor Xa activity assays)
- Blood glucose concentration <50 mg/dL (2.7 mmol/L)
- CT demonstrates multilobar infarction (hypodensity >1/3 cerebral hemisphere)
- Relative exclusion criteria

Relative contraindications
- Only minor or rapidly improving stroke symptoms (clearing spontaneously)
- Pregnancy
- Seizure at onset with postictal residual neurological impairments
- Major surgery or serious trauma within previous 14 days
- Recent gastrointestinal or urinary tract hemorrhage (within previous 21 days)
- Recent acute myocardial infarction (within previous 3 months)

The checklist includes some FDA-approved indications and contraindications for administration of IV rtPA for acute ischemic stroke. Recent guideline revisions have modified the original FDA-approved indications. A physician with expertise in acute stroke care may modify this list.

Onset time is defined as either the witnessed onset of symptoms or the time last known normal if symptom onset was not witnessed.

In patients without recent use of oral anticoagulants or heparin, treatment with IV rtPA can be initiated before availability of coagulation test results but should be discontinued if INR is >1.7 or PT is abnormally elevated by local laboratory standards.

In patients without history of thrombocytopenia, treatment with IV rtPA can be initiated before availability of platelet count but should be discontinued if platelet count is <100,000/mm.

Abbreviations: aPTT, activated partial thromboplastin time; ECT, ecarin clotting time; FDA, Food and Drug Administration; INR, international normalized ratio; IV, intravenous; PT, partial thromboplastin time; rtPA, recombinant tissue plasminogen activator; TT, thrombin time.

INCLUSION AND EXCLUSION CRITERIA FOR IV TPA UNDER 4.5 HOURS (IN ADDITION TO 3 HOURS)
Inclusion criteria   • Diagnosis of ischemic stroke causing measurable neurological deficit   • Onset of symptoms within 3 to 4.5 hours before beginning treatment   *Relative exclusion criteria*   • Age >80 years   • Severe stroke (NIHSS >25)   • Taking an oral anticoagulant regardless of INR   • History of both diabetes and prior ischemic stroke

Abbreviations: INR, international normalized ratio; IV, intravenous; NIHSS, National Institutes of Health Stroke Scale; rtPA, recombinant tissue plasminogen activator.

3. **Intra-arterial:** After a string of unsuccessful trails, five recent multiple-center trials have established the efficacy of mechanical thrombectomy using stent retriever technology, for patients presenting with ischemic stroke with large-vessel occlusion involving the anterior circulation. The American Heart Association and American Stroke Association updated their guidelines in 2015 as follows:

   a. Patients should receive endovascular therapy with a stent retriever if they meet all of the following criteria:

      i. Prestroke modified Rankin Scale score zero to one,

      ii. Acute ischemic stroke receiving intravenous tPA within 4.5 hours of onset

      iii. Causative occlusion of the ICA or proximal MCA (M1),

      iv. Age ≥18 years,

      v. NIHSS score of ≥6,

      vi. Alberta Stroke Program Early CT Score of ≥6, and

      vii. Treatment can be initiated (groin puncture) within 6 hours of symptom onset.

   b. Use of stent retrievers is indicated in preference to the Mechanical Embolus Removal in Cerebral Ischemia (MERCI) device

   c. The technical goal of the thrombectomy procedure should be a Thrombolysis In Cerebral Infarction grade 2b/3 angiographic result.

C. Secondary stroke prevention: for all ischemic stroke patients, aspirin should be initiated within 24 to 48 hours. Patients on statins or blood pressure medications can continue these unless there is concern for hypotension. Testing to evaluate etiology of the stroke should be undertaken, which should include cerebral and cervical arterial imaging, cardiac imaging, cardiac rhythm monitoring, and atherosclerosis risk factor evaluation.

D. Prevention of complication: admitted ischemic stroke patients are at a high risk for deep vein thrombosis (DVT), and aspiration. Early swallow evaluation and DVT prophylaxis are helpful.

E. Rehabilitation: once patient is medically stable, rehabilitation should be initiated.

X. Antiplatelets and Anticoagulants Approved for Use in Ischemic Stroke for Secondary Prevention

ANTIPLATELETS				
	ASPIRIN	CLOPIDOGREL	TICLOPIDINE	ASPIRIN AND EXTENDED-RELEASE DIPYRIDAMOLE
Mechanism	Irreversibly inhibits cyclooxygenase-1 and 2	Prevents activation of the GPIIb/IIIa receptor complex by blocking ADP receptor	Prevents activation of the GPIIb/IIIa receptor complex by blocking ADP receptor	Dipyridamole inhibits the uptake of adenosine into platelets (see Aspirin)
Dosage and frequency	75–325 mg once daily	75 mg once daily	250 mg twice daily	Dipyridamole extended-release 200 mg, aspirin 25 mg, twice daily
Side effects	Bleeding, gastrointestinal discomfort, Reye's syndrome, hypersensitivity	Bleeding, rash, thrombocytopenic thrombotic purpura (TTP)	Bleeding, elevated cholesterol, diarrhea, neutropenia (blackbox warning), rash, thrombocytopenic thrombotic purpura (TTP)	Bleeding, headache, gastrointestinal discomfort
Resistance and genetic testing	Higher resistance in enteric-coated aspirin; competitive inhibition when used with other nonsteroidal anti-inflammatory Polymorphisms affecting enzymes COX-1, COX-2, TXA2 synthase, and receptors GPIa/IIa, GPIba, GPIIIa, GPIIbIIIa, GPIb/V/IX, von Willebrand factor receptor	Inhibitors (calcium channel blockers, statins), CYP3A4 substrates CYP2C19 substrates and inhibitors (proton pump inhibitors) Polymorphisms affecting enzymes CYP3A4, CYP1A2, CYP2C19, and P2Y12 receptor	Not reported	Dipyridamole resistance has not been reported (see aspirin resistance)

Cilostazol: Phosphodiesterase three inhibitor mainly used for intermittent claudication from peripheral artery disease has shown to be noninferior to aspirin for stroke prevention in Asian population, with a lower rate of hemorrhagic events. However, it is not FDA approved for stroke in the United States.

ANTICOAGULANTS					
	DABIGATRAN	**APIXABAN**	**RIVAROXABAN**	**EDOXABAN**	**WARFARIN**
Mechanism	Direct thrombin inhibitor	Factor Xa inhibitor	Factor Xa inhibitor	Factor Xa inhibitor	Vitamin K antagonist
Dosage and frequency	150 mg twice daily	5 mg twice daily Reduce to 2.5 mg twice daily if at least 2 of the 3 following factors: a) ≥80 years; b) ≤60 kg; c) serum creatinine ≥1.5 mg/dl	20 mg once daily	60 mg once daily	Variable
Half-life	12–17 hours	12 hours	5–9 hours	6–10 hours	40 hours
Known reversal agent	Idarucizumab	None	None	None	Prothrombin complex concentrate, fresh frozen plasma, vitamin K
Monitoring	Ecarin level, PT	Xa level	Xa level	Xa level	PT, INR *Polymorphisms in the gene encoding vitamin K epoxide reductase complex (VKORC1) can affect dose requirements

Abbreviations: INR, international normalized ratio; PT, partial thromboplastin time.

XI. Infectious and Inflammatory Disease of Brain Arteries

A. **Infectious causes**

1. *Meningovascular syphilis, tuberculous meningitis, fungal meningitis, and subacute bacterial meningitis* may be accompanied by inflammatory changes and cause *occlusion of arteries or veins.*

2. *Mucormycosis* may *occlude ICA in diabetic* patients as part of the orbital and cavernous sinus infections.

A. **Infectious causes** (*cont'd*)

3. Angioinvasive aspergillosis can cause ischemic strokes as well as hemorrhagic stroke from ruptured mycotic aneurysms.

4. *Varicella zoster virus (VZV)*: causes a vasculopathy of intracranial vessels presenting usually as ischemic and less often as hemorrhagic stroke in gray–white matter junctions. Two-thirds may have history of zoster or varicella rash. Cerebrospinal fluid (CSF) studies show mild mononuclear pleocytosis, and diagnosis is confirmed by CSF VZV DNA or CSF VZV antibodies.

5. Infective endocarditis (IE): symptomatic cerebrovascular events occur in up to 30% of IE cases. Embolic events are highest during the first few weeks and dramatically reduce with successful antibiotic therapy. Risk of embolization is highest with anterior mitral valve involvement, *Staphylococcus aureus* IE, *Candida* IE, and HACEK group IE. Intracranial mycotic aneurysms occur in 1% to 5% of cases. CNS imaging should be performed in all IE cases who present with severe localized headache, neurological deficits, or meningeal signs. Anticoagulation is not recommended in native valve IE.

B. **Inflammatory causes**

1. *Giant cell arteritis*
   a. Incidence increases with age; women > men
   b. Medium and large arteries throughout the body, mainly aorta and branches
   c. Inflammation of arterial wall mononuclear cells and granulomas
   d. Symptoms: headache, polymyalgia rheumatic, vision loss
   e. Diagnosis: clinical suspicion in new-onset headache over 50, elevated erythrocyte sedimentation rate (ESR), and biopsy of temporal artery
   f. Treatment: glucocorticoids

2. *Primary angiitis of the central nervous system (PACNS)*
   a. Inflammation restricted to the cerebral circulation (and/or spinal vessels exclusively).
   b. Pathology: lymphocytes, plasma cells, granulomas with multinucleated giant cells, and, occasionally, neutrophils and eosinophils.
   c. Indolent course, heterogeneous presentations, out of proportion to systemic symptoms.
   d. Multifocal neurologic symptoms and signs may develop in a stepwise, progressive fashion, with episodes of quantitative and qualitative worsening, usually occurring after variable periods of stabilization.
   e. Cerebral angiographic results are sometimes abnormal, with alternating segments of concentric arterial narrowing and dilatation. Brain imaging with heterogeneous findings, but angiogram findings not diagnostic.
   f. Biopsy for diagnosis.
   g. Glucocorticoids and immunosuppressants.
   h. Must be differentiated from reversible cerebral vasoconstriction syndrome (see Section XII.B), which is a noninflammatory condition that is usually acute in presentation, with vascular imaging findings similar to PACNS, but is reversible with a benign CSF profile.

3. *Takayasu's disease*
   a. Young women
   b. Large-artery granulomatous arteritis that affects the aorta and its main branches, similar to giant cell arteritis
   c. Arm claudication and syncope
   d. Ischemic stroke in advanced disease
   e. Elevated ESR
   f. Treatment: steroids, cytotoxic agents, revascularization surgery

XII. Diseases Involving Cerebral Vasculature

A. **Cervical artery dissection**

1. Most are spontaneous (mostly idiopathic, less commonly with underlying Marfan's syndrome, Ehlers-Danlos syndrome [type IV], osteogenesis imperfecta, fibromuscular dysplasia [FMD] or other connective tissue disorder) and less commonly related to trauma (violent coughing, chiropractor manipulation, whiplash injury)

2. Intimal tear with intramural hematoma formation; mainly in extracranial internal carotid artery or extracranial vertebral artery

3. Subintimal dissections are more likely to cause luminal stenosis, whereas subadventitial dissections may cause dissecting aneurysm.

4. Symptoms: local pain, head or neck pain, ischemic stroke, partial Horner's syndrome, subarachnoid hemorrhage (intracranial dissection). Most stroke occur early, usually within 1 week of dissection occurrence.

5. Diagnosis can be made with vascular imaging. MRI can reveal crescent-shaped intramural hematoma. CT angiography can reveal focal stenosis in typical locations at skull base in internal carotid artery or vertebral artery around C1 to C2 vertebral bones. Angiogram reveals flame-shaped tapering occlusion (nonspecific finding) or dissection flap.

6. Treatment: the artery heals and re-endothelializes over weeks and months. There is little research to support efficacy of anticoagulation over antiplatelets. Neuroendovascular stenting may be an option for acute occlusion, persistent/recurrent symptoms, or expanding dissecting aneurysms.

B. **Reversible cerebral vasoconstriction syndrome (RCVS)**

1. Young to middle-aged patients presenting with recurrent thunderclap headache

2. Brain imaging may be normal, but can also show hemorrhagic stroke or ischemic stroke.

   a. Vascular imaging shows diffuse multifocal intracranial stenosis with reversibility on follow-up imaging around 8 to 12 weeks. Stenosis can progress over the first 2 weeks; arteries normalize after average of 1 month.

   b. CSF studies are normal to near normal.

   c. Associated with postpartum state, use of selective serotonin reuptake inhibitors, serotonin noradrenaline reuptake inhibitors, α-sympathomimetics, triptans, and illicit drugs (cocaine and cannabinoids).

   d. Treatment is usually conservative, with calcium channel blockers and headache control.

C. **Fibromuscular dysplasia (FMD)**

   a. *Nonatheromatous, noninflammatory vasculopathy with alternating fibrotic thickening and atrophy of the vessel wall*

   b. Women > male; ~20 to 50 years of age

   c. Medial fibroplasia is the most common form.

   d. "String of beads" appearance, in which the beads are larger than the normal vessel diameter, involving extracranial vessels mainly (carotid > vertebral)

   e. Asymptomatic, ischemic stokes, no-specific symptoms

   f. Intracranial aneurysms are seen in 7% to 8% of patients

   g. Treatment: conservative in most; antiplatelets in symptomatic patients; neuroendovascular procedures for nonresponders

   h. Surgical consideration for FMD-associated intracranial aneurysms are likely to be similar to those for all intracranial aneurysms.

D. **Moyamoya disease**

1. Nonatherosclerotic, noninflammatory vasculopathy

2. Pathology: intimal hyperplasia, smooth muscle proliferation, disruption of internal elastic lamina

3. Progressive stenosis and occlusion of bilateral distal internal carotid arteries and proximal middle cerebral arteries or anterior cerebral arteries with development of network of abnormal fine lenticulostriate collateral vessels

4. Childhood cases more common among males; adulthood cases more common among women

5. Ischemic stroke (hypoperfusion) or intracerebral or intraventricular hemorrhage (bleed from small collateral arteries) can occur.

6. 15% familial; RNF213 gene on chromosome 17 associated with majority of cases in East Asia

7. Association with Down syndrome, neurofibromatosis, cranial irradiation, and sickle cell disease (Moyamoya syndrome)

8. Digital subtraction angiography shows "puff of smoke" collateral appearance.

9. Medical treatment: antiplatelet therapy

10. Surgical treatment: superficial temporal artery to middle cerebral artery bypass, encephaloduroarteriosynangiosis, encephaloduroarteriomyosynangiosis

XIII. Genetic Syndromes in Cerebrovascular Disease

A. **Fabry disease**

1. X-linked lysosomal storage disease (α-galactosidase A)

2. Ischemic strokes, painful extremities with small-fiber neuropathy

3. Cardiac conduction defects, cardiomyopathy, renal failure

4. Imaging: hyperintensity in pulvinar on T1 sequences and dolichoectasia or large diameter of basilar artery

5. Diagnosis by measurement of α-galactosidase A activity

6. Treatment: enzyme replacement therapy appears to reduce MRI changes.

B. **Cerebral autosomal dominant arteriopathy with subcortical infarcts and leukoencephalopathy (CADASIL)**

1. Mutation in NOTCH3 gene on chromosome 19

2. Small-vessel arteriopathy

3. Migraines, recurrent ischemic stroke/TIA

4. MRI T2: hyperintensities of the white matter, typically involving of anterior temporal poles

5. Median age for ischemic stroke: ~50

6. Diagnosis: genetic testing, skin biopsy (granular, osmophilic materials in the arterial smooth muscle)

7. No specific treatment

C. **Cerebral autosomal recessive arteriopathy with subcortical infarcts and leukoencephalopathy (CARASIL)**

1. Stoke at ~30 years of age

2. Dementia ~50 years of age reported in Japan

3. Mutation in HTRA1 gene on chromosome 10

4. No specific treatment

D. **Mitochondrial encephalopathy, lactic acidosis, and stroke-like episodes (MELAS)**

1. Mitochondrial disorder

2. Onset of stroke before age 40

3. Encephalopathy: seizures or dementia

4. Ragged red fibers on Gomori trichome staining of skeletal muscle

5. Treatment: coenzyme Q10, levocarnitine, L-arginine, B vitamins

6. Avoid valproic acid and HMG CoA reductase inhibitors.

E. **Sickle cell disease**

1. Incidence is 0.61% to 0.76% per year during the first 20 years of life.

2. Asymptomatic patients should be followed with transcranial doppler ultrasound (TCD).

3. Red blood cell transfusion therapy reduces stroke risk. Given to keep the time-averaged mean velocity <200cm/s on TCD.

F. **Retinal vasculopathy with cerebral leukodystrophy (RVCL)**

1. Autosomal dominant; caused by mutation in TREX1 gene on chromosome 3p21

2. 30 to 50 years of age

3. Progressive visual loss, due to retinopathy, microaneurysms with telangiectasia, and capillary dropout

4. Ischemic strokes in deep white matter, irregular shape, mass effect, edema

5. No specific treatment

G. **COL4A1 Mutation**

1. Located on chromosome 13q34; expressed in basement membranes during early stages of development

2. In pediatric age groups causes porencephaly, infantile hemiparesis, and intracerebral hemorrhage

3. In adults can cause leukoaraiosis, microbleeds, lacunar infarctions, hemorrhagic strokes, retinal arteriolar tortuosity and dilated perivascular spaces

4. No specific therapy

H. **Hyperhomocysteinemia**

1. Homocysteine is derived from metabolism of methionine.

2. Increased levels are due to deficiencies in cystathionine β–synthase and methyltetrahydrofolate.

3. Vitamin deficiency of B_{12}, B_6, and folic acid can also cause hyperhomocysteinemia.

4. Hyperhomocysteinemia is associated with increased risk of strokes.

5. Vitamin supplementation reduces the levels of homocysteine, but does not prevent strokes.

XIV. Other Stroke Etiologies

A. **Thrombosis of cerebral veins and venous sinuses**

1. Anatomy: venous drainage of the brain is divided into superficial and deep system.

   a. Superficial cortical veins course over the surface of the brain, draining the majority of the cerebral cortex and eventually emptying into the superior sagittal sinus. Two large anastomotic veins, Trolard and Labbe, connect the superficial middle cerebral vein to the superior sagittal sinus and transverse sinus, respectively.

1. Anatomy (*cont'd*)

    b. The deep venous drains the deep white matter, corpus callosum, basal ganglia, and upper brainstem. The internal cerebral veins and basal veins of Rosenthal join to form the great cerebral vein of Galen, which drains into the straight sinus.

    c. The superior sagittal sinus, straight sinus, and transverse sinuses meet to form the torcular herophili at the internal occipital protuberance. The transverse sinuses drain into the sigmoid, which connects with the internal jugular vein.

2. 0.5% of all strokes

    a. Presents with headache, intracranial hypertension, seizures, focal neurological deficits, encephalopathy, hemorrhage

    b. Imaging: visualization of subacute thrombus or filling defect on imaging studies; magnetic resonance (MR) venogram, digital subtraction angiogram, CT venogram. Venous infarcts do not follow arterial distribution and may involve two arterial distributions.

    c. Etiology: hypercoagulable states, peripartum, ear or sinus infection, severe dehydration; risk factors are similar to those for systemic venous thrombosis.

    d. Treatment: anticoagulation for 3 to 6 months, even in the presence of intracerebral hemorrhage; progressive neurological deterioration calls for endovascular thrombolysis.

B. Antiphospholipid antibodies syndrome

1. Unexplained thrombosis, including ischemic stroke in young adult

2. Testing: lupus anticoagulant in plasma on two or more occasions at least 12 weeks apart

3. Related to systemic lupus erythematosus (SLE) in some

4. Treatment: anticoagulation with vitamin K antagonist

C. Sneddon syndrome

1. Young to middle-aged adults; usually neurological symptoms onset under 45 years of age

2. Deep-bluish-red lesions of *livedo reticularis and livedo racemosa in association with multiple recurrent strokes*

3. Associated with antiphospholipid antibodies, cardiac valvular lesions

4. MRI lesions are small, deep, and multiple.

5. Skin biopsy demonstrates an occlusive, noninflammatory vasculopathy involving medium-sized arteries along with focal and segmental intimal hyperplasia due to fibroelastic proliferation or subendothelial cell proliferation.

6. Treatment is anticoagulation in the presence of antiphospholipid antibody.

D. Susac's syndrome

1. Autoimmune microangiopathy presenting with triad of encephalopathy, branch retinal artery occlusion (BRAO), and hearing loss

2. Typically affects middle-aged women

3. MRI shows characteristic white-matter lesions in the central fibers of the corpus callosum and leptomeningeal enhancement.

4. Brain biopsy: microinfarctions and perivascular inflammation of small vessels

5. Fluorescein angiography: BRAO, leakage, arteriolar wall hyperfluorescence

6. Pure tone audiometry: bilateral sensorineural hearing loss in the low to moderate range of frequencies

7. Treatment: immunosuppressant and steroids

KEY WORDS

Dual antiplatelet therapy	Symptomatic intracranial stenosis
Facial nerve and abducens nerve palsy plus contralateral hemiplegia	Millard-Gubler syndrome
Finger agnosia, acalculia, right-left confusion, alexia with agraphia	Gerstmann syndrome
Ipsilateral CN III plus contralateral hemiplegia and tremor	Benedikt syndrome
Ipsilateral oculomotor palsy plus contralateral hemiplegia	Weber syndrome
Ischemic stroke symptoms presenting under 3 hours	Consider intravenous tissue plasminogen activator
Ipsilateral CN III plus contralateral cerebellar ataxia and tremor	Claude syndrome
Lateral medullary syndrome with ipsilateral hemiplegia	Opalski syndrome
NOTCH 3	CADASIL
Nystagmus, vertigo, nausea, vomiting, contralateral impairment of pain and thermal sense over one-half the body; ipsilateral Horner's; hoarseness, dysphagia, ipsilateral paralysis of palate and vocal cord, diminished gag; ipsilateral ataxia of limbs, impaired sensation on ipsilateral one-half of face	Wallenberg syndrome/lateral medullary syndrome
Oculomotor apraxia, optic ataxia asimultanagnosia	Balint's syndrome
Paralysis of upward gaze and accommodation, fixed pupils	Parinaud's syndrome
Postpartum stroke	Venous sinus thrombosis/RCVS
Recurrent thunderclap headache	RCVS
Stroke and painful peripheral neuropathy	Fabry's disease
Symptomatic carotid stenosis >70%	CEA or carotid stenting

Gerstmann syndrome	Finger agnosia, acalculia, right-left confusion, alexia
Kluver-Bucy syndrome	Docility, hyperorality, hypersexuality
Dejerine Roussy syndrome	Thalamic infarction contralateral pain syndrome
Balint's syndrome	Oculomotor apraxia, optic ataxia, asimultagnosia
Wallenberg syndrome	Lateral medulla infarction
Millard-Gubler syndrome	Pons; VI, VII and corticospinal tract (contra paresis)
Weber syndrome	III, corticospinal tract (contralateral paresis)
Claude syndrome	III, red nucleus, brachium conjunctivum (contra ataxia)
Benedikt syndrome	III, red nucleus, corticospinal
Nothnagel syndrome	III, sup cerebellar peduncular
Parinaud's syndrome	Paralysis upgaze, fixed pupils, retraction convergence nystagmus
Fabry's disease	X linked, alpha galactosidase, strokes, skin lesions, cardiac conduction defects
CADASIL	NOTCH3 mutation chromosome 19
CARASIL	Recessive, mutation HTRA1 gene chromosome 10
Sneddon syndrome	Recurrent strokes, livedo reticularis, antiphospholipid antibodies, cardiac valvular lesions

Suggested Readings

Cerebrovascular disease [Entire issue]. *Continuum* (Minneap Minn).2014;20(2).

Furie KL, Goldstein LB, Albers GW, et al. Oral antithrombotic agents for the prevention of stroke in nonvalvular atrial fibrillation: a science advisory for healthcare professionals from the American Heart Association/American Stroke Association. *Stroke*.2012;43(12):3442–3453.

Jauch EC, Saver JL, Adams HP, et al. Guidelines for the early management of patients with acute ischemic stroke: a guideline for healthcare professionals from the American Heart Association/ American Stroke Association. *Stroke*.2013;44(3):870–947.

Kernan WN, Ovbiagele B, Black HR, et al. AHA/ASA guidelines for the prevention of stroke in patients with stroke and transient ischemic attack. *Stroke*.2014;45:2160–2236.

Kernan WN, Ovbiagele B, Black HR, et al. Guidelines for the prevention of stroke in patients with stroke and transient ischemic attack: a guideline for healthcare professionals from the American Heart Association/American Stroke Association. *Stroke*.2014;45(7):2160–2236.

Meschia JF, Bushnell C, Boden-Albala B, et al. Guidelines for the primary prevention of stroke: a statement for healthcare professionals from the American Heart Association/American Stroke Association. *Stroke*.2014;45(12):3754–3832.

Mohr, JP, Grotta, JC, Wolf, PA, Moskowitz, MA, Mayberg, MR, Von Kummer, R. *Stroke: Pathophysiology, Diagnosis, and Management.* Philadelphia, PA: Elsevier Health Sciences;2011.

Mozaffarian D, Benjamin EJ, Go AS, et al. Heart disease and stroke statistics—2015 update: a report from the American Heart Association. *Circulation*.2015;131(4):e29.

Osborn, AG. *Diagnostic Cerebral Angiography.* Philadelphia, PA: Lippincott Williams & Wilkins;1999.

Powers WJ, Derdeyn CP, Biller J, et al. 2015 American Heart Association/American Stroke Association focused update of the 2013 guidelines for the early management of patients with acute ischemic stroke regarding endovascular treatment: a guideline for healthcare professionals from the American Heart Association/American Stroke Association. *Stroke*.2015;46(10):3020–3035.

Sacco RL, Kasner SE, Broderick JP, et al. An updated definition of stroke for the 21st century: a statement for healthcare professionals from the American Heart Association/American Stroke Association." *Stroke*.2013;44(7):2064–2089.

Wijdicks EFM, Varelas PN, Gronseth GS, et al. Evidence-based guideline update: determining brain death in adults. *Neurology*.2010;74:1911–1918.

CHAPTER 6

Head Trauma

I. Cranio-Cerebral Trauma

A. Overview

1. In persons up to 44 years old, trauma and injuries are the leading cause of death.

   a. Traumatic brain injury (TBI) is responsible for 30% of trauma-related deaths.

2. Eighty percent of head injury cases are first seen by a general physician in the emergency room.

   a. Seventy-five percent of TBI cases are mild in nature.

3. Less than 20% of TBI patients ever require neurosurgical intervention.

4. Men are more likely than women to suffer TBI (4:1).

5. Patients older than 75 years of age have the highest mortality from TBI.

B. Definitions

1. Concussion: violent shaking or jarring of the brain with resulting transient functional impairment

2. Contusion: bruising of the brain without interruption of its architecture

3. Coup injury: head is struck while immobilized; the focus of the injury is at the site of impact.

4. Contre-coup injury: focus of injury is opposite the site of impact due to the head not being immobilized (i.e., it was in motion, accelerating or decelerating).

5. Severe TBI: traumatic head injury leading to loss of consciousness, with a Glasgow Coma Scale (GCS) score of less than 9

C. Mechanisms of brain injury: About 1.7 million persons in the United States suffer a TBI every year.

1. Falls (35%)

2. Gunshot wound/assault to the head (10%)

3. Injury to the skull by objects (17%)

4. Motor vehicle accident (17%)

5. Sports-related injuries

6. Cranium distorted by forceps at birth

II. Approach to the Patient With Head Injury

A. Overview

1. As with all trauma, patients with head injury must be evaluated for airway and breathing compromise and circulatory distress. The "ABCs" must be intact. A full trauma survey should ideally be completed within the first minutes of arrival to a care center.

A. **Overview** (*cont'd*)

2. GCS and pupillary responses should be assessed repeatedly, especially during the first few hours, to establish neurological stability.

3. In some cases of mild and in all cases of moderate to severe head trauma, a **head CT scan** should be completed as soon as feasible.

4. Spine imaging should be considered if the patient shows any signs of new autonomic instability, motor weakness, or a sensory level.

5. Volume status should be ascertained and resuscitated as needed.

6. Oxygen saturation should remain above 90% at all times.

7. Currently, there is **no** evidence for adjunct steroid therapy in traumatic central nervous system (CNS) injury, and steroid therapy is not recommended.

8. Assess for skull fracture

   a. The fracture size and type can give a rough estimate of the force that caused the trauma.

   b. Skull fractures can also confer the extent of cerebral injury.

   c. The skull fracture site can lead to ingress of bacteria or air or egress of cerebrospinal fluid (CSF).

9. In patients with severe TBI with minimal neurological examination, an **intracranial pressure monitor should be considered**.

   a. Cerebral perfusion pressure is recommended at 50 to 70 mmHg

   b. Adjunct monitoring (cerebral oximetry and microdialysis) are currently being studied, but are not currently recommended in all TBI patients.

B. **Minor head injury**

1. Most head injuries are minor, and patients generally have not lost consciousness or are rapidly regaining consciousness; 90% of concussion do not involve loss of consciousness.

2. Little need for neurologic consultation for these injuries

3. Hospitalization is generally not required, provided that a family member is able to report changes

   a. 1-in-1000 chance of developing intracranial hemorrhage if without fracture and mentally clear

   b. 1 in 30 if with fractures and mentally clear

4. Family or caregivers should monitor for the following:

   a. Posttraumatic syndrome: headaches, giddiness, fatigability, insomnia, and nervousness

   b. Delayed fainting after head injury: a vasodepressor syncopal attack, related to pain and emotional upset—must be distinguished from a "lucid interval of epidural bleed"

   c. Transient traumatic paraplegia, blindness, and migrainous phenomena: both legs become temporarily weak, with bilateral Babinski sign, occasional sphincteric incontinence; symptoms disappear after a few hours.

   d. Delayed hemiplegia or coma: usually young adults after relatively minor athletic or road injury; massive hemiplegia, hemianesthesia, hemianopsia, aphasia—represents either dissecting aneurysm of internal carotid, late evolving epidural or subdural hematoma, intracranial hemorrhage (ICH), or preexisting arteriovenous malformation (AVM); with fracture of large bones and pulmonary symptoms 24 to 72 hours later, traumatic fat embolism should be considered.

C. **Moderate to severe head injury**

1. Monitor for increased intracranial pressure (ICP), cerebral contusions (with serial CT scans), lacerations, subarachnoid hemorrhage (SAH), zones of infarction, and scattered ICHs, and consider MRI with diffusion tensor imaging to assess for diffuse axonal injury.

2. Severe head injury: first step is to clear the airway and ensure adequate ventilation; perform careful search for other injuries; Glasgow Coma Score provides a means of evaluating state of consciousness; control factors that raise ICP, such as hypoxia, hypercarbia, hyperthermia, awkward head positions, and high mean airway pressure.

3. **NB:** brady-arrhythmia may be sufficient to damage brain.

4. Brain death evaluation should ideally be delayed for at least 24–48 hours post TBI and assessments for anoxia, drug or alcohol intoxication and hypotension should be made.

5. Traumatic delirium: when stupor gives way to a confusional state, may last for weeks; associated with aggressive behavior or uncooperativeness

6. Traumatic dementia: once the patient improves, he or she is slow in thinking and unstable in emotion, with faulty judgment.

7. Small groups are in a vegetative state: normal vital signs but do not speak and are capable only of primitive reflexes; this signals arousal without awareness. If this is persistent, it may become persistent vegetative state.

8. After moderate to severe head injury, several conditions should be monitored for:

   a. **A concussion followed by a lucid interval and serious cerebral damage:** initial and temporary loss of consciousness is generally due to concussion. If there is later deterioration, it is potentially because of delayed expansion of subdural hematoma, worsening brain edema, or epidural clot.

   b. **Acute epidural hemorrhage:** generally caused by a temporal or parietal fracture with laceration of the middle meningeal artery or vein; less often a tear in dural venous sinus; meningeal vessels may be torn without a fracture.

      i. CT: lens-shaped clot with a smooth inner margin

      ii. Treatment: burr hole excision of epidural hematoma (EDH); emergent craniotomy or drainage may be necessary if patient becomes unstable or if bleed is uncontrollable (prognosis is poor if patient develops bilateral Babinski sign and decerebrate posturing).

   c. **Acute subdural hematoma (SDH)**

      i. May be unilateral or bilateral.

      ii. Sometimes characterized by a lucid interval followed by a sudden deterioration.

      iii. More often, patient is stuporous from the time of injury, and mental status progressively worsens.

      iv. SDH is frequently combined with epidural hematoma.

      v. CT detects in more than 90% of cases; less acute hematomas may be isodense to the cortex and present only as a ventricular shift.

      vi. Treatment: burr hole excision of SDH after stabilization and liquification of clot material; craniotomy for more emergent expansion of bleed with neurological worsening.

   d. **Chronic subdural hematoma:**

      i. Generally due to traumatic injury that was trivial or forgotten

      ii. Period of weeks passes before onset of headaches, giddiness, slowness of thinking, confusion, apathy, drowsiness, or seizures

    d. **Chronic subdural hematoma** (*cont'd*)

        iii. CSF may be clear, bloody, acellular to xanthochromic

        iv. Subdural hygroma (collection of blood and CSF in subdural space) may form in the potential space created by the SDH

    e. **Cerebral contusion**

        i. Areas of brain parenchyma that suffer direct and indirect mechanical trauma due to impact—coup and coup contre-coup.

        ii. These can cause parenchymal shifts and increased ICP.

        iii. CT: appear as edematous areas of cortex and subcortical white matter admixed with areas of higher density (representing leaked blood); main concern is tendency of contused areas to swell or to develop hematomas, giving rise to delayed clinical deterioration; swelling may be precipitated by excessive administration of IV fluids.

D. Penetrating wounds of the head

  1. Bullets and fragments: air is compressed in front of the bullet so that it has an explosive effect upon entering tissue.

  2. If brain is penetrated at the lower brainstem level, death is instantaneous from respiratory or cardiac arrest.

  3. If vital centers are untouched, immediate problems are **bleeding, increased ICP, swelling.**

  4. Treatment:

    a. Rapid and radical debridement

    b. Control ICP with mannitol or hypertonic saline.

    c. Prevent systemic complications; epilepsy is the most troublesome sequelae (more than one-half of patients).

    d. Consider surgical decompression if there are compressive blood products causing neurological deficit.

SEQUELAE OF HEAD INJURY	SYMPTOMS	TREATMENT
Posttraumatic epilepsy	Focal or generalized seizures that occur shortly after TBI. This is the most common delayed sequela of craniocerebral trauma, although the interval between injury and epilepsy varies. The interval is generally longer in children. Earlier seizures are more likely to have complete remission	Antiepileptic medications
Autonomic dysfunction syndrome in the vegetative state ("diencephalic storming")	Extensor posturing, profuse diaphoresis, hypertension, tachycardia following TBI	Narcotics, benzodiazepines, bromocriptine, nonselective beta blockade

(continued)

SEQUELAE OF HEAD INJURY	SYMPTOMS	TREATMENT
Posttraumatic nervous instability (postconcussion syndrome)	Following TBI, symptoms of neurasthenia, dizziness, and generalized or localized headache of variable quality. Symptoms are precipitated by straining or emotion. Intolerance to noise, emotional excitement, crowds. Patients also experience tenseness, restless, decreased concentration, and resistance in doing varieties of treatment.	Relieved by rest, quiet room, and benzodiazepines. Some antidepressants can be of use in this population.
Posttraumatic Parkinson syndrome	Controversial syndrome; most patients likely had Parkinson's disease or postencephalitic parkinsonism brought to light by head injury (seen in boxers).	Some Parkinsonian medications can help treat underlying Parkinson's disease in this population.
Punch-drunk encephalopathy, "dementia pugilistica"	Dysarthric speech, forgetful, slow thinking; movements are slow, stiff, uncertain; legs with shuffling, wide-based gait; often with parkinsonian syndrome and ataxia. Other symptoms include enlargement of lateral ventricles, thinning of corpus callosum, widened cavum septum pellucidum; fenestration of septal leaves; diffuse plaques and Alzheimer's changes; no Lewy bodies.	No known treatments
Posttraumatic hydrocephalus	Adhesive basilar arachnoiditis	Shunt placement
Posttraumatic cognitive and psychiatric disorders	Long anterograde amnesia and permanent cognitive and personality changes	

III. Head Trauma Related to Sports

A. The American Academy of Neurology updated the evaluation, management and treatment guidelines for the management of concussion in sports in 2013. The following is a summary of the new recommendations.

   1. Greatest risk for concussion exists in

      a. Football

      b. Rugby

      c. Soccer

      d. Hockey

A. **The American Academy of Neurology** (*cont'd*)

2. Female athletes who play soccer and basketball have a predominance for head injury.

3. Athletes with history of concussion or mild TBI have a higher risk for further concussions, especially within the first 10 days of a previous concussion.

4. Wearing a helmet during contact sports reduces but does not eliminate risk of concussion and head injury.

5. Standard symptom checklists (postconcussion symptom scale/graded symptom checklist) and the standardized assessment of concussion are highly specific and sensitive for identifying concussion if completed early after a sports-related head injury.

6. Physicians and other health care providers who are knowledgeable on sideline assessment tools should train sideline health officials.

7. If an athlete suffers symptoms of concussion, a trained health official should complete the sideline assessment tool and provide the data to the treating physician for further assessment.

8. Athletes with suspected head injury or concussion should immediately be removed from play to avoid further injury.

9. The injured athlete should **not** return to play until assessed by an experienced care provider with training both in the diagnosis and management of concussion and in the recognition of more severe TBI.

10. **Imaging:** CT imaging should be considered to assess intracranial hemorrhage in athletes who have loss of consciousness, posttraumatic amnesia, persistently altered mental status (Glasgow Coma Scale <15), focal neurologic deficit, evidence of skull fracture on examination, or signs of clinical deterioration.

11. **Return to play:** Athletes with concussion should not return to play or practice **until the concussion has resolved** as confirmed by health care professional clinical examination and assessment. Athletes with concussion should be prohibited from playing until the concussion has resolved.

12. Early postconcussive symptoms and cognitive impairments last longer in younger athletes relative to older athletes and thus these patients should be managed more conservatively than older adults.

13. Concussion resolution is also predominantly a clinical determination made on the basis of a comprehensive neurologic history, neurologic examination, and cognitive assessment. There is moderate evidence that tests such as symptom checklists, neurocognitive testing, and balance testing are helpful in monitoring recovery from concussion.

14. Cognitive restructuring may be a useful form of brief psychological counseling that consists of education, reassurance, and reattribution of symptoms, often utilizing both verbal and written information, and has been shown to diminish the development of chronic postconcussion syndrome.

CHEAT SHEET

Concussion	Violent shaking or jarring of the brain with resulting transient functional impairment
Severe TBI	Traumatic head injury leading to loss of consciousness with GCS score of less than 9

(continued)

Acute epidural hematoma	Sometimes worsening after lucid interval; CT shows lens-shaped clot with smooth inner margin
Acute subdural hematoma	Usually stuporous from time of injury, CT detects in >90%
Chronic subdural hematoma	Often after trivial trauma; weeks of progressive symptoms

Suggested Readings

Cancelliere C, Cassidy JD, Li A, Donovan J, Côté P, Hincapié CA. Systematic search and review procedures: results of the International Collaboration on Mild Traumatic Brain Injury Prognosis. *Arch Phys Med Rehab.*2014;95(Suppl 3):S101–S131.

Giza CC, Kutcher JS, Ashwal S et al. Summary of evidence-based guideline update: Evaluation and management of concussion in sports. Report of the Guideline Development Subcommittee of the American Academy of Neurology. *Neurology.*2013;80(24):2250–2257.

Ryan ME, Palasis S, Saigal G, et al. ACR appropriateness criteria head trauma—child. *J Am Coll Radiol.*2014;11(10):939–947.

CHAPTER 7

Neurocritical Care

I. Critical Care Management of Acute Ischemic Stroke

A. Acute ischemic stroke management is discussed more extensively in Chapter 5. Majority of stroke patients are managed on a regular or step-down nursing floor. Approximately 15% to 20% of stroke patients are admitted to an intensive care unit, mainly for the following indications:

- Monitoring and treatment of malignant cerebral cytotoxic edema ("hemicraniectomy watch")
- Monitoring hemorrhagic transformation of an acute ischemic stroke
- Airway management due to neurological deficits of stroke
- Intractable seizure management
- Aggressive blood pressure (BP) augmentation/control
- Neurological monitoring post intra-arterial intervention or intravenous tissue plasminogen activator (tPA)

1. **Malignant cerebral edema management ("hemicraniectomy watch")**

   a. The definitive treatment of malignant cerebral edema due to large territory stroke is **hemicraniectomy** or **suboccipital decompression,** generally within 48 hours of infarction.

      i. Involves the surgical removal of the skull proximal to the affected area of brain for resolution of pressure and compression due to cerebral edema

      ii. Reduces mortality, not necessarily morbidity

      iii. Better functional outcomes in patients younger than 60 years of age

   b. Hyperosmolar therapy (medical management)—used to "shrink" **normal** (unaffected) brain by drawing water out of living brain cells into the vasculature

      i. Hypertonic saline

         (A) 2% hypertonic saline—can be given by peripheral access

         (B) 3% hypertonic saline—central access only (vesicant)

         (C) 23.4% hypertonic saline "bullet"—central access only (vesicant)

            (1) Given for neurological emergencies (e.g., herniation)

      ii. Mannitol push (0.5 g–1 g/kg)—can be given by peripheral access

   c. Other adjunct therapies to reduce intracranial pressure that may be considered

      i. Therapeutic hypothermia (systemic cooling generally from 32–36°C)

      ii. Elevating head of the bed

      iii. Hyperventilation (prolonged hyperventilation can cause further **ischemia**)

    c. Other adjunct therapies (*cont'd*)

        iv. Anesthetics (propofol, pentobarbital)

        v. Extraventricular device placement (in theory can lead to upward herniation)

2. **Hemorrhagic transformation management**

    a. Hemorrhage after ischemic stroke (hemorrhagic transformation) is common (20%–40%).

    b. It is more common in patients with microbleeds seen on gradient echo MRI, in patients treated with tPA, and in older patients.

    c. There is a higher predilection for hemorrhagic transformation if the patient has:

        i. **Hypertension** ($>$185/110 mmHg)

        ii. **Hyperglycemia** (especially $>$200 mg/dL)

        iii. **Anticoagulation**

        iv. A National Institute of Health Stroke Scale (NIHSS) score of greater than 20

        v. A larger stroke size ($>$1/3 territory)

        vi. Early venous filling discovered on angiography

    d. The current intensive care unit (ICU) management of hemorrhagic transformation is risk factor management of:

        i. **Refractory hypertension**: Aim to keep mean arterial pressure (MAP) less than 130, diastolic BP (DBP) less than 105, systolic BP (SBP) less than 220 mmHg.

            (A) Prehospitalization BP (baseline SBP/DBP) should be taken into consideration when aggressively lowering BP so as to not cause further ischemia.

            (B) Utilization of intravenous calcium channel blockers such as **nicardipine** or **hydralazine** or a mixed alpha and beta antagonist such as **labetalol** is recommended.

            (C) Nitroprusside, although effective at decreasing blood pressure rapidly, is uncommonly used because it leads to venodilation, which may lead to increased intracranial pressure (ICP).

        ii. **Hyperglycemia**: can be managed with long-acting insulins, short-acting insulins, and insulin drips. American Heart Association/American Stroke Association (AHA/ASA) recommends frequent monitoring of glucose, in all acute stroke patients, especially in known diabetics, with a goal of between 80 and 200 mg/dL and a strict goal to **avoid hypoglycemia**. Stroke patients with higher admission glucose levels have been shown to have poorer neurological outcomes. However, acute aggressive reduction has **not** been shown to be beneficial.

        iii. **Anticoagulation**: heparin drip, if needed due to high-risk conditions (e.g., mechanical valve prophylaxis, left ventricular thrombus) with close neurological monitoring.

3. **Seizure management of acute stroke patients**

    a. First-time seizures occur in **less than 5%** of stroke patients.

    b. Seizures in stroke patients are generally an indicator of a larger infarction, generally involving the cortex. Patients with larger strokes, cortical involvement, and hemorrhage are at higher risk for post-stroke seizures.

c. There are a number of abnormal movements that can result from stroke that are not related to seizures, and it is important to differentiate seizures from nonepileptiform movement disorders.

d. Antiepileptic drugs/medications (AEDs)

   i. AEDs **should not** be prescribed in the post-stroke setting if the patient does not have a seizure disorder (i.e., prophylactically) because they have been associated with worsened outcomes (e.g., phenytoin), increased sedation, cognitive impairment, and improper duration of therapy.

   ii. AEDs **should be** prescribed for at least a short term (3–6 months) in the post-stroke setting if the patient has a seizure within the first weeks after an acute ischemic stroke. Reassessment of the need for AEDs should be made in follow-up visits because a significant number of patients recover from their need for AED therapy.

   iii. Continuous EEG monitoring (cEEG) should be considered in post-stroke patients with impaired consciousness or altered mental status to assess for nonconvulsive seizure activity

   iv. After hemicraniectomy, AEDs can be considered for a short term (generally for up to a week) because there is a higher predilection to seizures in the immediate postoperative period.

4. **Blood pressure augmentation/reduction and cardiac considerations**: arterial line placement is ideal in the titration of vasoactive medications.

   a. **Augmentation**: patients may have symptomatic penumbral oligemia surrounding the core infarct ("perfusion-dependence") that can be theoretically salvaged by induced hypertension. Mean arterial pressures (MAPs) are generally augmented by normal saline boluses or vasopressive medications (e.g., phenylephrine, norepinephrine).

   b. **Reduction**: most patients should have a goal of MAP less than 130, DBP less than 105, and SBP less than 220 mmHg without aggressive reduction (no more than 10% reduction per hour). Utilization of calcium channel blockers (hydralazine, nicardipine) and/or alpha-beta blockade (labetalol) may be of use in the acute setting.

   c. **Other cardiac considerations**: Cardiopulmonary effects of acute ischemic stroke include neurogenic pulmonary edema (catecholamine release mediated), stunned myocardium, and myocardial infarction. Echocardiogram, electrocardiogram, and cardiac enzymes should be assessed on most if not all stroke patients to monitor for cardiac changes.

5. **Neurological monitoring after tPA and/or intra-arterial therapy:** during and immediately following tPA infusion, there is a heightened predilection for patients to have intracerebral and other bleeding diathesis. A number of assessments are required, including:

   a. Neurological assessments and vital sign checks every 15 min during tPA infusion

   b. Continued neurological monitoring every 15 min after infusion for the first hour

   c. Continued neurological monitoring every 30 min after infusion for the next 6 hours

   d. Hourly neurological assessments after infusion for the remaining hours until 24-hour CT scan is obtained

   e. Continuous monitoring for angioedema or other reactions, and minor or major bleeding, for first 24 hours after tPA infusion

II. Critical Care Management of Acute Intracerebral Hemorrhage

A. **General principles of intracerebral hemorrhage (ICH)**

   1. ICH constitutes 15% to 20% of new strokes annually, with an incidence of 15 per 100,000 people.

   2. Functional morbidity is seen in up to 80% of patients, and up to 50% of patients suffer mortality within 30 days.

      a. It is unknown if much of the morbidity and mortality is due to the primary effect of the ICH or the secondary inflammatory responses to blood degradation products, microglial infiltration, and cerebral edema.

      b. Hematoma volume at presentation is currently the best predictor of clinical outcome.

   3. Longstanding hypertension is the most common cause of ICH (about 50%).

      a. Hypertensive ICH is thought to arise mainly from lenticulostriate arteries, which stem from the major cerebral vessels but, unlike the larger vessels, do not benefit from cerebral autoregulation of blood pressure. Pathological changes can include liophyalinosis of small arterioles and microaneurysms of perforating arteries (Charcot-Bouchard aneurysms).

      b. Hypertensive ICH occurs mainly in deep brain structures such as the basal ganglia (especially putamen), thalamus, pons, and cerebellum.

   4. Anticoagulants, including the new oral anticoagulants (NOACs), and pathological processes such as cerebral amyloid angiopathy (lobar hemorrhage, often recurrent) and blood vessel malformations account for most of the remaining ICH etiologies. Statin use has also recently been implicated as a potential risk factor in the development of ICH.

Common Etiologies of Primary and Secondary Intracerebral Hemorrhage

ETIOLOGY OF ICH	GENERAL LOCATION/SIZE OF ICH	UNDERLYING PATHOLOGY	% OF ICH PATIENTS
Hypertensive (primary)	Basal ganglia, thalamus, cerebellum, and pons (generally <20–30 cc)	High pressure within vessels without cerebral autoregulation leads to smooth muscle cell proliferation, eventual smooth muscle cell death	Up to 50%
Cerebral amyloid angiopathy (primary)	Superficial, lobar (generally >30 cc)	Amyloid deposition within the parenchymal cortical vessels	Up to 25% (especially in elderly)
Anticoagulation related (secondary)	Varies, may see a fluid level on CT (separation of plasma and sedimented blood)	Coagulopathy	10%–20%

(continued)

Common Etiologies of Primary and Secondary Intracerebral Hemorrhage (continued)

ETIOLOGY OF ICH	GENERAL LOCATION/SIZE OF ICH	UNDERLYING PATHOLOGY	% OF ICH PATIENTS
Arteriovenous malformation (secondary)	Varies, can include all areas of the central nervous system (CNS), including the spine	Abnormal "direct" connection between cerebral artery and cerebral vein, appearing as tangles of arteries and veins that develop during embryonic/fetal development	<5% (especially in young)
Cavernous malformation (secondary)	White matter	Abnormal sinusoidal vessels carrying high pressure, which tend to leak and eventually rupture	<10%
Neoplasm related (secondary)	Gray–white junction, generally with vasogenic edema	Melanoma and renal cell carcinoma (more common) thyroid carcinoma, choriocarcinoma (less common)	<10%

Abbreviation: ICH, intracerebral hemorrhage.

B. **ICH expansion**

1. Nearly half of all ICHs will expand in size from initial presentation within the first few hours, and most if not all of these patients should be monitored in an appropriate ICU.

2. Hematoma expansion generally stabilizes within 24 hours and is more often observed in **hypertensive patients** and in patients with **poorly controlled diabetes**.

3. Antiplatelet use has **not** been shown to the increase risk for ICH expansion, and evidence for platelet transfusion in patients who have been using antiplatelet medications is currently lacking.

4. CT angiogram in the acute setting may be helpful in identifying a bleeding source ("**spot sign**"), which, if found, is a relatively strong predictor of hematoma expansion.

C. **Supportive treatment of ICH**

1. Intubation for rapidly declining neurological status or a Glasgow Coma Scale (GCS) score of less than 8

   a. For large hemorrhages, controlled hyperventilation to a partial pressure of carbon dioxide (PCO_2) of 25 to 30 mmHg for short periods of time may be beneficial.

2. Maintenance of **euvolemia**

3. Close glucose monitoring and electrolyte normalization

4. Prevention of deep venous thrombosis (DVT) with subcutaneous heparinoids (generally started 24–48 hours following ICH ictus) and compression stockings

5. Management of cardiopulmonary effects of ICH, including neurogenic pulmonary edema, troponin leak due to myocardial infarction, and stunned myocardium

C. **Supportive treatment of ICH** (*cont'd*)

6. Treatment of seizure disorder secondary to ICH

7. ICP monitoring (especially in patients with GCS <8) with intra-parenchymal or external ventricular device placement for patients with hydrocephalus and declining mental status; goal of ICP less than 20 mmHg and cerebral perfusion pressure (CPP) less than 50 mmHg

8. The use of tissue-dehydrating agents: *mannitol* (with osmolality kept between 295 and 305 mOsm/L and Na at 145–150 mEq), or hypertonic saline (generally 2% or 3%) for tissue swelling or impending herniation

9. Management of ICH-related fever

D. **Adjunctive treatments for ICH: in addition to the supportive treatment for ICH, there is increasing evidence that adjunctive therapies for ICH may be beneficial for patients with certain conditions.**

1. **Anti-epileptic medications/drugs**

   a. Clinical seizures are common after ICH (10%–30%).

   b. Continuous EEG monitoring may be beneficial in patients with fluctuating or depressed neurological exam.

   c. AEDs are controversially used for seizure prophylaxis as clinical studies have shown **limited benefit** and some observational studies have shown **worsened outcomes** with phenytoin.

   d. AEDs should **only be prescribed** for clinical or electrographic seizures due to ICH. The duration of AED therapy should be readdressed after the acute phase of ICH.

2. **Anticoagulant reversal**

   a. *Vitamin K antagonist*: warfarin

      i. **Fresh frozen plasma** and **intravenous vitamin K** are the current mainstay of therapy for warfarin-related ICH because they are effective in normalizing the prothrombin time/international normalized ratio (PT/INR). **Prothrombin complex concentrates** (PCCs) are becoming increasingly common because they have stronger therapeutic efficacy and faster effect; however, they are costly, and no difference in clinical outcomes have been proven.

   b. *Factor Xa inhibitors*: rivaroxaban, apixaban, edoxaban

      i. **Andexanet alfa** (rivaroxaban, apixaban, edoxaban antidote) is a therapeutic option that is currently being studied for the more immediate reversal of the Xa inhibitor NOACs. Dialysis, fresh frozen plasma, 4-factor prothrombin complex, anti-inhibitor coagulant complex (FEIBA), and cryoprecipitate have also been hypothesized to be beneficial in symptomatic hemorrhages.

   c. *Direct thrombin inhibitor*: dabigatran

      i. **Idarucizumab** (dabigatran antidote) has been shown in a recent study to reverse the activity of dabigatran and underwent fast-track approval by the U.S. Food and Drug Administration (FDA) for clinical use.

   d. *Antithrombin III activator/Xa inhibitor*: heparin, enoxaparin

      i. **Protamine sulfate** dosed at 1.0 to 1.5 mg per 100 IU of heparin (or per 1 mg of enoxaparin) if it can be dosed within the first 30 minutes since the cessation of heparin to a maximum of 50 mg protamine sulfate

ii. **Protamine sulfate** dosed at 0.5 to 0.75 mg per 100 IU of heparin (or per 1 mg of enoxaparin) if it can be dosed from 30 minutes to 1 hour after heparin cessation

3. **Aggressive blood pressure control**

   a. Initially a more debated topic, aggressive BP control was considered the mainstay of ICH therapy because it was thought to limit hematoma expansion and end-organ damage.

   b. Recently some evidence suggested that aggressive BP control may lead to increased hematoma expansion due to bleeding into peri-hematomal cerebral ischemia.

   c. Recent studies show that patients radiologically appear better with more aggressive BP lowering (SBP <140); however, further studies are ongoing to evaluate clinical outcomes.

4. **Surgical management of ICH**

   a. The surgical trial in ICH (STICH) failed to show benefit of surgical hematoma evacuation for supratentorial bleeds. There were some analyses showing that superficial cortical hemorrhages may benefit from surgery more than deeper ICHs.

   b. Catheter-based studies infusing tPA into the hemorrhage with clot aspiration have shown some outcome benefit.

   c. Surgical management is recommended for infratentorial ICH if larger than 3 cm to reduce morbidity and mortality.

   d. Patients suffering ICH with intraventricular component may benefit from tPA instillation via intraventricular catheter, although data for this are still being analyzed.

   e. The efficacy of endoscopic (minimally invasive) resection of blood products from ICH currently is being studied.

   f. Iron chelation from ICH-related blood currently is being studied.

E. **ICH scoring**

ELEMENT	SCORING
GCS	13–15 (0); 5–12 (1); 3–4 (2)
Age	<80 (0) ; > or = 80 (1)
Infratentorial	No (0) ; Yes (1)
Volume	<30 cc (0); >30 cc (1)
Intraventricular Blood	No (0) ; Yes (1)

Mortality by Score 1 (13%), 2 (26%), 3 (72%), 4 (97%), 5 (>99%), 6 (>99%)

F. **Diagnosing ICH etiology**

1. ICH and ICH stability are easily diagnosed on **plain head CT**.

2. CT angiogram can be used to determine if there is a "spot sign" (active extravasation), which is a strong predictor of hematoma expansion.

3. All patients with ICH under the age of 40 and/or without evidence of hypertension should undergo diagnostic digital subtraction angiography for detection of vessel abnormality (arteriovenous malformation [AVM], dural venous fistula, etc.).

F. **Diagnosing ICH etiology** (*cont'd*)

4. MRI should be completed on most patients with ICH to further clarify etiology utilizing gradient echo (GRE), T1 and T2 sequences.

   a. Cavernomas have a characteristic "popcorn" appearance on T2 sequences (low intensity on T2WI and GRE [hemosiderin] surrounding various circumscribed regions of hemorrhage [hyperintense on T1WI because of the presence of methemoglobin])

   b. Cerebral amyloid angiopathy shows up with numerous microbleeds as "Swiss-cheese brain" on gradient-echo or susceptibility weighted imaging.

   c. Tumors generally show up as contrast-enhancing lesions on post-contrast T1 imaging.

   d. Blood aging can also be better determined by MRI sequences:

	T1	T2
Hyperacute 0–24 hours (oxyhemoglobin)	Isointense	Hyperintense (bright)
Acute 1–3 days (deoxyhemoglobin)	Isointense	Hypointense (dark)
Early subacute 3–7 days (methemoglobin)	Hyperintense (bright)	Hypointense (dark)
Late subacute 7–30 days (extracellular methemoglobin)	Hyperintense (bright)	Hyperintense (bright)
Chronic >30 days (hemosiderin)	Hypointense (dark)	Hypointense (dark)

III. Critical Care Management of Subarachnoid Hemorrhage and Delayed Cerebral Ischemia

A. **General principles of unruptured intracranial aneurysms and subarachnoid hemorrhage:**

1. Subarachnoid hemorrhage (SAH) is a neurological disorder that is caused by the rupture of a cerebral artery, causing blood to collect in the subarachnoid space.

2. **Trauma** is the most common cause of SAH.

3. Up to 80% of nontraumatic SAH is caused by intracranial saccular aneurysm rupture, making it the most common cause of nontraumatic SAH.

4. About 2% of the general population harbors an unruptured intracranial aneurysm, and aneurysmal SAH occurs at an estimated rate of 6 to 16 per 100,000 population (30,000 people in the United States suffer an SAH annually).

5. Screening is recommended for family members with two or more first-degree relatives with history of SAH or brain aneurysm.

6. Common sites of aneurysm include:

   a. Anterior communicating artery (30%–40%),

   b. Internal carotid artery (30% including all cavernous and supraclinoid segment aneurysms),

   c. Middle cerebral artery (20%–30%)

   d. Vertebrobasilar arteries (10%).

7. Aneurysms occur more frequently in females (3:1)

8. Other risk factors associated with aneurysm formation include:

   a. Cigarette smoking

   b. Hypertension

   c. Age

   d. Inherited genetic conditions

      i. Autosomal dominant polycystic kidney disease

      ii. Vascular type Ehlers-Danlos syndrome

      iii. Hereditary hemorrhagic telangiectasia

      iv. Pseudoxanthoma elasticum

9. Aneurysm rupture risk is related to size, with larger aneurysms predicting a higher risk of rupture. Posterior circulation and posterior communicating aneurysms potentially are associated with a higher risk of rupture compared to anterior circulation aneurysms.

10. There is a high mortality rate (>30%) in the field on initial bleed. Of the patients who survive the ictal bleed, about one-third die in the hospital, one-third live with significant disability, and one-third recover with little disability.

11. One of the major complications that arises generally between 4 and 12 days post-SAH is **delayed cerebral ischemia** (DCI), which is the development of a secondary stroke or neurological deficit. DCI is the cause of nearly half of the disability and death in patients hospitalized for SAH.

   a. DCI has been rarely reported earlier than 3 days and later than 21 days post-SAH.

   b. **Transcranial Doppler** has been a standard monitoring modality to assess cerebral artery vasospasm, which is commonly thought to be associated with and potentially causative of DCI.

   c. It is important to note, however, that DCI and cerebral artery vasospasm are **independent entities** that occur after SAH, and **one may happen without the other**.

   d. Aneurysmal rupture is commonly associated with DCI, whereas traumatic SAH is less often associated with complications of DCI.

B. **Grading of subarachnoid hemorrhage**

GRADE	HUNT AND HESS CLASSIFICATION
Grade I	Asymptomatic or with slight headache
Grade II	Moderate to severe headache, nuchal rigidity, no focal or lateralizing signs
Grade III	Drowsy, confusion, mild focal deficit
Grade IV	Persistent stupor, semicoma, early decerebrate rigidity
Grade V	Deep coma and decerebrate rigidity

B. Grading of subarachnoid hemorrhage (*cont'd*)

GRADE	MODIFIED FISHER SCALE
Grade 0	No subarachnoid or intraventricular blood noted on CT scan
Grade I	Thin subarachnoid blood with no intraventricular component
Grade II	Thin subarachnoid blood with intraventricular component
Grade III	Thick subarachnoid blood with no intraventricular component
Grade IV	Thick subarachnoid blood with intraventricular component

C. Management of cerebral arterial vasospasm:

- Post-SAH vasospasm is specifically defined as symptomatic or asymptomatic delayed narrowing of the large cerebral arteries that is associated with clinical or radiographic signs of ischemia following a SAH.

- It is commonly found in patients generally 3 to 7 days following SAH, and the gold standard imaging modality for workup is the **digital subtraction (catheter) angiography**. However, monitoring is also done noninvasively (transcranial Doppler [TCD], CT angiography [CTA]/ CT perfusion [CTP], electroencephalogram, etc.).

1. **TCD monitoring:** very common, noninvasive technique to assess for vasospasm. Very specific but variable sensitivity for vasospasm and is proceduralist dependent. Important numbers indicating possible vasospasm:

    a. **Velocity >200 cm/s (severe in middle cerebral artery [MCA])**

    b. **Rapid rise between serial TCD measurements (>50 cm/s)**

    c. High ratio of MCA velocity to ipsilateral extracranial internal carotid artery (ICA) (Lindegaard Index)

    d. Cannot complete if thickened temporal bones

    e. Like other ultrasound studies, visualization is highly operator dependent.

2. **CTA/CTP:** Is moderately sensitive (>70%), very specific (>90%)

    a. Requires iodinated dye load and CT radiation

    b. Overcomes anatomical limitations of TCD

3. **Catheter angiogram**

    a. Gold standard, most invasive, requires iodinated dye load

    b. Confirm diagnosis of vasospasm

    c. Can offer endovascular therapy (intra-arterial [IA] vasodilators such as verapamil, nicardipine, or balloon angioplasty) for treatment of vasospasm

4. **Emerging adjunct ("multi-modality") monitoring for DCI in SAH patients:** includes electroencephalogram, brain tissue oximetry, microdialysis, near-infrared spectroscopy, thermal diffusion flowmetry

D. **Routine screening and management of high risk DCI in SAH patients in the critical care unit**

1. There are several clinical signs and symptoms that can lead a clinician to suspect DCI:

    a. The presence of a new neurological deficit on clinical exam

    b. A sudden increase in BP

    c. An increasing level of velocities on TCD (or increased ratio)

    d. New strokes on imaging

2. The following are some techniques that can help in the screening of DCI in the SAH patient:

    a. TCD every day for at least 14 days

    b. Frequent neurological checks (every 2 hours to every 4 hours)

    c. Consideration of multi-modality monitoring (see Section III.C.4)

3. **"Triple-H" therapy**: Many neurological ICUs employ the use of triple-H therapy in the treatment and prophylaxis of DCI. There is relatively weak evidence for this particular therapeutic approach, however. After the aneurysm is secured, the main goal is to **maintain cerebral perfusion**. Triple-H therapy employs the following:

    a. "Hemodilution"—theoretically improves rheology to increase brain tissue oxygen perfusion. However, studies have **not** shown that a lower hemoglobin (Hgb) is beneficial. Anemia is also associated with poorer outcomes in SAH patients. A **target Hgb of 8 g/dl to 10 g/dl** is considered by expert opinion to be most beneficial; however, increased phlebotomy to drop hemoglobin is not advised.

    b. "Hypertension"–permissive/induced (unless heart failure, myocardial infarct, etc.): in patients with DCI, can trial **induced hypertension** to a **MAP 10% above baseline** with fluid boluses, or to symptom resolution. If there is improvement, can consider norepinephrine or phenylephrine or other medication for the hemodynamic augmentation of BP.

    c. "Hypervolemia" (volume expansion)—goal is ideally for **euvolemia** with the avoidance of intravascular volume depletion. Hypervolemia has **not** shown improved outcomes. Fluid balance should be closely monitored, and routine placement of pulmonary artery catheters or other invasive methods should be avoided unless the balance is difficult to ascertain.

4. **Angioplasty/IA therapy**: patients who are refractory to or are unable to tolerate the previously discussed medical therapies should be considered for **endovascular spasmolytic therapies**. These therapies (usually angioplasty or IA calcium channel blocker) should be directed only at vessels that are thought to be causing clinical deficit.

5. **Nimodipine in the SAH patient**: nimodipine was initially used for its calcium-channel-blocking properties because the mechanism of vasospasm was thought to begin with cerebral smooth muscle contraction. SAH patients, however, had improved outcomes with nimodipine, but not with other calcium channel blockers, and patients receiving oral nimodipine continued to show angiographic vasospasm. The improved outcomes related to oral nimodipine are now thought to be possibly secondary to **protective effects on the neurovascular unit**. Additionally, due to its continued benefit seen in multiple large randomized studies, oral or nasogastric **nimodipine is strongly recommended** (level I-A) in post-aneurysmal SAH patients for 21 days. If the patient's BP does not tolerate a dose of 60 mg of nimodipine every 4 hours (i.e., not able to meet physiological or physician set MAP goals), a dose of 30 mg every 2 hours may be trialed.

IV. Other Intracranial Vascular Malformations

A. Arteriovenous malformations

1. Consists of multiple arteries and veins, connecting at a nidus without an intervening normal capillary bed. Pathogenesis is not well understood, but they are considered sporadic congenital developmental vascular lesions

2. Brain AVMs occur in about 0.1% of the population (one-tenth the incidence of intracranial aneurysms) Supratentorial lesions account for 90% of brain AVMs, and the remainder are in the posterior fossa. They usually occur as single lesions, but as many as 9% are multiple.

A. **Arteriovenous malformations** (*cont'd*)

   3. Brain AVMs usually present between the ages of 10 and 40 years, with ICH, seizure, headache, or focal neurologic deficits. Hemorrhage is the most common presentation, particularly in children.

   4. Overall, annual hemorrhage rates from brain AVMs are between 2% and 3%. After an initial hemorrhage, annual hemorrhage rates are approximately 6% to 17% in the first year, but then decrease.

   5. Diagnosis can be made by CT or MRI. MRI is more sensitive, particularly in the setting of an acute ICH. Digital subtraction angiography (DSA) is the gold standard for the diagnosis, treatment planning, and follow-up after treatment of brain AVMs

   6. Important considerations in the decision to treat and the choice of treatment are age, lesion size and location, and prior history of intracerebral hemorrhage.

   7. Surgery is the mainstay of treatment; radiosurgery is a useful option in lesions deemed at high risk for surgical therapy, and endovascular embolization can be a useful adjunct to these techniques.

B. **Cavernous malformations**

   1. Cavernomas are thin-walled dilated capillaries with a simple endothelial lining.

   2. May occur as a sporadic or familial condition

   3. Three genetic loci (CCM1, CCM2, and CCM3) responsible for familial cavernous malformations have been reported. Nearly all familial cases of cerebral cavernous malformation among Hispanic Americans have been linked to a founder mutation of CCM1 localized to 7q (**KRIT1 gene**)

   4. They can occur throughout the brain but are most common in the subcortical Rolandic and temporal areas.

   5. Clinical presentation can include hemorrhage, seizures, and/or progressive neurologic deficits. Annual bleeding rates are up to 1% per year for supratentorial lesions and up to 3% per year for brainstem lesions.

   6. Cavernous malformations are typically identified on MRI ("popcorn-like lesions") and are often angiographically occult.

   7. Asymptomatic cavernous malformations are followed without intervention. Surgical resection may be indicated for progressive neurologic deficits, intractable epilepsy, and/or hemorrhage. Stereotactic radiosurgery is an option for nonoperable lesions.

C. **Developmental venous anomaly**

   1. Developmental venous anomalies (DVAs) or venous angiomas are the most common congenital vascular malformation and consist of radially arranged medullary veins.

   2. Usually diagnosed as an incidental finding on MRI, DVAs are usually supratentorial and solitary but can be multiple and occur with cavernous malformations.

   3. DVAs rarely present with seizures or hemorrhage. Most patients are followed without intervention. Surgery is rarely required for hemorrhage or intractable epilepsy.

D. **Capillary telangiectasia**

   1. Small lesions that are usually found incidentally on MRI, in the pons, middle cerebellar peduncles, and dentate nuclei.

   2. Multiple lesions are common. They are not associated with morbidity, and intervention is not required.

V. The Critical Care Management of Status Epilepticus

A. General principles of status epilepticus

1. Status epilepticus (SE) is a major neurological emergency that, similar to stroke, should be managed in a very timely manner.

2. The official definition of SE is in a controversial state; however, most neurologists agree that SE is a serious condition characterized by **the presence of electrographic seizures with more than 30 minutes of uncontrolled seizure activity.**

3. As the duration of seizures increases, so does the number of neurons lost, and the likelihood of a successful treatment decreases.

4. If true seizure activity occurs for longer than 5 to 10 minutes, the likelihood of cessation of activity is unlikely without intervention.

5. Convulsive SE is seemingly more serious because there are a number of body systems involved; however, increasing evidence is showing that nonconvulsive SE may also necessitate early treatment, as some neuronal loss due to SE may be irreversible.

6. **The strongest predictor of outcome is cause and duration of the SE.**

7. **Mortality is 10% to 20% in SE, and up to 32% in refractory cases.**

B. Continuous EEG (cEEG) monitoring

1. EEG has been used in medical ICUs for decades to assess for nonconvulsive seizures in the comatose population and to further clarify alterations in mental status.

2. Technological improvements have allowed for the use of cEEG monitoring in the hospital. As the number of patients on cEEG monitoring increased, so did the detection of subclinical seizure activity.

3. The incidence of seizures in the neurological ICU patient population has been found to be roughly around 30%.

C. Common types of status epilepticus treated in the neurological ICU setting

1. **Generalized convulsive status epilepticus (GCSE):** continuous seizure activity associated with generalized tonic-clonic convulsions for an indefinite amount of time; tends to increase lactate and creatine kinase levels in the blood, and can elevate whole body temperature, which all can lead to further complications.

2. **Nonconvulsive status epilepticus (NCSE):** continuous seizure activity, most often noted on EEG record, without typical manifestations of motor activity as in GCSE; generally presents as an altered mental state

3. **Simple-partial status epilepticus:** Also known as epilepsy partialis continua (EPC), an electrographic phenomenon that can cause motor or sensory symptoms or alteration in mental status, or a combination of symptoms generally lateralized and/or localized to a certain brain area without spread to other brain regions. Because of their localization, these seizures generally do not affect awareness.

D. Managing SE in the ICU

1. Treatment initiation of SE in an expeditious manner is of utmost importance to improve outcomes.

2. Often the ABC (airway, breathing, circulation) method of therapy is indicated for SE patients upon arrival to secure the patient's airway and to provide immediate supportive care.

D. **Managing SE in the ICU** (*cont'd*)

   3. The management of SE in the ICU centers on stopping the electrographic seizures and determining etiology while avoiding complications and preventing recurrence.

     a. **Acute seizure management**

       i. **Imaging** should be completed as soon as possible, and a cEEG monitor should be placed on the patient immediately upon the suspicion of SE.

       ii. Initially **benzodiazepines** (IV lorazepam, IM midazolam, PR diazepam) are most useful as first-line pharmacological abortive therapies.

       iii. The clinician should be prepared to infuse **fosphenytoin** (fPHT) or **valproic acid** (VA) within the first few minutes if the seizures are refractory to benzodiazepine therapy.

       iv. Levetiracetam (LEV) and lacosamide (LCM) can be considered for abortive therapy; however, evidence for their use is currently lacking.

       v. Should the SE be refractory to fPHT or VA, consideration for anesthetic doses of **propofol, phenobarbital,** or **midazolam** should be made (mainly in cases of NCSE and GCSE).

       vi. **Pentobarbital** should be reserved for refractory cases.

       vii. Ketamine is also being researched as an SE abortive therapy.

     b. **Complication management**

       i. Patients with SE may be hypertensive; however, hypertension in the acute setting of SE rarely needs to be treated because anti-epileptic medications generally cause a drop in blood pressure.

       ii. The rise in creatine kinase and **rhabdomyolysis,** however, pose a threat to other organ systems and should be monitored.

       iii. Other ICU complications such as DVT, ventilator-associated pneumonia, catheter-associated urinary tract infection, and bloodstream infection should be monitored and treated accordingly.

       iv. Propofol-related infusion syndrome (PRIS) is a life-threatening condition characterized by acute refractory bradycardia progressing to asystole and one or more of the following: (1) metabolic acidosis, (2) rhabdomyolysis, (3) hyperlipidemia, (4) enlarged or fatty liver. Large dose for a long time ($>$4 mg/kg/hr for 48 hours) is a risk factor.

     c. **Etiology management:** the etiology of SE should be ascertained as soon as the seizure management algorithm is completed. The following SE etiologies are more commonly seen in the neurological critical care setting:

       i. **Bacterial meningitis:** treated with empiric antibiotics followed by de-escalated antibiotic therapy based on cultures. Steroid management can help, but its use is controversial. Continuation of AED is important while treating the underlying bacterial infection.

       ii. **Ethyl alcohol (ETOH) withdrawal:** generally seen no earlier than 24 to 48 hours since the last alcoholic drink; treat promptly with **benzodiazepine** or barbiturate agent. Phenytoin has not been shown to be very efficacious for ETOH withdrawal seizures.

       iii. **Viral meningitis/encephalitis:** generally secondary to Herpes simplex virus (HSV); treat with acyclovir and standard generalized anti-epileptic medications.

       iv. **Autoimmune encephalitis:** There are a number of autoimmune etiologies to SE (both paraneoplastic and idiopathic). Among them are limbic encephalitis and autoimmune encephalitis. Treatment is related to immune suppression combined with plasmapheresis and/or intravenous immunoglobulin therapy and steroids in addition to escalated anti-epileptic medication therapy. There is no current standard therapy for autoimmune-related encephalitis.

VI. Brain Herniation

A. Herniation syndromes

	PARENCHYMAL SHIFT	COMPLICATIONS OF HERNIATION SYNDROME	CHARACTERISTIC SYMPTOMS
Uncal herniation (supratentorial)	Medial temporal lobe (uncus) gets displaced into the midbrain region	Sudden blockage of parasympathetic input to the eye followed by efferent fibers from cranial nerve (CN) III **Kernohan's notch phenomenon (false-localizing) is a result of the compression of the contralateral cerebral peduncle against the tentorium cerebelli due to uncal herniation Left untreated, can also lead to ipsilateral **posterior cerebral artery** territory infarction due to its proximity to the artery	**Pupil dilation** ("**blown pupil**") followed by CN III palsy Hemiparesis ipsilateral to side of lesion (contralateral to Kernohan's notch) Cortical blindness
Subfalcine herniation (supratentorial)	Caused by brain parenchyma (most commonly the cingulate gyrus) being displaced laterally into the falx cerebri	Can cause minor to major compression of the reticular activation system May cause compression of the **anterior cerebral** and/or middle cerebral arteries, leading to ischemia A precursor to other herniation syndromes	Can cause alteration of mental status and **drowsiness**
Central herniation (transtentorial herniation)	The diencephalon and medial temporal lobes are displaced downward into and sometimes through the tentorium	Stretch and shearing of basilar pontine perforators can lead to fatal hemorrhages (Duret hemorrhages)	Downward herniation leads to upward gaze palsy and resultant downward gaze "**sunsetting eyes**"
Transcalvarial herniation	Herniation of brain parenchyma through a surgical, trauma-related, or other skull defect	Can lead to damage of the brain that is herniating through the skull defect	Symptomatology is related to the region of brain that is herniating
Tonsillar herniation	Herniation of cerebellar tissue downward through the foramen magnum	Causes compression of the lower brainstem (medulla, lower pons)	Sudden respiratory abnormalities (including apnea) with unstable vital signs, dysregulated blood pressure and heart rate ("**Cushing's triad**")

B. **"Neuro coding"**: The immediate treatment of herniation syndromes and/or high ICP through the use of the following:

1. Hypertonic saline

   a. 23.4% saline "bullet" (central line only)

   b. 3% saline bolus (central line only)

   c. 2% saline bolus (peripheral or central line)

2. Mannitol push (0.5– 1g/kg)

3. Hyperventilation

4. Elevation of the head of the bed

5. Pentobarbital or propofol

VII. Coma and Brain Death

A. **Coma:** There are some subtle semantic differences in the exact definition of coma; however, most describe a coma as a profound **unarousable** state of **unresponsiveness** and **unconsciousness** with little or no response to pain, voice, or other external stimulation and no spontaneous eye opening.

1. As such, the Glasgow Coma Scale (GCS) and the Full Outline of UnResponsiveness (FOUR) score were created to assess the level of responsiveness and awareness.

2. Etiologies for coma include severe bilateral hemispheric brain damage, injury to vital areas of the reticular activation system (brainstem, basal forebrain, thalamus and hypothalamus), and metabolic, septic, or drug effect.

3. It is important to note that **arousal** requires an **intact brainstem and subcortical function,** whereas **awareness** requires an **intact cerebral cortex.**

4. Management of coma requires standard airway, breathing, and circulation supportive therapy while determining etiology and the potential for reversibility.

5. FOUR score

PATTERN	SCORING
Eye response	4—Eyelids open, tracking or blinking 3—Eyelids open, but not tracking 2—Eyelids closed, but opens to loud voice 1—Eyelids closed, but opens to pain 0—Eyelids closed, even with pain
Motor response	4—Thumb's up, fist, or peace sign to command 3—Localizing to pain 2—Flexion to pain 1—Extension to pain 0—No movement to pain or generalized myoclonus status
Brainstem reflexes	4—Pupil and corneal reflexes present 3—One pupil wide and fixed 2—Pupil or corneal reflex absent 1—Pupil and corneal reflex absent 0—Absent pupil, corneal, and cough reflex
Respiration	4—Not intubated, regular breathing pattern 3—Not intubated, Cheyne-Stokes breathing pattern 2—Not intubated, irregular breathing pattern 1—Intubated, breathes above ventilator rate 0—Intubated, breathes at ventilator rate or apnea

6. Glasgow Coma Scale

Eye opening	Spontaneous	4
	To voice	3
	To pain	2
	None	1
Best motor response	Obeys commands	6
	Localizes pain	5
	Withdraws to pain	4
	Flexor posturing	3
	Extensor posturing	2
	None	1
Best verbal response	Conversant and oriented	5
	Conversant and disoriented	4
	Inappropriate words	3
	Incomprehensible words	2
	None	1

7. Respiratory patterns associated with coma

PATTERN	DESCRIPTION	LOCATION
Cheyne-Stokes	Hyperpnea (in a crescendo-decrescendo pattern) followed by apnea	Bilateral diencephalon or cerebrum
Central neurogenic hyperventilation	Regular, rapid, deep hyperpnea	Brainstem tegmentum
Apneustic	Hyperpnea pauses at full inspiration	Pons
Ataxic	Irregular rate and depth of respiration	Medullary reticular formation

8. Pupillary clues in the comatose state

DESCRIPTION	LESION
Small and reactive	Diencephalon
Ipsilateral pupillary constriction	Hypothalamus
Pinpoint but still reactive	Pons
Large and fixed	Tectum
Midposition and fixed	Midbrain
Dilated and fixed	Uncal herniation

B. **Brain death**

1. The difference between coma and brain death is that brain death is characterized by the total **irreversible loss** of all brain function to sustain life.

2. The term serves as a second legal declaration of death, the only other currently being cardiac death. Certain conditions must be met to make the declaration of death by neurological criterion:

   a. The cause must be known and must be irreversible.

   b. There must be no severe overlying medical condition (electrolytes, acid/base disturbances, endocrine abnormalities).

   c. There must be no drug intoxication or poisoning.

   d. The core temperature of the patient must be at least 90°F (32°C).

   e. There should be no recent administration or continued presence of neuromuscular blocking agents.

3. The neurological examination must demonstrate the following:

   a. The patient must be completely unresponsive (no motor response to pain).

   b. The patient must exhibit complete loss of brainstem reflexes.

      i. No pupillary response to light

      ii. No oculocephalic reflex (doll's eyes maneuver)

      iii. No caloric vestibular reflex ("**cold calorics**"): using 50 mL of cold water, instill water for 1 minute into each ear and allow for at least 5 minutes between ears. Eyes should turn slowly **toward** the ear being stimulated in the patient with intact reflexes.

      iv. No corneal reflex; no grimacing to pain

      v. No gag reflex; no cough or bradycardia with suction

   c. The patient must not be spontaneously breathing. To test for spontaneous breathing, an **apnea test** may be completed as follows:

      i. Patient's body temperature must be at least 97°F (36.5°C); systolic BP at least 90 mmHg; no diabetes insipidus or positive fluid balance in the past 6 hours.

      ii. Patient should be preoxygenated to achieve a PO_2 of at least 200 and PCO_2 of at least 40 or lower. Cannulated 100% oxygen can be delivered down the endotracheal tube to provide oxygenation.

      iii. The ventilator should be disconnected once the previous steps are complete. Patient will pass the apnea test (not deemed brain dead) if there are any respiratory movements. The apnea test should be stopped if the systolic BP drop to less than 90 mmHg, if the PO_2 significantly decreases, or there is SpO_2 desaturation or cardiac arrhythmia.

      iv. Serial arterial blood gases should be drawn while ventilator is disconnected: test is *positive for brain death* (patient fails apnea test) if **PCO_2 rises to 60 mmHg** or there is a **20-mmHg increase over baseline**; generally should not take longer than 8 minutes.

4. If the patient meets all of the previous criteria, generally on two separate occasions at least 6 hours apart, patient meets the legal definition of death by neurological criteria posed by most states. The apnea test only needs to be completed once over the two occasions. There are several confirmatory tests that can assist with the clinical examination if there is uncertainty of brain death:

   a. **Digital subtraction angiography** can be done, which in the brain-dead patient will demonstrate no filling above the level of carotid bifurcation (internal carotid artery), the intracranial vertebral arteries, or the circle of Willis.

   b. **Electroencephalography**: Brain death is indicated by electro-cerebral silence noted with **no EEG activity over 2 uV when recording from scalp electrode** pairs 10 cm or more apart with interelectrode impedances between 100 and 10,000 Ω. A minimum of eight electrodes is necessary. There should also be no electroencephalographic reactivity to somatosensory or audiovisual stimuli.

c. **Transcranial Doppler ultrasound**: total cerebral circulatory arrest will be seen in the patient with brain death. This will be indicated by a lack of diastolic flow and small sharp systolic peaks in early systole. Sensitivity is greater than 95% and specificity is 100% for brain death.

d. **Technetium 99 hexamethylpropyleneamine oxime brain scan**: this test is very sensitive and specific. It will show no radiotracer uptake within the cerebral vessels or parenchyma in the brain-dead patient.

e. **Somatosensory evoked potentials**: no response of N20 to P22, indicating a lack of communication between the body and the cortex.

CHEAT SHEET

ICH most common cause	Chronic hypertension
Hypertensive ICH locations	Basal ganglia (Putamen), thalamus, pons, cerebellum
Amyloid angiopathy ICH	Lobar, recurrent, microbleeds on GRE
Metastasis ICH	Melanoma, renal cell most common; at gray–white junction
SAH most common cause	Trauma, saccular aneurysm rupture for spontaneous
Cavernous malformations	"Popcorn" appearance on T2-weighted imaging, KRIT 1 gene
Status epilepticus	Cause and duration most important predictors of outcome
Uncal herniation	Parasympathetic oculomotor nerve palsy, Kernohan's notch, posterior cerebral artery (PCA) stroke
Subfalcine herniation	Anterior cerebral artery (ACA) stroke
Central herniation	Duret's hemorrhage
Tonsillar herniation	Cushing's triad

CHAPTER 8

Dementia

I. Definitions

A. **Delirium:** an acute confusional state, marked by decreased attention and prominent alterations in perception and consciousness and associated with vivid hallucinations, delusions, heightened alertness, and agitation; hyperactivity of psychomotor and autonomic functions; insomnia; and so forth. Symptoms often fluctuate. A hypoactive form may also be seen.

B. **Dementia:** a syndrome characterized by a progressive deterioration of function in memory, plus two other cognitive domains (e.g., executive functioning, praxis, language, visuospatial function, etc.) compared to previous baseline cognitive ability, and severe enough to interfere with usual social functioning and activities of daily life. Defined as longer than 12 months in progression. Less than 12 months in progression is known as rapidly progressive dementia.

C. **Mild cognitive impairment (MCI):** progressive cognitive impairment, in memory or other cognitive domains, not sufficient to cause significant impairment in activities of daily living. Can be separated into amnestic and nonamnestic forms. No specific pathological correlation. Not all patients with MCI progress to dementia; some return to normal cognition.

II. Dementia

A. **Etiologies of dementia.** NB: The most common types of dementia are Alzheimer's dementia (AD), vascular dementia, Lewy body dementia, and frontotemporal dementia.

Trauma	Chronic traumatic encephalopathy
	Chronic subdural hematoma (subacutely progressive)
Inflammatory/ infection	Chronic meningitis (tuberculosis, cryptococcus, cysticercosis)
	Syphilis *(general paresis of the insane, gumma, vasculitic)*
	HIV dementia and opportunistic infections
	Progressive multifocal leukoencephalopathy (subacute, usually focal or multifocal)
	Creutzfeldt-Jakob disease (CJD) (subacute, often with other neurological deficits (visual, motor, somatosensory, etc.)
	Lyme disease
	Cerebral sarcoidosis
	Subacute sclerosing panencephalitis (SSPE)
	Whipple's disease of the brain

(continued)

A. Etiologies of dementia *(cont'd)*

Neoplastic	Benign and malignant tumors
	Paraneoplastic limbic encephalitis
Metabolic	Hypothyroid
	Vitamin B$_1$ deficiency *(Wernicke-Korsakoff) (acute to subacute)*
	Vitamin B$_{12}$ deficiency
	Vitamin E deficiency *(neuropathy, ataxia, encephalopathy)*
	Nicotinic acid (niacin or vitamin B$_3$) deficiency *(pellagra)*
	Uremia/dialysis dementia
	Chronic hepatic encephalopathy
	Chronic hypoglycemic encephalopathy
	Chronic hypercapnia/hyperviscosity/hypoxemia
	Chronic hypercalcemia/electrolyte imbalance
	Cushing's disease (usually behavior change or psychosis)
Vascular	Multi-infarct dementia
	Binswanger's encephalopathy
	Specific vascular syndromes (thalamic, inferotemporal, bifrontal) (post-acute)
	Triple border-zone watershed infarction (post-acute)
	Diffuse hypoxic/ischemic injury (post-acute)
	Mitochondrial disorders (e.g., mitochondrial encephalomyopathy with lactic acidosis and stroke-like episodes [MELAS])
	Cerebral autosomal dominant arteriopathy with subcortical infarcts and leukoencephalopathy (CADASIL)
Autoimmune	Systemic lupus erythematosus (lupus cerebritis)
	Polyarteritis nodosa
	Temporal arteritis
	Wegener's granulomatosis
	Isolated angiitis of the central nervous system Autoimmune dementia (dementia with autoantibody markers)
Drugs/toxins	Medications: β-blockers, neuroleptics, antidepressants, histamine receptor blockers, dopamine receptor blockers
	Substances of abuse: alcohol, phencyclidine, mescaline, marijuana psychosis, etc.
	Toxins: lead, mercury, arsenic
	Bismuth containing medications
Demyelinating	Multiple sclerosis, Schilder's disease, Baló concentric sclerosis (usually MRI is diagnostic)
	Electric injury-induced demyelination (circumstances diagnostic)
	Decompression sickness demyelination (circumstances diagnostic)
	Adrenoleukodystrophy

(continued)

	Metachromatic leukodystrophy
	Other inflammatory/infectious processes
Cerebrospinal fluid (CSF) processes	Normal pressure hydrocephalus
	Obstructive hydrocephalus
Degenerative— adult	Alzheimer's dementia (AD)
	Parkinson's disease (PD)
	Huntington's disease
	Frontotemporal dementia (also known as frontotemporal lobar degeneration or FTLD)
	Progressive supranuclear palsy (PSP)
	Dementia with Lewy bodies (DLB)
	Multiple system atrophy (MSA)
	Corticobasal (ganglionic) degeneration (CBD or CBGD)
	Hallervorden-Spatz disease (now known as pantothenate kinase-associated neurodegeneration [PKAN] or neurodegeneration with brain iron accumulation–1 [NBIA1])
	Primary progressive aphasia (PPA)
Degenerative— pediatric	Mitochondrial diseases (myoclonic epilepsy with ragged red fibers [MERRF] and mitochondrial encephalomyopathy with lactic acidosis and stroke-like episodes [MELAS])
	Adrenoleukodystrophy
	Metachromatic leukodystrophy
	Kufs' disease *(neuronal ceroid lipofuscinosis)*
	GM_1 and GM_2 gangliosidoses
	Niemann-Pick II-C
	Krabbe's disease *(globoid cell leukodystrophy)*
	Alexander's disease
	Lafora's disease
	Cerebrotendinous xanthomatosis

B. Diagnostic workup

Basic	Blood tests may include: complete blood count (CBC), comprehensive metabolic panel (CMP), thyroid function tests, vitamin B_{12} level, serum folate, erythrocyte sedimentation rate (ESR) Urinalysis, chest X-ray. Brain imaging: either computed tomography (CT) of the head or brain MRI (with contrast if suspecting an enhancing lesion)
Expanded	Brain MRI with gadolinium
	Spinal tap—cells, protein, glucose, fungus, tuberculosis, virus, cytology, oligoclonal banding, immunoglobulin G, 14-3-3, lactate
	Electroencephalography

(continued)

B. Diagnostic workup (*cont'd*)

Expanded	Neuropsychology assessment for executive function, language, processing speed, visuospatial function, memory (recall, registration)
	Toxin screen (drugs, poisons, metals)
	Labs for infection: HIV, syphilis, others
	Vitamins B_1, B_3, B_6, E
	Quantitative plasma amino acids (in children and young adults)
	Quantitative urine amino acids (in children and young adults)
	Vasculitis workup: C-reactive protein (CRP), anti–double-stranded DNA, Ro, La, Sm, ribonucleoprotein, antineutrophil cytoplasmic antibodies, C3, C4, CH50
	Tumor screen, paraneoplastic serum antibodies
	Consider CSF for a beta 42/total and phosphorylated tau (May be helpful in diagnosing Alzheimer's disease with biomarker; however, does not change management.)
If necessary	PET/single-photon emission computed tomography (SPECT)
	Consider amyloid PET imaging (for Alzheimer pathology; does not change treatment, may not be covered by insurance)
	Cerebral angiography for vasculitis (low sensitivity, specificity)
	Genetic counseling and testing for Alzheimer's dementia (AD), frontotemporal dementia (FTD) dominant gene markers
	Biopsy: brain, meninges, nerve, muscle, skin, liver, kidney (rarely necessary, often nondiagnostic)

C. Suggested evaluations for dementia of undetermined cause (rare causes)

Low-serum ceruloplasmin and copper, high-urine and liver copper	*Wilson's disease*
Plasma very-long-chain fatty acids	*Adrenoleukodystrophy*
White blood cell arylsulfatase A	*Metachromatic leukodystrophy*
Serum hexosaminidase A and B	*Tay-Sachs disease (Hex A)*
	Sandhoff disease (Hex A and B)
Muscle biopsy (ragged red fibers on trichrome; polysaccharide non-membrane-bound structures)	*Mitochondrial encephalomyopathy with lactic acidosis and stroke-like episodes(MELAS)*
	Myoclonic epilepsy with ragged red fibers (MERRF)
	Lafora disease
White blood cell count for galactocerebroside β-galactosidase	*Krabbe's disease*
Serum cholestanol or urine bile acids	*Cerebrotendinous xanthomatosis*
White blood cell for β-galactosidase	*GM_1 gangliosidosis*
Skin biopsy for biochemical testing of fibroblasts	*Niemann-Pick II-C*

(continued)

X-ray of hands for bone cysts, bone or skin biopsy for fat cells	*Polycystic lipomembranous osteodysplasia with sclerosing leukoencephalopathy*
Urine mucopolysaccharides elevated, serum α-N-acetyl glucosaminidase deficient	*Mucopolysaccharidoses*
Indications for biopsy	*Focal, relevant lesion(s) of undetermined etiology*
	Central nervous system vasculitis
	Subacute sclerosing panencephalitis, Creutzfeldt-Jakob disease (CJD), progressive multifocal leukoencephalopathy
	Krabbe's disease (periodic acid-Schiff–positive histiocytes)
	Kufs' disease (intranuclear fingerprint pattern)
	Neuronal intranuclear (eosinophilic) inclusion disease

D. **Alzheimer's dementia:** the most common degenerative disease of the brain; incidence increases sharply with age after 65; age is the most important and common risk factor (10% of people >65 years old [y/o], 50% of people >85 y/o); other risk factors: Down syndrome (patient 30–45 y/o shows similar pathologic changes), midlife obesity, diabetes mellitus, current tobacco use, head injury, apolipoprotein E4 genotype; reported protective factors: education, Mediterranean-type diet, low or moderate alcohol intake, physical activity, inheritance of apolipoprotein E2 allele. Dominant AD can occur with multiple genetic mutations (presenilin-1 [PS1] most common, presenilin-2 [PS2], amyloid precursor protein [APP], C9 open reading frame 72, Trem2, etc.)

> **NB:** The Clinical Dementia Rating (CDR) Scale is a dementia staging instrument with an impairment range from none to maximal (0, 0.5, 1, 2, 3) in six domains: memory, orientation, judgment and problem solving, function in community, home and hobbies, and personal care.

> **NB:** Recent update in diagnosis of Alzheimer's disease includes three phases: preclinical (patients with biomarker or dominant gene but no clinical symptoms, up to 20 years before onset of dementia), prodromal (patients with cognitive symptoms and impairment not meeting dementia criteria with biomarker data for AD), and Alzheimer's dementia.

1. Alzheimer's dementia—*clinical features:* characteristically impaired recall, repeated questions to family. Tasks, places, and events are forgotten; remote memory is also affected, difficulty remembering words, echolalia (repetition of spoken phrase), difficulty balancing checkbook; may progress to acalculia, difficulty parking car, getting lost on way to home; initially little change in behavior but later with paranoid delusions, anxiety, phobias, akinesia, mutism; day–night pattern

1. Alzheimer's dementia—*clinical features* (*cont'd*)

    changes; parkinsonian look; rigidity and fine tremor; myoclonus (late). Gait disorder may accompany dementia or may precede dementia.

2. Variants:

    a. Frontal variant: presenting with frontal behavioral change (impulsiveness, conduct disorder, apathy, sexual disinhibition) simulating behavioral variant frontotemporal dementia (bvFTD)

    b. Posterior cortical atrophy (PCA): patients with prominent visuospatial deficits early, relative sparing of insight and memory, pathology appears more posterior initially then spreads to more typical AD locations

    c. Logopenic aphasia: patients presenting with prominent language disorder, sparser speech, word finding difficulty, with AD pathology

    d. Early-onset AD: onset prior to age 65; more likely to have genetic causation

> **NB:** Early in the disease, AD patients are characterized by impaired word recall and normal digit span. Word recall worse for semantic (e.g., four-legged animals) than phonemic (e.g., words beginning with *F*).

3. *Pathology:* brain *volume is decreased* in advanced case up to 20% or more; ventricles enlarge proportionally; extreme *hippocampal atrophy;* atrophic process involves temporal, parietal, and frontal, but cases vary a lot; microscopically: *senile or neuritic plaques, neurofibrillary tangles, granulovacuolar degeneration* of neurons most prominent in pyramidal cell layer of hippocampus; *Hirano bodies.*

    a. *Cholinergic neurons of the nucleus basalis of Meynert* (substantia innominata), *medial septal nuclei, and diagonal band of Broca are reduced;* with resulting deficiency of acetylcholine. Locus ceruleus degeneration and loss of cortical noradrenergic innervation have also been described early in AD.

    b. *Neurofibrillary tangles* are composed of clusters of abnormal tubules, and *senile plaques contain a core of amyloid;* tangles and plaques are found in all association cortex; *CA1 zone of the hippocampus* disproportionately affected.

> **NB:** Amyloid starts as an amyloid precursor protein (APP), normally cleaved by a series of enzymes into a short version that can be easily excreted by the body. In AD, APP is incorrectly cleaved by beta-secretase and gamma-secretase (assisted by presenilin-1). This abnormal cleaving results in amyloid aggregation that ultimately leads to plaque formation.

4. *Genetics: familial in 10%*

    a. A defective gene was identified on *chromosome 21* near the β-amyloid gene, which codes for an errant *APP gene.*

    b. *Chromosome 14,* for the protein called *presenilin-1;* **accounts for 80% of the familial cases**

    c. Gene mutation on *chromosome 1* for the protein *presenilin-2;* age of onset for all familial cases is earlier.

    d. *Apolipoprotein E4 on chromosome 19* is associated with increased *risk* of acquiring AD.

5. *Treatment*

> **NB:** There is no treatment that halts the progression of AD pathology or that prevents worsening of dementia or delays onset of dementia.

a. Cholinesterase inhibitors: pharmacologic characteristics

	TACRINE	DONEPEZIL	RIVASTIGMINE	GALANTAMINE
Year available	1993	1996	2000	2001
Brain selectivity	No	Yes	Yes	Yes
Reversibility	Yes	Yes	Yes/slow	Yes
Chemical class	Acridine	Piperidine	Carbamate	Phenanthrene alkaloid
Enzymes inhibited				
Acetylcholinesterase	Yes	Yes	Yes	Yes
Butyrylcholinesterase	Yes	Negligible	Yes	Negligible
Nicotinic receptor modulation	No	No	No	Yes
Doses per day	4	1	2	2
Initial dose (mg/day)	40	5	3	8
Maximum dose (mg/day)	160	10	12	24
Given with food	No, unless nausea occurs	No	Yes	Yes
Plasma half-life (hrs)	2–4	~70	~1	~6
Elimination pathway	Liver	Liver	Kidney	50% Kidney
				50% Liver
Metabolism by cytochrome P450	Yes	Yes	Minimal	Yes

b. *Memantine:* a *noncompetitive N-methyl-D-aspartate (NMDA) receptor anta-gonist* (NMDA receptors, by the excitatory amino acid glutamate, have been hypothesized to contribute to the symptomatology of AD); approved by the U.S. Food and Drug Administration (FDA) for the treatment of moderate to severe dementia in AD; titrate doses up to 20 mg/day.

> **NB:** There is lack of definitive evidence that ginkgo biloba, estrogen, statins, or nonsteroidal anti-inflammatory drugs can prevent or treat AD.

> **NB: Long-acting forms or transdermal forms of medication available for treatment:** Aricept 23 mg; Exelon patch (4.6, 9.5, 13.3 mg/day); Namenda SR 28 mg per day.

> **NB:** At a severity of CDR 0.5, driving is mildly impaired, and a referral for a driving performance evaluation should be considered. At a severity of CDR 1, driving is potentially dangerous, and discontinuation of driving should be strongly considered.

E. **Multi-infarct (vascular) dementia:** history of one or more strokes is usually clear; deficit increases with strokes (usually in a stepwise fashion), and focality of deficits may indicate the type and location of strokes; multiple lacunar infarcts may also give rise to a pseudobulbar palsy with a history of stroke; Binswanger's disease: multi-infarct state of cerebral white matter associated with dementia; cerebral autosomal-dominant arteriopathy with subcortical infarcts and leukoencephalopathy. Treatment: may respond to cholinesterase inhibitors.

> **NB:** *Many patients with dementia have a mixed dementia, a combination of Alzheimer pathology and vascular pathology.*

F. **Diffuse Lewy body disease, also known as dementia with Lewy bodies (DLB):** characterized by the clinical triad of fluctuating cognitive impairment (especially attention; alertness), recurrent visual hallucinations, and spontaneous motor features of parkinsonism; in an attempt to define DLB as a distinct clinical syndrome, separate from AD and Parkinson's disease (PD) with dementia, a consensus workshop established a new set of diagnostic criteria:

Mandatory	Presence of dementia, PLUS
	Core features (at least two out of three for probable DLB):
	Fluctuation of cognition, function, or alertness
	Visual hallucinations
	Parkinsonism
Supporting features	Repeated falls
	Syncope
	Transient loss of consciousness
	Neuroleptic sensitivity
	Systematized delusions
	Nonvisual hallucinations
	Depression
	Rapid eye movement (REM) sleep behavior disorder

1. *Clinical:* the degree to which an individual patient exhibits cognitive impairment, behavioral problems, and parkinsonian features is variable.

2. *Pathology:* the essential hallmark of DLB pathology is *the Lewy body (LB); these LBs are observed in the brainstem nuclei, subcortical regions, and cerebral cortices;* in the brainstem, pigmented neurons often present with the classic morphology of intracellular LBs, comprising an eosinophilic core with a peripheral halo; immunohistochemistry using antibodies against ubiquitin or α-synuclein has been shown to be more sensitive and specific in the detection of cortical LB; the clinical overlap of AD, DLB, and PD with dementia similarly extends to their pathology—most cases of DLB have varying degrees of AD pathology, including deposits of β-amyloid protein and neurofibrillary tangles.

3. *Neurochemistry:* substantial *loss of cholinergic neurons* in the nucleus basalis of Meynert, suggesting a cholinergic mechanism of cognitive impairment in DLB, similar to that of AD; *deficits in γ-aminobutyric acid (GABA), dopamine, and serotonin* neurotransmission have also been described in DLB; neocortical choline acetyltransferase, a synthetic enzyme for acetylcholine, is decreased significantly, similar to that seen in AD or PD with dementia; reduced dopamine and its metabolites have been shown in DLB brains, possibly accounting for its parkinsonian features.

4. *Treatment:* must be individualized

   a. Although there are no officially approved drugs for DLB, limited experience from clinical trials and past experience with treatment of AD and PD patients provide some basis for making drug choices; the cholinergic deficit seen in DLB makes *cholinesterase inhibitor* drugs the mainstay of treatment for cognitive impairment; this class of drugs has also shown therapeutic benefit in reducing hallucinations and other neuropsychiatric symptoms of the disease.

b. Patients with DLB are exquisitely prone to the extrapyramidal side effects of neuroleptic medications; thus, only *atypical antipsychotic agents,* such as quetiapine, should be considered as alternative treatment for psychosis.

c. Anxiety and depression are best treated with *selective serotonin reuptake inhibitors* (SSRIs), whereas rapid eye movement (REM) sleep behavior disorder may be treated with low-dose *clonazepam.*

d. Parkinsonism responds to dopaminergic agents; however, precipitation or aggravation of hallucinosis may occur; *levodopa* is preferred over dopamine agonists owing to its lower propensity to cause hallucinations and somnolence.

G. **Frontotemporal dementia (FTD):** syndrome characterized by prominent frontal lobe symptoms, in contrast to the more pronounced amnestic symptoms in AD; reduced frontal cerebral blood flow; frontal and anterior temporal atrophy with frontal ventricular enlargement; striatum, amygdala, or hippocampus is usually spared. Major clinical variants: behavioral variant FTD (bvFTD), semantic dementia (SD), progressive nonfluent aphasia (PNFA).

> **NB:** Serotonergic deficit has been consistently reported in FTD such that some experts will treat with SSRIs even in the absence of depression. There is no evidence of significant cholinergic deficit in FTD.

1. **Behavioral variant FTD (bvFTD):** Clinically: gradual onset of confusion with personal neglect, apathy, focal disturbances (such as aphasia and apraxia), personality changes, abulia, frontal release signs, and sometimes Klüver-Bucy syndrome; incidence of depression is much less compared to PD, Huntington's disease (HD), or multiple sclerosis; atrophy in frontal and anterior temporal regions.

2. Semantic dementia (SD) is characterized by insidiously progressive yet relatively focal disease until late in the course of their illness. These patients have fluent yet empty speech, with naming impairment and failure to understand the meaning of the words; atrophy in left anterior temporal lobe.

3. Progressive nonfluent aphasia (PNFA): progressive aphasia; word-finding difficulty; telegraphic, sparse speech; MRI and CT may show focal atrophy in the left inferior frontal and insular regions.

> **NB:** ALS-*FTD (FTD with motor neuron disease):* previously described clinical and neuropathologic findings are *coupled with motor neuron degeneration; motor neuron loss is most severe in the cervical and thoracic segments.*

a. Frontotemporal lobar degeneration (FTLD) pathology: varies; three main histologic subtypes—FTD-tau, FTD-TDP43, FTD-FUS

b. Genetic mutations identified in FTD patients (minority): GNR, MAPT, C9orf72

> **NB:** FTD refers to the clinical syndrome, which may have a variety of pathological substrates. FTLD refers to the pathological diagnosis.

H. Other dementias

1. Chronic traumatic encephalopathy (CTE) (prior name was *dementia pugilistica*): initially found in boxers, CTE may be seen in others, usually after contact-sport history with concussive injury. Characteristics include progressive dementia, memory loss, aggression, confusion, and depression. CTE appears years or decades after trauma; often postmortem diagnosis. Pathology: atrophy, enlarged lateral and third ventricles, neuron loss, tau deposition, TDP 43 beta amyloid deposition, neurofibrillary tangles. Beta amyloid deposits are rare; rarely associated with motor neuron symptoms.

2. *Primary progressive aphasia:* a linguistic syndrome of *progressive aphasia without initial dementia;* may exhibit neuropathologic features identical to FTD of the frontal lobe degeneration type, except that speech areas are more heavily involved; progressive aphasia has also been described in the context of AD, CJD, and corticobasal ganglionic degeneration. Specific pathology cannot adequately be predicted by clinical presentation.

3. *Prion disorders: CJD, Gerstmann-Straussler-Scheinker, Fatal familial insomnia (FFI)*

   a. CJD: degenerative disorder; rapidly progressive prion disease (misfolding proteins that replicate by causing misfolding in other proteins). Patient presents with rapidly progressive dementia, presenting variably: memory loss, personality change, hallucinations, anxiety, psychosis, ataxia, gait disorder, visual loss, weakness due to motor neuron loss. Although myoclonus occurs, it is not part of the diagnostic criteria because it may be seen in other dementias.

   b. Pathology: spongiform change in brain.

   c. Diagnosis: clinical + MRI (cortical ribboning on diffusion weighted imaging [DWI], altered signal in basal ganglia); CSF 14-3-3 protein consistent with diagnosis, but not specific; rarely brain biopsy; no treatment

4. *Hydrocephalic dementia:* normal-pressure hydrocephalus—dementia, gait disturbance (magnetic gait), and urinary incontinence

5. *Hippocampal sclerosis dementia:* rare FTLD variant with atrophy of hippocampus, amygdala, entorhinal cortex with FTLD pathology; usually amnesia at onset, sometimes psychiatric disorder or abnormal conduct.

CHEAT SHEET

Disorder	Genetic mutation	Chromosome	Comment
AD	PS1	14q24.2	
AD	PS2	1q42.13	
AD	APP	21q21.3	
FTD	GRN	17q21.31	
FTD	MAPT	17q21.31	
FTD	C9orf72	9p21.2	Families may have AD, PD, and FTD members
FTD-ALS	C9orf72	9p21.2	

Suggested Readings

Latoo J, Jan F. Dementia with Lewy bodies: clinical review. *BJMP*.2008;1:10–14.

Levine DA, Langa KM. Vascular cognitive impairment: disease mechanisms and therapeutic implications. *Neurotherapeutics*.2011;8:361–373.

McKhann GM, Knopman DS, Chertkow H, et al. The diagnosis of dementia due to Alzheimer's disease: recommendations from the National Institute on Aging-Alzheimer's Association workgroups on diagnostic guidelines for Alzheimer's disease. *Alzheimers Dement*.2011;7:263–269.

Mesulam MM. Primary progressive aphasia-a language-based dementia. *NEJM*.2003;349: 1535–1542.

Murray K. Creutzfeldt-Jacob disease mimics, or how to sort out the subacute encephalopathy patient. *Postgrad Med J*.2011;87:369–378,

Warren JD, Rohrer JD, Rossor MN. Clinical review. Frontotemporal dementia. *BMJ*.2013;347: f4827.

CHAPTER 9

Headache Syndromes

I. Headache Syndromes

A. The International Headache Classification (ICHD) of primary and secondary headaches

1. *Primary headaches*

   a. Migraine

      i. Migraine without aura

      ii. Migraine with aura

      iii. Childhood periodic syndromes that are commonly precursors to migraine

      iv. Retinal migraine

      v. Complications of migraine

      vi. Probable migraine

   b. Tension-type headache

      i. Infrequent episodic tension-type headache

      ii. Frequent episodic tension-type headache

      iii. Chronic tension-type headache

      iv. Probable tension-type headache

   c. Cluster headache and other trigeminal autonomic cephalgias

      i. Cluster headache

      ii. Paroxysmal headache

      iii. Short-lasting unilateral neuralgiform headache attacks with conjunctival injection and tearing (SUNCT)

      iv. Probable trigeminal autonomic cephalgia

   d. Other primary headaches

      i. Primary stabbing headaches

      ii. Primary cough headaches

      iii. Primary exertional headaches

      iv. Primary headache associated with sexual activity

      v. Hypnic headache (with sleep)

      vi. Primary thunderclap headache

      vii. Hemicrania continua

      viii. New daily persistent headaches

2. *Secondary headaches*

   a. Headache attributed to head and/or neck trauma

   b. Headache attributed to cranial or cervical vascular disorder

   c. Headache attributed to nonvascular intracranial disorder

   d. Headache attributed to substance or its abuse

2. *Secondary headaches (cont'd)*

    e. Headache attributed to infection

    f. Headache attributed to disorders of homeostasis

    g. Headache of facial pain attributed to disorder of cranium, neck, eyes, ears, nose, sinuses, teeth, mouth, or other facial or cranial structures

    h. Headache attributed to psychiatric disorder

> **NB:** Migraines are more likely to be frontal than unilateral in children. Benign paroxysmal vertigo is a frequent precursor of migraine in children. Ibuprofen is more efficacious than triptans in children.

B. **International Headache Classification, 2nd Edition (ICHD-II) diagnostic criteria for migraine without aura**

1. At least five attacks fulfilling criteria 2 through 4

2. Headache attacks lasting 4 to 72 hours

3. Headache has at least two of the following characteristics:

    a. Unilateral location

    b. Pulsating quality

    c. Moderate or severe pain intensity

    d. Aggravation by or causing avoidance of routine physical activity

4. During headache, at least one of the following:

    a. Nausea and/or vomiting

    b. Photophobia and phonophobia

5. Not attributed to another disorder

> **NB:** Caffeine withdrawal is a common cause of acute severe headache among patients with migraine.

C. **ICHD-II diagnostic criteria for migraine with typical aura**

1. At least two attacks fulfilling criteria 2 through 4

2. Aura consisting of one or more of the following but no motor weakness:

    a. Fully reversible visual symptoms including positive features (e.g., fiickering lights, spots, or lines) and/or negative features (i.e., loss of vision)

    b. Fully reversible sensory symptoms including positive features (i.e., pins and needles) and/or negative symptoms (i.e., numbness)

    c. Fully reversible dysphasic speech disturbance

3. At least two of the following characteristics:

    a. Homonymous visual symptoms and/or unilateral sensory symptoms

    b. At least one aura symptom develops gradually over greater than or equal to 5 minutes, and/or different aura symptoms occur in succession over greater than or equal to 5 minutes

    c. Each symptom lasts greater than or equal to 5 minutes and not longer than 60 minutes

4. Headache fulfilling criteria 2 through 4 for migraine without aura; begins during the aura or follows aura within 60 minutes

5. Not attributed to another disorder

D. **ICHD-II diagnostic criteria for frequent episodic tension-type headache**

1. At least 10 episodes occurring on 1 or more but less than 15 days per month for at least 3 months and fulfilling criteria 2 through 4

2. Headache lasting from 30 minutes to 7 days

3. Headache has at least two of the following characteristics:

   a. Bilateral location

   b. Pressing/tightening (nonpulsating) quality

   c. Mild or moderate intensity

   d. Not aggravated by routine physical activity such as walking or climbing stairs

4. Both of the following:

   a. No nausea or vomiting (anorexia may occur)

   b. No more than one of photophobia or phonophobia

5. Not attributed to another disorder

E. **ICHD-II diagnostic criteria for cluster headache**

1. At least five attacks fulfilling criteria 2 through 4

2. Severe or very severe unilateral orbital, supraorbital, and/or temporal pain lasting 15 to 180 minutes if untreated

3. Headache is accompanied by at least one of the following:

   a. Ipsilateral conjunctival injection and/or lacrimation

   b. Ipsilateral nasal congestion and/or rhinorrhea

   c. Ipsilateral eyelid edema

   d. Ipsilateral forehead and facial sweating

   e. Ipsilateral miosis and/or ptosis

   f. A sense of restlessness or agitation

4. Attacks have a frequency of one every other day to 8 per day.

5. Not attributed to another disorder

> **NB:** Cluster headaches may be triggered by vasodilating substances such as nitroglycerin, histamine, and ethanol. They will often respond acutely to oxygen inhalation at a flow rate of 8 to 10 L/min via face mask. Dihydroergotamine (DHE) is an alternative. Preventive treatments include verapamil, lithium, and methysergide.

F. **ICHD-II diagnostic criteria for SUNCT and short-lasting unilateral neuralgiform headache with cranial autonomic features (SUNA)**

1. *SUNCT*

   a. At least 20 attacks fulfilling criteria b through d

   b. Attacks of unilateral orbital, supraorbital, or temporal stabbing or pulsating pain lasting 5 to 240 seconds

   c. Pain is accompanied by ipsilateral conjunctival injection and lacrimation.

   d. Attacks occur with a frequency of 3 to 200 per day.

   e. Not attributed to another disorder

2. *SUNA*

   a. At least 20 attacks fulfilling criteria b through e

   b. Attacks of unilateral orbital, supraorbital, or temporal stabbing pain lasting 5 seconds to 10 minutes

   c. Pain is accompanied by one of the following:

      i. Conjunctival injection and/or tearing

      ii. Nasal congestion and/or rhinorrhea

      iii. Eyelid edema

   d. Attacks occur with a frequency of greater than or equal to one per day for more than half the time.

   e. No refractory period follows attacks from trigger areas.

   f. Not attributed to another disorder

> **NB:** *Paroxysmal hemicrania* is a disorder, more common in women, characterized by frequent episodes of unilateral, severe, but short-lasting headaches associated with autonomic manifestations. Indomethacin is the treatment of choice.

> **NB:** *Pseudotumor cerebri* has been linked to the use of isotretinoin and other vitamin A–containing compounds (and also vitamin D). It is much more common in women and is characterized by normal cerebrospinal fluid (CSF) composition and normal ventricles on imaging. Neuro exam is typically normal, but sixth-nerve palsies and enlarged blind spots may be seen.

G. Medications associated with probable medication-overuse headache

   1. Opioid intake for more than 10 or more days per month

   2. Nonopioid/over-the-counter (OTC) analgesic intake for more than 15 days per month

   3. Use of triptans for more than 10 days per month

   4. Use of ergotamine for more than 10 days per month

   5. Combination of analgesic medications, or combination of ergotamine, triptans, nonopioid/OTC analgesics, or opioids for more than 10 days per month

H. Activity-induced headaches

Primary cough headache	Occurs with coughing or in conjunction with other Valsalva maneuvers Sharp, stabbing, or splitting pain Usually bilateral, sudden onset, short duration Most have underlying cause (i.e., Chiari I malformation, aneurysm, etc.)
Primary exertional headache	Occurs with exercise or other forms of exertion Usually bilateral, pulsating, or throbbing Lasts for minutes to days Young onset (early 20s)

(continued)

Headache associated with sexual activity	Subclassified further into: preorgasmic (dull, aching pain that increases in severity during orgasm) or orgasmic (maximal and severe during orgasm) Lasts less than 3 hours

I. Symptomatic and preventive therapies for migraine

RECOMMENDATION	PREVENTIVE TREATMENT	SYMPTOMATIC/ABORTIVE TREATMENT
First line	Amitriptyline Divalproex sodium Propranolol Topiramate	All triptan medications (naratriptan, rizatriptan, sumatriptan, zolmitriptan) DHE +/− antiemetic ASA + caffeine ASA/ibuprofen/naproxen/ butorphanol IN Prochlorperazine IV
Second line	Atenolol/metoprolol/nadolol Verapamil ASA/naproxen Ketoprofen Fluoxetine Gabapentin	Acetaminophen + caffeine Butalbital, ASA, caffeine + codeine Chlorpromazine Metoclopramide IV Isometheptene Prochlorperazine IM, PR Ketorolac IM Lidocaine IN Meperidine IM, IV Methadone IM
Third line	Bupropion Imipramine Mirtazapine Nortriptyline Paroxetine/sertraline/ venlafaxine Cyproheptadine (especially in children) Indomethacin	Butalbital, ASA + caffeine, metoclo-pramide IM, PR ergotamine + caffeine PO, ergotamine PO

CHEAT SHEET

SUNCT—short-lasting unilateral neuralgiform headache associated with conjunctival injection and tearing	Attacks of unilateral orbital, supraorbital, or temporal stabbing or pulsating pain lasting 5 to 240 seconds; attacks occur with a frequency from 3 to 200 per day
SUNA—short-lasting unilateral neuralgiform headache with cranial autonomic features	Attacks of unilateral orbital, supraorbital, or temporal stabbing pain lasting 5 seconds to 10 minutes; attacks occur with a frequency of greater than or equal to one per day for more than half the time
Paroxysmal hemicranias	Indomethacin responsive
Cough headache	May be related to Chiari I malformation, aneurysm, etc.

HEADACHE Red Flags: (Mnemonic—"SNOOP")

A. **S**ystemic symptoms or illness

1. Fever

2. Altered level of consciousness

3. Anticoagulation

4. Pregnancy

5. Cancer

6. HIV infection

B. **N**eurologic symptoms or signs

1. Papilledema

2. Asymmetric cranial nerve function

3. Asymmetric motor function

4. Abnormal cerebellar function

C. **O**nset recently or suddenly

D. **O**nset after age 40 to 50 years

E. **P**rior headache history that is different or progressive

1. Different location is less useful as predictor of serious cause.

2. Pain response to standard headache therapy is not predictive of serious cause.

Suggested Readings

International Headache Classification, 2nd Ed. (IHS-ICHD-II) website: http://ihs-classification .org/en/

Queiroz, LP. Unusual headache syndromes. *Headache*.2013;53(1):12–22.

Tepper, SJ, Tepper, DE. *The Cleveland Clinic Manual of Headache Therapy*. New York, NY: Springer;2011.

CHAPTER 10

Neuromuscular Disorders

I. General Evaluation

A. **History**

1. Chief complaint

   a. Weakness/motor versus sensory

   b. Acute versus subacute versus chronic

   c. Symmetric versus asymmetric

2. Contributing history

   a. Family history

   b. Medications, toxins

   c. Trauma

   d. Infections

   e. Vaccinations

   f. Diet

   g. Concurrent medical conditions (i.e., autoimmune, rheumatologic, endocrinopathies, cardiovascular)

3. Neurophysiologic/electrodiagnostic studies (see Chapter 17)

B. **Types of muscle fibers**

	TYPE 1	TYPE 2A	TYPE 2B
Axon innervating	Smaller	Larger	Larger
Type	Tonic	Phasic	Phasic
Color	Dark	Dark	Pale
Fiber diameter	Small	Larger	Largest
Twitch speed	Slow	Fast	Fast
Fatigability	Low	Low	High

C. **Electromyography (EMG) of neuropathic, neuromuscular junction, and myopathic processes**

	MUPs	RECRUITMENT
Myopathy	Low amplitude, short duration, polyphasic	"Early" pattern
Neuromuscular junction disorder	Motor unit instability; possibly low amplitude, short duration, polyphasic (when severe)	Normal (typically)

(continued)

C. Electromyography (EMG) of neuropathic, neuromuscular junction, and myopathic processes (*cont'd*)

	MUPs		RECRUITMENT
Denervation (with reinnervation from collateral sprouting of intact axons)	High amplitude, long duration (and polyphasia, marked in early chronic stage)		Decreased
Denervation with reinnervation (with no intact axons for collateral sprouting)	I = low amplitude, short duration, polyphasic in EARLY stages of reinnervation ("nascent units")		Decreased (without "early" pattern)

Abbreviation: MUPs, motor unit potentials.

D. Pathologic differentiation between myopathic and neurogenic processes

MYOPATHIC	NEUROGENIC
Marked irregularity of fiber size	Nests of atrophic fibers
Rounded fibers	Angular fibers
Real increase in number of muscle nuclei	Pseudo-increase of nuclei due to cytoplasmic atrophy
Centralized nuclei	Centralized nuclei not present
Necrotic and basophilic fibers	Necrotic and basophilic fibers not present
Cytoplasmic alterations	Target fibers
Copious interstitial fibrosis at times	Minimal interstitial fibrosis
Inflammatory cellular infiltrate (with myositis)	Inflammatory cellular infiltrate not present

II. Peripheral Neuropathic Syndromes

A. Classification and degrees of peripheral nerve injury

1. **Segmental demyelination**

    a. Conduction block

    b. Segmental conduction velocity slowing

    c. Temporal dispersion

    d. Prolongation of distal latencies

    e. Normal compound muscle action potential (CMAP) and sensory nerve action potential (SNAP) at DISTAL stimulation sites.

2. **Neurapraxia:** *localized conduction loss along a nerve without axon loss, caused by a focal lesion, typically demyelinating in nature, and followed by a relatively rapid and complete recovery*

3. **Axonotmesis:** *nerve injury characterized by disruption of the axon and myelin sheath but with sparing of the connective tissue components, resulting in degeneration of the axon distal to the site of damage; regeneration of the axon is typically successful, with good functional recovery.*

4. *Wallerian degeneration: (e.g., for L5–S1 radiculopathy) complete in 10 to 14 days for nerves supplying proximal areas such as paraspinal muscles and up to 5 to 6 weeks in the distal leg and foot muscles.*

	1ST DEGREE	2ND DEGREE	3RD DEGREE	4TH DEGREE	5TH DEGREE
Pathology	Segmental demyelination; neurapraxia	Loss of axons with intact supporting structures; axonotmesis	Loss of axons with disrupted endoneurium; neurotmesis	Loss of axons with disrupted endoneurium and perineurium	Loss of axons with disruption of all supporting structures (discontinuous)
Prognosis	Excellent; usually complete recovery in 2–3 mos	Slow recovery dependent on sprouting and reinnervation	Protracted, and recovery may fail because of misdirected axonal sprouts	Recovery unlikely without surgical repair	Recovery not possible without surgical repair

B. **Mononeuropathies**

1. **Sciatic mononeuropathy**

   a. *Common causes*

      i. Hip replacement/fracture/dislocation

      ii. Femur fracture

      iii. Acute compression (coma, drug overdose, intensive care unit [ICU], prolonged sitting)

      iv. Gunshot or knife wound

      v. Infarction (vasculitis, iliac artery occlusion, arterial bypass surgery)

      vi. Gluteal contusion or compartmental syndrome (during anticoagulation)

      vii. Gluteal injection or compartment syndrome

      viii. Endometriosis (catamenial sciatica)

> **NB:** The sciatic nerve is composed of a peroneal division and tibial division. *The only muscle above the knee supplied by the peroneal division is the short head of the biceps femoris.*

2. **Footdrop**

   a. *Common causes*

      i. Deep peroneal mononeuropathy

      ii. Common peroneal mononeuropathy

      iii. Sciatic mononeuropathy

      iv. Lumbosacral plexopathy (especially of the lumbosacral trunk)

      v. Lumbar radiculopathy (L5 or, less commonly, L4)

      vi. Motor neuron disease/spinal cord lesion

      vii. Parasagittal cortical or subcortical cerebral lesion

> **NB:** **To differentiate a peroneal nerve lesion from an L5 lesion in a patient with a footdrop, test the foot invertors. Peroneal nerve lesions should not involve the foot invertors.** Foot evertors will be involved with damage to the superficial peroneal nerve. *The majority of the peroneal palsies occur at the level of the fibular head.*

Clinical Assessment of Footdrop

	PERONEAL NEUROPATHY	L5 RADICULOPATHY	LUMBAR PLEXOPATHY	SCIATIC NEUROPATHY
Common causes	Compression/ trauma	Disk herniation, spinal stenosis	Pelvic surgery, hematoma, prolonged labor	Hip surgery, injection injury
Ankle inversion	Normal	Weak	Weak	Normal or mildly weak
Plantar flexion	Normal	Normal	Normal	Normal or mildly weak
Ankle jerk	Normal	Normal	Normal	Normal or depressed
Sensory loss	Peroneal only	Poorly demarcated except big toe	Poorly demarcated, often L5 dermatome	Peroneal and lateral cutaneous of calf

3. **Piriformis syndrome**

   a. Clinically: *buttock and leg pain worse during sitting without low back pain;* exacerbated by internal rotation or abduction and external rotation of the hip; local tenderness in the buttock; soft or no neurologic signs

   b. EMG/nerve conduction studies (NCS): *denervation seen in branches after the piriformis muscle, but normal in branches before the piriformis muscle*

4. **Femoral mononeuropathy**

   a. Clinically: *acute thigh and knee extension weakness; numbness of anterior thigh;* absent knee jerk; normal thigh adduction

   b. Common causes

      i. *Compression in the pelvis:* retractor blade during pelvic surgery (iatrogenic), abdominal hysterectomy, radical prostatectomy, renal transplantation, and so forth; iliacus or psoas retroperitoneal hematoma; pelvic mass

      ii. *Compression in the inguinal region:* inguinal ligament during lithotomy position (vaginal delivery, laparoscopy, vaginal hysterectomy, urologic procedures); inguinal hematoma; during total hip replacement; inguinal mass

      iii. *Stretch injury* (hyperextension)

      iv. Others: radiation; laceration; injection

> **NB:** The pain in femoral mononeuropathy due to psoas hematoma is markedly worse with forced hyperextension of the hip (stretches the psoas muscle).

5. **Tarsal tunnel syndrome:** compression of the tibial nerve or any of its three branches under the flexor retinaculum

   a. *Clinically:* sensory impairment in the sole of the foot; Tinel's sign; muscle atrophy of the sole of the foot; rarely weak (long toe flexors are intact); ankle reflexes normal; sensation of the dorsum of the foot normal; note: not associated with footdrop

> **NB:** Nocturnal pain is common, such as in carpal tunnel syndrome (CTS). There is an anterior tarsal tunnel syndrome caused by compression of the deep peroneal nerve at the ankle that results in paresis of the extensor digitorum brevis alone.

  b. Differential diagnosis

    i. Plantar fasciitis

    ii. Stress fracture

    iii. Arthritis

    iv. Bursitis

    v. Reflex sympathetic dystrophy

    vi. High tibial or sciatic mononeuropathy

    vii. Sacral radiculopathy

    viii. Peripheral neuropathy

6. **Meralgia paresthetica**

  a. Anatomy

    i. Entrapment of the *lateral femoral cutaneous nerve,* which is a pure sensory branch via L2 and L3 nerve roots

    ii. Enters through the opening between the inguinal ligament and its attachment to the anterior superior iliac spine

  b. Etiologies

    i. Obesity

    ii. Wearing tight belt or girdle

    iii. Pregnancy

    iv. Prolonged sitting

    v. More common in diabetics

    vi. Abdominal or pelvic mass

    vii. Metabolic neuropathies

  c. Clinical: *burning paresthesia in the anterolateral aspect of the upper thigh just above the knee;* may be exacerbated by clothing contact; may improve with massage; bilateral in 20% of cases

  d. Differential diagnosis

    i. Femoral neuropathy

    ii. L2 or L3 radiculopathy

    iii. Nerve compression by abdominal or pelvic tumor

  e. Treatment: usually spontaneous improvement; nonsteroidal anti-inflammatory drugs for 7 to 10 days for pain; avoid tight pants/belts; use suspenders, if able

7. **Ulnar nerve mononeuropathy**

  a. Localization of ulnar neuropathy

    i. Guyon's canal (wrist) entrapment: sensory loss of the palmar surface of the little and ring fingers and the ulnar side of the hand

    ii. Sensory loss of medial half of the ring finger that spares the lateral half (pathognomonic of ulnar nerve lesion; not seen in lower trunk or C8 root lesion)

    iii. *If flexor carpi ulnaris and flexor digitorum profundus are both abnormal with axonal loss features, the lesions are localized at or proximal to the elbow.*

    a. Localization of ulnar neuropathy (*cont'd*)

        iv. *Purely axonal lesions with normal flexor carpi ulnaris and flexor digitorum profundus suggest lesions at the distal forearm or wrist.*

        v. Ulnar entrapment syndromes at the elbow

            (A) *Cubital tunnel syndrome:* proximal edge of the flexor carpi ulnaris aponeurosis (arcuate ligament)

            (B) Subluxation of the ulnar nerve at the ulnar groove: often caused by repetitive trauma

            (C) *Tardy ulnar palsy:* may occur years after a distal humeral fracture in association with a valgus deformity

            (D) Idiopathic ulnar neuropathy at the elbow

            (E) Other causes of compressive ulnar neuropathy at the elbow: pressure; bony deformities; chronic subluxation

        vi. *Martin-Gruber anastomosis: patients with apparent conduction block of the ulnar motor fibers at the elbow should undergo further investigation to rule out the presence of anomalous nerves (Martin-Gruber anastomosis), which occur in 20% to 25% of the normal population. This is an anatomical variant in which branches cross over from the median to the ulnar nerve in forearm.*

    b. Clinical signs of ulnar neuropathy: Tinel's sign at the elbow; sensory exam may be normal despite symptoms; ulnar claw hand (caused by weakness or by flexion of the interphalangeal joints of the 3rd and 4th lumbricals); *Froment's sign;* when the patient is asked to adduct the thumb in a pincer-type grip (such as grasping a sheet of paper), there will be hyperflexion of the thumb interphalangeal (IP) joint (flexor pollicis longus, median innervated) to compensate for loss of the ulnar-dependent adductor strength.

> **NB:** Ulnar nerve lesions do not typically cause sensory symptoms proximal to the wrist. If such symptoms are present, consider a proximal lesion (e.g., root or plexus).

LESION SITE	NERVE AFFECTED	CLINICAL
Guyon's canal	Main trunk of ulnar nerve	Ulnar palmar sensory loss and weakness of all ulnar intrinsic hand muscles
	Ulnar cutaneous branch	Ulnar palmar sensory loss only
Pisohamate hiatus **NB:** Pure motor lesion!	Deep palmar branch (distal to branch to the abductor digiti minimi)	Weakness of ulnar intrinsic hand muscles with sparing of the hypothenar muscles and without sensory loss
Midpalm (rare)	Deep palmar branch (distal to hypothenar)	Weakness of adductor pollicis, the 1st, 2nd, and possibly the 3rd interossei only, sparing the 4th interossei and hypothenar muscles, without sensory loss

8. **Radial nerve mononeuropathy**

   a. Anatomy

      i. Arises from *posterior divisions* of three trunks of the brachial plexus

      ii. Receives contribution from C5 to C8

      iii. Winds laterally along spiral groove of the humerus

      iv. Distinguished from brachial plexus posterior cord injury by sparing deltoid (axillary nerve) and latissimus dorsi (thoracodorsal nerve)

   b. Etiologies and localization

      i. *Spiral groove* (most common)

      ii. *Saturday night palsy:* acute compression at the spiral groove

      iii. Humeral fracture

      iv. Strenuous muscular effort

      v. Injection injury

      vi. Trauma

   c. Clinical

      i. *Axillary compression:* less common than compression in the upper arm; etiologies: secondary to misuse of crutches or during drunken sleep; clinical: weakness of triceps and more distal muscles innervated by radial nerve

      ii. *Mid–upper-arm compression:* site of compression: spiral groove, intermuscular septum, or just distal to this site; etiologies: Saturday night palsy, under general anesthesia; clinical: weakness of wrist extensors (wristdrop) and finger extensors; triceps normal

      iii. *Forearm compression:* radial nerve enters anterior compartment of the arm above the elbow and gives branches to brachioradialis and extensor carpi radialis longus before dividing into posterior interosseous nerve and the superficial radial nerve; the posterior interosseous nerve goes through the supinator muscle via the *arcade of Frohse* (fibrous band between the two heads of the supinator muscle).

> **NB:** The posterior interosseous nerve is purely motor. A lesion results in fingerdrop. The superficial radial nerve is mainly sensory.

   (A) *Posterior interosseous neuropathy*

      (1) Etiologies: lipomas, ganglia, fibromas, rheumatoid disease

      (2) Clinical: extensor weakness of thumb and fingers (fingerdrop)—**distinguished from radial nerve palsy by less to no wrist extensor weakness; no sensory loss.**

> **NB:** Posterior interosseous syndrome spares the supinator, which receives innervation proximal to the site of compression.

   (B) *Radial tunnel syndrome (supinator tunnel syndrome)*

      (1) Contains radial nerve and its two main branches, including posterior interosseous nerve and superficial radial nerve

      (2) Etiologies: mass lesion, local edema, inflammation (including that of the supinator muscle), hand/wrist overuse through repetitive movements, blunt trauma to the proximal forearm

      (3) Clinical: pain in the region of common extensor origin at the lateral epicondyle (mimicking "tennis elbow"); tingling in distribution of superficial radial nerve; usually no weakness

> **NB:** Cheiralgia paresthetica (Wartenburg syndrome) is a pure sensory syndrome caused by lesion of the superficial cutaneous branch of the radial nerve in the forearm. It causes paresthesia and sensory loss/disturbance in the radial part of the dorsum of the hand and the dorsal aspect of the thumb and index fingers.

9. **Median nerve entrapment**

   a. The two most common sites of entrapment of the median nerve: transverse carpal ligament at the wrist *(carpal tunnel syndrome; CTS);* and upper forearm by pronator teres muscle *(pronator teres syndrome)*

   b. Anatomy

      i. Contribution from C5 to T1 (but mostly C8–T1).

      ii. In the upper forearm, it passes through the pronator teres, supplying this muscle, and then branches to form the purely motor anterior interosseous nerve (AIN), which supplies the lateral half of flexor digitorum profundus, flexor pollicis longus, and pronator quadratus; it emerges from the lateral edge of the flexor digitorum superficialis and later passes under the transverse carpal ligament.

      iii. The transverse carpal ligament attaches medially to the pisiform and hamate.

      iv. The palmar cutaneous branch arises from the radial aspect of the nerve proximal to the transverse carpal ligament and crosses over the ligament to provide sensory innervation to the base of the thenar eminence.

   c. **Carpal tunnel syndrome (CTS)**

      i. Etiologies

         (A) *Trauma:* repetitive movement; repetitive forceful grasping or pinching; awkward positioning of hand or wrist; direct pressure over carpal tunnel; use of vibrating tools

         (B) *Systemic conditions:* obesity; diabetes mellitus; pregnancy; hypothyroidism; amyloidosis; mucopolysaccharidosis V; tuberculous tenosynovitis

         (C) Other: dialysis shunts

      ii. Differential diagnosis

         (A) Cervical radiculopathy, especially C6/C7

         (B) Neurogenic thoracic outlet syndrome: sensory manifestations are in C8/T1 distribution but motor deficits are typically in the thenar eminence.

         (C) Peripheral polyneuropathy: manifestations in the distal lower limbs; hyporeflexia/areflexia

         (D) *High median mononeuropathy: for example, pronator syndrome, compression at the ligament of Struthers in the distal arm; will have weakness in the lateral long finger flexors*

         (E) Cervical myelopathy

      iii. Clinical

         (A) Paresthesias with numb hand that may awaken patient at night: palm side of lateral 3½ fingers, including thumb, index, middle, and lateral half of ring finger; dorsal side of the same fingers distal to the proximal interphalangeal joint; radial half of palm

         (B) Weakness of hand: particularly thumb abduction

  (C) *Phalen's test:* 30 to 60 seconds of complete wrist flexion reproduces pain in 80% of cases.

  (D) *Tinel's sign:* paresthesia or pain in median nerve distribution produced by tapping carpal tunnel in 60% of cases

  (E) Shake sign: patients show that they shake out their hands at night when they fall asleep.

 iv. *EMG/NCS*

  (A) The electrophysiologic hallmark of CTS is *focal slowing of conduction at the wrist.*

  (B) Normal in ~15% of cases of CTS (sensitivity increases by obtaining palmar mixed nerve responses)

  (C) *Sensory latencies are more sensitive than motor latencies.*

 v. Lab testing (informed by clinical suspicion)

  (A) Fasting blood glucose, 2 hour oral glucose tolerance test (OGTT), HbA1C (diabetes)

  (B) Thyroid function tests (TFTs) (thyroid disease/myxedema)

  (C) Complete blood count, serum immunofixation (monoclonal gammopathy)

 vi. Treatment

  (A) Nonsurgical: rest; neutral position wrist splint at nights; nonsteroidal anti-inflammatory drugs; local steroid injection

  (B) Surgical: carpal tunnel release

  (C) Short-term low dose oral steroids

d. **Pronator teres syndrome**

 i. *Etiologies:* direct trauma; repeated pronation with tight handgrip

 ii. Nerve entrapment between two heads of pronator teres

 iii. Clinical: vague aching and fatigue of forearm with weak grip; not exacerbated during sleep; pain in palm distinguishes this from CTS because median palmar cutaneous branch transverses over the transverse carpal ligament

C. Radiculopathies

 1. Clinical

  a. **Lumbosacral radiculopathy**

   i. *L5 radiculopathy:* most common radiculopathy

Clinical Presentations in Lumbosacral Radiculopathy

	S1	L5	L4	L2/L3
Pain radiation	Buttock	Buttock	Hip	Groin
	Posterior thigh and leg	Posterior thigh and leg	Anterior thigh Knee	Anteromedial thigh
	Lateral foot	Dorsal foot	Medial leg	

(continued)

a. **Lumbosacral radiculopathy** (*cont'd*)

	S1	L5	L4	L2/L3
Sensory impairment	Posterior thigh	Lateral leg	Anterior thigh	Groin
		Dorsal foot	Medial leg	Medial thigh
	Lateral foot	Big toe		
	Little toe			
Weakness	Plantar flexion	Toe dorsiflexion	Knee extension	Hip flexion and knee extension
	Toe flexion	Ankle dorsiflexion	Ankle dorsiflexion	
		Inversion		
		Eversion		
Diminished reflexes	Ankle jerk	None	Knee jerk	Knee jerk

b. *Cervical radiculopathies*

Clinical Presentations in Cervical Radiculopathy

	C5	C6	C7	C8
Pain	Parascapular area, shoulder	Shoulder Arm	Posterior arm, forearm	Medial arm
	Upper arm	Forearm, Thumb/index finger	Index/middle fingers	Forearm, little/ring fingers
Sensory impairment	Upper arm	Lateral arm	Index/middle fingers	Medial arm
		Forearm		Forearm
		Thumb/index finger		Little finger
Weakness	Scapular fixators	Shoulder abduction	Elbow extension	Hand intrinsics and long finger flexors
	Shoulder abduction	Elbow flexion	Wrist and finger extension	and extensor of index finger
		Forearm pronation		
	Elbow flexion			
Diminished reflexes	Biceps brachioradialis	Biceps brachioradialis	Triceps	None

2. Differential diagnosis of radiculopathies

    a. Congenital

        i. Meningeal cyst

        ii. Conjoined nerve root

    b. Acquired/degenerative

        i. Spinal stenosis

        ii. Spondylosis

iii. Spondylolisthesis

iv. Ganglion cyst of facet joint

c. Infectious

i. Diskitis

ii. Lyme disease, other inflammatory syndromes

d. Neoplastic

e. Vascular (including that seen in diabetic amyotrophy)

f. Referred pain syndromes

i. Kidney infection

ii. Nephrolithiasis

iii. Cholelithiasis

iv. Appendicitis

v. Endometriosis

vi. Pyriformis syndrome

3. Electrodiagnostic studies in radiculopathies

a. *Needle EMG: the most sensitive electrodiagnostic test for diagnosis of radiculopathy in general*

b. Goals of EMG in radiculopathy: confirm root involvement; exclude more distal lesion; localize the lesion to either a single root or multiple roots; assess severity of injury; assess whether chronic and/or active denervation.

c. Differential diagnosis of lumbosacral plexopathy versus lumbosacral radiculopathy—depends on electrodiagnostic findings, for example: *needle exam of paraspinal muscles → abnormal in radiculopathy; SNAP → abnormal in plexopathy*

> **NB:** Intraspinal canal lesions that are typically proximal to the dorsal root ganglion will manifest clinically with sensory loss, but sensory NCS responses will be normal.

d. *Criteria for diagnosing radiculopathy require: denervation in a segmental/myotomal distribution, and normal SNAP*

e. SNAP-correlated levels

i. L4: saphenous

ii. S1: sural

iii. L5: superficial peroneal

D. **Plexopathies**

1. **Brachial plexopathy**

a. Etiologies

i. Tumor (Pancoast's syndrome): usually lower plexus

ii. Idiopathic brachial plexitis/plexopathy (neuralgic amyotrophy or Parsonage-Turner syndrome): usually upper plexus or diffuse; antecedent respiratory tract infection occurs in ~25% of cases; one-third have bilateral involvement; **predominant symptom is acute onset of intense pain with sudden weakness,** typically within 2 weeks.

iii. Viral

iv. After **radiation** treatment (**myokymia is a typical needle exam finding**)

a. Etiologies (*cont'd*)

   v. Diabetes

   vi. Vasculitis

   vii. Hereditary (hereditary neuralgic amyotrophy, associated with autosomal-dominant mutations in gene septin 9 [SEPT9])

   viii. Traumatic

b. Clinical:

   i. **Erb-Duchenne palsy** *(upper radicular syndrome): upper roots (C4, C5, and C6) or upper trunk of the brachial plexus;* blow to neck or birth injury; clinical: *Waiter's/bellhop's tip; weak arm abduction/elbow flexion, supination, and lateral arm rotation*

   ii. **Klumpke's palsy** (lower radicular syndrome): *C8 and T1 lesion* (clinically, as if combined median and ulnar damage); sudden arm pull or during delivery; clinical: weak thenar, hypothenar muscles and finger flexors; flattened simian hand

   iii. **Middle radicular syndrome:** *C7 or middle trunk lesion; crutch injury;* clinical: loss in radial innervated muscles (except brachioradialis and part of triceps)

> **NB:** In a patient with breast cancer and history of radiation, the plexus may be affected by carcinomatous invasion of the plexus versus radiation-induced plexopathy. Carcinomatous invasion is usually painful, whereas radiation-induced plexopathy is usually painless and may present with myokymic discharges on EMG.

2. **Lumbosacral plexopathy**

   a. *Etiologies*

      i. *Pelvic masses:* malignant neoplasms (lymphoma; ovarian, colorectal, and uterine cancer); retroperitoneal lymphadenopathy; abscess

      ii. *Pelvic hemorrhage:* iliacus hematoma (only femoral nerve); psoas hematoma; extensive retroperitoneal hematoma

      iii. *Intrapartum*

      iv. Pelvic fracture

      v. Radiation injury

      vi. Diabetes

      vii. Idiopathic lumbosacral plexitis

   b. *Anatomy and clinical findings*

      i. Lumbar plexus

         (A) From ventral rami of L1, L2, L3, and most of L4 roots, which divide into dorsal (femoral nerve without L1) and ventral (obturator nerve without L1) branches

         (B) Plexus also posteriorly gives rise directly to iliacus, psoas muscles.

      ii. *Lumbosacral trunk (lumbosacral cord)*

         (A) Primarily L5 root

         (B) Travels adjacent to the sacroiliac joint while being covered by psoas muscle, except the terminal portion at the pelvic rim where the S1 nerve root joins

         (C) *Lesion will cause weakness of ankle inversion and eversion in addition to footdrop; may have variable hamstring and gluteal muscle weakness.*

iii. *Sacral plexus*

  (A) Fusion of lumbosacral trunk and ventral rami of S1, S2, S3, and S4 roots

  (B) Gives rise to sciatic nerve and superior and inferior gluteal nerves

  (C) *Lesion will cause sciatica-like symptom with gluteal muscle involvement.*

E. **Cauda equina syndrome and conus medullaris syndrome**

	CONUS MEDULLARIS SYNDROME	CAUDA EQUINA SYNDROME
Onset	Sudden	Gradual
Localization	Typically bilateral	Typically unilateral
Spontaneous pain	Symmetric in perineum > thighs	Prominent, asymmetric, severe radicular-type pain
Sensory deficit	Bilateral symmetric, more perianal	Saddle distribution sensory reduction
Motor loss	Symmetric and more upper motor neuron type	Asymmetric and more lower motor neuron type
Reflexes	Ankle jerk affected	Both ankle and knee jerks affected
Sphincter dysfunction	Urinary/fecal incontinence presents early	Urinary retention (90%), usually presents later; diminished anal tone
Erectile dysfunction	Common	Less common

F. **Diabetic neuropathies**

  1. *Pathophysiology:* diabetes mellitus is the most common cause of neuropathy; seen in up to 50% of patients with diabetes; most common after age 50 years.

  a. *Pathology: loss of myelinated fibers is the predominant finding; segmental demyelination-remyelination along with axonal degeneration.*

  b. *EMG/NCS: both demyelinating and axonal findings may be present.*

  2. *Classification of diabetic neuropathy*

  a. **Distal symmetric polyneuropathy**

  i. Mixed sensory-motor-autonomic

  ii. Predominantly sensory

  (A) Types: small fiber (including autonomic); large fiber; mixed

  (B) Signs/symptoms: symmetric; lower extremities affected more than upper extremities; presents with pain, paresthesia, and dysesthesia; chronic and slowly progressive; accelerated loss of distal vibratory sensation

  b. **Asymmetric polyradiculoneuropathy:** proximal asymmetric motor-predominant neuropathy (diabetic amyotrophy); thoracoabdominal polyradiculopathy

  c. **Cranial mononeuropathy:** typically pupil-sparing cranial nerve III lesion; cranial nerves VI and VII may also be involved; spontaneous recovery possible in approximately 2 to 3 months.

  d. **Entrapment mononeuropathy:** median mononeuropathy at the wrist (CTS); ulnar mononeuropathy; peroneal mononeuropathy

  e. **Diabetic amyotrophy** (diabetic lumbosacral radiculoplexus neuropathy)

  i. Usually older than 50 years with mild type 2 diabetes

e. **Diabetic amyotrophy** (*cont'd*)

   ii. Two-thirds have associated predominantly sensory polyneuropathy but minimal sensory loss in distribution.

   iii. Recovery usually occurs in less than 3 to 4 months but may take up to 3 years.

   iv. Recurrent episodes may occur in up to 20%.

   v. Abrupt onset of asymmetric pain in hip, anterior thigh, knee, and sometimes calf

   vi. Weakness of quadriceps, iliopsoas, and occasionally thigh adductors

   vii. Loss of knee jerk

   viii. Weakness is usually preceded by weight loss.

   ix. EMG shows involvement of paraspinals but no evidence of myopathy.

f. **Autonomic neuropathy**

   i. Often superimposed on sensorimotor polyneuropathy

   ii. Symptoms: involves bladder, bowel, circulatory reflexes; orthostatic hypotension; erectile dysfunction; diarrhea; constipation

   iii. Pathology: degeneration of neurons in sympathetic ganglia; loss of myelinated fibers in splanchnic and vagal nerves; loss of neurons and intermediolateral cell column

   iv. Treatment of orthostatic hypotension: elevate head of bed; liberalized sodium in diet; elastic stockings; fludrocortisone; midodrine; pyridostigmine.

> **NB:** Midodrine may also be used for the treatment of orthostatic hypotension without mineralocorticoid effects.

G. **Mononeuritis multiplex**

1. *Diabetic neuropathies (see Section II.F)*

2. *Vasculitis*

   a. Multiple systemic symptoms, including weight loss, fever, and malaise, with potential multiple organ involvement

   b. Elevated sedimentation rate

   c. NCS/EMG shows sensory and motor axon loss changes in multiple nerve distributions, classically asymmetric but confluent presentations commonly seen.

   d. Diagnosis often confirmed by sural nerve biopsy

   e. Treatment with immunosuppressive agents

   f. Etiologies

      i. Polyarteritis nodosa

      ii. Rheumatoid arthritis

      iii. Systemic lupus erythematosus

      iv. Wegener's granulomatosis

      v. Progressive systemic sclerosis

      vi. Sjogren's syndrome

      vii. Churg-Strauss syndrome (allergic granulomatosis and angiitis)

      viii. Temporal arteritis

      ix. Behcet's disease

      x. Hypersensitivity vasculitis

      xi. Lymphomatoid granulomatosis

3. *Multifocal motor neuropathy*

    a. *Subacute to chronic progression typically involving upper extremities*

    b. *Pure motor involvement is present in 50% of cases, but mild sensory symptoms and signs can be present.*

    c. Tendon reflexes are usually reduced or absent.

    d. Controversy over whether this is a variant of chronic inflammatory demyelinating polyradiculoneuropathy (CIDP)

    e. Males affected more than females

    f. *Asymmetric distal upper extremity weakness, particularly in three-fourths of cases*

    g. Progresses slowly

    h. Mimics motor neuron syndromes

    i. *Elevated anti-GM1 antibody (Ab) titers in 40% to 60% of cases; the importance of GM1 Ab in the diagnosis and treatment of multifocal motor neuropathy is not compelling.*

    j. Presence of conduction block appears to correlate with pathologic alteration in sural and motor nerves and is a better guide to management.

    k. NCS: demyelinating neuropathy with multifocal conduction block in motor nerves, but relatively normal sensory conduction

    l. *Pathology: demyelination with remyelination ± inflammation*

    m. Treatment: intravenous immunoglobulin (IVIg); plasma exchange (PE); cyclophosphamide; prednisone relatively ineffective (may actually cause worsening)

> **NB:** **The characteristics of a demyelinating polyneuropathy (acquired type) include segmental conduction velocity slowing, conduction block, and temporal dispersion of the CMAP.**

4. *Sarcoidosis*

    a. *5%—nervous system involvement*

    b. *3%—central nervous system (CNS) findings without systemic manifestations*

    c. Organs commonly involved include lungs, skin, lymph nodes, bones, eyes, muscle, and parotid gland; hypothalamic involvement may produce diabetes insipidus.

    d. Pathology: primarily involves leptomeninges, but parenchymal invasion may occur; noncaseating granulomas with lymphocytic infiltrate

    e. Predilection for posterior fossa

    f. May produce basilar meningitis

    g. Clinical

        i. *Mononeuritis multiplex:* most common; usually large and irregular areas of sensory loss can be distinguishing feature

        ii. *Cranial neuropathies* (particularly facial palsies)

> **NB:** **In a patient with bilateral facial nerve palsies, consider Lyme disease, sarcoidosis, or Guillain-Barré syndrome (GBS).**

        iii. *Polyneuropathy*

        iv. *Mononeuropathy* (usually early on course)

4. *Sarcoidosis (cont'd)*

    h. Serum testing: angiotensin-converting enzyme is elevated in 80% with active pulmonary sarcoidosis, but only in 11% with inactive disease. Soluble interleukin 2 may be helpful, but is not specific.

    i. Cerebrospinal fluid (CSF): subacute meningitis with elevated pressure, mild pleocytosis (10–200 cells) that are mainly lymphocytes, elevated protein, and reduced glucose; CSF angiotensin-converting enzyme level elevated in some patients with neurosarcoidosis; however, sensitivity and specificity unclear.

    j. NCS/EMG: axonal involvement

    k. Treatment: steroids or other immunosuppressants if steroids ineffective

5. *Lyme disease*

    a. Pathophysiology: *caused by* Borrelia burgdorferi; *vector: via* Ixodes immitis *tick;* early summer most common

    b. Clinical: acute form: more severe signs and symptoms and often with cranial nerve palsy (facial palsy most common); presentations: erythema chronicum migrans; headache; myalgias; meningismus; cranial neuropathy (cranial nerve VII most common); radiculopathy; mononeuritis multiplex; peripheral neuropathy (one-third have neuropathies)

    c. Diagnosis: *sural biopsy demonstrates perivascular inflammation and axonal degeneration*

    d. Treatment

        i. *Facial palsy: doxycycline, 100 mg bid for 3 weeks*

        ii. *CNS involvement: third-generation intravenous cephalosporin (e.g., ceftriaxone, 2 mg intravenously q12h); penicillin, 3.3 million units intravenously q4h; treatment for 2 to 3 weeks*

6. *Leprosy*

7. *HIV*

H. Multiple cranial nerve palsies

1. Differential diagnosis

    a. Congenital (e.g., *Möbius' syndrome):* facial diplegia; affects cranial nerve VI in 70%; external ophthalmoplegia in 20%; ptosis in 10%; voice paralysis in 15% to 20%

    b. Infectious: chronic meningitis (e.g., spirochete, fungal, mycoplasma, viral, including HIV, tuberculous [cranial nerve VI most frequent])

    c. Lyme disease

    d. Neurosyphilis

    e. Acute fungal infection (cryptococcus, aspergillosis, mucormycosis)

    f. Traumatic (particularly skull base fracture)

    g. Tumor: for example, meningioma, adenocarcinoma, glomus jugular tumors, carcinomatous meningitis, primary CNS lymphoma

    h. Wegener's granulomatosis

    i. Sarcoidosis

    j. Inflammatory

    k. Acute inflammatory demyelinating polyneuropathy (AIDP)

    l. Entrapment syndromes, for example, Paget's disease, fibrous dysplasia

I. Chronic sensorimotor polyneuropathy

1. Diabetic neuropathy (see Section II.F)

2. CIDP
3. Nutritional
   a. Mechanism of production of the nutritional neuropathies
      i. Chronic alcoholism
      ii. Food/nutritional dietary fads
      iii. Malabsorption
      iv. Drugs
   b. Neuropathic beriberi
      i. *Disease of the heart and peripheral nerves*
      ii. Clinical features: slow onset and evolution of a generalized peripheral neuropathy with weakness and wasting affecting the lower extremities distally, followed by involvement of the upper extremities distally; similar distribution of sensory loss involving all methods of sensation; reflexes are absent or reduced; vagal involvement; cranial neuropathies (rare); subacute loss of vision (rare).
      iii. Pathology: axonal degeneration affecting the distal segments of lower more than upper extremities; vagus and phrenic nerves often affected (late); chromatolytic changes occur in the dorsal root ganglion and alpha motor neuron cell bodies; secondary degeneration of dorsal columns may occur; accumulation of membrane-bound sacs and depletion of neurotubules and neurofilaments of the distal ends of motor and sensory axons.
   c. Strachan's syndrome: amblyopia; painful neuropathy; orogenital dermatitis; caused by deficiency of the B vitamins
   d. Burning feet syndrome: subacute onset of a neuropathy characterized by severe burning pain in the extremities with hyperhidrosis of the feet; may be associated with deficiencies of the B vitamins, including pantothenic acid, thiamine, nicotinic acid, and riboflavin
   e. Vitamin B_{12} deficiency
      i. Pathogenesis: pernicious anemia with absence or marked reduction of intrinsic factor; posterior column involvement more significant than peripheral neuropathy.
      ii. *Clinical:* slowly progressive; numbness and paresthesias of the feet followed by ataxia, weakness, and wasting of distal lower extremities (upper extremities become involved in severe); *loss of vibration and position sense is prominent early, followed by a distal loss of pain and temperature perception.*
      iii. Lab testing: reduced vitamin B_{12} levels; if uncertain, *Schilling test* or test for intrinsic factor blocking Ab may be done. Elevated methylmalonic acid and homocysteine may be confirmatory.
      iv. Treatment: *vitamin B_{12}, 1000 mcg intramuscularly daily for 7 days, followed by the same dosage q weekly × 1 month, then monthly*

> **NB:** Vitamin B_{12} deficiency may involve the dorsal columns as well as pyramidal tracts, causing subacute combined degeneration of the spinal cord.

   f. Vitamin E deficiency: chronic axonal sensory neuropathy; clinical: increased creatine phosphokinase (CPK) possible; ataxia; ophthalmoplegia
   g. Alcoholic polyneuropathy
      i. Pathogenesis: likely secondary to dietary deficiency and alcoholic gastritis; significant weight loss may also be contributory; thiamine deficiency has a major role and may cause axonal degeneration in experimental models.

   g. *Alcoholic polyneuropathy (cont'd)*

    ii. Clinical: chronic slowly progressive neuropathy; distal weakness and wasting affecting mainly the lower extremities; mild pansensory impairment distally; ankle jerks usually absent; *peripheral neuropathy occurs in 80% of patients with Wernicke-Korsakoff syndrome;* NCS/EMG with axon loss motor and sensory nerve changes.

    iii. Pathology: axonal degeneration

    iv. Treatment: balanced high-calorie diet; supplemental B vitamins daily (thiamine 25 mg, niacin 100 mg, riboflavin 10 mg, pantothenic acid 10 mg, pyridoxine 5 mg)

  4. Connective tissue disease

  5. Paraneoplastic

  6. *Multiple myeloma*

   a. *Uncontrolled proliferation of plasma cells that infiltrate in bone and soft tissues*

   b. May be a hyperviscosity state due to paraproteinemia, renal failure, hypercalcemia, and amyloidosis, all of which affect nerve excitation and conduction, or cause fiber degeneration

   c. Clinical

    i. Neuropathy due to direct effect of neoplastic tissue: root compression due to deposits or from vertebral collapse produces radicular pain, which is the most common neurologic symptom in multiple myeloma; cauda equina syndrome; sensorimotor polyneuropathy.

    ii. Neuropathy due to compression with amyloid deposits

    iii. Amyloid generalized neuropathy

    iv. Neuropathy due to remote effect of multiple myeloma

    v. Osteosclerotic myeloma with polyneuropathy

> **NB:** POEMS syndrome may occur: <u>p</u>olyneuropathy, <u>o</u>rganomegaly, <u>e</u>ndocrinopathy, <u>m</u>onoclonal gammopathy, <u>s</u>kin changes (also known as Crow-Fukase syndrome).

  7. *Monoclonal gammopathy of undetermined significance*

   a. *50% of neuropathies associated with M-protein*

   b. *Anti-MAG Ab in 50% of cases*

   c. Typically men greater than 50 years old [y/o]

   d. Slow progressive ascending demyelinating (+ axonal) sensory-predominant neuropathy with weakness

   e. May be associated with Raynaud's phenomenon, ataxia, and intentional tremor

   f. Treatment with immunosuppressive agents: PE; IVIg: steroids

  8. *Waldenström's macroglobulinemia*

   a. *Usually affecting elderly with fatigue, weight loss, lymphadenopathy, hepatosplenomegaly, visual disturbances, and bleeding diathesis, and, hematologically, by a great excess of 19S IgM macroglobulin in the blood*

   b. May occur in association with chronic lymphocytic leukemia, lymphosarcoma, carcinoma, cirrhosis of the liver, collagen vascular diseases, and in hemolytic anemia of the cold Ab type; in these conditions, symptoms are caused by involvement of nerve, CNS, and systemic manifestations.

   c. IgM M-protein class is usually κ light chain.

      d. Slowly progressive neuropathy

         i. Early stage may be asymmetric.

         ii. In later stages, there is a typical sensorimotor neuropathy.

         iii. Sensory symptoms consisting of paresthesia, pain, and objective sensory loss, and there may also be marked weakness and wasting extremities.

         iv. Myopathy can also occur because of IgM binding to decorin.

      e. Treatment with immunosuppression: PE, chemotherapy

9. *Cryoglobulinemia*

      a. *Characterized by the presence in the serum of a cryoglobulin that precipitates on cooling and redissolves on rewarming to 37°C*

      b. Types of cryoglobulinemia

         i. *Idiopathic: monoclonal gammopathy such as myeloma, macroglobulinemia, and lymphomas; M component is cryoprotein.*

         ii. Secondary: *collagen vascular disorders, chronic infections (hepatitis C), mesothelioma, and the polyclonal gammopathies*

      c. Neuropathy occurs in 7%.

      d. Usually, gradually progressive axonal neuropathy

      e. Patients present with Raynaud's phenomenon, cold sensitivity, purpuric skin eruptions, and ulceration of the lower limbs.

      f. Over years, eventually develop asymmetric sensorimotor neuropathy (lower > upper extremities) accompanied by pain and paresthesia

      g. Necessary to work up for a collagen vascular disorder, hematologic causes of an M protein, and for hepatitis C (50% of patients with chronic hepatitis C have cryoglobulinemia)

      h. Treatment: avoidance of cold, plasmapheresis, cytotoxic agents, corticosteroids; in hepatitis C, neuropathy may respond to interferon-α.

10. *Uremic polyneuropathy*

      a. *Two-thirds of dialysis patients*

      b. *May begin with burning dysesthesias*

      c. Painful distal sensory loss followed by weakness (lower > upper extremities)

      d. Uremia is also associated with CTS and ischemic monomelic neuropathy.

      e. Treatment: hemodialysis improves signs/symptoms; renal transplant: complete recovery in 6 to 12 months

11. *Leprosy*

      a. *Classic most common cause of neuropathy globally but rare in the United States*

      b. *Laminin-2 has been identified on the Schwann cell-axon unit as an initial neural target for the invasion of* Mycobacterium leprae.

      c. *Trophic ulcers, Charcot joints, and mutilated fingers are common due to anesthesia.*

      d. *Tuberculoid leprosy:* causes mononeuritis multiplex; skin lesions consist of asymmetric hypesthetic macules; superficial nerve fibers are always affected and may be palpable as skin; sensory loss is earliest for pain and temperature; ulnar, median, peroneal, and facial nerves are especially prone; superficial cutaneous radial, digital, posterior auricular, and sural are the commonly affected sensory nerves.

      e. *Lepromatous leprosy:* hematogenous spread to skin, ciliary bodies, testes, nodes, and peripheral nerves; lesions tend to occur on other cooler parts of the body: the dorsal surface of hands, dorsomedial surface of forearm, dorsal surface of feet, and anterolateral aspects of legs, with loss of pain and temperature.

11. *Leprosy (cont'd)*

   f. Pathology: segmental demyelination

   g. Treatment: combination of dapsone, 100 mg daily, and rifampin, 600 mg monthly, for 6 months

12. *Critical illness polyneuropathy*

   a. 50% of critically ill ICU patients (length of stay > 1 week), particularly if patient has concurrent sepsis and multiorgan failure

   b. Primarily axonal degeneration (motor > sensory)

> **> NB:** There is also a critical care myopathy known as myosin-losing myopathy.

13. *HIV neuropathy*

   a. Clinical

      i. *IDP*

         (A) Acute inflammatory demyelinating polyradiculoneuropathy (AIDP) and CIDP have been associated with HIV-1 infection.

         (B) Main features that distinguish HIV-1–infected individuals from HIV-1–seronegative patients with IDP

            (1) HIV-1–infected patients with IDP frequently have a lymphocytic CSF pleocytosis of 20 to 50 cells.

            (2) HIV-1 infected individuals have polyclonal elevations of serum immunoglobulins.

         (C) Electrodiagnostic features of IDP in HIV-1–seropositive individuals are not different.

      ii. *Mononeuritis multiplex:* with and without necrotizing vasculitis

      iii. *Distal predominantly sensory polyneuropathy:* several factors involved, including age, immunosuppression, nutritional status, and chronic disease

      iv. *Distal symmetric polyneuropathy associated with neurotoxic drugs:* dose-dependent neuropathy (e.g., zalcitabine, didanosine, stavudine, lamivudine)

      v. *Autonomic neuropathy:* more frequently in the late stage

      vi. ***Polyradiculoneuropathy associated with cytomegalovirus:*** patients have low CD4 lymphocyte counts; clinical: stereotypic development of a rapidly progressive cauda equina syndrome; upper extremities are usually spared until late in the course; rapidly fatal if untreated.

J. **Carcinomatous/paraneoplastic neuropathy**

   1. Syndromes

      *a. Antineuronal nuclear Ab type 1 (**ANNA-1**)*

         i. ***Also known as anti-Hu Ab syndrome***

         ii. Panneuronal Ab binding to both nucleus and cytoplasm of neurons of both the peripheral nervous system and CNS

         iii. Associated with *small-cell lung carcinoma* and more recently found to be associated with the gastroenterologic neuropathy typically presenting as a pseudo-obstruction syndrome; may also be associated with prostate and breast cancer

         iv. Two-thirds of cases are female.

         v. Tumor may not be discovered for up to 3 years after onset of signs/symptoms or not until autopsy.

vi. Antigen reactive with ANNA-1 has been identified in homogenized small-cell lung carcinoma tissue.

vii. Clinical: subacute sensory neuropathy (most common); motor neuron disease; limbic encephalopathy; cerebellar dysfunction; brainstem dysfunction; autonomic dysfunction

b. *ANNA-2*

   i. *Also known as anti-Ri and anti-Nova Ab syndrome*

   ii. Associated with carcinoma of the breast

   iii. Antigens are 55- and 80-kDa CNS proteins.

   iv. Clinical: cerebellar ataxia; opsoclonus; myelopathy; brainstem dysfunction

c. *Anti-Purkinje cytoplasmic Ab type 1 (PCAb1)*

   i. *Also known as anti-Yo Ab syndrome*

   ii. Ab reacts with the cytoplasm of cerebellar Purkinje cells, particularly rough endoplasmic reticulum, and also cytoplasm of cerebellar molecular neurons and Schwann cells.

   iii. PCAb1 is a serologic marker for *ovarian carcinoma and, less often, breast carcinoma.*

   iv. Clinical: subacute cerebellar syndrome (most common); neuropathy (rare)

AB	STRUCTURE	CANCER	NEUROLOGIC SYNDROME
ANNA-1 (antI-Hu)	Panneuronal	Small-cell lung	Sensory neuronopathy
		Cancer	Pseudo-obstruction syndrome
ANNA-2 (anti-Ri or anti-Nova)	Neuronal nucleus	Breast cancer	Cerebellar ataxia; myelopathy
PCAb1 (anti-Yo)	Purkinje cytoplasmic	Ovarian and breast cancer	Subacute cerebellar dysfunction

2. *Clinical patterns of neuropathies associated with cancer*

   a. *Sensory neuronopathy*

      i. Approximately 20% of the paraneoplastic neuropathies

      ii. Underlying malignancy is almost always a lung carcinoma and usually small (oat) cell; other causes include esophageal and cecal carcinoma.

      iii. Affects females more than males.

      iv. Mean age of onset is 59 years.

      v. Neuropathy usually precedes diagnosis of the tumor by approximately 6 months to 3 years.

      vi. Subacute onset and slow progression

      vii. Sensory symptoms predominate, including numbness and paresthesia of the extremities, aching limb pains, and a sensory ataxia.

      viii. Motor weakness and wasting are minimal until more advanced.

      ix. Pseudoathetosis may develop due to sensory dysfunction.

      x. Removal of the underlying tumor does not usually alter course.

      xi. Mean duration from onset of neuropathy to death is approximately 14 months.

      xii. Pathology: dorsal root ganglia cells degenerate and are replaced by clusters of round cells *(residual nodules of Nageotte);* dorsal root fibers and

   a. *Sensory neuronopathy (cont'd)*

   the dorsal columns are degenerated; perivascular lymphocytic infiltration affecting the dorsal root ganglia and also the hippocampus, amygdaloid nucleus, brainstem, and spinal cord.

   b. *Mild terminal sensorimotor neuropathy:* little disability; malignant disease was known to have been present for 6 months or longer in 70% of patients and for 2 years in 40%; mean interval from onset of the neuropathy to death was 11 months.

   c. *Acute and subacute sensorimotor neuropathy*

   d. *Remitting and relapsing neuropathy*

   e. *Pandysautonomia:* sympathetic and parasympathetic dysfunction resulting in orthostatic hypotension and anhidrosis, among other possible autonomic features

K. **Neuropathy associated with lymphoma, lymphoproliferative, and Hodgkin's disease**

   1. Cranial neuropathies by local compression, leptomeningeal involvement, or direct invasion; *cranial nerves III, IV, VI, and VII are the most commonly affected.*

   2. Root compression occurs from extension of vertebral deposits or from vertebrae collapse; may present as cauda equina syndrome.

   3. Other presentations: plexopathy; lumbosacral greater than cervical; mononeuropathies

L. **Neuropathy associated with myeloma**

   1. *Multiple myeloma*

M. **Medication-induced neuropathies**

   1. *Amiodarone:* 5% to 10% of patients have symptomatic peripheral neuropathy invariably associated with a static or intention tremor and possible ataxia (possible cerebellar dysfunction); +/- demyelinating features; slowly progressive symmetric distal sensory loss and motor neuropathy with areflexia.

   2. *Cisplatin:* predominantly sensory neuropathy often occurs when dose exceeds a total of 400 mg/m^2; axonal; Lhermitte's phenomenon; distal paresthesia in lower and upper extremities followed by progressive sensory ataxia; loss of all sensory modalities in glove and stocking distribution but more prominent loss of vibration and joint position sense; areflexia; differential diagnosis is paraneoplastic sensory neuropathy.

   3. *Colchicine:* binds tubulin and interferes with mitotic spindle formation and axonal transport; chronic axonal sensorimotor neuropathy; association with an acute myopathy that superficially resembles acute polymyositis (PM).

   4. *Dapsone:* chronic distal axonal motor neuropathy; sparing of sensory function

   5. *Disulfiram (Antabuse®):* chronic distal axonal sensorimotor neuropathy; begins with distal paresthesia and pain and progresses to distal sensory loss and weakness; more common in patients taking 250 to 500 mg/day of disulfiram; treatment: discontinuing disulfiram or lowering it to less than 125 mg/day typically results in gradual but complete recovery.

   6. *Isoniazid:* chronic distal axonal sensory greater than motor neuropathy; begins with symmetric distal paresthesia in the feet and hands, progressing to include painful distal sensory loss; relative preservation of proprioception; treatment: pyridoxine (15–50 mg/day) appears to prevent the neuropathic side effects of isoniazid.

   7. *Lithium:* chronic axonal sensorimotor neuropathy

   8. *Metronidazole:* chronic axonal sensory greater than motor neuropathy

   9. *Nitrofurantoin:* chronic axonal sensorimotor neuropathy

   10. *Phenytoin:* chronic axonal sensory greater than motor neuropathy

11. *Pyridoxine:* chronic axonal sensory neuropathy: usually taking megadoses (1–5 g/day), but minimum dose of pyridoxine that has been associated with neuropathic symptoms is 50 mg/day; neuropathic symptoms may begin with ataxia in combination with Lhermitte's phenomenon (may be misdiagnosed as multiple sclerosis); motor or autonomic involvement is rare; treatment: limit pyridoxine to less than 50 mg/day.

12. *Vincristine:* chronic axonal sensorimotor neuropathy

N. Heavy metal–induced neuropathies

1. *Arsenic*

   a. Clinical

      i. Acute axonal sensory greater than motor neuropathy begins 5 to 10 days after ingestion.

      ii. Most typical history is that of an acute gastrointestinal illness followed by burning painful paresthesia in the hands and feet with progressive distal muscle weakness.

      iii. CNS symptoms may develop rapidly in acute poisoning, with drowsiness and confusion progressing to stupor or psychosis and delirium.

      iv. Hyperkeratosis and sloughing of the skin on the palms and soles may occur several weeks after ingestion and be followed by a more chronic state of redness and swelling of the hands and feet.

      v. Nail changes *(Mees' lines)*

      vi. With chronic poisoning, may have aplastic anemia

   b. Diagnosis

      i. Acute intoxication: renal excretion greater than 0.1 mg arsenic in 24 hours

      ii. Chronic intoxication: hair concentrations greater than 0.1 mg/100 g of hair; slow-growing hair, such as pubic hair, may be elevated as long as 8 months after exposure.

   c. Treatment: acute oral ingestion—gastric lavage with 2 to 3 L of water followed by instillation of milk or 1% sodium thiosulfate; British anti-Lewisite (BAL) is given parenterally in a 10% solution.

   d. Prognosis: mortality in severe arsenic encephalitis: greater than 50% to 75%; once neuropathy occurs, treatment is usually ineffective.

2. *Gold*

   a. Pathophysiology: used in the treatment of arthritis, lupus erythematosus, and other inflammatory conditions

   b. Clinical: chronic distal axonal sensory greater than motor neuropathy; painful, producing burning or itching in the palms of the hands or soles of the feet; possibly myokymia; brachial plexopathy; AIDP

   c. Pathology: loss of myelin as well as active axonal degeneration

   d. Treatment: chelation therapy with BAL has been used but is usually unnecessary.

3. *Mercury*

   a. Clinical

      i. Acute: stomatitis, salivation, and severe gastrointestinal disturbances followed by hallucinations and delirium

      ii. Chronic

         (A) Chronic axonal sensory-predominant neuropathy

         (B) Constriction of visual fields, ataxia, dysarthria, decreased hearing, tremor, and dementia

ii. Chronic (*cont'd*)

(C) Parkinsonism

(D) In children: *acrodynia*

b. Treatment: chelating agents (e.g., D-penicillamine, BAL, ethylenediaminetetraacetic acid)

4. *Thallium*

a. Clinical

i. **Hallmark: *alopecia***

ii. Acute

(A) Gastrointestinal symptoms develop within hours of ingestion.

(B) Large doses (>2 g) produce cardiovascular shock, coma, and death within 24 hours.

(C) Moderate doses produce neuropathic symptoms within 24 to 48 hours, consisting of limb pain and distal paresthesia with increasing distal-to-proximal limb sensory loss accompanied by distal limb weakness.

(D) May produce AIDP-like syndrome.

iii. Chronic: chronic axonal sensorimotor neuropathy

b. Treatment: chelating agents such as Prussian blue (potassium ferric hexacyanoferrate, BAL, dithizone, diethyldithiocarbamate); if acute, can also perform gastric lavage

5. *Lead*

a. Pathophysiology

i. Passes placental barriers

ii. Diminishes cerebral glucose supplies

iii. The brain is also unusually sensitive to the effects of triethyl lead.

iv. Triethyl lead chloride intoxication decreases the incorporation of labeled sulfate into sulfatides, resulting in inhibition of myelin synthesis and demyelination.

v. Adults: use of exterior paints (less common today) and leaded gasoline; more likely to present with neuropathy

vi. Children: pica and eating lead-based paints (less common today); more likely to present with encephalopathy

b. Clinical

i. Neuropathy

(A) Chronic axonal motor neuropathy

(B) Classic neurologic presentation: radial neuropathy with wristdrop

(C) Typical clinical triad: abdominal pain and constipation; anemia; neuropathy

ii. CNS toxicity

(A) Adult: prodrome: progressive weakness and weight loss; ashen color of the face; mild persistent headache; fine tremor of the muscles of the eyes, tongue, and face; progression into encephalopathic state; may have focal motor weakness

(B) Children: prodrome usually nonspecific, evolving into encephalopathic state (50%); if large amounts of lead are ingested, prodrome symptoms may be present.

c. Treatment: chelating agents such as BAL, ethylenediaminetetraacetic acid, penicillamine

d. Prognosis

    i. Mild intoxication: usually complete recovery

    ii. Severe encephalopathy: mortality high but lessened by the use of combined chelating agent therapy

    iii. Residual neurologic sequelae: blindness or partial visual disturbances, persistent convulsions, personality changes, and mental retardation

    iv. Prognosis worse in children than in adults

O. Hereditary polyneuropathy

1. *Inherited axonal neuropathies*

    a. *Predominantly motor axonal neuropathies*

        i. *Hereditary motor and sensory neuropathy type 2 (Charcot-Marie-Tooth type 2)*

            (A) Pathophysiology: autosomal dominant (AD): three types: types 2a, 2b, 2c, with some linkage to chromosome 1p

            (B) Clinical: symptoms start in early adulthood; stork leg appearance (peroneal muscular atrophy); rarely totally incapacitated; on NCS—mildly slowed conduction velocity with decreased sensory and motor amplitudes.

        ii. *Acute intermittent porphyria*

            (A) Pathophysiology: actually an inborn error of metabolism; AD

            (B) Clinical: 90% never have symptoms; symptoms begin at puberty; *motor neuropathy develops in proximal distribution (arms > legs); 50% of patients with neuropathy can have mild sensory involvement in the same distribution.*

    b. *Predominantly sensory axonal neuropathies*

        i. *Hereditary sensory and autonomic neuropathies (HSAN)*

MAJOR CLINICAL FEATURES OF HSAN II, HSAN III, AND HSAN IV			
CLINICAL FEATURES	**HSAN TYPE II**	**HSAN TYPE III**	**HSAN TYPE IV**
Onset	Birth	Birth	Birth
Initial symptoms (from birth to age 3 years)	Swallowing problems	Swallowing problems	Fevers
	Self-mutilation (65%)	Aspiration pneumonia	Self-mutilation (88%)
	Delayed development	Breech presentation (37%)	
		Hypothermia	
		Delayed development	
Unique features	No axon flare	No axon flare	No axon flare
	Lack of fungiform papilla	Lack of fungiform papilla	Anhidrosis
	Hearing loss (30%)	Alacrima	Consanguinity 50%

(continued)

MAJOR CLINICAL FEATURES OF HSAN II, HSAN III, AND HSAN IV			
CLINICAL FEATURES	HSAN TYPE II	HSAN TYPE III	HSAN TYPE IV
Sensory dysfunction			
Depressed DTR	Frequent (71%)	Almost consistent (99%)	Infrequent (9%)
Pain perception	Absent	Mild to moderate decrease	Absent
Temperature perception	Severe decrease	Mild to moderate decrease	Absent
Vibration sense	Normal	Normal	Normal to moderate decrease
Autonomic			
Gastroesophageal reflux	Frequent (71%)	Frequent (67%)	Uncommon (24%)
Postural hypotension	Uncommon (25%)	Almost consistent (99%)	Uncommon (29%)
Episodic hypertension	Rare	Frequent	Rare
Ectodermal features			
Dry skin	No	No	Consistent
Fractures	29%	40%	71%
Scoliosis	59%	85%	23%
Intelligence			
IQ <65	Common (38%)	Uncommon (10%)	Common (33%)
Hyperactivity	Common (41%)	Uncommon	Common (54%)
Rare <1% Infrequent <10% Uncommon <30% Common 30–65% Frequent >65% DTR = deep tendon reflexes			

Source: Adapted from Axelrod and Gold-von Simson, *Orphanet Journal of Rare Diseases.* 2007;2:39. doi:10.1186/1750-1172-2-39

    c. Sensorimotor axonal neuropathies

        i. *Giant axonal neuropathy*

            (A) Pathophysiology: rare; AR; affects both central and peripheral axons

            (B) Clinical; usually presents by age 3 years with gait problems, distal leg atrophy, and severely impaired vibration and proprioception; diagnosis: *sural nerve biopsy with enlarged axons with disrupted neurofilaments that are surrounded by a thin or fragmented myelin sheath (secondary demyelination)*

        ii. *Familial amyloid neuropathy*

            (A) Pathophysiology: *AD; chromosome 18; associated with gene for prealbumin*

            (B) Clinical: involves sensation, then autonomic function, and then motor late in course; marked autonomic dysfunction: erectile dysfunction, incontinence, anhidrosis, and cardiac involvement; death within 15 years; Portuguese heritage: young adulthood and predominantly involves the legs; Swiss heritage: less severe form affecting predominantly the arms; nerve conduction studies show axonal sensory motor polyneuropathy; diagnosis: amyloid on sural biopsy

   iii. **Friedreich's ataxia:** *AR;* primarily affects the *corticospinal tracts, dorsal columns, and spinocerebellar tracts;* late in the disease course, can affect peripheral nerves (dorsal root ganglion); EMG/NCS: absent SNAPs and normal motor conduction studies

2. *Inherited demyelinating neuropathies* Patients with inherited demyelinating neuropathies have **uniform slowing** of the conduction velocities of all nerves without signs of conduction block, whereas acquired demyelinating neuropathies will tend to have multifocal/segmental slowing (with conduction block and temporal dispersion).

   a. **Charcot-Marie-Tooth type 1 (hereditary motor and sensory neuropathy type 1)**

      i. Pathophysiology

         (A) Most common

         (B) *AD mostly but can also be AR or X-linked*

         (C) *Genetically heterogeneous group*

         (D) *Three gene products have been identified as abnormal:*

            (1) Peripheral myelin protein 22 (PMP22)

            (2) Myelin protein zero (MPZ)

            (3) Connexin 32

         (E) *Men affected more severely and more commonly*

         (F) *Demyelination with onion bulb formation*

      ii. Clinical: symptoms begin in 2nd decade; foot deformity with hammertoes and high arches followed with atrophy of the peroneal musculature; atrophy later involves upper leg and upper extremities; characteristic gait abnormality results from bilateral footdrop; have palpable nerves and loss of vibration and proprioception, then ankle jerks, and then diffuse reflex loss; NCS: slow with limited/no temporal dispersion.

> **NB:** In CMT type 1A, there is *duplication* of the PMP 22 gene; in hereditary neuropathy with liability to pressure palsies (HNPP), there is *deletion* of PMP 22 gene. CMT 2 is the *axonal* phenotype!

   b. **Dejerine-Sottas (hereditary motor and sensory neuropathy type 3)**

      i. Pathophysiology: *AR; defect: PMP22 and point mutation of MPZ; demyelination with onion bulb formation*

      ii. Clinical: delayed motor milestones in infancy; pes cavus; muscle cramps; palsies of the 6th and 7th cranial nerves; adults—severe truncal ataxia; nerve conduction velocities (NCV): severe slowing

   c. **Hereditary neuropathy with liability to pressure palsies (HNPP) (tomaculous neuropathy)**

      i. Pathophysiology: *AD, chromosome 17; deletion of PMP22*

      ii. Clinical: asymmetric; associated with minor nerve compression or trauma; NCS: conduction block in areas not typically associated with

    c. **Hereditary neuropathy with liability to pressure palsies (HNPP) (tomaculous neuropathy)** (*cont'd*)

        entrapment; biopsy (teased nerve preparation) reveals tomacula (focal myelin swellings).

    d. **Congenital hypomyelinating neuropathy**

        i. Pathophysiology: *AR; MPZ point mutation; severe hypomyelination or complete lack of myelination of peripheral nerves*

        ii. Clinical: biopsy: lack onion bulbs; hypotonia; severe distal weakness; difficulty with respiration and feeding; may be associated with arthrogryposis congenita; NCS: extremely slow conduction velocities

3. **Multiple endocrine neoplasia type 2B**

    a. Pathophysiology: rare; *AD; gene linked to chromosome 10q11.2*

    b. *Clinical: medullary carcinoma of the thyroid (can metastasize); pheochromocytoma; ganglioneuromatosis; abnormalities of bony and connective tissue elements; peroneal muscular atrophy and pes cavus foot deformity with or without hammer toes; multiple endocrine disturbances develop.*

III. Acute and Chronic IDP

A. AIDP

1. Epidemiology: aka Guillain-Barré syndrome; 1 to 2 cases per 100,000 in North America; progressive increase with age, reaching 8.6/100,000 in individuals 70 to 79 y/o; affects males more than females; antecedent respiratory and enteric infections (especially *Campylobacter*) present in one-half to two-thirds of cases.

2. Clinical

    a. Core features: acute onset; *ascending predominantly motor polyradiculoneuropathy typically beginning in the lower limbs;* CSF changes of elevated protein with normal cell count (albuminocytological dissociation); areflexia

    b. Onset within 1 to 3 weeks after a benign upper respiratory or gastrointestinal illness

    c. Associated with AIDP

        i. Antecedent viral infection: cytomegalovirus, Epstein-Barr virus, HIV, smallpox-vaccinia viruses, hepatitis B

        ii. Antecedent bacterial infections: *Campylobacter jejuni: 20% of AIDP cases, Mycoplasma pneumoniae, Borrelia burgdorferi* (Lyme disease)

        iii. Vaccines: rabies vaccine, tetanus toxoid vaccine, polio vaccine

        iv. Drugs

        v. Surgery

        vi. Pregnancy

        vii. Lymphoma

    d. Maximal weakness over the course of a few days to 6 weeks

    e. Facial weakness to some degree occurs in more than 50% of patients.

    f. May also have development of sensory loss

    g. Dysautonomia, mainly cardiovascular, manifested as tachycardia and orthostatic hypotension and associated with increased mortality

    h. CSF: increase in protein associated with a cell count less than 10

> **NB:** The H-reflex is the most sensitive test for early GBS. Absent H response, abnormal F wave, and abnormal upper extremity SNAP combined with a normal sural SNAP are characteristic of early GBS.

> **NB:** There is an axonal form of the disease—acute motor axonal neuropathy (AMAN), which has a poorer prognosis.

> i. *Electrodiagnostic findings: conduction slowing/block; prolonged distal latency; prolonged F-wave latencies; may be delayed for several weeks (usually 10–14 days, depending on severity of clinical symptoms)*

  i. Clinical variants

  > i. *Autonomic variant:* core features: acute or subacute onset; widespread sympathetic and parasympathetic failure; relative or complete sparing of somatic fibers; sympathetic: orthostatic hypotension; anhidrosis; parasympathetic: dry eyes; dry mouth; bowel and bladder dysfunction; Schirmer test confirms reduced tear secretion.

  > ii. *Miller-Fisher variant:* triad: *ophthalmoplegia; ataxia; areflexia;* 5% of AIDP cases; many cases are associated with motor involvement; associated with a particular serotype of *C. jejuni* (GQ1b epitope); CSF protein increased; EMG/NCS: demyelinating neuropathy; patients may respond to plasmapheresis better than IVIg.

3. Differential diagnosis

   a. Periodic paralysis

   b. Neuromuscular transmission disorder (myasthenia gravis [MG], botulism, tick paralysis)

   c. Peripheral nerve disorder (porphyria, toxins)

   d. Anterior horn cell disorder (e.g., poliomyelitis)

   e. Acute myelopathy

   f. Drugs/toxins

   > i. Acute hexacarbon neuropathy from volatile solvents (paint lacquer vapors, glue sniffing)

   > ii. Nitrofurantoin

   > iii. Dapsone

   > iv. Organophosphates

   g. Saxitoxin

   h. Infection

   > i. Cytomegalovirus

   > ii. Diphtheria

   > iii. Lyme disease

   > iv. HIV: AIDP develops as patients seroconvert or have AIDS-related complex; usually have CSF pleocytosis (>40 cells)

4. Mechanisms

   a. Demonstration of IgM Abs that bind to carbohydrate residues of peripheral nerve in 90% of patients with AIDP at the onset of the disease

   b. Abs may induce demyelination by binding to C1q and activating the complement cascade or potentially bind to the Fc receptor on macrophages.

   c. Therapeutic IVIg is capable of neutralizing Abs in AIDP by an Ab-mediated mechanism.

5. Prognosis

   a. Monophasic, but 3% to 5% of cases may relapse; onset to peak in excess of 4 weeks may have a greater risk of relapse

   b. 75% have full functional recovery, and 10% have significant functional deficit

5. Prognosis (*cont'd*)

    c. Factors indicating good prognosis

       i. Young age

       ii. Mild disease

       iii. Acute (onset to peak at 1–3 weeks) but not hyperacute (onset to respirator support at 1–3 days) evolution

       iv. Improvement within 1 week of peak severity

    d. Factors indicating poor prognosis

       i. Old age

       ii. Hyperacute onset

       iii. Severe illness

       iv. Marked reduction in CMAP in more than 80% on NCS

       v. Delayed onset of recovery

    e. Mortality rate: 5% to 8%; most commonly resulting from ventilator-associated pneumonia

6. Treatment

    a. Supportive care

       i. Forced vital capacity (FVC), maximal inspiratory pressure (MIP), maximal expiratory pressure (MEP), and hemodynamic measures checked regularly.

       ii. ICU setting due to potential for rapid evolution/deterioration

       iii. **FVC greater than 20 mL/kg, MIP less than 30 cm H_2O, and MEP less than 40 cm H_2O (the "20/30/40 rule") or a reduction in any of these readings greater than 30% is associated with progression to respiratory failure and the need for intubation.**

    b. Interventions

       i. Plasma exchange (PE)

          (A) Patient who is deteriorating or has severe disease

          (B) Mechanism of action of PE is not known but may be due to the removal of Ab, complement components, immune complexes, lymphokines, and acute-phase reactants.

          (C) Regimen: six PEs over 2 weeks, with 3.0 to 3.5 L exchanged per treatment

          (D) Adverse effects: transient hypotension, hypocalcemia, slightly increased bleeding risk

       ii. IVIg

          (A) 0.4 g/kg per treatment

          (B) Five treatments over 3 or 6 days

          (C) Adverse effects: 5% of patients; congestive heart failure, hypotension, deep vein thrombosis, acute renal failure, anaphylaxis, aseptic meningitis, cerebral infarction, encephalopathy

       iii. Oral corticosteroids are not recommended.

    c. Rehabilitation

       i. Needed in 40%

       ii. More likely to require rehabilitation:

          (A) Ventilator support

          (B) Dysautonomia

          (C) Increased acute and total length of hospital stay

          (D) Cranial nerve dysfunction

B. CIDP

1. Pathophysiology and epidemiology; inflammatory (macrophage-dependent) demyelination of nerve roots and peripheral nerves; immune-mediated disease possibly triggered by an influenza-like infection or other viral infections; prevalence 1 to 2 per 100,000 (6–7 per 100,000 in those >70 y/o); affects males more than females; 30% to 50% have relapsing-remitting course.

2. Clinical
   a. Two courses
      i. Monophasic course: slow, stepwise, or steady dysfunction
      ii. Relapsing course
   b. *Symmetric, affecting both motor and sensory fibers with muscle weakness and sensory loss*
   c. Weakness of both proximal and distal muscles ± atrophy
   d. Sensory symptoms include numbness and paresthesias.
   e. Decreased or absent deep tendon reflexes (DTRs)
   f. Cranial nerve involvement far less common than in AIDP
   g. CSF: *protein elevated between 60 and 200 mg;* CSF pleocytosis uncommon and should exclude other conditions (HIV, Lyme disease, and lymphoproliferative disorders)
   h. NCS/EMG: multifocal demyelination; motor conduction velocities less than 80% of normal; temporal dispersion of the CMAP; variable degree of conduction block; EMG needle study: chronic denervation

3. Prognosis
   a. 10%: die due to complications
   b. 5%: recover completely
   c. 60%: work with residual deficits
   d. 10%: confined to a wheelchair
   e. Patients with significant denervation/axon loss features do worse.

4. Treatment
   a. Prednisone: both progressive and relapsing course improved
   b. PE: be wary of long-term costs and difficulty maintaining venous access.
   c. IVIg: 0.4 g/kg per treatment; three to five treatments over 7 to 14 days

Comparison of AIDP and CIDP

	AIDP	CIDP
Viral infection	Common	Uncommon
Onset to peak	<6 wks	>6 wks
Relapses	Uncommon (<5-7%)	More common
Facial weakness	>50%	<50%
Respiratory failure	Common	Uncommon
Sensory loss	Minimal	Moderate +
Abnormal electrodiagnostic findings	Patchy May be normal for initial 2 wks	Diffuse
Treatment	PE	Prednisone
	IVIg	PE IVIg
Prognosis	Good	Variable

Comparison of Chronic Acquired Immune-Mediated Demyelinating Polyneuropathies

DISORDER	CIDP	DISTAL ACQUIRED DEMYELINATING SYMMETRIC NEUROPATHY	MULTIFOCAL ACQUIRED DEMYELINATING SENSORY AND MOTOR NEUROPATHY	MULTIFOCAL MOTOR NEUROPATHY
Clinical features				
Distribution of weakness	Symmetric; proximal and distal	Symmetric; predominantly distal; sometimes no weakness	Asymmetric; distal > proximal; upper > lower limbs	Asymmetric; distal > proximal; upper > lower limbs
Reflexes	Symmetrically reduced	Symmetrically reduced	Reduced (multifocal or diffuse)	Reduced (multi-focal or diffuse)
Sensory deficits	Symmetric	Symmetric	Multifocal	None
Lab findings				
CSF protein	Usually elevated	Usually elevated	Usually elevated	Usually normal
Monoclonal protein	Occasionally present; IgG or IgA	IgM-**K** present in the majority; 50%–70% are positive for myelin-associated glycoprotein	Rare	Rare
Anti-GM1 Abs	Rare	Absent	Rare	Present 50% of the time
Electrodiagnostics				
Abnormal CMAPs	Usually symmetric	Usually symmetric; prolonged distal latencies	Asymmetric; multifocal	Asymmetric; multifocal
Abnormal SNAPs	Usually symmetric	Usually symmetric	Asymmetric; multifocal	Normal SNAPs
Conduction block	Frequent	Rare	Frequent	Frequent
Treatment				
PE	Good	Poor[a] or Good	Unclear	Poor
Prednisone	Good	Poor[a] or Good	Good	Poor
Cyclophosphamide	Good	Poor[a] or Good	Unclear	Good
IVIg	Good	Poor[a] or Good	Good	Good

[a]*Treatment response when associated with IgM-monoclonal gammopathy of undetermined significance.*

IV. Neuromuscular Junction Disorders

A. Myasthenia gravis (MG)

1. Pathophysiology

   a. Abnormal production of *acetylcholine (ACh) receptor Abs in thymus gland*

   b. Thymus gland *with lymphoid hyperplasia in more than 65% to 75% of MG cases and 15% with thymomas;* the thymus gland in patients with MG contains an increased number of B cells, and thymic lymphocytes in tissue culture secrete ACh receptor Abs.

   c. ACh receptor Abs interferes with ACh binding and decreases the number of ACh receptors.

   d. 2 to 10 per 100,000

   e. Bimodal distribution

      i. In those less than 40 y/o, 3 times more women than men

      ii. In those greater than 50 y/o, more men than women and more frequently have thymomas

   f. Passive transfer of MG from humans to mice using patient IgG

   g. Normal number of quanta of ACh released from the presynaptic membrane of the terminal axon at the neuromuscular junction in response to a nerve action potential, and each quantum contains a normal number of ACh molecules; miniature end-plate potential frequency in MG is normal, whereas amplitude is decreased (approximately 80%), related to the decreased number of available ACh receptors.

   h. *Normal-amplitude CMAP (Note: small CMAP seen in the Lambert-Eaton syndrome and in botulism)*

2. Clinical

   a. Three cardinal signs/symptoms

      i. Fluctuating weakness: worse with increased activity

      ii. Distribution of weakness: ocular and facial weakness in 40% to 50% at presentation and 85% at some point

      iii. Response to cholinergic agents

   b. Initial symptoms/signs of MG

      i. Extraocular muscles (ptosis, diplopia): 50%

      ii. Leg weakness: 10%

      iii. Generalized fatigue: 9%

      iv. Dysphagia: 6%

      v. Slurred/nasal speech: 5%

      vi. Difficulty chewing: 5%

      vii. Weakness of the face: 3%

      viii. Weakness of neck: 3%

      ix. Weakness of arms: 3%

   c. *Transient neonatal myasthenia*

      i. *12% of infants born to mothers with MG*

      ii. *At birth, hypotonia with respiration and feeding dysfunction*

      iii. *Symptoms usually begin during the first 24 hours after birth and may last for several weeks.*

      iv. May have fluctuating ptosis

  c. *Transient neonatal myasthenia (cont'd)*

   v. Arthrogryposis multiplex congenita as a result of lack of fetal movement in utero

   vi. Difficulty in feeding, generalized weakness, respiratory difficulties, weak cry, and facial weakness

   vii. Some improvement with edrophonium

   viii. EMG: repetitive nerve stimulation abnormal in weak muscles; repetitive nerve stimulation abnormal after sustained activity for 5 minutes in strong muscles; increased jitter

  d. *Slow channel syndrome: AD;* weakness in facial and limb musculature; muscle can be atrophic; usually after infancy in childhood, but onset may delay to adulthood; EMG: decrement on repetitive nerve stimulation, but not in all muscles

  e. *Congenital acetylcholinesterase (AChE) deficiency*

   i. Clinical: neonatal generalized weakness; sluggish pupillary reactivity; develop postural problems and fixed spinal column deformities; no response to AChE inhibitors

   ii. EMG: repetitive nerve stimulation at 2 Hz; demonstrates decrement in all muscles; single stimuli elicit repetitive CMAPs for 6 to 10 milliseconds after the initial response; these fade quickly during repetitive stimulation, even at rates as low as 0.2 Hz.

> **NB:** Congenital myasthenic syndromes such as slow channel syndrome and congenital AChE deficiency/end-plate deficiency of AChE are *not* related to an immune process but are caused by genetic defects affecting the neuromuscular junction (NMJ).

  f. *Limb-girdle (myasthenic) syndrome:* clinical onset during adolescence; progressive weakness responds to AChE inhibitors.

  g. *Exacerbation of MG*

   i. Etiologies

    (A) Medications

     (1) D-penicillamine

     (2) Aminoglycosides

     (3) Quinidine

     (4) Procainamide

     (5) Beta blockers

     (6) Synthroid

     (7) Lithium

     (8) Chlorpromazine

    (B) Infection

   ii. Myasthenic crisis

    (A) ICU setting to monitor FVC

    (B) **FVC less than 20 mL/kg, MIP less than 30 cm H_2O, and MEP less than 40 cm H_2O (the "20/30/40 rule") or a reduction in any of these readings greater than 30% is associated with progression to respiratory failure and the need for intubation.**

    (C) Often provoked by medications or infection

   iii. Cholinergic crisis

    (A) Overmedication resulting in miosis, increased salivation, diarrhea, cramps, and fasciculations

(B) Treatment: withdrawal of anticholinesterase medications under close observation

iv. If unsure if myasthenic crisis versus cholinergic crisis, use Tensilon® (edrophonium chloride) test challenge.

h. Differential diagnosis of MG

   i. Psychogenic neurasthenia

   ii. Progressive external ophthalmoplegia

   iii. Oculopharyngeal dystrophy

   iv. Amyotrophic lateral sclerosis (ALS)

   v. Progressive bulbar palsy

   vi. Lambert-Eaton syndrome

   vii. Botulism

   viii. Intracranial mass lesions compressing cranial nerves

   ix. Intranuclear ophthalmoplegia of multiple sclerosis

3. Diagnosis

  a. History

  b. Physical exam: ptosis with prolonged upgaze or decremental weakness after repetitive activity (particularly proximal muscles)

  c. Tensilon® test

    i. Short-acting AChE inhibitor

    ii. Procedure

      (A) Determine weak muscles (i.e., ptosis).

      (B) *Edrophonium chloride, 10 mg intravenously; normal saline (maintain atropine, 1 mg, at bedside for side effects such as bradycardia, hypotension, or arrhythmias).*

      (C) Inject 2 mg edrophonium chloride and observe.

      (D) Inject 2 mg normal saline and observe (for assessment of functional patients).

      (E) If no response, inject 4 to 8 mg edrophonium chloride and observe.

  d. Cooling (ice pack) test

    i. Place ice on muscles affected and observe.

    ii. Cooling muscles (particularly eyelid muscles) will improve weakness.

  e. Repetitive nerve stimulation testing (Jolly test): slow repetitive nerve stimulation at 2 to 3 Hz produces a decremental response of the CMAP that is maximal with the third or fourth stimulus.

  f. ACh receptor Ab test: generalized MG: 80% to 90% positive; ocular MG: 30% to 50% positive; does not correlate to severity of MG

> **NB:** Anti-MuSK antibody is found to be positive in ~50% patients considered "seronegative" for *ACh receptor Abs.*

  g. Antistriated muscle Ab: positive in 85% of patients with thymomas

  h. Single-fiber EMG: *increased jitter and blocking;* should only be performed by experienced electromyographers; 90+% of MG positive; may be positive for other conditions

    i. Other testing for differential diagnosis

    ii. Autoimmune battery (antinuclear Ab, erythrocyte sedimentation rate, rheumatoid factor, double-stranded DNA)

    h. Single-fiber EMG (*cont'd*)

      iii. Thyroid function test

      iv. Chest x-ray ± chest CT

      v. Purified protein derivative of tuberculin (before initiating immunosuppressant treatment)

      vi. Pulmonary function tests/FVC

4. Treatment

    a. General

      i. Pace activities

      ii. Get plenty of rest

      iii. Avoid exacerbation of weakness caused by infections, fever, heat, cold, pain, overexertion, emotional stress, and medications that can exacerbate MG.

    b. Continued scheduled treatment

      i. AChE inhibitors

        (A) *Pyridostigmine (Mestinon®)*

          (1) Onset: 30 minutes

          (2) Peak: 2 hours

          (3) Duration: 4 to 6 hours ± 1 hour

          (4) Side effects: diarrhea, nausea/vomiting, sweating, increased salivation, miosis, bradycardia, hypotension (glycopyrrolate 1–2 mg q8h to reduce diarrhea and salivation; also can use to decrease salivation in ALS)

          (5) May induce cholinergic crisis if too much is taken by patient

      ii. Immunosuppression

        (A) *Prednisone*

          (1) May hospitalize due to risk of acute exacerbation of MG induced by steroids ("steroid dip")

          (2) 1 to 1.5 mg/kg (60–100 mg) per day until clinical stabilization followed by slow outpatient taper

          (3) If minimal symptoms, outpatient prednisone, 10 to 20 mg, followed by 5-mg dose increase every 3 to 5 days until clinical stabilization or max of 60 mg/day (riskier due to risk of exacerbation)

          (4) Side effects: insomnia, hyperglycemia, peripheral edema due to fluid retention, peptic ulcer disease, osteoporosis, psychosis, avascular necrosis

        (B) *Azathioprine (Imuran®):* use when steroids are contraindicated and/or for steroid-sparing effect; begin 50 mg/day for 1 week and titrate up to 2 to 3 mg/kg/day if complete blood count stable; may take 6 to 12 months for benefit; side effects: *leukopenia, bone marrow suppression, macrocytic anemia, elevated liver function tests, pancreatitis. Alternative medication is CellCept® (mycophenolate mofetil).*

        (C) *Cyclosporine: a* second-line immunosuppressive agent; 5 mg/kg/day divided into twice-per-day dosing with meals (100–200 mg bid); more rapid onset than azathioprine; side effects: kidney and liver toxicity, leukopenia, gingival hyperplasia, hypertension, tremor, hirsutism

      iii. Immune modulation

        (A) *Plasma exchange (PE)*

        (B) *IVIg, 0.4 g/kg/day*

iv. *Thymectomy:* in patients with or without the presence of thymoma (but with other thymic abnormalities such as hyperplasia); typically recommended between ages 8 and 55 years; maximal response 1 to 4 years after thymectomy

c. Myasthenic exacerbation

    i. Supportive care

      (A) *FVC q4h (intubate if* $\underline{FVC}$ <20 mL/kg, MIP <30 cm H_2O, and MEP <40 cm H_2O [the "20/30/40 rule"] *or a reduction in any of these readings* >30%; *arterial blood gas may be misleading)*

      (B) Neurologic checks q2 to 4h (if increased bulbar signs/symptoms, consider intubation)

    ii. PE should be used because it has a faster rate of effect compared with IVIg.

d. *Cholinergic crisis*

    i. Overmedication resulting in miosis, increased salivation, diarrhea, cramps, fasciculations

    ii. Treatment: withdrawal of anticholinesterase medications under close observation

B. Lambert-Eaton syndrome

1. Pathophysiology

  a. Autoimmune response with **autoantibodies directed against voltage-gated calcium channels on the presynaptic nerve terminal** of the neuromuscular junction and autonomic synapses, resulting in decreased presynaptic ACh release

  b. Two types

    i. Paraneoplastic condition: 50% to 66% have cancer, particularly small-cell (oat) lung carcinoma; *onset of Lambert-Eaton typically precedes diagnosis of cancer by 9 to 12 months.*

    ii. Primary autoimmune form: associated with various autoimmune disorders, including pernicious anemia, hypothyroidism, hyperthyroidism, Sjogren's syndrome, rheumatoid arthritis, systemic lupus erythematosus, vitiligo, celiac disease, psoriasis, ulcerative colitis, juvenile diabetes mellitus, and MG

2. Clinical

  a. Symmetric proximal weakness without atrophy

  b. Decreased or absent reflexes

  c. Oculo-orophrayngeal symptoms far less common than in MG

  d. Increased strength with repetitive effort

  e. Dysfunction of the autonomic nervous system

    i. Dry mouth (most common)

    ii. Erectile dysfunction, decreased lacrimation and sweating, orthostatism, and abnormal pupillary light reflexes also present

  f. EMG/NCS/single-fiber EMG: small CMAP (as low as 10% of normal); decreased response to 3- to 5-Hz stimulation of muscle; facilitation after activation or during repetitive stimulation rates greater than 20 Hz; EMG demonstrates markedly unstable motor unit action potentials (typical); NCS is typically normal but may be abnormal if associated with underlying malignancy; single-fiber EMG: jitter with frequent blocking.

  g. Differential diagnosis

    i. MG

    ii. AIDP

      g. Differential diagnosis (*cont'd*)

         iii. Polymyositis

         iv. Peripheral neuropathy

         v. Plexopathy

         vi. Multiple radiculopathies

3. Treatment

    a. Poor response to AChE inhibitors

    b. Improvement with treatment of tumor

    c. Prednisone, 60 to 80 mg qod, with azathioprine, 2 to 3 mg/kg/day

    d. Other treatment

       i. Guanidine HCl: raises the intracellular calcium concentration, resulting in an increase in ACh

       ii. **3,4-diaminopyridine:** inhibits the neuronal voltage-gated K^+ ion conductance, which prolongs action potential, allowing increased Ca^{2+} and increased neurotransmitter

       iii. Immunomodulation

         (A) PE

         (B) IVIg

C. Toxin-induced: botulism

1. Pathophysiology

    a. Caused primarily by *Clostridium botulinum, which is gram-positive anaerobe*

    b. Three forms

       i. Food-borne botulism: 1,000 cases per year worldwide; usually *home-canned vegetables; most associated with type A spores*

       ii. Wound botulism: injection drug use with black tar heroin; posttraumatic

       iii. *Infant botulism:* most common in children *aged 1 week to 11 months:* usually neurotoxins types A and B; death in less than 2% of cases in the United States, but higher worldwide

> **NB:** Sluggish and fatiguable pupils are a characteristic finding in botulism (when accompanied by acute- or subacute-onset descending paralysis involving the cranial nerves, neck, and shoulder girdle).

    c. The most common form is wound botulism and then that associated with subcutaneous heroin use.

    d. Neurotoxins types A, B, and E are the usual cause, but, rarely, types F and G can also be symptomatic.

    e. Irreversible binding to the presynaptic membrane of peripheral cholinergic nerves, blocking ACh release at the neuromuscular junction

       i. Three-step process

         (A) Toxin binds to receptors on the nerve ending.

         (B) Toxin molecule is then internalized.

         (C) Within the nerve cell, the toxin interferes with the release of ACh.

       ii. *Cleavage of one of the soluble N-ethylmaleimide–sensitive factor attachment protein receptor (SNARE) proteins by botulinum neurotoxin inhibits the exocytosis of ACh from the synaptic terminal.*

2. Clinical
    a. Blurred vision, dysphagia, dysarthria, pupillary response to light, dry mouth, constipation, and urinary retention

> **NB:** Blurred vision is secondary to paresis of accommodation.

    b. Tensilon® test: positive in 30% of cases
    c. Infant botulism: constipation, lethargy, poor sucking, weak cry
    d. Electrophysiologic criteria for botulism
        i. ↓CMAP amplitude in at least two muscles
        ii. Greater than or equal to 20% facilitation of CMAP amplitude with repetitive stimulation
        iii. Persistent facilitation for ≥2 minutes after activation
        iv. No postactivation exhaustion
        v. Single-fiber EMG: ↑ jitter and blocking
    e. Prognosis: most patients recover completely in 6 months.
3. Treatment
    a. Supportive care
    b. Antibiotics
        i. Wound botulism: penicillin G or metronidazole
        ii. Antibiotics are not generally recommended for infant botulism because cell death and lysis may result in the release of more toxin.
    c. Horse serum antitoxin
        i. Types A, B, and E
        ii. Side effects of serum sickness and anaphylaxis
D. **Differential diagnosis of neuromuscular junction disorders**
    1. ALS
    2. Syringomyelia
    3. Polio
    4. Polyneuropathy
    5. Myopathies
    6. Oculocraniosomatic myopathy
        a. Like ocular MG clinically, but slowly progressive
        b. Tensilon® test negative
        c. Single-fiber EMG: ↑ jitter in facial muscles; EMG reveals myopathic findings in muscle in shoulders.
        d. Biopsy: ragged red fibers
    7. Hypermagnesemia
        a. Interferes with action of calcium in the release of ACh
        b. Seen in renal disorders patients who receive laxatives, and preeclampsia
        c. Treated with magnesium
        d. Severe weakness occurs with levels of Mg greater than 10 mEq/L
        e. Clinically resembles Lambert-Eaton syndrome
        f. Tensilon® test positive
        g. Neurophysiologic testing resembles botulism

D. **Differential diagnosis of neuromuscular junction disorders** (*cont'd*)

8. Organophosphates

   a. Pathophysiology: *irreversible ACh inhibitors;* organophosphates are found in insecticides (*e.g., parathion, malathion*), pesticides, and chemical warfare agents (*e.g., tabun, sarin, soman*); highly lipid soluble; may be absorbed through the skin, mucous membranes, gastrointestinal tract, and lungs

   b. Clinical

      i. Symptoms occur within a few hours of exposure.

      ii. Neuromuscular blockade; autonomic and CNS dysfunction, including headache, miosis, muscle fasciculations, and diffuse muscle cramping; weakness; excessive secretions; nausea; vomiting; and diarrhea; excessive exposure may lead to seizures and coma.

      iii. May cause a delayed neuropathy or myelopathy beginning 1 to 3 weeks after acute exposure

      iv. Electrodiagnostics: resembles slow channel syndrome and congenital AChE deficiency: increased spontaneous firing rate and amplitude of the miniature end-plate potential; depolarization block

   c. Treatment

      i. Remove clothing and clean exposed skin.

      ii. Gastric lavage

      iii. Supportive care

      iv. Atropine, 1 to 2 mg: antagonizes excessive ACh at muscarinic receptor sites, autonomic ganglia, and CNS synapses, but not at the neuromuscular junction

      v. Pralidoxime, 1 g intravenously: cholinesterase reactivator

9. Envenomation by snakes (see Chapter 15)

V. Motor Neuron Diseases

A. ALS

1. Epidemiology: aka Lou Gehrig disease; male-to-female ratio is 2:1; onset is usually after 6th decade; *5% to 10% of ALS is familial; mutations in the C9orf72 gene are responsible for 30% to 40% of familial ALS in the United States and Europe. Approximately 20% is due to a defect in the superoxide dismutase (SOD) gene on chromosome 21.*

2. Pathology: *degeneration of the anterior horn cells and corticospinal tracts; Bunina bodies:* intracytoplasmic, eosinophilic inclusions in anterior horn cells; muscle biopsy: fascicular atrophy, neurogenic atrophy (small angulated fibers)

3. Clinical features

   a. Weakness, atrophy, fasciculations (lower motor neuron signs)

   b. Increased reflexes, spasticity, upgoing toes (upper motor neuron signs)

   c. Hands may be affected early, usually asymmetrically, and then the disease generalizes to involve the legs and bulbar muscles (dysphagia, dysarthria, sialorrhea).

   d. Muscle cramps due to hypersensitivity of denervated muscle

   e. Weight loss

   f. Sensation, extraocular muscles, and sphincter function are spared.

   g. Death within 3 to 5 years (mean)

   h. Variants: *hemiplegic (Mills) variant—starts with weakness on one side of the body; bulbar ALS—starts with bulbar weakness*

      i. Emotional lability/pseudobulbar affect has been described in many ALS patients.

4. *Electrodiagnostic findings:* NCSs may be normal; EMG shows widespread dener-vation in at least three limbs, with giant motor unit potentials (MUPs), polyphasic MUPs, and fasciculations.

5. Treatment

   a. *Riluzole,* a glutamate presynaptic inhibitor, has a slight effect of prolonging sur-vival of ALS patients by approximately 2 to 3 months. A study in an Irish ALS population over a 5-year period showed that riluzole reduced mortality rate by 23% and 15% at 6 and 12 months, respectively, and prolonged survival by 4 months. Survival benefit was more marked in the bulbar-onset disease.

   b. A double-blind, placebo-controlled, randomized study *of vitamin E plus rilu-zole versus riluzole alone* showed no effect on survival after 12 months of treat-ment, but patients given vitamin E were less likely to progress from the milder to the more severe state.

   c. *Anti-epileptic drugs with mild glutamate inhibitory properties* (such as gabapen-tin and topiramate) have been ineffective in well-designed trials.

   d. Results of *creatine* trials on improving strength in ALS patients are mixed.

   e. *Noninvasive positive pressure ventilation* improves survival among ALS patients who can tolerate its use.

   f. Placement of percutaneous endoscopic gastrostomy tube may improve survival rate and quality of life.

B. **Progressive spinal muscular atrophy (SMA)**

   1. General description: spinal muscular atrophies, types 1 to 3, are *all AR and linked to chromosome 5 (mutation in the SMN gene);* pure lower motor neuron syndrome.

   2. Pathology: *degeneration of the anterior horn cells; in Fazio-Londe syndrome, there is loss of motor neurons in the hypoglossal, ambiguus, facial, and trigeminal motor nuclei.*

   3. Clinical

      a. *Werdnig-Hoffmann syndrome (SMA type 1)*

         i. Symptoms are evident at birth or before 6 months of age.

         ii. A common etiology for floppy infant syndrome

         iii. Proximal muscles are first affected, but flaccid quadriplegia eventually ensues.

         iv. Tongue fasciculations

         v. Absent reflexes

         vi. Extraocular muscles are spared.

         vii. 85%: die by age 2 years

      b. *SMA type 2*

         i. Onset is from age 6 months to 1 year.

         ii. Patients may survive past age 2 years.

         iii. Otherwise, clinical features are similar to SMA type 1.

      c. *Kugelberg-Welander disease (SMA type 3)*

         i. Onset in late childhood or adolescence

         ii. Slowly progressive gait disorder

         iii. Proximal arm weakness/wasting

         iv. Absent reflexes

         v. Fasciculations of the tongue and limb muscles

         vi. More benign course and may have a normal life span

         vii. Sensation, bulbar muscles, and intellect are generally spared

3. Clinical (*cont'd*)

    d. *Fazio-Londe syndrome (childhood bulbar muscular atrophy)*

        i. Onset is late childhood to adolescence.

        ii. Selective dysarthria, dysphagia, and facial diplegia

        iii. Tongue wasting with fasciculations

        iv. Weakness of the arms and legs can develop later, but symptoms may also remain restricted for years.

    e. *Kennedy's disease (adult bulbar muscular atrophy)*

        i. *X-linked recessive and trinucleotide (CAG) repeat disease.*

        ii. Symptoms generally begin after age 40 years.

        iii. Dysarthria and dysphagia appear first, followed by limb weakness; tongue fasciculations are present along with absent reflexes.

        iv. *Gynecomastia* is present in most cases.

4. Denervation is seen on NCS/EMG and muscle biopsy; creatine kinase is usually elevated.

5. Treatment: a placebo-controlled trial of gabapentin in adults with SMA showed no benefit in slowing down the progression of weakness using quantitative strength testing.

C. **Primary lateral sclerosis**

1. Epidemiology: rare and accounts for less than 5% of all motor neuron disorders

2. Pathology: degeneration is confined to the corticospinal tracts; MRI is usually normal.

3. Clinical features: age of onset is usually after 40 years; usually starts as a slowly progressive spastic gait that later stabilizes; patients rarely lose the ability to walk with a cane or some other assistance; sphincter is usually preserved, but spastic bladder can occur rarely.

4. Differential diagnosis

    a. Multiple sclerosis (MS)

    b. ALS

    c. Cervical cord compression

    d. Adrenoleukodystrophy

    e. Tropical spastic paraparesis

    f. HIV-associated myelopathy

    g. Vitamin B_{12} deficiency

    h. Paraneoplastic myelopathy

D. **Postpolio syndrome:** patients often complain of fatigue, as well as a decline in functional abilities, decades after the initial poliovirus infection; pyridostigmine has been previously studied, with mixed results.

E. **West Nile poliomyelitis**

1. First recognized in the United States in 1999; the infection is caused by a *flavivirus that is transmitted from birds to humans through the bite of mosquitos.*

2. In addition to meningoencephalitis, **West Nile virus is associated with a lower motor neuron paralytic syndrome**.

3. Clinically and pathologically appears to be a form of poliomyelitis.

4. Most of the cases had fever, meningitis, or encephalitis, and one-half had flaccid weakness that progressed over 3 to 8 days; the weakness tended to be proximal and asymmetric.

5. CSF typically showed pleocytosis and elevated protein—positive for West Nile virus–specific IgM Abs.

6. Pathology: anterior horn cell loss and perivascular inflammation.

VI. Myopathy

A. Degenerative muscular dystrophy (MD)

1. General

   a. MD has five essential characteristics:

   i. Myopathy by clinical, EMG, and pathologic processes; no evidence of denervation or sensory loss

   ii. All symptoms are effects of limb or cranial muscle weakness.

   iii. Symptoms become progressively worse.

   iv. Histology implies degeneration and some regeneration but no evidence of abnormal storage products.

   v. Heritable (even if no other evidence in other family members)

   b. Features of the most common MDs:

	DUCHENNE'S	FACIOSCAPULOHUMERAL	MYOTONIC
Age of onset	Childhood	Adolescence (rarely childhood)	Adolescence or later
Sex	Male	Either	Either
Pseudohypertrophy	Common	Never	Never
Location of onset	Pelvic	Shoulder	Distal limbs
Weakness of face	Rare and mild	Always	Common
Rate of progression	Relatively rapid	Slow	Slow (variable)
Contracture deformities	Common	Rare	Rare
Cardiac disorders	Usually late	Rare	Common (conduction)
Inheritance	X-linked	Dominant	Dominant
Expressivity	Full	Variable	Variable
Genetic heterogeneity	Duchenne's/Becker's	None	Proximal limb weakness

2. **X-linked MD**

   a. *Duchenne's MD*

   i. Pathophysiology: *deletion or duplication at Xp21 in 60% to 70% of cases; abnormality of dystrophin (a cytoskeletal protein located in or near the plasma membrane and seems to be associated with membrane glycoproteins that link it to laminin on the external surface of the muscle fiber; when dystrophin is absent, the sarcolemma becomes unstable with subsequent excessive influx of calcium due to damage, which causes muscle necrosis)*

   ii. Clinical

   (A) *X-linked recessive trait* with females as carriers

   (B) Some carriers have mild manifestations.

   (C) Begins with difficulties walking and running followed by difficulty climbing and rising from chairs *(Gowers' sign)*

   (D) Calf hypertrophy

   (E) Often have exaggerated lordosis to maintain upright posture

ii. Clinical (*cont'd*)

    (F) As disease progresses, arms and hands affected with slight facial weakness (but speech, swallowing, and ocular muscles are spared).

    (G) Iliotibial and heel cord contractures

    (H) By age 12 years, usually wheelchair bound

    (I) By age 20 years, usually respirator dependent

    (J) Heart spared, but abnormal electrocardiogram (ECG) (change in RS amplitude in V1 and deep narrow Q waves in left precordial leads)

    (K) Developmental delay in one-third of cases

  b. Becker's MD: essentially the same as Duchenne's MD except for two aspects—later age of onset (usually after 12 years) and lower rate of progression (still walking at age 20 years)

3. Facioscapulohumeral MD (Landouzy-Dejerine syndrome)

  a. Pathophysiology: *AD; chromosome 4q35-qter*

  b. Clinical

    i. Associated disorders in childhood include deafness, oropharyngeal disorders, and, possibly, mental retardation; may have tortuous retinal vessels and Coats' disease (exudative telangiectasia of retina).

    ii. Initially involves the muscles of the face and trapezius, pectoralis, biceps, and triceps; muscles of the lower extremities are affected much later.

    iii. EMG: may show low-amplitude, short-duration, polyphasic MUPs recruited out of proportion to the degree of muscle force.

4. *Limb-girdle MD*

  a. Pathophysiology: *AR;* several variants; men and women affected equally

  b. Clinical

    i. Somewhat diagnosis of exclusion

    ii. Lower extremities usually affected first, followed by the upper extremities

    iii. Cranial nerves usually spared

    iv. Typically begins in the 2nd to 3rd decade with pelvic involvement and soon spreads to involve shoulders (face spared)

    v. Pseudohypertrophy may or may not occur in calves or deltoids.

    vi. Slightly increased CPKs

    vii. Usually normal life span

    viii. Subdivided into myopathic and "neurogenic" forms

    ix. Conditions that simulate limb-girdle MD:

      (A) Inflammatory (PM, dermatomyositis [DM], inclusion body myositis [IBM], sarcoid)

      (B) Toxic myopathies (chloroquine, steroid, vincristine, lovastatin, ethanol, phenytoin)

      (C) Endocrinopathies (hyper- and hypothyroid, hyperadrenocorticism, hyperparathyroidism, hyperaldosteronism)

      (D) Vitamin deficiency (vitamins D and E)

      (E) Paraneoplastic (Lambert-Eaton, carcinomatous myopathy)

      (F) MG

      (G) Metabolic disorders (late-onset acid maltase deficiency or carnitine deficiency)

      (H) SMA

5. *Myotonic dystrophy (DM)*

   a. *Myotonic dystrophy Type 1 (DM1)*

      i. Pathophysiology: characterized by muscle wasting and weakness associated with myotonia and a number of other systemic abnormalities; AD; incidence: 1:8,000; prevalence: 3 to 5 per 100,000; sodium conductance is altered as a result of abnormal opening of the channels at potentials that have no effect in normal muscle; this results in increased intracellular sodium concentrations.

      ii. Genetic diagnosis

         (A) *Chromosome 19q13.3*

         (B) *Amplified CTG repeat located in the 3' untranslated region of the gene that encodes myotonin protein kinase*

         (C) Amplification in successive generations yields increasing severity.

	NORMAL	BORDERLINE	"CARRIERS"	FULL MUTATION
Number of CTG repeats	5–37	38–49	50–99	>100
Clinical phenotype	Normal	Normal	Mild or no symptoms	Symptomatic

      iii. Clinical features

         (A) Primary form

            (1) Myotonia —delayed muscle relaxation after contraction

            (2) Weakness and wasting affecting facial muscles and distal limb muscles (Hatchet Facies)

            (3) Long face with wasting of the masseter and temporal muscles

            (4) Thin neck with wasting of the sternocleidomastoids

            (5) Frontal balding in males

            (6) Cataracts

            (7) Cardiomyopathy with conduction defects

            (8) Gastrointestinal motility disturbances—cholecystitis, dysphagia, constipation, urinary tract symptoms

            (9) *Multiple endocrinopathies*

               (a) Hyperinsulinism, rarely diabetes

               (b) Adrenal atrophy

               (c) Infertility in women

               (d) Testicular atrophy: growth hormone secretion disturbances

            (10) Low intelligence or dementia

            (11) Excessive daytime sleepiness

         (B) Congenital form

            i. Children born to mothers with myotonic dystrophy

            ii. Significant hypotonia

            iii. Facial diplegia

            iv. Feeding and respiratory difficulties

            v. Skeletal deformities (e.g., clubfeet)

            vi. Delayed developmental progression during childhood

            vii. EMG myotonic discharges may NOT be seen in child but will typically be seen in mother.

iii. Clinical features (*cont'd*)

    (C) EMG/NCS: myotonic discharges: bursts of repetitive potentials that wax and wane in both amplitude and frequency ("dive bomber" potentials).

    (D) *Muscle biopsy: random variability in the size of fibers and fibrosis; multiple nuclei throughout the interior of the fibers and type 1 fiber atrophy; ring fibers*

    (E) Treatment: rarely required unless symptoms are severe; phenytoin: membrane-stabilizing effect

b. *Myotonic dystrophy type 2 (DM2)*: previously named "proximal myotonic myopathy" or "PROMM" due to pattern of weakness. **CNBP (formerly ZNF9),** the gene encoding cellular nucleic acid-binding protein (zinc finger protein 9), is the **only gene in which mutation is known to cause DM2. Expansion of the CCTG repeat causes DM2.**

    i. Characterized by myotonia (90% of affected individuals) and muscle symptoms—weakness, pain, and stiffness (82%), and less commonly by cardiac conduction defects, iridescent posterior subcapsular cataracts ("Christmas tree" cataracts), insulin-insensitive type 2 diabetes mellitus, and testicular failure. Although myotonia has been reported during the first decade in some cases, onset is typically in the third decade, most commonly with fluctuating myalgia and with weakness of the neck and finger flexors. Subsequently, weakness occurs in the elbow extensors and the hip flexors and extensors. Notably, facial weakness and weakness of the ankle dorsiflexors are less commonly seen. In DM2, myotonia rarely causes marked symptoms.

6. *Oculopharyngeal dystrophy*

a. Pathophysiology: rare form of progressive ophthalmoplegia; *AD inheritance in French-Canadian families*

b. Clinical

    i. Progressive ptosis and dysphagia develop late in life, with or without extraocular muscle weakness.

    ii. EMG: Polyphasic MUPs are recruited early in proximal muscles of the upper extremities.

    iii. NCSs are normal, except low CMAPs.

    iv. Differential diagnosis: MG (difficult to differentiate clinically) differentiated with ACh receptor Ab, Tensilon® test, NCS/EMG with repetitive nerve stimulation (RNS), single-fiber EMG (SFEMG).

c. Pathology: muscle biopsy—variation of fiber size, occasional, internal nuclei, small angulated fibers, and an intermyofibrillary network with moth-eaten appearance when stained with oxidative enzymes

7. *Hereditary distal myopathy*

a. Rare AD disorder

b. Clinical

    i. Adult onset

    ii. Unlike most dystrophies, predominantly affects distal muscles of upper extremities and lower extremities

    iii. Weakness typically begins in intrinsic hand muscles, followed by dorsiflexors of the wrist and foot.

    iv. Typically spares proximal muscles

    v. EMG: low-amplitude, short-duration MUPs during mild voluntary contraction *c.* Pathology: muscle biopsy—vacuolar changes

  8. *Emery-Dreifuss syndrome*

       a. Pathophysiology: most have *X-linked inheritance* (but rare families have autosomal dominance).

       b. Clinical: weakness develops in humeroperoneal muscles; early contractures with marked restriction of neck and elbow flexion; also cardiac abnormalities causing atrial fibrillation and a slow ventricular rate.

       c. Pathology: mixed pattern of myopathic and neurogenic change; absent emerin

B. Infectious forms of myopathy

  1. *Trichinosis* (only one that occurs relatively frequently)

       a. Infection due to undercooked pork containing encysted larvae of *Trichinella spiralis*

       b. Post-initial gastroenteritis may have invasion of skeletal muscles, but weakness is mainly limited to muscles innervated by cranial nerves (tongue, masseters, extraocular muscles, oropharynx, and so on).

       c. Rarely, may have cerebral symptoms in acute phase due to emboli from trichinella myocarditis

       d. Labs: eosinophilia, bentonite flocculation assay, and muscle biopsy

       e. Treatment: symptoms usually subside spontaneously; if severe, thiabendazole, 25 mg/kg bid, plus prednisone, 40 to 60 mg/day.

  2. *Other infectious causes*

       a. Toxoplasmosis

       b. Cysticercosis

       c. Trypanosomiasis

       d. Mycoplasma pneumoniae

       e. Coxsackie group B (pleurodynia or Bornholm disease)

       f. Influenza

       g. Epstein-Barr virus

       h. Schistosomiasis

       i. Chagas disease

       j. Legionnaire's disease

       k. Candidiasis

       l. Acquired immunodeficiency syndrome

      m. Influenza

       n. Rubella

       o. Hepatitis B

       p. Behcet's

       q. Kawasaki

       r. Echovirus

C. Endocrine processes

  1. Thyroid disease

       a. Hyperthyroid myopathy

          i. In frequency of causative factor: hyperthyroid (thyrotoxic myopathy) greater than hypothyroid

          ii. Myopathy affects men more frequently than women (although thyrotoxicosis affects women more than men in general).

a. *Hyperthyroid myopathy* (*cont'd*)

   iii. Clinical: some proximal weakness; typical weakness involves muscles of shoulder girdle more than pelvic girdle; usually normal DTRs but can be hyperactive; spontaneous muscle twitching and myokymia may develop.

   iv. EMG: myopathic features; quantitative EMG reveals low-amplitude, short-duration MUPs.

   v. Other neurologic conditions associated with thyrotoxicosis include exophthalmic ophthalmoplegia, MG, and hypokalemic periodic paralysis.

b. *Hypothyroid myopathy*

   i. Clinical: proximal muscle weakness, painful muscle spasm, and muscle hypertrophy; features of myxedema, delayed muscle contraction—best demonstrated on eliciting an ankle reflex (brisk reflex with slow return to original position)

> **NB:** Tapping the muscle causes a ridge of muscle contraction (aka myoedema). This may elevate creatine kinases and produce painful cramps.

   ii. EMG: increased insertional activity with possibly some complex repetitive discharges (CRDs) (but no myotonia)

2. *Adrenal and pituitary disease*

a. Similar weakness occurs with steroids/adrenocorticotropic hormone because steroids reduce the intracellular concentration of potassium.

b. Dysfunction of the retinaculum or mitochondria may also contribute to the pathogenesis.

c. Preferential weakness of pelvic girdle and thigh muscles (difficulty arising from a chair or climbing stairs)

d. Muscle biopsy reveals type 2 atrophy, but neither necrosis nor inflammatory changes.

e. *Cushing's disease*: hyperadrenalism with associated myopathic symptoms

f. *Acromegaly*: elevated growth hormone levels, increasing hand and foot size, thickened heel pad, frontal bossing, prognathism, macroglossia, hypertension, soft tissue swelling, headache, peripheral nerve entrapment syndrome, sweating

3. Parathyroid disease

a. *Hypoparathyroidism causes hypocalcemia, which results in tetany.*

   i. Normally, influx of calcium into the axon terminal facilitates the release of ACh at the neuromuscular junction, resulting in excitation–contraction coupling; a reduction of calcium results in increased conductance for Na^+ and K^+, which causes instability and hyperexcitability of the cell membrane.

   ii. *EMG of tetany: doublets or triplets of MUPs; low-amplitude, short-duration MUPs recruit early in weak muscles; no abnormal spontaneous activity.*

   iii. NCS may reveal reduced amplitude of CMAP, but normal sensory and motor NCVs.

b. *Hyperparathyroidism*

   i. Less frequently, neuromuscular symptoms in hypercalcemia—may also result from osteolytic metastatic disease, multiple myeloma, or chronic renal disease

   ii. Varying proximal muscle weakness occurs in hyperparathyroidism (usually affecting the pelvic girdle more than the shoulder) with brisk DTRs, occasional Babinski, and axial muscle wasting.

D. **Congenital disorders of the muscle**

  1. *Myotonia congenita (Thomsen's disease)*

    a. Pathophysiology: *chromosome 7q35; almost always AD inheritance; dysfunctional chloride channel (mutations in the CLCN1 gene) with decreased Cl⁻ conductance*

    b. Clinical

        i. Symptoms are only caused by myotonia or consequences thereof.

       ii. Differs from myotonic dystrophy because there is typically no muscle weakness or wasting, and also systemic manifestations, such as no cataracts, ECG abnormalities, Endocrinopathies, and so forth, but the myotonia tends to be more severe.

      iii. Due to isometric contractions of myotonia, muscles tend to hypertrophy and make the patient look athletic (*mini-Hercules appearance*).

       iv. Myotonia may affect:

          (A) Limbs: difficulty with grip; may often predominate in the lower extremities, causing difficulty with ambulation

          (B) Oropharyngeal muscles (dysphagia)

          (C) Orbicularis oculi

          (D) Does not affect respiratory muscles

        v. Myotonia worse on initiation of activity, but decreases with gradually increasing exercise ("warming-up" phenomenon) in the individual limb.

       vi. Movements begin slowly and with difficulty, especially after prolonged rest.

      vii. Diagnosis

          (A) Depends on signs and symptoms (including percussion myotonia) and positive family history

          (B) In equivocal cases, exposure to cold can be a provocative test.

          (C) NCS/EMG helpful, in that progressive nerve stimulation may cause progressive decline in successive evoked CMAPs due to increased muscle refractoriness (this may occur in any type of myotonic disorder).

     viii. Muscle biopsy: reveals absence of type 2B fibers and presence of internal nuclei

    c. Treatment: *myotonia relieved with:*

        i. *Mexiletine*

       ii. *Phenytoin or quinine sulfate* (200–1,200 mg/day).

      iii. *Acetazolamide occasionally effective.*

       iv. *Procainamide may ameliorate myotonia but may induce lupus.*

  2. *Paramyotonia congenita*

    a. AD; male = female; sodium Channelopathy—mutations in the SCN4A gene

    b. Clinical

        i. Begins at birth or early childhood, without improvement with age

       ii. Paradoxically, the myotonia intensifies (instead of remits) with exercise.

      iii. *In cold, patient may have stiffness of tongue, eyelids, face, and limb muscles.*

       iv. EMG: discharges disappear with cooling despite increased muscle stiffness.

        v. Clinically, similar to hyperkalemic periodic paralysis in that there may be episodes of flaccid weakness

       vi. May have elevated levels of serum K^+

> **NB:** Substantial decrease in the amplitude of the CMAP occurs with exposure to cold in paramyotonia congenita.

3. *Congenital myopathy*
   a. **Nemaline rod myopathy**
      i. *AD inheritance*
      ii. Clinical
         (A) Nonprogressive hypotonia that begins in early childhood
         (B) May be benign if onset is in childhood or adulthood, but fatal in newborn/neonate
         (C) Diffuse weakness
         (D) Dysmorphism with reduced muscle bulk and slender muscles, resulting in elongated face, high-arched palate, high-arched feet, kyphoscoliosis, and occasional scapuloperoneal distribution of weakness
         (E) Slightly elevated CPK
         (F) Muscle biopsy: patients and carriers have type 1 fiber predominance; *Gomori's trichrome stain shows typical rod-shaped bodies near sarcolemma staining bright red (not noted with other stains) that contain material identical to Z-bands of muscle fibers, involving either type 1 or 2, or both; rods may be found in other disorders as nonspecific finding.*
         (G) EMG: low-amplitude, short-duration, polyphasic MUPs with early recruitment

> **NB:** Most common presentation is congenital hypotonia.

   b. **Centronuclear (or myotubular) myopathy**
      i. Pathophysiology: linked *to chromosome Xq28; inheritance varies (X-linked recessive, infantile-juvenile AR, and milder AD); fetal myotubules persist into adult life; histology: the nuclei are positioned centrally instead of the normal sarcolemmal distribution and are surrounded by a pale halo.*
      ii. Clinical: most have hypotonia, ptosis, facial weakness, and extraocular movement palsy at birth; may also affect proximal and distal muscles; course varies from death in infancy/childhood to mild progression with survival into adulthood.
         (A) *Muscle biopsy*
            (1) *Type 1 fiber atrophy and central nuclei (considered characteristic of fetal muscle)*
            (2) *The central part of the fiber is devoid of myofibrils and myofibrillar adenosine triphosphate (ATP) and, therefore, stains poorly with ATPase.*
            (3) *Oxidative enzymes may show decreased or increased activity in central region.*
         (B) NCS/EMG: excessive number of polyphasic, low-amplitude MUPs, fibs, positive sharp waves, +/– CRDs

> **NB:** Centronuclear (myotubular) myopathy is the only congenital myopathy consistently associated with abnormal spontaneous activity.

c. **Central core disease**

    i. Pathophysiology: histology: an amorphous area in the middle of the fiber stains blue with Gomori trichrome and contrasts with the peripheral fibrils that stain red; the cores are devoid of enzyme activity; *on electron microscopy, there are no mitochondria; AD—chromosome 19q13.1.*

    ii. Clinical

        (A) Hypotonia shortly after birth, developmental delay, and occasional hip dislocations

        (B) Proximal muscle weakness but no distinct muscle atrophy

        (C) May have skeletal deformities (lordosis, kyphoscoliosis, foot abnormalities)

        (D) Malignant hyperthermia occurs in association with central core disease.

        (E) *Muscle biopsy: marked type 1 fiber predominance; central region of muscle fiber contains compact myofibrils devoid of oxidative and phosphorylase enzymes because of virtual absence of mitochondria (these central areas are referred to as* cores*); common in type 1 and less common in type 2 fibers; resemble target fibers, which indicate denervation and reinnervation, suggesting that central core disease may be a neurogenic process.*

        (F) NCS/EMG: suggest mixed myopathic–neurogenic process; usually insertional activity is normal with no spontaneous discharges, small MUPs with recruitment.

d. **Cytoplasmic body myopathy**

    i. Histology: accumulation of desmin

    ii. Clinical

        (A) Weakness characteristically involves the face, neck, and proximal limb muscles, as well as respiratory, spinal, and cardiac muscles; may have scoliosis; elevated CPK; abnormal ECG.

        (B) Muscle biopsy: central nuclei, necrosis, fibrosis, and cytoplasmic bodies

        (C) EMG: typical myopathic findings—low-amplitude, short-duration, polyphasic MUPs with early recruitment

E. **Inflammatory myopathy**

  1. **Polymyositis (PM)**

    a. Pathogenesis: presumed to be cell mediated (unlike presumed humoral mediation in DM)

    b. Clinical

        i. Primarily affects adults with underlying connective tissue disease or malignancy

            (A) Male—bowel, stomach, or lung cancer

            (B) Female—ovary or breast cancer

        ii. Usually no pain, fever, or initiating event; usually general systemic manifestations

        iii. Proximal weakness (lower > upper extremities) with head lolling due to neck flexor (anterior compartment) weakness

        iv. Affected muscles are typically nontender.

        v. No significant decrease in DTRs and no significant muscle atrophy

    c. EMG: *"Myopathic changes" with small-amplitude, short-duration, polyphasic potentials and early recruitment; features of muscle inflammation/irritability may be noted with fibs and positive waves but no fasciculations; CRDs may be present.*

      d. Pathology: *infiltration around normal muscle by CD8$^+$ T lymphocytes; muscle necrosis and regeneration may be present (but differs from DM in that, with PM, there are no vascular lesions or perifascicular atrophy and differs from inclusion body myositis by lack of vacuoles or inclusions).*

2. **Dermatomyositis (DM)**

    a. Pathogenesis

        i. Believed to be autoimmune but no direct evidence; most likely humorally mediated due to evidence of presence of more B cells than T cells in infiltrated muscle and a vasculopathy that deposits immune complexes in intramuscular blood vessels

        ii. Tends to be associated with Raynaud's phenomenon, systemic lupus erythematosus, polyarteritis nodosa, Sjögren's syndrome, or pneumonitis

    b. Clinical

        i. Usually begins with nonspecific systemic manifestations, including malaise, fever, anorexia, weight loss, and features of respiratory infection

        ii. Skin lesions may precede, accompany, or follow myopathic process and vary from scaly eczematoid dermatitis to diffuse exfoliative dermatitis or scleroderma; characteristic heliotropic "lupus-like" facial distribution and on extensor surfaces of the extremities—Gottron's papules = discrete erythematous papules overlying the metacarpal and interphalangeal joints.

        iii. Also may have mild perioral and periorbital edema

        iv. Usually proximal limb weakness, but cranial nerve musculature may also be involved with dysphagia in one-third of cases

        v. Occurs in all decades of life, with peak before puberty and around age 40 years

        vi. More common in females than males

        vii. Higher incidence of associated connective tissue diseases and occurs in conjunction with tumors with approximately 10% of cases of women greater than 40 y/o having an associated malignancy (lung, colon, breast, etc.)

    c. **Pathology: *perifascicular atrophy (not seen in PM); inflammatory cells are found in the perimysium rather than within the muscle fiber itself.***

    d. Childhood variant: in conjunction with DM, may have pain, fever, melena, hematemesis, and possible gastrointestinal perforation

    e. Treatment

        i. Prednisone, 60 mg/day (higher doses may be necessary in children)

        ii. Other immunosuppressant/steroid-sparing medications

        iii. IVIg

        iv. Plasmapheresis ineffective

3. **Inclusion body myositis**

    a. Pathogenesis: idiopathic; like PM, low association with malignancy

    b. Clinical: more common in males, especially those greater than 50 y/o; disproportionate affliction of distal limbs in conjunction with proximal limb involvement; weakness of hands may be early symptom and is one of only a few myopathies that affect the long/deep finger flexors (together with quadriceps); dysphagia is rare; only slight increase in CPK

    c. Pathology: *muscle biopsy (distinctive)—intranuclear and intracytoplasmic inclusions composed of masses of filaments and sarcolemmal whorls of membranes, combined with fiber necrosis, cellular infiltrates, and regeneration; also may have rimmed vacuoles*

    d. Treatment: poor response to treatment such as steroids or other immunotherapies

F.   Familial periodic paralysis

	HYPOKALEMIC PERIODIC PARALYSIS	HYPERKALEMIC PERIODIC PARALYSIS	PARAMYOTONIA CONGENITA
Age of onset	1st–2nd decade	1st decade	1st decade
Sex	Predominantly male	Equal	Equal
Incidence of paralysis	Interval of weeks to months	Interval of hours to days	May not be present
Degree of paralysis	Usually severe	Usually mild (occasionally severe)	Usually mild (occasionally severe)
Duration	Hours to days	Minutes to hours	Hours
Effect of cold	May induce attack	May induce attack	Usually induces attack
Effect of glucose	May induce attack	Relieves attack	Relieves attack
Effect of activity	Triggered by rest	Triggered by rest	Triggered by exercise
Serum potassium	Low	High	Normal but may be high
Oral potassium	Prevents attack	Precipitates an attack	Precipitates an attack
Myotonia	None	Occasional	Prominent
Genetics	AD	AD: Chromosome 17q13.1	AD
Channel	Calcium	Sodium	Sodium

1. **Hypokalemic periodic paralysis**
   a. Pathophysiology: K^+ less than 3.0 mg/dL (often accompanied by high Na^+ levels); may be induced by injections of insulin, epinephrine, fluorohydrocortisone, or glucose; may follow high-carbohydrate diet; very rare; male:female 3:1
   b. Clinical
      i. Attack usually begins after resting (commonly present at night or on awakening)
      ii. Weakness varies from mild to complete paralysis of all muscles of limbs and trunk (oropharyngeal and respiratory muscles are usually spared even in severe attacks).
      iii. Duration varies from few hours to 48 hours.
      iv. Some patients have improved strength with activity.
      v. Weakness especially likely on morning after ingesting high-carbohydrate meal
      vi. Rarely, it is associated with peroneal muscle atrophy.
      vii. DTRs and motor NCS amplitudes are reduced proportionally to the severity of the attack (sensory NCSs are normal).
      viii. Not associated with any general medical problems.
      ix. Frequency of attacks tends to decrease as patient gets older and may cease after age 40 to 50 years.
      x. Fatalities are rare but may occur due to respiratory depression.
      xi. Diagnosis made during attack: *low K^+ and high Na^+; induction during glucose (100 g) or insulin (20 units) infusion*

   b. Clinical (*cont'd*)

    xii. Correlation with hyperthyroidism (especially in those of Asian descent)

    xiii. EMG: reduced recruitment of MUPs and decreased muscle excitability

    xiv. Repetitive stimulation may result in incremental response.

   c. Pathology: light microscopy reveals few abnormalities; electron microscopy—vacuoles arising from local dilation of the transverse tubules and sarcoplasmic reticulum.

> **NB:** Vacuole formation in muscle fibers is the most common change in hypokalemic periodic paralysis. They are most prominent during the attacks.

   d. Treatment

    i. Acute attack: 20 to 100 mEq of KCl

    ii. Prophylactic therapy: *carbonic anhydrase inhibitors (acetazolamide, 250–1,000 mg/day) help prevent attacks in 90% of patients; if acetazolamide ineffective, may be treated with triamterene or spironolactone.*

  2. **Hyperkalemic periodic paralysis**

   a. Pathophysiology: *autosomal dominance with almost complete penetrance;* at the cellular level, extracellular Na^+ influx causes K^+ efflux from the cell.

   b. Clinical

    i. Early age of onset (usually $<$10 years)

    ii. Attacks usually occur during the day and are shorter and less severe.

    iii. Myotonia demonstrable on EMG but usually not clinically relevant

    iv. Myotonic lid-lag and lingual myotonia may be the only traits noted.

    v. *Elevated serum K^+ (may be due to leak from muscles)*

    vi. *Precipitated by hunger, rest, or cold and by KCl ingestion*

   c. Treatment

    i. Acute attack: may be terminated by *calcium gluconate, glucose, or insulin*

    ii. Prophylactic: *acetazolamide, 250 to 1,000 mg/day, and thiazides or fludrocortisone*

  3. **Paramyotonia congenita** (see Section D.2)

 G. **Necrotizing polymyopathy (rhabdomyolysis) with myoglobinuria**

  1. Crush/infarction

  2. PM or DM with necrosis

  3. Toxic (alcohol, resins, poisoned fish [Haff disease])

  4. Hereditary disorders of glycolysis

   a. Myophosphorylase deficiency (McArdle's disease)

   b. Phosphofructokinase deficiency (Tarui's disease)

   c. Lipid storage myopathy

   d. Carnitine palmityltransferase deficiency

   e. Phosphoglycerate deficiency

  5. Excessive exercise

  6. Familial paroxysmal myoglobinuria

  7. *Malignant hyperthermia*

   a. Pathogenesis: *AD (rare); defect of phosphodiesterase; reduced reuptake of Ca^+ by the sarcoplasmic reticulum; highly susceptible to anesthetics including halothane* *and succinylcholine; the hyperthermia is thought to be secondary to abnormal depolarization of skeletal muscle by halothane.*

   b. Clinical

      i. After anesthetic induction, the patient develops fasciculations and increased muscle tone, followed by an explosive increase in temperature coinciding with muscle rigidity and necrosis.

      ii. If untreated, patient will die of hyperthermia (up to 42°C), acidosis, and recurrent convulsions, and, possibly, circulatory collapse.

   c. Treatment: stop anesthetic; cool the patient; intravenous dantrolene.

H. **Medications/agents associated with myopathy**

   1. Alcohol

   2. Colchicine

   3. Lovastatin

   4. Diazacholesterol

   5. Clofibrate

   6. Steroids

   7. Rifampin

   8. Kaliuretics

   9. Zidovudine (AZT)

   10. Chloroquine

> **NB:** **AZT inhibits mitochondrial DNA polymerase, producing mitochondrial DNA depletion. Muscle biopsy shows ragged red fibers, reflecting abnormal mitochondrial proliferation.**

> **NB:** Statin myopathy is a necrotizing myopathy due to the effects of the drug in inhibiting the synthesis of mevalonic acid, a precursor of several essential metabolites, including CoQ10.

> **NB:** Chronic steroid myopathy may develop in Cushing's disease or during chronic steroid treatment. There is moderate to severe atrophy of type 2 fibers.

I. **Inherited metabolic disorders**

   1. *Glycogen storage diseases*

      a. **Acid maltase deficiency (type 2 glycogenosis, Pompe's disease)**

         i. *AR*

         ii. *Acid maltase deficiency leads to accumulation of glycogen in tissue lysosomes.*

         iii. Clinical

            (A) Infantile (Pompe's disease): children develop severe hypotonia after birth and die within the first year of cardiac or respiratory failure.

            (B) Childhood: in less severe childhood and adult forms, symptoms mimic those of limb-girdle MD or PM with onset in childhood;

iii. Clinical (*cont'd*)

results in proximal limb and trunk muscle weakness with variable progression; may die of respiratory failure by end of 2nd decade; increased net muscle protein catabolism has a role because this condition improves with a high-protein diet.

(C) Adulthood: begin with insidious limb-girdle weakness during 2nd to 3rd decade followed by respiratory difficulty

(D) Elevated CPKs

(E) EMG: increased insertional activity, fibrillation potentials, positive sharp waves, CRDs (possibly due to anterior horn cells involvement); myotonic potentials, especially in paraspinal muscles

iv. Pathology

(A) Histologically, anterior horn cells contain deposits of glycogen particles (as do other organs, including the heart, liver, and tongue [an enlarged tongue and cardiac abnormalities differentiate Pompe's from Werdnig-Hoffman disease]).

(B) Muscle biopsy: vacuolar myopathy affecting type 1 more than type 2 fibers

b. **Debrancher enzyme deficiency (type 3 glycogenosis)**

i. Pathogenesis: *AR; absence of debrancher enzyme prevents breakdown of glycogen beyond the outer straight glucosyl chains;* consequently, glycogen with short-branched outer chains (aka phosphorylase-limit-dextrin) accumulates in the liver and striated and cardiac muscle; despite the generalized enzymatic defect, skeletal muscles may show little weakness.

ii. Clinical

(A) Child with hypotonia and proximal weakness with failure to thrive

(B) Accumulation of glycogen within the liver causes *hepatomegaly, episodic hypoglycemia, and elevated CPK.*

(C) Clinical features of myopathy may develop after hepatic symptoms have abated.

(D) Patients may improve in adolescence but may later develop distal limb weakness and atrophy (similar to motor neuron disease).

(E) EMG: fibs, CRDs, and short-duration, small MUPs

iii. Pathology: muscle biopsy—subsarcolemmal periodic acid-Schiff–positive vacuoles in type 2 fibers without histologic signs of denervation

c. **Myophosphorylase deficiency (McArdle's disease; type 5 glycogenosis)**

i. Pathogenesis: male:female 4:1; *usually AR (rarely AD);* myophosphorylase deficiency blocks the conversion of muscle glycogen to glucose during heavy exercise under ischemic conditions; abnormality is confined to skeletal muscle.

ii. Clinical

(A) Usually begins in childhood/adolescence; initially only causes muscle fatigability and weakness, but exercise intolerance develops by adolescence.

(B) Repetitive contraction causes cramping (which may improve if patient slows down and performs nonstrenuous activity due to **mobilization of free fatty acids as an alternative energy source** = *second-wind phenomenon*).

(C) Associated breakdown of muscle **causes myoglobinuria.**

(D) Neurologic exam between bouts demonstrates only mild proximal muscle weakness.

(E) Differential diagnosis

(1) Phosphofructokinase deficiency: recurrent myoglobinuria and persistent weakness

(2) Brody's disease: caused by deficiency of calcium ATPase in sarcoplasmic reticulum

(F) Confirmation study: ischemic exercise test (causing severe cramping); no rise in serum lactate with exercise.

d. **Phosphofructokinase deficiency (type 7 glycogenosis, Tarui's disease)**

i. Pathogenesis: due to *defect of muscle phosphofructokinase, which is necessary for the conversion of F-6-phosphate to 1-6 diphosphate*

ii. Clinical

(A) Painful muscle contracture and myoglobinuria (similar to McArdle's) usually in infancy

(B) Infant usually has limb weakness, seizures, cortical blindness, and corneal opacities.

(C) Differentiated from McArdle's by evaluation of phosphofructokinase activity in muscle.

> **NB:** Myophosphorylase deficiency and phosphofructokinase deficiency do not have a normal rise in serum lactate with the ischemic exercise test.

2. *Lipid storage disease*

a. *Carnitine deficiency*

i. Pathogenesis

(A) Whereas glycogen serves as the main energy source of muscle during rapid strenuous activity, circulating lipid in the form of free fatty acids maintains the energy supply at rest and during prolonged low-intensity activity.

(B) Carnitine palmitoyltransferase catalyzes the reversible binding of carnitine to plasma fatty acids; once carnitine is bound to the fatty acids, it can then transport the fatty acids across the mitochondrial membrane for oxidation.

(C) AR (probable)

(D) Two types:

(1) Restricted type: develops lipid storage predominantly in muscle, causing a lipid storage myopathy; probably develops due to decreased ability of muscle to uptake carnitine (despite normal serum carnitine levels)

(2) Systemic type: insufficient synthesis lowers carnitine levels in liver, serum, and muscle.

ii. Clinical

(A) A congenital and slowly progressive myopathy of limb-girdle type and episodic hepatic insufficiency

(B) Severe defect may cause bulbar and respiratory defects, with early death.

(C) NCS/EMG: low-amplitude, short-duration, polyphasic MUPs

iii. Pathology: muscle biopsy: excess lipid droplets, mainly in type 1 fibers (which depend on the oxidation of long-chain fatty acids to a greater extent than type 2 fibers)

2. *Lipid storage disease (cont'd)*

   b. *Carnitine palmitoyltransferase deficiency*

      i. Pathogenesis: *AR;* oxidation of lipid substrates is impaired because long-chain fatty acids (not coupled to carnitine) cannot move across the inner mitochondrial membrane.

      ii. Clinical

         (A) Painful muscle cramps; on prolonged exercise or fasting, recurrent myoglobinuria (first episode of myoglobinuria is usually in adolescence)

         (B) Muscle is strong between attacks, but cramping is elicited with exercise.

         (C) NCS/EMG: normal

      iii. Pathology: muscle biopsy—no abnormalities, or only slight increase in intrafiber lipid droplets next to the mitochondria in type 1 fibers

3. *Mitochondrial encephalomyopathy*

   a. **Kearns-Sayre ophthalmoplegia** *(aka oculocraniosomatic neuromuscular disease)*

      i. Pathogenesis: most common type of mitochondrial myopathy; occurs sporadically (almost never familial)—believed to be due to a mutation in the ovum or somatic cells

      ii. Clinical

         (A) Triad

            (1) Age of onset less than 20 years

            (2) Progressive external ophthalmoplegia

            (3) Pigmentary retinopathy

         (B) Plus at least one of the following:

            (1) Heart block

            (2) Cerebellar dysfunction

            (3) CSF protein greater than 100 mg/dL

            (4) MRI/CT = leukoencephalopathy or basal ganglia calcification

         (C) May also commonly have lactic acidosis and dementia

         (D) Typical presentation: ptosis and extraocular muscle palsies appearing during childhood and adolescence; progressive weakness of extraocular muscles, cardiac abnormalities, and somatic complaints; progressive weakness and fatigue occur with a wide variety of neurologic deficits (including pigmentary degeneration of the retina, sensorineural deafness, cerebellar degeneration, endocrine abnormalities, sensorimotor neuropathy, and demyelinating polyradiculopathy).

         (E) Labs

            (1) Increased serum levels of lactate and pyruvate

            (2) Increased CSF protein greater than 100 mg/dL

      iii. Pathology: muscle biopsy— ragged red fibers

   b. **Myoclonic epilepsy with ragged red fibers (MERRF)**

      i. Pathogenesis: *point mutation of nucleotide pair 8344 (nt-8344, or nt-8356): both are found in mitochondrial DNA gene for transfer RNA for lysine.*

      ii. Clinical

         (A) Essential features

            (1) Myoclonic epilepsy

            (2) Cerebellar dysfunction

            (3) Myoclonus

      (B) Other features

         (1) Short stature

         (2) Ataxia

         (3) Dementia

         (4) Lactic acidosis

         (5) Weakness

     (C) MRI/CT: leukoencephalopathy and cerebellar atrophy

   iii. Pathology: muscle biopsy—ragged red fibers

  c. **Mitochondrial encephalopathy, lactic acidosis, and stroke-like episodes (MELAS)**

    i. Pathogenesis: *point mutation at locus nt-3243 (affected gene is the transfer RNA for leucine)*

    ii. Clinical

     (A) Age of onset less than 40 years

     (B) Short stature

     (C) Seizures

     (D) Dementia

     (E) Lactic acidosis

     (F) Recurrent headache

     (G) Stroke-like episodes

     (H) CT/MRI: lesions do not conform to normal vascular distributions.

   iii. Pathology: muscle biopsy—*ragged red fibers*

  d. *Respiratory chain defects (complex I, III; complex IV [cytochrome-c oxidase])*

  e. **Leigh's disease (subacute necrotizing encephalomyelopathy)**

    i. Pathogenesis: *cytochrome oxidase and pyruvate dehydrogenase deficiency*

    ii. Clinical

     (A) Age of onset usually less than 2 years

     (B) Developmental delay

     (C) Ataxia

     (D) Failure to thrive

     (E) Ophthalmoplegia

     (F) Hypotonia

     (G) Irregular respiration

     (H) Weakness

     (I) MRI: abnormality of brainstem and basal ganglia nuclei

     (J) Labs: increased serum pyruvate and lactate (which may also be increased in CSF)

J. **Muscle cramps and stiffness**

  1. *Myotonia*

    a. Once muscle membrane is activated, it tends to fire repetitively, inducing delayed muscle relaxation.

    b. Causes no pain, unlike cramping or spasm

    c. During movement, myotonia may worsen initially but improve with warm-up period.

    d. Percussion myotonia elicited after muscle tap.

1. *Myotonia (cont'd)*

    e. Cold exacerbates both postactivation and percussion myotonia.

    f. Myotonic discharges with or without clinical myotonia occur with:

        i. Hyperkalemic periodic paralysis

        ii. Acid maltase deficiency

        iii. Hyperthyroidism

        iv. Familial granulovacuolar lobular myopathy

        v. Malignant hyperthermia

        vi. Diazacholesterol

    g. Underlying process unknown but may be associated with sarcolemmal membrane; K^+ ions accumulate in the transverse tubules, resulting in negative afterpotentials; may also be associated with low chloride conductance.

2. **Neuromyotonia (Isaacs' syndrome)**

    a. Typically occurs sporadically

    b. Clinical

        i. Affects any age group

        ii. Begins insidiously and slowly progresses

        iii. *Spontaneous continuous muscle activity—myokymia*

        iv. Due to myokymia, may have abnormal postures of limbs

        v. May also have pseudomyotonia (caused by relapsing and remitting of myotonic bursts—not seen on EMG) and no percussion myotonia

        vi. Liability to cramps (failure to relax) with hyperhidrosis

        vii. Reduced/absent DTRs

        viii. Stiffness and myokymia are present at rest and persist in sleep and anesthesia.

        ix. EMG

            (A) *Prolonged, irregular discharges of action potentials that are variable in amplitude and configuration (and some may resemble fibs)*

            (B) *Voluntary contraction produces more intense discharges that persist on relaxation.*

            (C) *A marked decrement of successive amplitude results from inability of the motor unit to follow rapidly recurring nerve stimuli.*

        x. Occasionally associated with paraneoplastic process

        xi. May have an increased level of γ-aminobutyric acid (GABA) in CSF

    c. Treatment: carbamazepine or phenytoin often controls symptomatology.

3. **Tetany**

    a. Pathophysiology

        i. *Caused by hypocalcemia and alkalosis*

        ii. *Decreased extracellular calcium increases sodium conductance, which leads to membrane depolarization and repetitive nerve firing.*

        iii. *Hypo-Mg^{2+} and hyper-K^+ also induce carpopedal spasm.*

        iv. *Tetanic contraction stops with infusion of curare (but not with peripheral nerve block); therefore, spontaneous discharges tend to occur at some point along the length of the nerve, which can be demonstrated with Chvostek's sign by tapping the facial nerve and Trousseau's sign by inducing ischemia.*

    b. Clinical

        i. Characterized by seizures, paresthesias, prolonged contraction of limb muscles, or laryngospasm

        ii. Accompanied by signs of excitability of peripheral nerves

iii. Occurs in hypo-Ca^{2+} (which, if latent, may produce tetany after hyperventilation), hypo-Mg^{2+}, or alkalosis; typical carpopedal spasms

iv. If spasm is severe, it may proceed to involve proximal limbs and axial muscles.

v. In tetany, nerves are hyperexcitable, as manifested by ischemia (Trousseau's sign) or percussion (Chvostek's sign).

vi. Spasms are due to spontaneous firings of peripheral nerves (starting in the proximal portions of the longest nerves).

vii. EMG: individual motor units discharging independently at a rate of 5 to 25 Hz; each discharge consists of a group of two or more identical potentials.

c. Treatment: correcting metabolic disorder

4. **NB:** Stiff-person syndrome (Moersch-Woltman syndrome)

a. Pathophysiology

i. *Unknown but postulated that α and γ motor neurons are hyperactive by excitatory influences descending from the brainstem*

ii. May involve autoimmunity with Abs to glutamate decarboxylase found in serum and CSF

iii. *Abs have been demonstrated against glutamic acid decarboxylase (GAD), which is the rate-limiting enzyme for the synthesis of the inhibitory GABA.*

iv. Occasionally paraneoplastic

b. Clinical

i. Progressive muscular rigidity and painful spasms

ii. Slow progressive course over months to years

iii. Aching mainly in axial and proximal limb muscles

iv. Stiffness decreases in sleep and under general anesthesia.

v. Later, painful reflex spasm occurs in response to movement, sensory stimulation, startle, or emotion.

vi. Co-contraction of agonist and antagonist muscles may immobilize extremity in unnatural position.

vii. Spasms may lead to joint deformities and may be powerful enough to tear muscle or cause fractures.

viii. Passive muscle stretch produces an exaggerated reflex contraction that lasts several seconds.

ix. Normal sensory and motor findings otherwise; seizures sometimes occur.

x. Continuous muscle activity relieved by benzodiazepines

xi. Aka *stiff-man syndrome,* but changed because 80% are female.

xii. **EMG: continuous discharges of MUPs similar to voluntary contraction**

xiii. Differentiated clinically from Isaacs' by the fact that Isaacs' affects mainly distal upper extremities and lower extremities, and stiff-person affects the trunk.

c. Treatment

i. GABAergic drugs

(A) Diazepam

(B) Clonazepam

(C) Baclofen

(D) Vigabatrin

(E) Tiagabine

ii. Immunomodulation: IVIg—most successful immunomodulation

5. *Myokymia*

   a. *Consecutive repetitive contractions of adjacent muscle bands 1 to 2 cm in width*

   b. *Due to lesion of peripheral branches of motor nerve causing continuous activity of motor units*

   c. *Rest and sleep do not change myokymia.*

   d. Lidocaine (Xylocaine®) infusion of peripheral nerve trunk will block myokymic discharges.

   e. EMG: caused by brief tetanic contractions of repetitively discharging single or multiple motor units; typically occur alone without fibs or positive sharp waves

   f. Facial myokymia

      i. Usually suggests multiple sclerosis or pontine glioma, but also occurs in Bell's palsy, polyradiculoneuropathy, cardiopulmonary arrest, and, occasionally, metastatic tumor that interrupts the supranuclear pathway to the facial nerve

      ii. Two EMG discharges characterize facial myokymia:

         (A) Continuous type—rhythmic single or paired discharges of one or a few motor units recur at regular intervals of 100 to 200 milliseconds; tends to be more commonly associated with MS.

         (B) Discontinuous type—bursts of single motor unit activity at 30 to 40 impulses per second last for 100 to 900 milliseconds and repeat regularly; more commonly associated with brainstem glioma

   g. Treatment: carbamazepine

   h. **Miscellaneous**

K. **Channels associated with neuromuscular disorders**

DISORDER	CHANNEL
Hypokalemic periodic paralysis	Calcium
Hyperkalemic periodic paralysis	Sodium
Paramyotonia congenita	Sodium
Myotonia congenita	Chloride
Malignant hyperthermia	Calcium
Central core disease	Calcium
Episodic ataxia and myokymia	Potassium
Barium-induced periodic paralysis	Barium blocks potassium channels

CHEAT SHEET

The sciatic nerve is composed of a peroneal division and tibial division. The only muscle above the knee supplied by the peroneal division is the short head of the biceps femoris.

Intraspinal canal lesions that are typically proximal to the dorsal root ganglion will manifest clinically with sensory loss, but sensory NCS responses will be normal.

After radiation treatment, myokymia is a typical needle exam finding.

(continued)

CHEAT SHEET (continued)

The characteristics of a demyelinating polyneuropathy (acquired type) include segmental conduction velocity slowing, conduction block, and temporal dispersion of the CMAP.
In a patient with bilateral facial nerve palsies, consider Lyme disease, sarcoidosis, or Guillain-Barré syndrome (GBS).
In CMT type 1A, there is duplication of the PMP 22 gene; in hereditary neuropathy with liability to pressure palsies (HNPP), there is deletion of PMP 22 gene. CMT 2 is the axonal phenotype!
The H-reflex is the most sensitive test for early GBS. Absent H response, abnormal F wave, and abnormal upper extremity SNAP combined with a normal sural SNAP are characteristic of early GBS.
Indications for intubation in neuromuscular respiratory failure: FVC less than 20 mL/kg, MIP less than 30 cm H_2O, and MEP less than 40 cm H_2O (the "20/30/40 rule") or a reduction in any of these readings greater than 30%.
Sluggish and fatiguable pupils are a characteristic finding in botulism (when accompanied by acute or subacute onset descending paralysis involving the cranial nerves, neck, and shoulder girdle).
Cleavage of one of the SNARE proteins by botulinum neurotoxin inhibits the exocytosis of ACh from the synaptic terminal.
Malignant hyperthermia occurs in association with central core disease.
Myophosphorylase deficiency and phosphofructokinase deficiency do not produce a normal rise in serum lactate with the ischemic exercise test.

Suggested Readings

Katirji B, Kaminski HJ, Ruff RJ. *Neuromuscular Disorders in Clinical Practice.* 2nd ed. New York, NY: Springer;2014.

Preston DC, Shapiro BE. *Electromyography and Neuromuscular Disorders.* 3rd ed. New York, NY: Elsevier Saunders;2012.

CHAPTER 11

Epilepsy and Related Disorders

I. Miscellaneous

A. Definitions

1. *Seizure: reflects a sudden, sustained, and simultaneous discharge of very large numbers of neurons, either within a region of the brain or throughout the brain*

   a. *Partial:* focal cortical onset of epileptiform activity

      i. *Simple:* no definitive loss of awareness

      ii. *Complex:* loss of awareness at some level

   b. *Generalized:* diffuse cortical epileptiform activity

      i. *Primary:* immediate onset of diffuse cortical epileptiform activity

      ii. *Secondary:* spread of focal discharges throughout cortex

2. *Epilepsy: a tendency toward recurrent seizures unprovoked by systemic or neurologic insults*

B. Incidence and prevalence

1. Seizure: incidence: approximately 80/100,000 per year; *lifetime prevalence: 9% (one-third are benign febrile convulsions)*

2. Epilepsy

   a. Incidence: approximately 45/100,000 per year

   b. Point prevalence: 0.5 to 1.0% (2.5 million)

      i. Less than or equal to 14 years old (y/o): 13%

      ii. 15 to 64 y/o: 63%

      iii. Greater than or equal to 65 y/o: 24%

   c. Cumulative risk of epilepsy: 1.3% to 3.1%

C. Impact of epilepsy in the United States

1. Economic: the total cost to the nation for seizures and epilepsy is approximately $12.5 billion; direct costs: $1.7 billion (medical costs); indirect costs: $10.8 billion (productivity).

2. Psychosocial: self-esteem and behavior issues; depression and anxiety disorder; *sudden unexplained death in epilepsy (annual risk: 1/200–1/500;* cause unknown but suspected to be cardiopulmonary arrest)

D. Experimental protocols to induce epilepsy in animal models

1. Aluminum gel

2. Freezing

3. Penicillamine

4. Cobalt

5. Stimulation

6. Kainic acid

E. Etiologies

1. Metabolic

   a. Inborn errors: for example, gangliosidoses, glycogen storage diseases

   b. Acquired: hyponatremia, hypocalcemia, hypomagnesemia, hypophosphate-mia, hypoglycemia or hyperglycemia, hyperthyroidism/thyrotoxicosis, uremia, hyperammonemia

2. Toxic

   a. Alcohol toxicity or withdrawal

   b. Barbiturate toxicity or withdrawal

   c. Benzodiazepine toxicity or withdrawal

   d. Cocaine

   e. Phencyclidine

   f. Amphetamines

   g. Common medications that cause seizures

      i. Antidepressants (tricyclic antidepressants, bupropion)

      ii. Antipsychotics (chlorpromazine, thioridazine, trifluoperazine, perphena-zine, haloperidol)

      iii. Analgesics (fentanyl, meperidine, pentazocine, propoxyphene, tramadol [Ultram®])

      iv. Local anesthetics (lidocaine, procaine)

      v. Sympathomimetics (terbutaline, ephedrine, phenylpropanolamine)

      vi. Antibiotics (penicillin, ampicillin, cephalosporins, metronidazole, isonia-zid, pyrimethamine)

      vii. Antineoplastic agents (vincristine, chlorambucil, methotrexate, bis-chloroethylnitrosourea, cytosine arabinoside)

      viii. Bronchodilators (aminophylline, theophylline)

      ix. Immunosuppressants: cyclosporine, ornithine-ketoacid transaminase 3

      x. Others (insulin, antihistamines, atenolol, baclofen, cyclosporine)

3. Neoplasm (metastasis, primary)

4. Infection

   a. Meningitis

   b. Encephalitis

      i. Herpes simplex virus 1: most commonly causes temporal lobe seizures

      ii. Herpes simplex virus 2: infection acquired in birth canal

      iii. HIV

      iv. Epidemic encephalitides

   c. Brain abscess

5. Vascular: stroke (ischemia, hemorrhage), subarachnoid hemorrhage, arteriove-nous malformation, cavernous malformation, venous sinus thrombosis, amyloid angiopathy

6. Trauma: closed-head injury: subdural hematoma, contusion nonlesional; open-head injury

7. Eclampsia

8. Idiopathic: mesial-temporal sclerosis

9. Congenital

10. Perinatal insults

11. Phakomatoses: tuberous sclerosis, Sturge-Weber syndrome

12. Neuronal migration disorders

13. Autoimmune: systemic lupus erythematosus; central nervous system (CNS) vasculitis; autoimmune encephalitis (including LGI1, GABAa, GABAb encephalitis and others)

F. **Febrile seizures**

  1. *Uncommon before age 6 months and after age 6 years*

  2. *13% incidence of epilepsy if at least two of the following factors*

      a. *Family history of nonfebrile seizures*

      b. *Abnormal neurologic examination or development*

      c. *Prolonged febrile seizure*

      d. *Focal febrile seizure with Todd's paralysis*

G. **Genetic basis for idiopathic epilepsies**

CLINICAL PHENOTYPE	LINKAGE
Benign familial neonatal convulsions	8q; 20q
Benign familial infantile convulsions	19q
Autosomal-dominant nocturnal frontal lobe epilepsy (FLE)	20q
Partial epilepsy with auditory features	10q
Juvenile myoclonic epilepsy (JME)	6p
Generalized epilepsy with febrile seizures plus	19q; 2q
Febrile seizures	19p; 8q

H. **Differential diagnosis of seizures**

  1. Hypoglycemia

  2. Syncope (convulsive syncope common, often misinterpreted as seizure)

  3. Asterixis

  4. Tremor

  5. Cerebrovascular accident/transient ischemic attack

  6. Myoclonus

  7. Dystonia

  8. Narcolepsy

  9. Panic attack/anxiety

  10. Migraine

  11. Psychogenic seizures

  12. Malingering

  13. Breath-holding spells

> **NB:** Breath-holding spells occur in up to 5% of infants, often triggered by frustration or sudden pain. Consciousness is lost prior to (occasional) brief clonic jerking.

I. **Emergent evaluation of a patient with seizures**

1. Airway, breathing, and circulation: protect airway by turning patient on side to reduce risk of aspiration

2. Examination

Examination	Assess for focal deficits that may indicate a lesion (i.e., tumor, infections, stroke)
	Short-term memory deficits suggestive of temporal lobe epilepsy
	Frontal lobe executive dysfunction suggestive of frontal lobe epilepsy
History	History of seizures (type, duration, frequency)
	Intake of antiepileptic drugs (AEDs) and other medications that may cause seizures
	Family history of seizures
	History of head trauma with loss of consciousness >30 mins or penetrating head injury
	History of febrile seizures
	History of central nervous system infections
	History of substance abuse (especially ethyl alcohol [ETOH] and barbiturate; either intoxication or withdrawal)

3. Basic labs

  a. Electrolytes: $\downarrow Na^+$, Ca^{2+}, Mg^{2+}

  b. $\uparrow$ or $\downarrow$ glucose

  c. Platelets (thrombotic thrombocytopenic purpura, disseminated intravascular coagulopathy)

  d. Toxicology screen (especially ETOH and barbiturate intoxication or withdrawal)

  e. Antiepileptic drug (AED) levels

  f. Erythrocyte sedimentation rate (if vasculitis suspected)

  g. Infection: urinalysis, chest x-ray, $\pm$ lumbar puncture (LP) (perform if recent fever, atypical mental status changes)

4. Diagnostic tests

  a. Radiographic: MRI preferred over CT (either should be acquired with or without contrast); evaluate for tumor, stroke, and/or infectious process; if patient stable, MRI preferred; if focal deficit, CT emergently followed by MRI.

  b. LP: if there is any suggestion of fever, meningeal signs (nuchal rigidity), elderly, or behavioral signs → perform LP; once LP is performed, treat empirically if any suggestion of infection clinically even before results are known; if LP cannot be performed and infection suspected, always treat patient and do not await availability of LP or results; may want to treat empirically with acyclovir, 10 mg/kg q8h, and third-generation cephalosporin.

  c. Electroencephalography (EEG): obtain within 24 to 48 hours (increased epileptiform potentials are noted postictally within 24–48 hours); if persistent mental status changes, stat EEG to rule out nonconvulsive status epilepticus (SE).

5. *Treatment*
    a. Single seizure
        i. None (unless SE)
        ii. *Recurrence risk after a first unprovoked seizure*
            (A) *Year 1: 14%*
            (B) *Year 2: 29%*
            (C) *Year 3: 34%*
        iii. **AEDs have no effect on risk or disease course.**
    b. Recurrent seizure or abnormality on evaluation
        i. Recommend, in most cases, to load with fosphenytoin, which provides rapid therapeutic effect (unless phenytoin [PHT] or rapid loading dose is contraindicated; may then convert patient to another AED of choice once patient is stabilized)
        ii. If recurrent self-limited seizures in emergency room, 1 to 2 mg of lorazepam (Ativan®) intravenously to max of 10 mg (or respiratory compromise significantly increases)
    c. If there is any history of alcohol (ETOH) abuse, administer thiamine, 100 mg intravenously, before glucose administration.
    d. *If AED level is low, use volume of distribution to calculate bolus dose:*
        Bolus dose (in mg) = $V_d \times$ (desired concentration – current concentration)
        V_d is in L/kg × body weight in kg.
        Concentration is in mg/L.
        V_d: PHT = 0.6 L/kg
        Valproic acid (VA) = 0.1–0.3 L/kg
        Phenobarbital (PB) = 0.6 L/kg
        Carbamazepine (CBZ) = 1–2 L/kg

II. Classifications

A. **International classification of epileptic seizures**
    1. *Partial seizures*
        a. *Simple partial seizures*
            i. With motor signs
            ii. With somatosensory or special sensory symptoms
            iii. With autonomic symptoms or signs
            iv. With psychic symptoms
        b. *Complex partial seizures (CPSs)*
            i. Simple partial onset
            ii. With impairment of consciousness at onset
        c. *Partial seizures evolving to secondary generalized seizures*
            i. Simple partial seizures evolving to generalized seizures
            ii. CPS evolving to generalized seizures
            iii. Simple partial seizures evolving to CPS evolving to generalized seizures
    2. *Generalized seizures*
        a. Absence seizures
            i. Typical absence
            ii. Atypical absence

2. *Generalized seizures (cont'd)*

    b. Myoclonic seizures

    c. Clonic seizures

    d. Tonic seizures

    e. Tonic-clonic seizures

    f. Atonic seizures

3. *Unclassified seizures*

B. **Revised international classification of epilepsies, epileptic syndromes, and related seizure disorders**

1. *Localization related*

    a. Idiopathic (primary)

       i. Benign childhood epilepsy with centrotemporal spikes

       ii. Childhood epilepsy with occipital paroxysm

       iii. Primary reading epilepsy

    b. Symptomatic (secondary)

       i. Temporal lobe epilepsies

       ii. Frontal lobe epilepsies

       iii. Parietal lobe epilepsies

       iv. Occipital lobe epilepsies

       v. Chronic progressive epilepsia partialis continua of childhood

       vi. Reflex epilepsies

    c. Cryptogenic

2. *Generalized*

    a. Primary

       i. Benign neonatal familial convulsions

       ii. Benign neonatal convulsions

       iii. Benign myoclonic epilepsy in infancy

       iv. Childhood absence epilepsy

       v. Juvenile absence epilepsy

       vi. Juvenile myoclonic epilepsy

       vii. Epilepsy with generalized tonic-clonic (GTC) convulsions on awakening

    b. Cryptogenic or symptomatic

       i. West's syndrome

       ii. Lennox-Gastaut syndrome

       iii. Epilepsy with myoclonic astatic seizures

       iv. Epilepsy with myoclonic absences

    c. Symptomatic

       i. Nonspecific etiology

          (A) Early myoclonic encephalopathy

          (B) Early infantile epileptic encephalopathy with suppression burst

       ii. Specific syndromes

3. *Epilepsies undetermined, whether focal or generalized*

    a. With both focal and generalized seizures

       i. Neonatal seizures

       ii. Severe myoclonic epilepsy in infancy

iii. Epilepsy with continuous spike waves during slow-wave sleep

iv. Acquired epileptic aphasia (Landau-Kleffner syndrome)

  b. Special syndromes

  c. Situation-related seizure

  d. Febrile convulsions

  e. Isolated seizures or isolated SE

  f. Metabolic or toxic events

C. **Primary generalized epilepsy**

1. *Absence*

  a. *Typical*

   i. No aura or warning

   ii. Motionless with blank stare

   iii. Short duration (usually < 10 seconds)

   iv. If seizure prolonged, eyelid fluttering or other automatisms may occur

   v. Little or no postictal confusion

   vi. 70% of cases: precipitated by hyperventilation

   vii. EEG: 3-Hz spike and wave

  b. *Atypical*

   i. Similar to simple absence with motor activity or autonomic features

   ii. May have clonic, atonic, and tonic seizures

   iii. Longer duration

   iv. More irregular spike wave with 2.5- to 4.5-Hz spike and wave, and poly-spike discharges

2. *Tonic*

3. *Atonic*

  a. Typical in children with symptomatic or cryptogenic epilepsy syndromes, such as Lennox-Gastaut syndrome

  b. Duration: tonic mean, 10 seconds; atonic, usually 1 to 2 seconds

4. *Tonic-clonic*

5. *Myoclonic seizures*

  a. Brief, shock-like muscle contractions of head or extremities

  b. Usually bilaterally symmetric but may be focal, regional, or generalized

  c. Consciousness preserved unless progression into tonic-clonic seizure

  d. Precipitated by sleep transition and photic stimulation

  e. May be associated with a progressive neurologic deterioration

  f. EEG: generalized polyspike-wave, spike-wave complexes

  g. Subtypes of myoclonic epilepsy

   i. **NB:** Juvenile myoclonic epilepsy (JME)

    (A) Onset is often *late adolescence (12–16 y/o) with myoclonic events followed by tonic-clonic seizures; within a few years, myoclonic events are more common in the morning shortly after awakening.*

    (B) *Genetically localized to chromosome 6p*

    (C) *Most common seizure induced by photic stimulation; also precipitated by alcohol intake and sleep deprivation*

    (D) May have severe seizures if missed AEDs

> **NB:** Treatment of choice for JME is valproic acid (VA); recurrence is likely if treatment is stopped.

    g. Subtypes of myoclonic epilepsy (*cont'd*)

        ii. *Progressive myoclonic epilepsy*

            (A) Unverricht-Lundborg disease (Baltic myoclonus)

                (1) Pathophysiology

                    (a) Mediterranean ancestry

                    (b) Autosomal recessive (AR)

                    (c) Genetic localization to chromosome 21q22.3, but may also occur sporadically

                    (d) Mutation is a dodecamer-repeat rather than a triplet-repeat disorder.

                    (e) Gene for cystatin B is the responsible gene.

                    (f) Two to 17 repeats is a normal finding, but more than 30 repeats is positive for this disease.

                (2) Clinical

                    (a) Relatively severe myoclonic-like events

                    (b) Typically begin between 6 and 16 y/o

                    (c) Progressive ataxia and dementia

                    (d) EEG: diffuse background slowing in the θ frequency with a 3- to 5-Hz polyspike and wave discharge; may also have sporadic focal spike and wave discharges

                    (e) Diagnosis is made by skin biopsy with a notation in sweat glands of vacuoles in one small series; pathology also demonstrates neuronal loss and gliosis of cerebellum, medial thalamus, and spinal cord.

                    (f) Athena Diagnostics also has a lab test that is approximately 85% sensitive for genetic profile.

            (B) Lafora's body disease

                (1) Pathophysiology: *AR; localized to chromosome 6q24*

                (2) Clinical

                    (a) Significant myoclonus

                    (b) Age of onset *is adolescence (10–18 y/o).*

                    (c) Tend not to have severe ataxia or myoclonus, but do have relatively severe dementia

                    (d) Death by early to mid-20s

                    (e) EEG demonstrates occipital spikes and seizures in approximately 50% of cases.

                    (f) Abnormal somatosensory-evoked potentials

                    (g) Diagnosis: *skin biopsy reveals Lafora bodies (polyglucosan neuronal inclusions in neurons and in cells of eccrine sweat gland ducts).*

                    (h) Prognosis is poor.

            (C) Neuronal ceroid lipofuscinosis: pathophysiology: AR; defined by histology—by light microscope, neurons are engorged with periodic acid-Schiff–positive and autofluorescent material, and electron

microscopy demonstrates that ceroid and lipofuscin are noted in abnormal cytosomes, such as curvilinear and fingerprint bodies that are diffusely distributed throughout the body (although only have CNS manifestations).

(1) *Infantile (Santavuori's disease)*

    (a) *AR; association with genomic marker HY-TM1, located on short arm of chromosome 1*

    (b) Begins at approximately 8 months with progressive vision loss, loss of developmental milestones, severe myoclonic jerks, and microcephaly

    (c) Also have optic atrophy and macular degeneration with no response on electroretinogram

(2) *Late infantile (Bielschowsky-Jansky disease)*

    (a) Onset between ages 2 and 7 years

    (b) *AR; localized to chromosome 15q21-q23*

    (c) Progressive vision deterioration with abolished electroretinogram and retinal deterioration

    (d) Myoclonus, ataxia, and dementia are relatively severe, with rapid progression to vegetative state; death usually by 5 to 7 years.

(3) *Juvenile (Spielmeyer-Vogt-Sjögren-Batten disease)*

    (a) *AR*

    (b) *Localized to chromosome 16p12.1*

    (c) Most common neurodegenerative disorder of childhood

    (d) Storage material contains large amounts of adenosine triphosphate synthase subunit C protein.

    (e) Variable onset usually between ages 4 and 12 years begins with progressive vision loss between ages 5 and 10 years due to pigmentary degeneration of the retina

    (f) Variable progression of myoclonus, ataxia, and dementia, but death usually by 2nd decade

    (g) Diagnosis: skin biopsy reveals curvilinear inclusions.

(4) *Adult (Kufs' disease)*

    (a) Onset typically between ages 11 and 34 years

    (b) *Autosomal dominant and recessive forms*

    (c) *More slowly progressive myoclonus, ataxia, and dementia, but usually severe by 10 years after initial diagnosis*

    (d) No retinal degeneration and therefore no visual impairment

    (e) Diagnosis: *fingerprint profiles noted on skin biopsy.*

(D) *Mitochondrial disorders*

    (1) **Myoclonic epilepsy with ragged red fibers**

        (a) *Point mutation of nucleotide pair 8344 (nt-8344 or nt-8356): both are found in mitochondrial deoxyribonucleic acid gene for transfer ribonucleic acid for lysine.*

        (b) *Clinical:* age of onset: 3 to 65 years; essential features: myoclonic epilepsy, cerebellar dysfunction, myoclonus; other features: short stature, ataxia, dementia, lactic acidosis, weakness, and sensory deficits

(1) **Myoclonic epilepsy with ragged red fibers** (*cont'd*)

    (c) MRI/CT: leukoencephalopathy and cerebellar atrophy

    (d) Diagnosis: muscle biopsy—ragged red fibers; genetic testing via Athena Diagnostics

(2) **Leigh disease (subacute necrotizing encephalomyelopathy)**

    (a) Incidence: 1/40,000

    (b) Inheritance: autosomal and X-linked recessive

    (c) Metabolic defect: pyruvate dehydrogenase complex, electron transport chain complexes

    (d) Clinical pattern: usually appears in early infancy or childhood; characterized by a myriad of neurologic manifestations that may include lethargy or coma, swallowing and feeding difficulty, hypotonia, ataxia and intention tremor, involuntary movements, peripheral neuropathy, external ophthalmoplegia, ophthalmoplegia, optic atrophy and vision loss, impaired hearing, vascular-type headaches, and seizures

(E) Sialidosis type 1

(1) *AR; chromosome 20*

(2) *Decrease in α-neuraminidase; measured most reliably in cultured skin fibroblasts*

(3) Pathology: *diffuse cortical atrophy with neuronal storage as well as vacuolar inclusions in liver*

(4) Onset in adolescence

(5) Severe myoclonus, visual impairment with disproportionate night blindness or loss of color vision, ataxia, cherry-red spots; death within 2 to 30 years

(6) Myoclonus is generalized and may be stimulus-sensitive or increased by stress, excitement, smoking, or menses; GTC seizures are noted with disease progression; EEG shows progressive slowing of background activity and appearance of bilateral fast-spike and wave activity, which is photosensitive.

(F) Schindler disease

(1) Incidence: very rare, with less than 10 described; *AR*

(2) *Pathology: axonal spheroids are present in axons of cerebral cortex and myenteric plexus; α-β-Acetylgalactosaminidase deficiency.*

(3) Clinical

    (a) Acute form: onset in infancy, severe psychomotor deterioration; chronic form: adult onset, mild cognitive impairment

    (b) Psychomotor deterioration rapid, leading to marked spasticity, cortical blindness, and myoclonic epilepsy; exaggerated startle response at onset

(G) Biotinidase deficiency disease

(1) Usually appearing in infancy *between 3 and 6 months of age*

(2) Features include *hypotonia, GTC and myoclonic seizures, skin rash (seborrheic or atopic dermatitis), and alopecia.*

(3) *EEG shows multifocal spikes and slow waves.*

(4) *Treatment: oral biotin (5–20 mg/day); skin and neurologic features improve, whereas hearing and vision problems are more resistant.*

(H) GM$_2$ gangliosidosis

	TYPE I TAY-SACHS	TYPE II SANDHOFF
Inheritance	AR	AR
Onset	4–12 mos	4–12 mos
Enzyme defect	Hexosaminidase A	Hexosaminidase A and B
Clinical	Developmental delay, cherry-red spot maculae; startle seizures	Developmental delay, cherry-red spot maculae; startle seizures

(I) **Treatment of myoclonic epilepsies**

   (1) Clonazepam: may also improve ataxia

   (2) VA

   (3) Topiramate

   (4) Zonisamide: anecdotal reports reveal that zonisamide may slow the deterioration of progressive myoclonic epilepsies.

(J) **Differential diagnosis of myoclonus**

   (1) Hypneic jerks

   (2) Exercise-induced (benign)

   (3) Benign infantile myoclonus

   (4) Photosensitive myoclonus

   (5) Infantile spasms

   (6) Lennox-Gastaut syndrome

   (7) Aicardi's infantile myoclonic epilepsy

   (8) JME

   (9) Progressive myoclonic epilepsy

   (10) Friedreich's ataxia

   (11) Ataxia telangiectasia

   (12) Wilson's disease

   (13) Hallervorden-Spatz disease

   (14) Huntington's disease

   (15) Mitochondrial encephalopathies

   (16) Sialidosis

   (17) Lipidoses

   (18) Alzheimer's disease

   (19) Multiple system atrophy

   (20) Progressive supranuclear palsy

   (21) Drugs: selective serotonin reuptake inhibitors, tricyclic antidepressants, lithium, levodopa, valproic acid (VA), carbamazepine (CBZ), phenytoin (PHT)

   (22) Metabolic: hepatic failure, renal failure, hypoglycemia, hyponatremia, dialysis, nonketotic hyperglycemia

   (23) Toxins: bismuth, heavy metals, methyl bromide, dichlorodiphenyltrichloroethane

   (24) Posthypoxic

   (25) Post-traumatic

   (26) Electric shock

(J) **Differential diagnosis of myoclonus** (*cont'd*)

    (27) Focal CNS lesions affecting the cortex, thalamus, brainstem (palatal myoclonus), or spinal cord (segmental or spinal myoclonus)

    (28) Infectious: viral, subacute sclerosing panencephalitis, Creutzfeldt-Jakob disease, postinfections

    (29) Psychogenic

6. **West's syndrome**

    a. Onset: *age 3 months to 3 years*

    b. Prenatal causes are most common, including tuberous sclerosis (most common) and chromosomal abnormalities.

    c. Truncal flexion, mental retardation, myoclonus

    d. EEG: *hypsarrhythmia*

    e. Treatment: *adrenocorticotrophin hormone; vigabatrin is approved by the U.S. Food and Drug Administration (FDA) with black-box warning.*

7. **Aicardi's syndrome**

    a. X-linked dominant

    b. Onset at birth with infantile spasms, hemiconvulsions, coloboma, chorioretinal lacunae, agenesis of corpus callosum, and vertebral anomalies

    c. EEG: *bursts of synchronous slow waves, spike waves, and sharp waves alternating with burst suppression*

    d. Treatment: *adrenocorticotropic hormone*

8. **Lennox-Gastaut syndrome**

    a. Onset: *age 1–10 years*

    b. Multiple seizure types, particularly atonic seizures, developmental delay

    c. EEG: slow spike-wave complex at 1.0 to 2.5 Hz (usually approximately 2 Hz), multifocal spikes and sharp waves, generalized paroxysmal fast activity

    d. Treatment: lamotrigine, VA, vagal nerve stimulation

D. **Partial seizures**

1. Simple partial seizures: no loss of awareness

2. CPS

    a. Impaired consciousness/level of awareness (staring)

    b. Clinical manifestations vary with origin and degree of spread

    c. Presence and nature of aura

    d. Automatisms (manual, oral)

    e. Dystonic motor activity

    f. Duration (typically 30 seconds to 3 minutes)

    g. Amnesia for event

3. Localization of partial seizures

    a. Temporal (Figure 11.1)

        i. *Approximately 70% of partial seizures*

        ii. Aura of déjà vu, epigastric sensation (rising), fear/anxiety, or olfactory sensation

        iii. Stare and nonresponsive

        iv. Oral and manual automatisms

        v. Usually 60 to 90 seconds

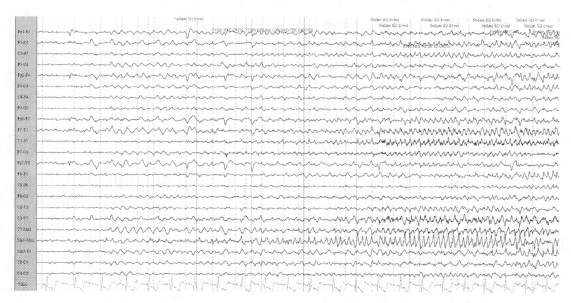

Figure 11.1 Temporal lobe complex partial seizure.

      vi. Contralateral, early dystonic upper extremity posturing has lateralizing value.

     vii. Postictal language disturbance when seizures originate in dominant hemisphere.

  b. *Frontal*

       i. *Approximately 20% of partial seizures*

      ii. Unilateral or bilateral (asymmetric) tonic posturing (bicycling and fencing posture)

     iii. Short duration (20–30 seconds) with minimal postictal confusion

     iv. Awareness and memory may be retained unless temporal spread is present.

      v. Localization: usually posterior-mesial-frontal gyrus/supplementary motor area (SMA)

     vi. Dorsolateral and orbitofrontal partial seizures may appear more similar to temporal lobe seizures, with staring, nonresponsiveness, and automatisms.

    vii. Posterior frontal may have focal clonic movements but no loss of awareness (consistent with simple partial seizures); SMA seizures are typically very brief (1–20 seconds), with dystonic posturing, fencing posture, or bicycling movements,

        (A) Diagnostic features *of SMA seizures*

           (1) *Short duration (<30 seconds)*

           (2) *Stereotypical events*

           (3) *Tendency to occur predominantly during sleep*

           (4) *Tonic contraction of arms in adduction*

           (5) *Note: scalp recordings of SMA seizures are frequently unremarkable.*

    viii. Prominent nocturnal pattern—often 5 to 10 or more seizures in one night

  c. *Parietal and occipital*

       i. Approximately 10% of partial seizures

    c. *Parietal and occipital* (*cont'd*)

        ii. Parietal: aura consists of sensory manifestations.

          (A) Anterior parietal: somatosensory sensation

          (B) Inferior posterior temporal parietal: formed hallucinations

        iii. Occipital: aura: nonspecific bright or colored objects

        iv. Spread often to ipsilateral (more likely) or contralateral temporal lobes, with resultant loss of awareness

  4. *Secondary generalized seizures*

    a. Assumed or observed to begin as simple and/or CPS

    b. Variable symmetry, intensity, and duration of tonic (stiffening) and clonic (jerking) phases

    c. Usual duration: 30 to 120 seconds; tonic phase: 15 to 60 seconds; clonic phase: 60 to 120 seconds

    d. If seizure duration is longer than 5 minutes, risk for continued development into SE is 40% to 70%.

    e. Postictal confusion, somnolence, with or without transient focal deficit (Todd's paralysis)

E. Psychogenic nonepileptic paroxysmal events

  1. Represent genuine psychiatric disease

  2. 10% to 45% of refractory epilepsy at tertiary referral centers

  3. Females affected more than males

  4. Psychiatric mechanism

    a. Dissociation

    b. Conversion

    c. Unconscious (unlike malingering)

  5. Association with physical, verbal, or sexual abuse in approximately 50% to 60% of cases

  6. Epileptic seizures and nonepileptic seizures may coexist in 10% to 20% of patients with pseudoseizures

  7. Video-EEG monitoring required to clarify the diagnosis

  8. Once recognized, approximately 50% respond well to specific psychiatric treatment

F. Other: Hereditary hyperekplexia: linked to long arm of chromosome 5; point mutation of gene encoding the α-1 subunit of the glycine receptor

III. Pediatric and Neonatal Seizures

A. Neonatal seizures

  1. Etiology

    a. Hypoxic-ischemic encephalopathy (50%–60%); usually occur within first 24 to 48 hours

    b. Intracranial hemorrhage (10%)

        i. Subarachnoid hemorrhage: healthy baby; seizures after 24 to 48 hours

        ii. Subdural hemorrhage: focal seizures; within first 24 to 48 hours of birth

        iii. Germinal matrix hemorrhage: premature infants, particularly less than 27 weeks of gestational age; seizures begin after 48 to 72 hours

   c. Metabolic: hypoglycemia; hypocalcemia; hypomagnesemia

   d. Infection (meningitis, encephalitis)

   e. Toxic (drug withdrawal of intoxication)

   f. Developmental

B. Pediatric seizures

  1. Etiology

   a. Idiopathic or genetic: 76%

   b. Development-related epilepsy: 13%

   c. Infection: 5%

   d. Head trauma: 3%

   e. Other causes: 2%

  2. **NB: Benign rolandic epilepsy**

   a. Onset between ages 18 months and 13 years; typically spontaneously ends by age 16 years

   b. *40%: family history of epilepsy or febrile seizures*

   c. Accounts for 10% of all childhood epilepsies

   d. Clinical: nocturnal seizures with somatosensory onset involving the tongue, lips, and gums followed by unilateral jerking that involves the face, tongue, pharynx, and larynx, causing speech arrest and drooling; no loss of awareness unless evolves into a secondary GTC seizure

   e. EEG: *centrotemporal spikes*

   f. Treatment: AEDs are typically unnecessary owing to isolated occurrence of seizures and overall cognitive effects of AEDs, but may be necessary if recurrent GTC seizures; *CBZ is the treatment of choice, if necessary.*

C. Rasmussen's encephalitis

  1. Rare, progressive neurologic disorder characterized by frequent and severe seizures, loss of motor skills and speech, hemiparesis (paralysis on one side of the body), encephalitis (inflammation of the brain), dementia, and mental deterioration

  2. Affects a single brain hemisphere; generally occurs in children less than 10 y/o

  3. Treatment

   a. AEDs usually not effective in controlling the seizures

   b. When seizures have not spontaneously remitted by the time hemiplegia and aphasia are complete, *the standard treatment for Rasmussen's encephalitis is hemispherectomy.*

   c. Alternative treatments may include plasmapheresis, IV immunoglobulin, ketogenic diet, and steroids.

D. Treatment of pediatric epilepsy

  1. Greater degree of pharmacokinetic variability and unpredictability in pediatric patients.

  2. Average clearance of antiepileptic medications during childhood is 2 to 4 times adult; adult levels are reached between ages 10 and 15 years.

  3. *Phenobarbital in children may cause paradoxical excitation and agitation.*

  4. *Levetiracetam has a significantly higher risk for hallucinations in children.*

  5. *VA has a markedly increased risk of hepatotoxicity in children less than 5 y/o, particularly those on multiple AEDs.*

D. Treatment of pediatric epilepsy (*cont'd*)

6. *Ketogenic diet*

   a. Predominantly used in children between age 2 years and adolescence

   b. The purpose of the diet is to establish and maintain ketosis and acidosis along with partial dehydration.

   c. Often initiated in the hospital with starvation until ketosis occurs and then food is introduced

   d. *Efficacy greatest for atonic, myoclonic, and atypical absence seizures; other seizure types (infantile spasms, tonic-clonic, secondarily GTC) and syndromes (Lennox-Gastaut syndrome) also respond.*

   e. Adverse effects

      i. During initiation, dehydration with metabolic acidosis may develop, requiring intervention.

      ii. Renal stones (5%–8%)

      iii. The long-term impact of hypercholesterolemia is unknown.

      iv. Cardiac abnormalities and death (rare)

IV. Women and Epilepsy

A. NB: AEDs that reduce oral contraceptive (OC) levels: CBZ, PHT, PB, topiramate (doses >200 mg/day), oxcarbazepine, and lamotrigine; however, levetiracetam, gabapentin, tiagabine, vigabatrin, zonisamide, and topiramate have no effect on OC concentration.

B. Epileptic women: 0.4% of pregnancies

C. Birth rates are reduced 30% to 60% by psychosocial and endocrine factors; optimization of management must be done preconceptually.

D. The percentage of women with epilepsy with children is lower than the average for the general population.

> **NB:** Valproic acid and CBZ (and epilepsy itself) have been associated with an increased frequency of polycystic ovary syndrome.

1. Psychosocial factors

2. Difficulties with conception

3. Higher risk for spontaneous miscarriage

4. Birth defects

5. Valproic acid has been linked to decreased IQ scores in children whose mothers took it in pregnancy.

E. **Risk for congenital malformations is 2 to 3 times normal risk; but continuing AEDs during pregnancy is recommended because the risk of seizures off medication is higher.**

1. VA: higher incidence of congenital malformation (6%–17%) compared with other AEDs (3%–6%); third-trimester exposure may result in lower IQ.

2. Carbamazepine: 5% rate of major malformations

3. Lamotrigine: has most data among newer AEDs; 3% rate of malformation; 25 times higher rate of cleft palate

4. Levetiracetam: 2% to 4% rate of malformation

F. Seizure frequency may increase during pregnancy.

G. Advise patient about risks and strategies to minimize risk factors.

1. *Appropriate anticonvulsant drug therapy*

2. *Monotherapy*

3. *Lowest acceptable dose*

4. *Follow anticonvulsant levels every 4 to 6 weeks*

5. *Initiate folic acid, 4 mg/day, preconceptually*

H. *Breastfeeding is not contraindicated, with the exception of sedation to the infant.*

V. Treatment

A. AEDs

> **NB:** *AEDs increase the risk of suicidal thoughts or behavior in patients. Patients, their caregivers, and families should be informed of the risk and advised to monitor and report any emergence or worsening of depression, suicidal thoughts or behavior, or any unusual change in mood or behavior or thoughts of self-harm.*

1. PHT (Dilantin®)

PHARMACOKINETICS	
Mechanism	Sodium channel blocker
Range of daily maintenance dose	5–15 mg/kg/day
Minimum dose	Adult: once daily
	Child: bid
Time to peak serum concentration	4–12 hrs (oral)
Percent protein bound	90
Volume of distribution	0.45 L/kg
Half-life	9–140 hrs (average, 22 hrs); saturation kinetics
Time to steady state (SS)	7–21 days
Metabolism	Hepatic
Serum levels	10–20 µg/mL
Major metabolites	5-(p-hydroxy phenyl)-5-phenylhydantoin (inactive)
Absorption	Acid-form poorly soluble in water but sodium salt is more so; do not give intramuscularly, owing to crystallization of drug and possibility of necrosis (Purple Glove syndrome); use fosphenytoin if IV access is questionable
Metabolism	Metabolized extensively by hepatic hydroxylase enzymes; <5% excreted unchanged in the urine; African descent may metabolize PHT slower; zero-order kinetics—the liver cannot increase rate of metabolism of PHT, and, therefore, only a fixed amount of drug can be removed regardless of the serum concentration

(continued)

1. PHT (Dilantin®) (*cont'd*)

PHARMACOKINETICS		
Drug interaction	Effect of PHT on other drugs	
	Potent inducer of hepatic enzymes: decrease coumadin, OCs, CBZ, benzodiazepine, other drugs	
	Effect of other drugs on PHT	
	Inhibition of PHT metabolism: increase PHT: VA	
	Induction of PHT metabolism: decrease PHT: CBZ/ chronic ETOH VA: results in increased free PHT but decreased total PHT	
Adverse effects	Dose-dependent	
	Neurologic: ataxia, nystagmus, diplopia, vertigo, tremor, dysarthria, headache, dyskinesias, peripheral neuropathy	
	Hepatic: toxicity rare and usually within first 6 wks and accompanied by rash, fever, and lymph-adenopathy and eosinophilia, suggestive of a hypersensitivity reaction	
	Endocrine: accelerate cortisol metabolism; decrease free thyroid hormones and increase conversion of T_4 to T_3; long-term treatment may cause hypocalcemia and affect vitamin D metabolism, resulting in osteoporosis	
	Hematologic: megaloblastic anemia, aplastic anemia, leukopenia, and lymphadenopathy	
	Pregnancy: must give mother vitamin K at end of pregnancy and infant vitamin K at birth owing to increased risk of hemorrhage	
	Dental: gingival hyperplasia	
	Skin: hirsutism	
	Teratogenicity: 2–3x normal level; cleft lip and palate; congenital heart defect; fetal hydantoin syndrome has been disputed; genetic defect in arene oxide detoxification may increase susceptibility to PHT birth defects	
Pathophysiology	Reduces post-tetanic potentiation	
Indications	CPS	
	GTC	
	Ineffective in absence seizure	

2. **Sodium VA (Depakote®)**

PHARMACOKINETICS	
Mechanism	Sodium channel blocker
Range of daily maintenance dose	Adult: 20–40 mg/kg/day
	Child: 10–40 mg/kg/day
Serum concentration	50–150 µg/mL
Time to peak serum level	1–4 hrs (plain tabs)
	2–8 hrs (enteric coated)
Oral absorption	>95%
Percent bound to plasma protein	Approximately 90
Volume of distribution	0.1–0.4 L/kg
Elimination half-life	9–21 hrs
Time to SS after initiation	4 days
Major metabolites	ω, ω-1 oxidation products
Dose frequency	Depakote®: once daily to three times daily (tid)
	Depakote ER®: once daily
Distribution	Binding is reduced by free fatty acids, liver disease, hypoalbuminemia, and renal disease
Metabolism	Almost completely metabolized (97%–99%) before excretion
	Major elimination path via conjugation with glucuronic acid (20%–70%), with remainder via oxidative paths
	2-en metabolite of VA has antiepileptic activity, approximately 10% with parent compound having approximately 90% therapeutic effect
Half-life	Between 2 and 21 hrs with mean 12–13 hrs but may be shortened by other AEDs that induce oxidation of VA
	Half-life in neonate between 20 and 66 hrs but falls rapidly in first few months of life
Drug interaction	Effect of VA on other AEDs
	PB: VA increases PB levels (possibly owing to inhibition of metabolism of PB)
	PHT: VA displaces PHT from plasma protein and inhibits PHT metabolism; results in either increased free PHT or unchanged total levels
	Effect of other AEDs on VA
	PHT, CBZ, or PB decrease VA serum concentration owing to enzyme induction
	Salicylates possibly displace VA from plasma protein

(continued)

2. Sodium VA (Depakote®) (*cont'd*)

PHARMACOKINETICS	
Adverse effects	Gastrointestinal: anorexia, nausea/vomiting, dyspepsia, diarrhea, constipation
	Weight gain
	Skin: rash (rare)
	Reversible hair loss
	Hematologic: thrombocytopenia and bruising; reports of abnormal platelet function
	Neurologic: tremor (benign essential tremor and reversible)
	Hepatotoxicity: severe with occasional fatal outcome as idiosyncratic reaction that usually occurs within first 6 mos of treatment and most often in kids—1/50,000 risk overall (black-box warning)
	Hyperammonemia: rare; may cause encephalopathy
	Teratogenicity: spina bifida in approximately 1% of infants of mothers on VA due to depletion of folate; therefore, supplement with folic acid
NB: *Polycystic ovary syndrome and fatal hemorrhagic pancreatitis may also occur with VA.*	
Indications	Absence seizures (up to 100% efficacy)
	Photosensitive epilepsy: drug of choice
	GTC
	Myoclonic epilepsy
	CPS (less effective for GTC but probably as efficacious as PHT/CBZ)
	Migraine headache (FDA approved)
Other	Passes through placenta and via breast milk (0.17%–5.40% of maternal concentration)

3. CBZ (Tegretol®/Tegretol XR®/Carbatrol®)

PHARMACOKINETICS	
Mechanism	Sodium channel blocker
Range of daily maintenance	Adult: 15–40 mg/kg/day
	Child: 10–30 mg/kg/day
Serum concentration	4–12 µg/mL
Peak serum level	4–8 hrs
Percent protein bound	CBZ: 75
	Epoxide metabolite: 50
Volume of distribution	1.2 L/kg
Half-life	Single dose: 20–55 hrs
	Chronic
	Adult 10–30 hrs
	Child: 8–20 hrs

(continued)

PHARMACOKINETICS	
Time to SS after initiation	Up to 10 days (may increase with autoinduction)
Metabolism	Hepatic
Major metabolite	10,11-epoxide
Dose frequency	
Generic CBZ/standard Tegretol®	tid
Tegretol XR® and Carbatrol®	bid
Absorption	Slow and erratic; enhanced by taking with food
Bioavailability	75%–85%
Distribution/binding	Highly lipid soluble; binding not influenced by other AEDs; brain concentration similar to serum
Metabolism	Mainly metabolized to 10,11-epoxide; 3–4 wks for maximal autoinduction of hepatic microsomal enzymes
Special situations	Transplacental transfer causes induction of fetal enzymes
Drug interaction	Effect of CBZ on other drugs
	Induce metabolism of other drugs, including VA, ethosuximide, PHT, clonazepam, OCs, coumadin
	Effect of other drugs on CBZ
	PHT/PB/myasthenia syndrome: decrease CBZ levels (but may increase epoxide levels)
	Enzyme-inhibiting drugs (cimetidine, propoxyphene, verapamil): increase CBZ levels
Adverse effects	Neurologic: nystagmus with blurred vision, dizziness, and diplopia and/or ataxia
	Hematologic: rare; bone marrow suppression with leukopenia, anemia, and/or thrombocytopenia; more rarely proliferative effects, such as eosinophilia and leukocytosis; incidence of aplastic anemia is 0.5/100,000/yr; 10% of patients have transient leukopenia usually within 1st mo
	Gastrointestinal: anorexia, nausea, and vomiting
	Hepatic toxicity: very rare
	Skin: rash in 3%–5%; alopecia rarely occurs
	Endocrine: hyponatremia and decreased plasma osmolality; induces hepatic enzymes, resulting in increased risk of OC failure
	Teratogenicity: increased risk for spina bifida
Pathophysiology	CBZ suppresses seizures by limiting sustained repetitive firing of neurons
Indications	CPS
	GTC

4. **Phenobarbital**

PHARMACOKINETICS	
Mechanism	γ-Aminobutyric acid-receptor agonist
Maintenance	Adult: 2–6 mg/kg/day
	Child: 3–8 mg/kg/day
Minimum dose frequency	Once daily
Time to peak serum level	1–6 hrs
Percent protein bound	45
Volume of distribution	0.5 L/kg
Half-life	Adult: 50–160 hrs
	Child: 30–70 hrs
Time to SS	Up to 30 days
Metabolism	Hepatic
Major metabolite	Para-hydroxy phenobarbitone
Therapeutic serum level	10–40 µg/mL
Distribution	Absorption rapid, but penetration of the brain is slow; PB sensitive to changes in the plasma pH because it has a pKa (7.3) close to physiologic pH; acidosis causes a shift of PB from plasma to tissues, and alkalosis results in higher plasma concentrations
Protein binding	45% bound (less susceptible to changes in plasma proteins)
Metabolism	11%–55% excreted unchanged and remainder hydroxylated in the para position to para-hydroxy phenobarbitone; child metabolizes PB faster than adult and requires higher doses
Drug interactions	Potent inducer of hepatic mixed function oxidase enzymes but is also highly unpredictable in regard to the magnitude; VA reduces PB metabolism: increases PB levels
Adverse effects	Neuropsychiatric (decreased cognition/sedation/paradoxical effect in children; may cause insomnia and hyperactivity in elderly); dependence occurs with withdrawal symptoms
	Hematologic: megaloblastic anemia and macrocytosis
	Endocrine: vitamin K-dependent coagulopathy; osteomalacia
Indications	CPS
	GTC

5. **Primidone (Mysoline®)**

PHARMACOKINETICS	
Mechanism	γ-Aminobutyric acid-receptor agonist
Daily maintenance	Adult: 250–1,500 mg/day
	Child: 15–30 mg/kg/day
Minimum dose frequency	bid
Time to peak serum level	2–5 hrs
Percent protein bound	<20
Metabolism	Hepatic
Volume of distribution	0.6 L/kg
Major active metabolites	PB and phenylethylmalonamide
Elimination half-life	Primidone: 4–12 hrs
	Derived PB: 50–160 hrs
	Phenylethylmalonamide: 29–36 hrs
Time to SS after initiation	Up to 30 days for derived PB
Indications	CPS
	GTC

6. **Ethosuximide (Zarontin®)**

PHARMACOKINETICS	
Mechanism	T-type calcium channel blocker
Daily maintenance	Adult: 500–1,500 mg/day
	Child: 10–15 mg/kg/day
Minimum dose frequency	Once daily
Time to peak concentration	1–4 hrs (faster with liquid)
Percent protein bound	Negligible
Volume of distribution	0.7 L/kg
Major metabolites (inactive)	Methyl succinimide derivatives
Half-life	Adult: 40–70 hrs
	Child: 20–40 hrs
Time to SS after initiation	Adult: up to 14 days
	Child: up to 7 days
Distribution	Rapidly crosses placenta, and 94% of serum level crosses into breast milk
Metabolism	Excreted as glucuronidase, with only 10%–20% excreted unchanged
Indications	Typical absence seizures only

7. Oxcarbazepine (Trileptal®)

PHARMACOKINETICS	
Daily maintenance	600–2,400 mg/day
Minimum dose frequency	bid
Time to peak concentration	3–8 hrs
Percent protein bound	50
Half-life	10–13 hrs
Time to SS after initiation	3 days
Major metabolites	Advantage is that it does not metabolize to the epoxide metabolite, which subsequently reduces side effects
Adverse effects	Side effects are milder than for CBZ and no definitive levels to follow, but may cause significant hyponatremia (free water restriction and increased use of salt may be helpful; worsened by sodium depleters, e.g., diuretics, selective serotonin reuptake inhibitors, etc.)
Drug interactions	OCs only
Indications	CPS
	GTC seizures

8. Lamotrigine (Lamictal®)

PHARMACOKINETICS	
Mechanism	Voltage-gated sodium channel blocker
Daily maintenance	50–400 mg/day
Dose frequency	bid to tid
Time to peak concentration	2–3 hrs
Serum levels	2–12 µg/mL
Percent protein bound	55
Volume of distribution	1.1 L/kg
Half-life	Monotherapy: 10–13 hrs
	Concurrent with inducer: 8–33 hrs
	Concurrent with VA: 30–90 hrs

(continued)

PHARMACOKINETICS	
Time to SS after initiation	3–15 days
Major metabolites	Glucuronide (inactive)
Adverse effects	If rash develops, must stop (black-box warning) because cannot tell if rash will be minor or evolve into Stevens-Johnson syndrome or toxic epidermal necrolysis; may also rarely have systemic organ failure
Indications	CPS Lennox-Gastaut Primary generalized (moderately effective but may worsen myoclonic seizures)

9. Gabapentin (Neurontin®)

PHARMACOKINETICS	
Mechanism	Unknown
Daily maintenance	600–4,800 mg/day
Minimum dose frequency	tid to qid
Time to peak concentration	2–3 hrs
Percent protein bound	0
Volume of distribution	0.7 L/kg
Metabolism	Renal excretion
Half-life	5–7 hrs
Time to SS after initiation	2 days
Major metabolites	None
Dosing	Gastrointestinal absorption markedly reduced at single doses > 1,200 mg
Drug interactions	None
Indications	CPS
	Neuropathic pain (FDA approved)

10. Zonisamide (Zonegran®)

PHARMACOKINETICS	
Daily maintenance	100–400 mg/day (adults)
Minimum dose frequency	bid or once daily
Time to peak concentration	2.5–6.0 hrs
Percent protein bound	40–50
Half-life	50–70 hrs

(continued)

10. **Zonisamide (Zonegran®)** (*cont'd*)

PHARMACOKINETICS	
Time to SS after initiation	5–12 days
Major metabolites	Many (probably inactive)
Adverse effects	Kidney stones (1.5% annual risk; increase fluid intake)
Metabolism	>90% hepatic (CYP3A4)
Indications	CPS
	GTC
	Progressive myoclonic epilepsy (anecdotal reports of slowing progression)

11. **Levetiracetam (Keppra®)**

PHARMACOKINETICS	
Mechanism	Unknown
Daily maintenance	1,000–3,000 mg/day
Minimum dose frequency	bid
Percent protein bound	<10
Half-life	6–8 hrs (effective concentration longer in brain)
Metabolism	65% is renally excreted unchanged, 10% is metabolized by P450 system, and 25% is hydrolyzed by undetermined liver mechanisms
Drug interactions	None
Indications	CPS
	GTC
Adverse effects	Hallucinations in kids
	Moodiness and irritability in children and adults

12. **Topiramate (Topamax®)**

PHARMACOKINETICS	
Mechanism	Unknown; possible sodium channel blocker
Daily maintenance	100–200 mg/day
Minimum dose frequency	bid
Percent protein bound	15
Half-life	18–23 hrs
Metabolism	55–65% renal excretion

(continued)

PHARMACOKINETICS	
Drug interactions	None at low dose; OCs at >200 mg/day
Indications	CPC
	GTC
	Primary generalized seizures except absence
	seizure
Adverse effects	Kidney stones (1.5% annual risk); paresthesias; naming and other cognitive dysfunction; elevated bicarbonate (likely clinically insignificant); *weight loss;*
	NB: can cause hypohydrosis and hyperthermia, esp. in children who exercise in hot weather

13. **Rufinamide (Banzel®)**

PHARMACOKINETICS	
Mechanism	Unknown; possible sodium channel modulator
Daily maintenance	In children daily dose 10mg/kg/day in bid dose in children max dose 45 mg/kg/day not to exceeed 3,200 mg per day. In Adults increase by 400-800 mg every other day, max dose 3200 mg. Taken with food.
Minimum dose frequency	bid
Percent protein bound	25-35%
Half-life	6-10 hrs
Metabolism	Hepatic
Drug interactions	P450 inducers (PB, PRM, PHT, CBZ) increase clearance. VA increases levels.
Indications	Adjunctive treatment of Lennox-Gastaut syndrome in pediatric patients 1 year of age and older and in adults.
Adverse effects	Contraindicated with Familial Short QT syndrome
	Central nervous system adverse effects including headache, dizziness, fatigue, somnolence, nausea. Rarely causes multi-organ hypersensitivity syndrome

14. **Clobazam (Frisium®)**

PHARMACOKINETICS	
Mechanism	Binding to GABA receptor; a 1,5 benzodiazepine
Daily maintenance	10–20 mg in 2 divided doses; initially 5 mg pediatric, 10 mg adult
Minimum dose frequency	bid
Percent protein bound	80
Half-life	36–42 hrs
Metabolism	Hepatic
Drug interactions	Alcohol increased bioavailability; cimetidine increases effects; VA increases levels
Indications	Lennox-Gastaut syndrome, adjunct; approved for other indications outside United States
Adverse effects	Common: ataxia, somnolence, diplopia, dysarthria.
	Rare: gelastic seizures, Stevens-Johnson, toxic epidermal necrolysis, urticarial, rashes
Contraindications	Myasthenia gravis, sleep apnea, severe liver disease, respiratory problems

15. **Lacosamide (Vimpat®)**

PHARMACOKINETICS	
Mechanism	Believed to act through voltage-gated sodium channels
Daily maintenance	Initial dose 50 mg bid, increased by 100 mg per day up to 200–400 mg per day
Minimum dose frequency	bid
Percent protein bound	Low
Half-life	12–16 hours
Metabolism	95% renal
Drug interactions	Limited
Indications	Adjunct for partial seizures
Adverse effects	Dizziness, ataxia, vomiting, diplopia, nausea, vertigo, blurred vision; less commonly, forgetfulness
	May have higher teratogenicity than lamotrigine, levetiracetam, and ethosuximide; pregnancy category C

16. **Vigabatrin (Sabril®)**

PHARMACOKINETICS	
Mechanism	Inhibition of breakdown of gamma aminobutyric acid by acting as a suicide inhibitor of GABA transaminase
Daily maintenance	Adults 500 mg po q12h initially, titrate weekly by 500 mg target dose of 1.5 g q12 h maintenance
	Infantile spasms: 1 month to 2 years: 50 mg/kg/day PO divided q12hr initially; if needed, may increase dose by 25- to 50-mg/kg/day increments every 3 days; not to exceed 150 mg/kg/day
Minimum dose frequency	bid
Percent protein bound	15
Half-life	18–23 hrs
Metabolism	55%–65% renal excretion
Drug interactions	None at low dose; OCs at >200 mg/day
Indications	Children monotherapy in patients 1 mo to 2 years of age with infantile spasms where benefits outweigh potential risk of vision loss
	Adjunct use in adults with refractory complex partial seizures who have inadequately responded to several alternative treatment and in whom risk outweighs benefits
Adverse effects	Common: weight gain, permanent bilateral concentric visual field constriction (>30%), fatigue, somnolence, headache, dizziness, convulsion, hyperactivity
	Black-box warning for permanent vision loss NB: Available through restricted distribution program SHARE: 1-888-45-SHARE

17. **Eslicarbazepine (Aptiom®)**

PHARMACOKINETICS	
Mechanism	Affects voltage-gated sodium channels
Daily maintenance	Begin 400 mg OD; may increase to max 1,600 mg per day
Minimum dose frequency	OD
Percent protein bound	<40
Half-life	13–20 hrs
Metabolism	Hepatic metabolism; metabolites excreted in urine
Drug interactions	Multiple
Indications	Adjunctive for epilepsy
Adverse effects	Suicidal behavior; serious dermatologic reactions; drug reaction with eosinophilia and systemic symptoms (DRESS); anaphylaxis and angioedema; hyponatremia; neurological side effects; drug-induced liver injury; abnormal thyroid tests

American Academy of Neurology Guidelines for Use of AEDs for Newly Diagnosed Epilepsy

AED	NEWLY DIAGNOSED MONOTHERAPY PARTIAL/MIXED	NEWLY DIAGNOSED ABSENCE
Gabapentin	Yes[a]	No
Lamotrigine	Yes[a]	Yes[a]
Topiramate	Yes[a]	No
Tiagabine	No	No
Oxcarbazepine	Yes	No
Levetiracetam	No	No
Zonisamide	No	No

[a]Not FDA approved for this indication.

American Academy of Neurology Guidelines for Use of AEDs for Refractory Epilepsy

AED	PARTIAL ADJUNCTIVE-ADULT	PARTIAL MONOTHERAPY	PRIMARY GENERALIZED	SYMPTOMATIC GENERALIZED	PEDIATRIC PARTIAL
Gabapentin	Yes	No	No	No	Yes
Lamotrigine	Yes	Yes	Yes[a] (only absence)	Yes	Yes
Levetiracetam	Yes	No	No	No	No
Oxcarbazepine	Yes	Yes	No	No	Yes
Tiagabine	Yes	No	No	No	No
Topiramate	Yes	Yes[a]	Yes	Yes	Yes
Zonisamide	Yes	No	No	No	No

[a]Not FDA approved for this indication.

Adjunctive Use of AEDs for Comorbid Conditions

MOOD STABILIZATION	HEADACHE	NEUROPATHIC PAIN	OBESITY	PLMS	TREMOR INSOMNIA
Oxcarbazepine	Topiramate[a]	Gabapentin[a]	Topiramate	Clonazepam	PB Tiagabine
VA	VA[a]	Oxcarbazepine	Zonisamide	Gabapentin	Primidone
Lamotrigine	Zonisamide	CBZ		Topiramate	Clonazepam
Topiramate	Oxcarbazepine	Topiramate		Zonisamide	Levetiracetam
CBZ					Topiramate

Abbreviation: PLMS, periodic limb movements of sleep.
[a]FDA approved for this indication.

Summary of Serious and Nonserious Adverse Events of the Newer AEDs

AED	SERIOUS ADVERSE EVENTS	NONSERIOUS ADVERSE EVENTS
Gabapentin	None	Weight gain, peripheral edema, behavioral changes
Lamotrigine	Rash, including Stevens-Johnson and toxic epidermal necrolysis (increased risk for children, also more common with concomitant VA use and reduced with slow titration); hypersensitivity reactions, including risk of hepatic and renal failure, diffuse intravascular coagulation, and arthritis	Tics and insomnia
Levetiracetam	None	Irritability/behavior change
Oxcarbazepine	Hyponatremia (more common in elderly), rash	None
Tiagabine	Stupor or spike-wave stupor	Weakness
Topiramate	Nephrolithiasis, open-angle glaucoma, hypohidrosis (predominantly children)	Metabolic acidosis, weight loss, language dysfunction
Zonisamide	Rash, renal calculi, hypohidrosis (predominantly children)	Irritability, photosensitivity, weight loss
Rufinamide	Multiorgan hypersensitivity syndrome	CNS adverse effects
Clobazam	Stevens-Johnson; gelastic seizures	Ataxia, somnolence
Lacosamide		Dizziness, ataxia, diplopia
Vigabatrin	Black-box warning for permanent vision loss	Weight gain, fatigue, somnolence
Eslicarbazepine	Drug reaction with eosinophilia and systemic symptoms	Abnormal thyroid tests

Major Drug–Drug Interactions of the Anticonvulsants

MEDICATION	ANTICONVULSANT	RESULTANT SERUM EFFECT
Analgesics		
Aspirin	PHT	Transient increase of PHT level
	VA	Transient increase in VA level
Propoxyphene	CBZ	Increased CBZ level
Antibiotics		
Erythromycin	CBZ	Increased CBZ level
Sulfa drugs	PHT	Increased PHT level
Isoniazid	CBZ	Increased CBZ level
Gastrointestinal		
Cimetidine	CBZ, PHT	Increased PHT > CBZ level
Antacids	PHT, VA	Unpredictable effects

(continued)

Major Drug–Drug Interactions of the Anticonvulsants (*cont'd*)

MEDICATION	ANTICONVULSANT	RESULTANT SERUM EFFECT
Bronchial agents		
Theophylline	CBZ, PHT	Decreased theophylline level
Cardiovascular		
Digoxin	PHT	Decreased digoxin level
Diltiazem	CBZ	Increased CBZ level
Verapamil	CBZ	Increased CBZ level
Warfarin	CBZ	Decreased effect of warfarin
	PHT	Increased effect of warfarin
Immunosuppressants		
Cyclosporine	PHT, CBZ	Decreased cyclosporine level
	VA	No significant effect on cyclosporine level
Contraceptives	PHT, CBZ	Decreased contraceptive level
Psychotropics		
Chlorpromazine	PHT, VA	Increased PHT and VA level
Haloperidol	CBZ, PHT	Decreased haloperidol level
	VA	No effect
Imipramine	PHT	Increased PHT levels
Anticonvulsants		
PHT	CBZ	Decreased CBZ level
	VA	Decreased PHT level
CBZ	PHT	Decreased PHT level
	VA	Decreased VA level
VA	PHT	Decreased PHT level
	CBZ	Increased CBZ level
Gabapentin	PHT, CBZ, VA	No effect
Lamotrigine	VA	Increased lamotrigine level
	PHT, CBZ	Decreased lamotrigine level
Tiagabine	PHT, CBZ, PB	Decreased tiagabine level

    B. **Epilepsy surgery**

        1. Types

           a. Proven efficacy

               i. Resective

               ii. Multiple subpial transection

               iii. Vagal nerve stimulator

           b. Experimental

               i. Deep brain (thalamic) stimulator

               ii. Stereotactic radiosurgery

    C. **Other treatments of refractory epilepsy**

        1. Ketogenic diet (see Section III.D.6)

VI. **Status Epilepticus (SE)**

A. **Clinical**

1. Definition: continuous seizure activity or recurrent seizures without regaining awareness that persist for more than 20 minutes

2. Most generalized seizures are self-limited to 2 to 3 minutes. If seizure activity extends beyond 4 to 5 minutes, begin treatment for SR, because a majority of these patients, if left untreated, will reach the criteria for the clinical diagnosis of SE.

3. Mean duration of SE without neurologic sequelae is 1.5 hours (i.e., must institute barbiturate coma by approximately 1 hour of onset).

4. SE is relatively common; 50,000 to 200,000 cases per year; approximately 10% of patients with epilepsy go into SE at some point in their lives; SE most common among children less than 5 y/o (~74% of cases), and next most common is elderly; approximately 30% to 50% of cases of SE are the patients' first seizures.

5. Etiologies

   a. Idiopathic: one-third of cases of SE

   b. Most common cause: AED noncompliance most common in adults

   c. In children: febrile seizures and meningitis (especially *Haemophilus influenzae* and *Streptococcus pneumoniae*) are common.

   d. Electrolyte imbalance (especially hyponatremia)

   e. Drug intoxication (especially cocaine) or drug withdrawal

   f. Systemic effects of convulsive SE

      i. Cyanotic appearance may be due to tonic contraction, desaturation of hemoglobin, or impedance of venous return due to increased intrathoracic pressure.

      ii. Cardiovascular system: stressed by repeated tonic contractions of skeletal muscles; tachycardia is invariable; bradycardia may occur owing to vagal tone modulation by the CNS; hyperkalemia may cause arrhythmia.

      iii. Endocrine: may have elevation of prolactin, glucagon, growth hormone, and corticotropin; serum glucose may initially increase to 200 to 250 mg/dL, but, if seizure activity is persistent, hypoglycemia may develop.

      iv. Rhabdomyolysis: due to tonic-clonic activity; may lead to renal damage; important to maintain hydration

      v. Metabolic-biochemical complications: respiratory and metabolic acidosis, hypokalemia, and hyponatremia

      vi. Autonomic disturbance due to activation of sympathetic and parasympathetic systems, including excessive sweating, hyperpyrexia, and salivary and tracheobronchial hypersecretion

      vii. Cerebrospinal fluid may demonstrate pleocytosis.

6. *Classification* (Figure 11.2)

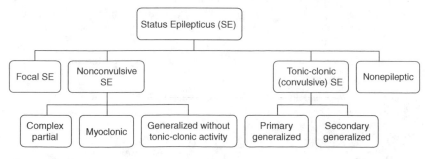

Figure 11.2 Classification of status epilepticus.

7. *Typical features of SE*

	CLINICAL MANIFESTATIONS	EEG PATTERN	TYPICAL SETTING	PROGNOSIS
Complex partial	Recurrent or continuous changes in mental status	Focal	History of seizures or focal brain lesion	Good
Myoclonic	Nonresponsive with myoclonic jerks	Generalized or burst suppression; EEG corresponds to myoclonus	Severe diffuse brain insult	Poor
Subtle generalized	Coma with subtle or no motor manifestations	Generalized	Severe diffuse brain insult	Variable, depending on underlying etiology
Absence	Recurrent or continuous changes in mental status	Generalized spike and wave pattern	History of seizures	Good
Focal (SE partialis)	Focal motor	Focal	Focal brain lesion	Variable, depending on underlying etiology but usually poor
Generalized convulsive	Bilateral tonic-clonic motor activity	Generalized or burst suppression; EEG corresponds to clonic movements	History of seizures with AED noncompliance, meningitis, encephalitis, electrolyte imbalance, or toxicity	Poor

B. **Morbidity and mortality**

1. Related to three factors: CNS damage due to underlying insult, CNS damage from repetitive electric discharges, systemic and metabolic effects of repeated GTC seizures

2. Increased duration of SE correlates to increased morbidity and mortality.

3. Convulsive SE

    a. Mortality: 8% to 12% acutely; up to 40% to 50% within 3 years (with large number due to underlying factors causing SE)

        i. Pediatric: 2.5%

        ii. Adult: 14%

        iii. Elderly: 38%

  b. In animal studies, neuronal death occurs after 60 minutes of seizure activity (despite paralyzing the animal to eliminate metabolic variables).

  c. In nonparalyzed primates in areas three, five, and six, cerebellum, hippocampus, amygdala, and certain thalamic nuclei; in paralyzed primates to minimize systemic effects, mainly the hippocampus is damaged with only partial involvement of other areas (this supports theory that nonconvulsive SE may produce hippocampal neuronal damage); mechanism of neuronal damage is uncertain but may involve decreased inhibition by γ-aminobutyric acid system, enhanced glutaminergic excitatory activity with increased intracellular concentration of calcium and sodium, and calcium-mediated cell damage.

C. EEG: initially EEG shows discrete seizures with interictal slowing; as SE continues, the seizures wax and wane, eventually evolving into continuous ictal discharges; if seizures persist, ictal discharges are interrupted by flat periods; in the final stage, paroxysmal bursts of epileptiform discharges arise from a flat background.

D. Motor systems: initially, motor activity correlates to epileptiform discharges, but if seizures persist for more than 1 hour, motor activity may diminish, although EEG activity continues; in final stages, may have electromechanical dissociation with no motor activity and periodic epileptiform discharges.

E. Systemic and metabolic effects

  1. Phase 1: ↑ blood pressure/↑ serum lactate and glucose/↓ pH (indicative of acidosis)

  2. Phase 2: blood pressure normalizes or hypotension develops; blood pressure no longer increases with each seizure.

F. Treatment of SE

TIME (MINS)	BASIC LIFE SUPPORT	PHARMACOLOGIC TREATMENT
0–3	ABCs (airway, breathing, and circulation); evaluate respiration and give 2–4 L oxygen per nasal cannula (intubate if needed) IV access: thiamine, 100 mg intravenously followed by 50 cc 50% dextrose in water intravenously and continue normal saline or 5% dextrose in water; attain 2nd line for administration of treatment; ± naloxone (Narcan®), 0.4 mg intravenously Draw blood for electrolytes, metabolic profile, complete blood cell count, toxicology, arterial blood gas, and AED levels Obtain urinalysis and chest x-ray	—
5	—	Lorazepam, 4- to 10-mg (0.1-mg/kg) bolus, or diazepam, 10-mg (0.2-mg/kg) bolus at 1–2 mg/min

(continued)

F. Treatment of SE (*cont'd*)

TIME (MINS)	BASIC LIFE SUPPORT	PHARMACOLOGIC TREATMENT
8–10	Pyridoxine, 100–200 mg IV, in children < 18 mos if seizures persist	Fosphenytoin (20 PE/kg) intravenously infused at a rate of no more than 0.75 mg/min/kg (max of 50 mg/min in adults)[a]
	Monitor electrocardiography and blood pressure during PHT administration	
10–15	Start continuous EEG monitoring	Benzodiazepine may be repeated up to max doses
45	CT scan LP	PB (20 mg/kg) infused at a rate of no more than 0.75 mg/min/kg of body weight (max of 50 mg/min in adults)
60–90		Pentobarbital: load with 3–5 mg/kg given over 3–5 mins followed by continuous infusion at 1 mg/kg/hr and increase continuous infusion at 1 mg/kg/hr with additional smaller loading doses until EEG shows burst-suppression
		or
		Midazolam (versed): 0.1- to 0.3-mg/kg bolus followed by continuous infusion at 0.05 mg/kg/hr and increasing by 0.05 mg/kg/hr q15mins up to 1 mg/kg/hr; if SE not controlled within 1 hr, start pentobarbital
		or
		Diazepam: 0.1 mg/kg IV bolus (if benzodiazepine not previously given) followed by 0.2 mg/mL at 0.5 mg/kg/hr up to 40 mg/hr to get a level of 0.2–0.8 mg/L; wean slowly over 8–12 hrs
		Note: Go to pentobarbital or another treatment if SE not controlled within 30–45 mins
		or
		Propofol drip: 1- to 2-mg/kg bolus followed by continuous infusion of 2–10 mg/kg/hr
		Note: Go to pentobarbital or another treatment if SE not controlled within 30–45 mins

Abbreviation: PE, PHT equivalents.
[a]PHT (20 mg/kg) diluted in 300–500 cc saline can be substituted if fosphenytoin not available; IV PHT has risk of extravasation and tissue necrosis.

1. Fosphenytoin: should be substituted for IV PHT (Dilantin®); administration should not exceed 150 mg/minute because fosphenytoin can cause cardiac arrhythmias, prolongation of the QT interval, and hypotension; if IV access not available, may be given intramuscularly.

2. Approximately 80% of prolonged seizures are brought under control with the combination of a benzodiazepine and PHT; if the seizure persists for more than 30 minutes, the patient should be transferred to an intensive care unit for probable intubation (likely secondary to decreased respiratory rate associated with barbiturate administration).

3. Comparison of commonly used AEDs in SE

TIME	DIAZEPAM	LORAZEPAM	PHT	PB
To reach brain	10 secs	2 mins	1 min	20 mins
To peak brain concentration	<5 mins	30 mins	15–30 mins	30 mins
To stop SE	1 min	<5 mins	15–30 mins	20 mins
Half-life	15 mins	6 hrs	>22 hrs	50 hrs

4. If on PHT, VA, or PB, give appropriate IV dose to achieve high or supratherapeutic serum level:

Bolus dose = [(V_d)(body weight)(desired serum

concentration – current serum concentration)]

Bolus dose (mg)

V_d: PHT = 0.6 L/kg   PB = 0.6 L/kg   VA = 0.1–0.3 L/kg Body weight (kg)

Serum concentration (mg/L)

VII. Sleep and Epilepsy

A. Mechanisms

1. Interictal discharges and seizures occur exclusively or primarily in non–rapid eye movement (NREM) sleep.

2. Neuronal synchronization with thalamocortical networks during NREM sleep results in enhanced neuronal excitability, facilitating seizures, and interictal epileptiform discharges in partial epilepsy.

B. Timing of seizures in the sleep–wake cycle

1. Peak times for seizures

   a. Wake—three peaks

      i. 1 to 2 hours after awakening (7–8 a.m.)

      ii. Afternoon (3 p.m.)

      iii. Early evening (6–8 p.m.)

   b. Nocturnal—two peaks

      i. Early sleep (~10–11 p.m.)

      ii. 1 to 2 hours before awakening (~4–5 a.m.)

   c. Awakening seizures

      i. Associated with arousal (including awakening from daytime naps)

      ii. Typically are primary generalized seizures, including primary GTC, myoclonic, and absence seizures disorders

C. Epileptiform activity during sleep

1. *More frequent in NREM than in wake and REM sleep*

2. In generalized seizures, epileptiform discharges are sometimes facilitated by K complexes.

3. NREM also facilitates focal spikes in partial seizures.

4. In benign rolandic epilepsy, may have 20 to 60 spikes per minute in stages 1 and 2 sleep.

D. **Effect of sleep deprivation: increased interictal epileptiform discharges and ictal events**

E. Epileptic syndromes associated with sleep

EPILEPSY SYNDROMES	AGE OF ONSET
Temporal lobe epilepsy	Late childhood to early adulthood
FLE	Late childhood to early adulthood
Benign rolandic epilepsy	3–13 yrs (peak 9–10)
Epilepsy with GTC seizures on awakening	6–25 yrs (peak 11–15)
JME	12–18 yrs (peak 14)
Absence seizures	3–12 yrs (peak 6–7)
Lennox-Gastaut syndrome	1–8 yrs (peak 3–5)
Electrical status of sleep	8 mos to 11.5 yrs

F. Partial seizures ± secondary GTC seizures

1. Thirty percent of partial epilepsies have both day and nocturnal seizures.

2. Forty percent of partial seizures with secondary GTC seizures have exclusively sleep epilepsy.

3. Fifteen percent to forty percent of partial seizures without secondary GTC seizures have exclusively sleep epilepsy.

4. *FLE: may occur primarily or predominantly during sleep; may be autosomal dominant with clustering of nocturnal motor seizures*

5. *Benign epilepsy of childhood with centrotemporal spikes (also known as benign rolandic epilepsy)*

   a. Common childhood epilepsy accounting for 15% to 20% of childhood epilepsy

   b. Peak onset between ages 4 and 13 years; 60% males to 40% females; significant hereditary predisposition

   c. Neurologic examination normal

   d. 75%: occur during sleep (most often in NREM sleep)

   e. Clinical ictal features: oropharyngeal signs, including hypersalivation and guttural sounds, are common features; focal clonic activity also is prominent with facial contractions or hemiconvulsions; consciousness is preserved in most cases (unless there is secondary generalization).

f. EEG: frequent focal rolandic/midtemporal spikes (5–10 per minute) remaining focal in wake and sleep

G. Primary generalized seizures

1. *Primary GTC seizures on awakening*

    a. Clinical: more than 90% of GTC seizures occur at or immediately after awakening (sleep or nap) or in the evening when relaxing; myoclonic and absence seizures may coexist in 40% to 50%, suggesting that the same gene in JME may also be involved.

    b. Photosensitivity and sleep deprivation are common precipitators.

    c. Account for 2% to 4% of adult epilepsy

    d. EEG: generalized spike and wave discharges at 3 to 4 Hz and polyspike-wave complexes, which may be associated with K complexes

2. *Absence epilepsy*

    a. Drowsiness and sleep activate spike and wave discharges that are most marked during the first cycle, max in NREM, and rare/absent in REM.

    b. Morphology also affected in NREM, with irregular polyspike and wave discharges predominating

3. *Lennox-Gastaut syndrome:* NREM sleep is associated with increased 2.0- to 2.5-Hz spike-and slow-wave complexes and rhythmic 10-Hz spikes that may be accompanied by tonic seizures.

4. *JME*

    a. Begins in 2nd to 3rd decade with myoclonic and generalized seizures

    b. 15% to 20%: also have absence seizures

    c. Genetic basis: isolated to chromosome 6p; concordance rate of 70% in monozygotic twins, and 50% of first-degree relatives have primary generalized seizures.

    d. EEG: generalized 4- to 6-Hz polyspike wave discharge most prominent on awakening and at sleep onset; may be frequent in REM and deeper stages of NREM

H. Other epilepsies associated with sleep

1. *Electrical SE of sleep*

    a. Almost continuous spike and wave complexes during NREM sleep (2.0- to 2.5-Hz generalized spike and wave discharges occurring in >85% of NREM sleep); in REM and wakefulness → spike and wave complexes are less continuous and more focal

    b. Occurs in 0.5% of children with epilepsy

    c. Average age onset: 8 to 9 years (range: 4–14 years) with spontaneous remission in 10 years

    d. Some have Landau-Kleffner syndrome: acquired aphasia with seizures, progressive language loss, and inattention to auditory stimuli

I. Differential diagnosis

1. Epileptic seizures

    a. Frontal lobe epilepsy

    b. Temporal lobe epilepsy

    c. Generalized

    d. Benign rolandic epilepsy

I. **Differential diagnosis** (*cont'd*)

   2. Nocturnal paroxysmal dystonia

   3. Sleep disorders

      a. Confusional arousals: body movement, automatic behaviors, mental confusion, fragmentary recall of dreams

      b. Night terrors

      c. Somnambulism

      d. REM sleep behavior disorder

      e. Periodic leg movements of sleep

      f. Sleep-onset myoclonus (hypnic jerk)

      g. Bruxism

      h. Rhythmic movement disorder

   4. Psychiatric disorders

      a. Nocturnal panic disorder

      b. Posttraumatic stress disorder

      c. Psychogenic seizures: patient is noted to be awake or drowsing on video-EEG.

VIII. EEG "Mini-Atlas"

A. Normal EEG

   1. Normal background

      a. Normal adult awake EEG

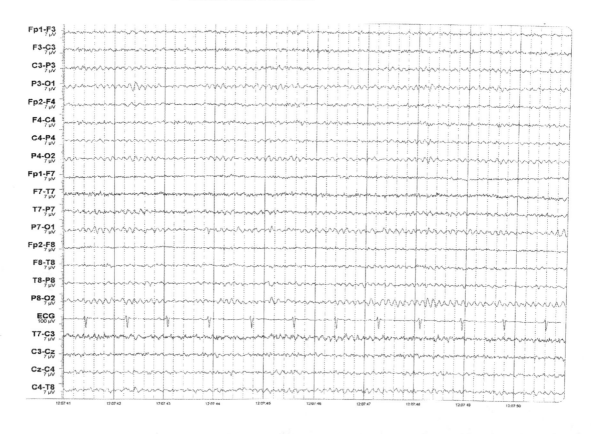

b. Normal light sleep (vertex wave)

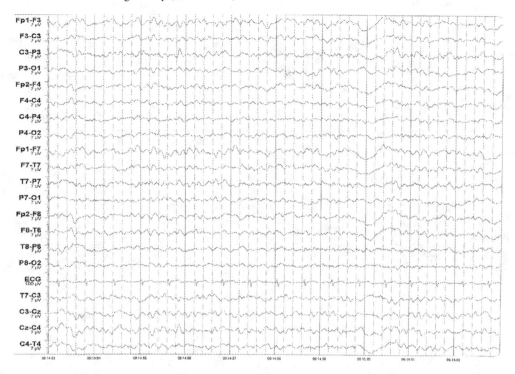

c. Normal light sleep (K complex) (Note that tech sneezed, which may precipitate K complex.)

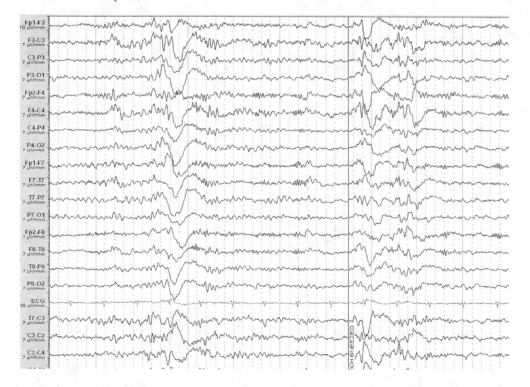

1. Normal background (*cont'd*)

   d. Normal deep sleep

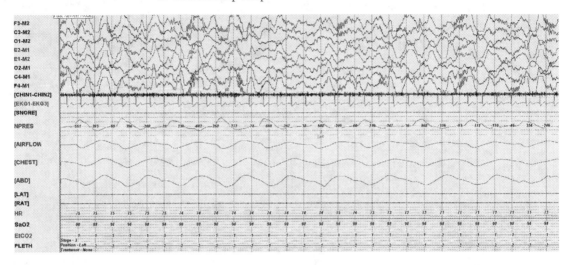

   e. Normal REM sleep

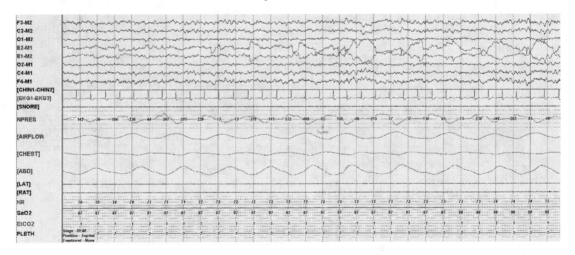

2. Normal variants

   a. Benign epileptiform transients of sleep (BETS): benign transients during sleep that occur typically in those between 30 and 60 years old and in children younger than 10 y/o

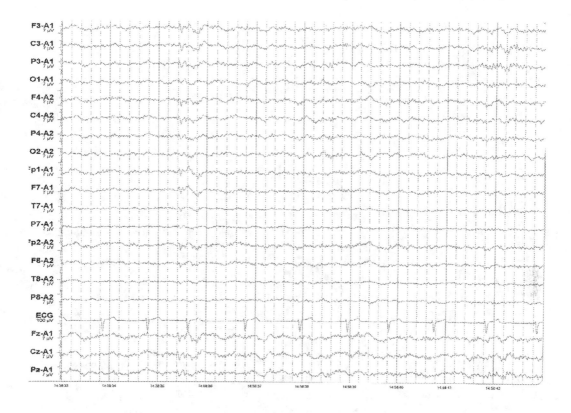

B. Abnormalities

1. Diffuse slowing after anoxic brain injury

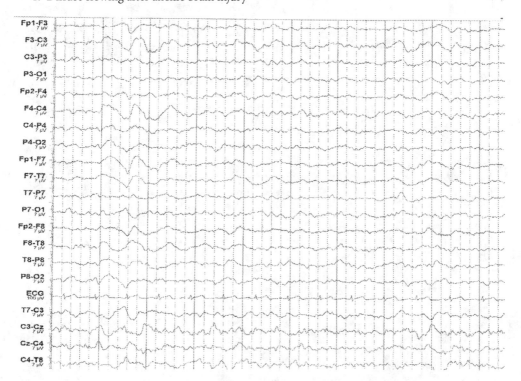

B. **Abnormalities** (*cont'd*)

    2. Alpha coma: seen in comatose patients; in anoxic encephalopathy, signifies poor prognosis

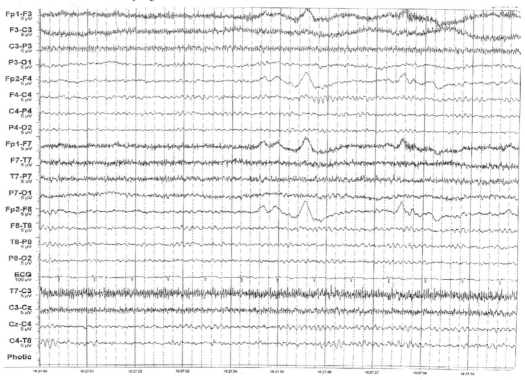

    3. Breech: 35-year-old following right anterior temporal lobectomy; due to craniotomy, cortical activity will have higher amplitude.

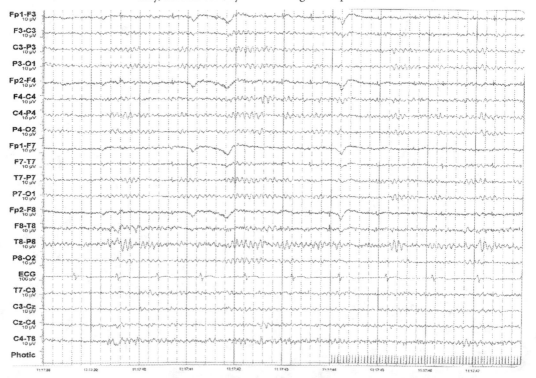

4. Burst suppression: 55-year-old with uncontrolled seizures placed in burst-suppression with pentobarbital to control seizures; suppression of seizure activity is to control epileptiform activity that may damage neurons.

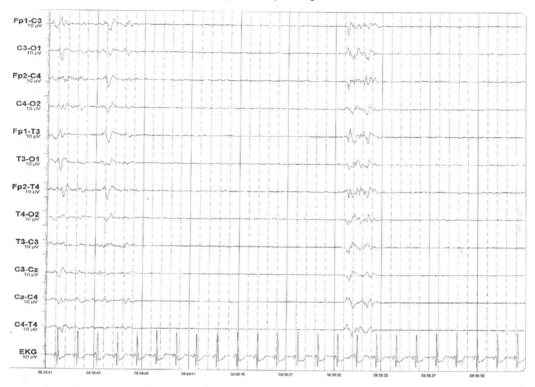

5. Focal slowing associated with left central parietal tumor.

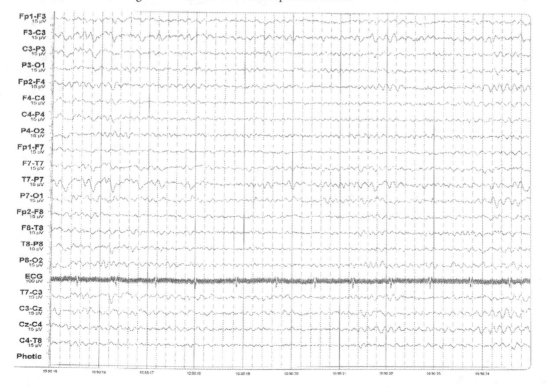

B. Abnormalities (*cont'd*)

6. Periodic lateralized epileptiform discharges in patient with old stroke 6 months prior and no clinical symptoms

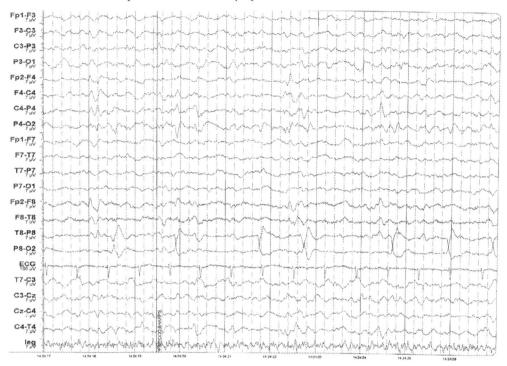

7. Frontal intermittent rhythmical delta activity (FIRDA): seen in multiple encephalopathies, including mild anoxic brain injury, metabolic dysfunction, and normal variants

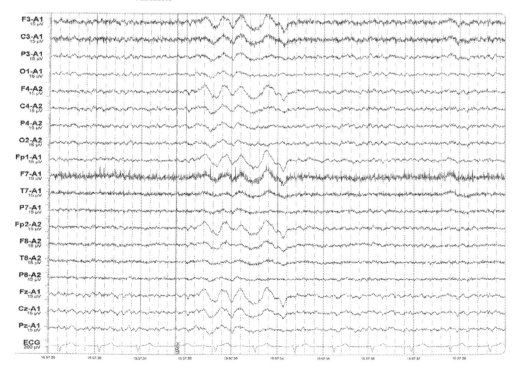

8. Triphasic waves in patient with renal failure

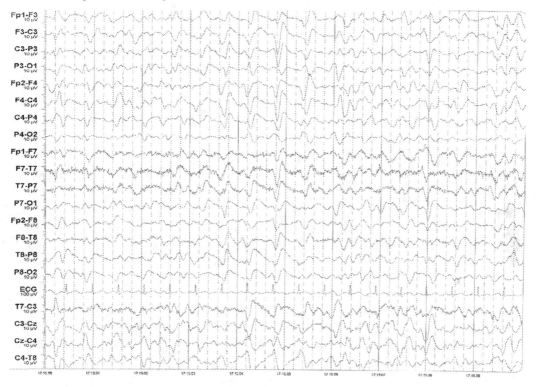

9. Seizure activity

    a. Temporal lobe interictal seizure activity

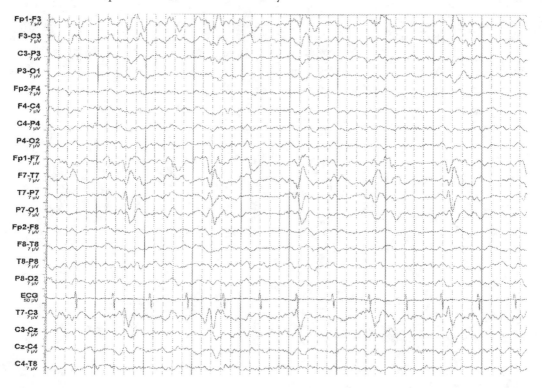

9. Seizure activity (*cont'd*)

   b. Polyspike wave generalized seizure activity

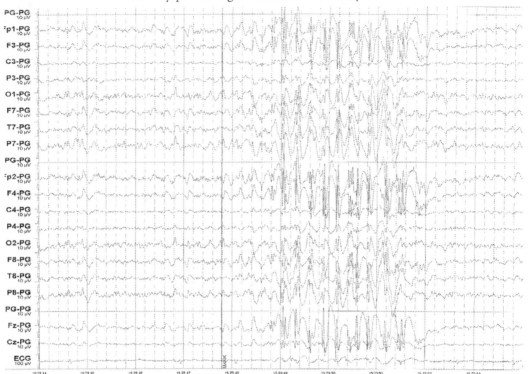

   c. Temporal lobe ictal seizure activity and nonconvulsive status epilepticus due to herpes simplex encephalitis

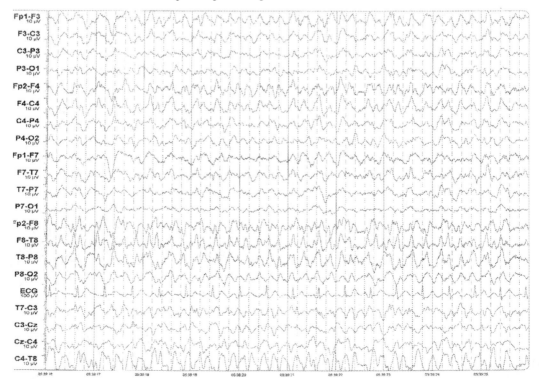

d. Frontal lobe ictal seizure

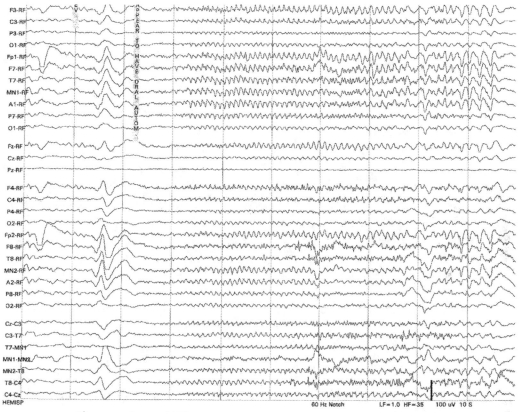

e. Absence seizure activity

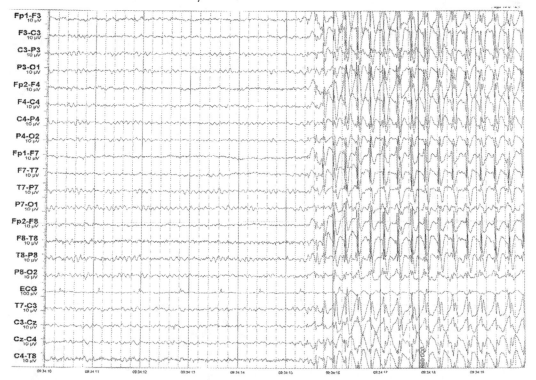

9. Seizure activity (*cont'd*)

f. Generalized atonic seizure

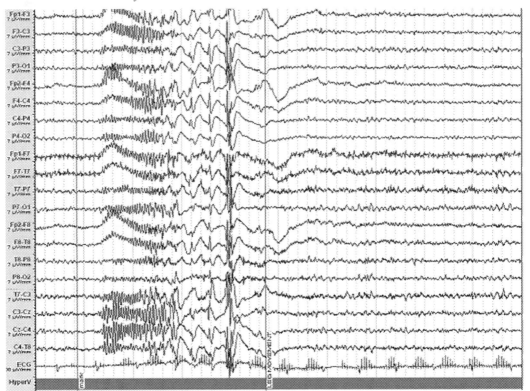

g. Generalized tonic-clonic seizure activity

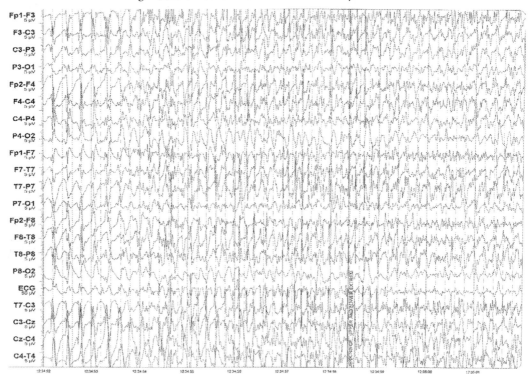

h. Postictal slowing

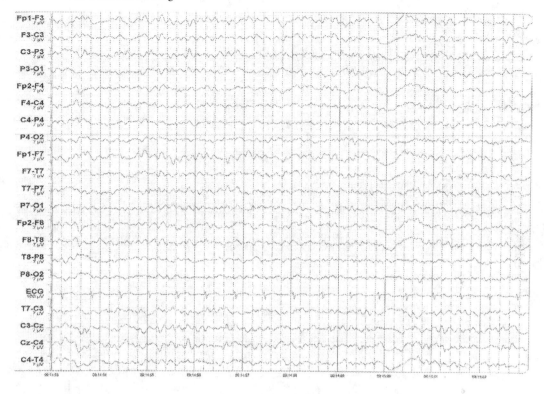

10. Artifact

a. Electrode pop (four-point star) due to poor impedance and EKG artifact (arrows)

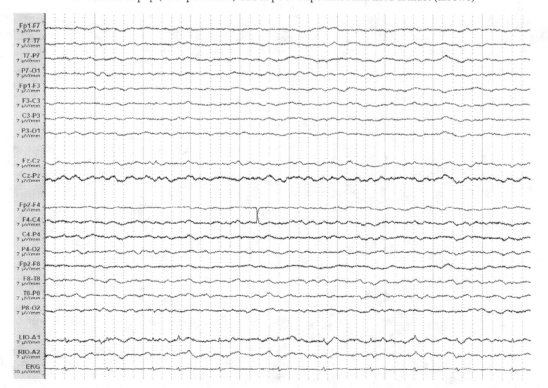

10. Artifact (*cont'd*)

b. Muscle artifact

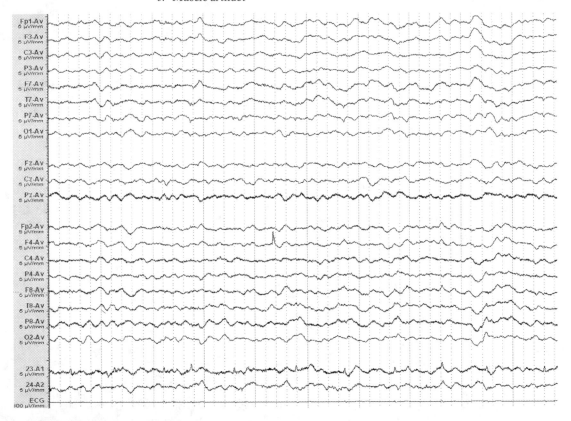

CHEAT SHEET

West's syndrome	Infantile spasms; hypsarrhythmia
Lennox-Gastaut	Multiple seizure types; atonic, tonic GTCs
Landau-Kleffner syndrome	Acquired epileptic aphasia
Juvenile myoclonic epilepsy	Adolescent, tonic-clonic, morning myoclonus, atypical absence; chromosome 6p
Unverricht-Lundborg	Baltic myoclonus, progressive myoclonus and ataxia
Rasmussen's encephalitis	Frequent severe seizures, loss of motor skills, affects single hemisphere

Suggested Readings

Brophy GM, Bell R, Claassen J, et al. Guidelines for the evaluation and management of status epilepticus. *Neurocrit Care*. doi:10.1007/s12028-012-9695-z

Go CY, Mackay MT, Weiss SK, et al. Evidence-based guideline update: medical treatment of infantile spasms. *Neurology*.2012;78:1974–1980.

Krumholz A, Wiebe S, Gronseth GS, et al. Evidence-based guideline: management of an unprovoked first seizure in adults. *Neurology*.2015;84:1705–1713.

CHAPTER 12

Movement Disorders

I. Definition

A. Motor disorders are defined as a group of neurological disorders characterized by paucity of movement (hypokinesia), excessive movement (hyperkinesia), or sometimes a combination of both.

B. Speed, amplitude, and quality of movement are affected in these disorders.

C. Classification

HYPOKINETIC MOVEMENTS	HYPERKINETIC MOVEMENTS
Parkinsonism *Hypothyroid slowness* *Stiff muscles* *Catatonia* *Psychomotor depression* *Cataplexy and drop attacks*	*Tremors* (an oscillatory, usually rhythmic and regular movement affecting one or more body parts) *Dystonia* (sustained or intermittent muscular contractions resulting in repetitive abnormal movements and/or postures) *Chorea* (involuntary, irregular, purposeless, nonrhythmic, abrupt, rapid, unsustained movements that seem to flow from one body part to another) *Ballism* (large-amplitude choreic movements of the proximal parts of the limbs, causing flinging and flailing of limbs) *Athetosis* (slow, writhing, continuous, involuntary movement) *Myoclonus* (sudden, brief, shock-like involuntary movements caused by muscular contractions or inhibitions [negative myoclonus]) *Ataxia (incoordination characterized by jerky movement or posture)* *Restless legs* (unpleasant crawling sensation of the legs, particularly when sitting and relaxing in the evening, which then disappears on walking) *Tics* (consist of abnormal movements or sounds; can be simple or complex) *Stereotypy* (coordinated movement that repeats continually and identically) *Hemifacial* spasm (unilateral facial muscle contractions) *Hyperekplexia* (excessive startle reaction to a sudden, unexpected stimulus) *Akathisia* (feeling of inner, general restlessness, which is reduced or relieved by walking about) *Myokymia* (fine persistent quivering or rippling of muscles) *Myorhythmia* (slow-frequency, prolonged, rhythmic or repetitive movement without the sharp wave appearance of a myoclonic jerk) *Paroxysmal dyskinesias* (recurrent episodes of chorea, dystonia, athetosis, ballism, or a combination of these movements with normal neurologic examination in between the episodes)

II. Parkinsonism: Core features: resting tremor, rigidity, bradykinesia akinesia, loss of postural reflexes (TRAP)

A. Etiologies

Idiopathic parkinsonism *Parkinson-plus* *syndromes*	Parkinson's disease (PD) Dementia with Lewy bodies (DLB) Multiple-system atrophy (MSA) Progressive supranuclear palsy (PSP) Corticobasal degeneration (CBD) Frontotemporal dementia with parkinsonism (FTD-P)
Secondary *parkinsonism*	Drug induced (antiemetics, neuroleptics, reserpine, tetrabenazine, lithium, flunarizine, cinnarizine, diltiazem) Vascular Structural (hydrocephalus, especially normal-pressure hydrocephalus; trauma; tumor) Hypoxia Toxins (1-methyl-4-phenyl-1,2,3, 6-tetrahydropyridine [MPTP], CO, manganese, cyanide, methanol) Infections (fungal, AIDS, subacute sclerosing panencephalitis, postencephalitic parkinsonism, Creutzfeldt-Jakob disease) Metabolic (hypo-/hypercalcemia, chronic hepatocerebral degeneration, Wilson's disease) Paraneoplastic parkinsonism Psychogenic
Heredodegenerative *disease*	Alzheimer's disease (AD) Huntington's disease Machado-Joseph disease Hallervorden-Spatz disease X-linked dystonia-parkinsonism (Lubag)

B. PD: neurodegenerative disorder characterized by the gradual and progressive onset of parkinsonism in the absence of known causes

1. *Clinical diagnosis: unilateral onset with asymmetry of clinical signs; bradykinesia, which is the most important clinical sign for the diagnosis of parkinsonism; rest tremor (in 80%, usually low frequency [4–7 Hz] with classic pronation-supination and pill-rolling pattern); rigidity of a lead pipe quality and in later stages of the disease postural instability;* insidious, often unilateral onset of subtle motor features; rate of progression varies; eventually symptoms worsen and become bilateral; *with* absence of other neurologic signs (spasticity, Babinski signs, atypical speech); absence of lab or radiologic abnormalities (e.g., strokes, tumors);

slowly progressive with significant and sustained response to dopaminergic ther-apy; classically or traditionally defined by motor features, it is now known to be associated with a host of nonmotor symptomatology, including autonomic dys-function (constipation, impotence, seborrheic dermatitis, bladder dyssynergia); *neuropsychiatric dysfunction* (**NB**: *depression* in up to 50%, *dementia* in up to 20%; *anxiety, panic attacks, hallucinations, delusions*); nearly all PD patients suf-fer from sleep disorders (e.g., insomnia, sleep fragmentation, excessive daytime sleepiness, nightmares, REM behavior disorder); treatment must be individual-ized and continually adjusted as the disease evolves. Nonmotor symptoms are now known to cause more impairment in quality of life and cause more care-giver stress than motor features.

2. *Epidemiology of PD:* estimated prevalence: *500,000 to 1 million* patients in United States; incidence: 40,000 to 60,000 new cases per year; average age of onset is 60 years; affects up to 0.3% of general population, but 1% to 3% of those over 65 years old (y/o); PD is largely a disease of older adults: only *5% to 10% of patients have symptoms before 40 y/o (young-onset PD).*

3. *Genetic factors:* autosomal dominant (AD) and recessive patterns of inheritance have been identified.

    a. *Park 1/Park 4: chromosome 4q21-23;* alanine-53-threonine mutation in the α *synuclein gene; AD;* earlier disease onset (mean age 45 years), faster progres-sion, some with fluent aphasia; central hypoventilation

    b. *Park 2: chromosome 6q25.2-27; the parkin gene;* parkin; autosomal *recessive (AR);* relatively young-onset parkinsonism; dystonia at onset; symmetric in-volvement; good levodopa response; slow disease progression; *absence of Lewy bodies* at autopsy

    c. *Park 3: chromosome 2p13; AD* but with 40% penetrance; all from northern Ger-many and southern Denmark; nigral degeneration and Lewy bodies at autopsy; dementia may be more common.

    d. *Park 5: mutation in ubiquitin carboxy-terminal hydrolase L1 on chromosome 4p14; AD;* late-onset progressive parkinsonism

    e. *Park 6: mutation of the PINK1 gene on chromosome 1p35-36; AR;* early-onset parkinsonism; phenotype similar to Parkin-PD but with cognitive and psychi-atric features; slow progression, and marked response to levodopa

    f. *Park 7: mutation of DJ-1 gene on chromosome 1p36;* early-onset *AR* parkin-sonism, slow progression, with levodopa responsiveness; mostly from the Netherlands

    g. *Park 8: mutation of the LRRK2 gene on chromosome 12q12; AD;* age of onset in the 60s with variable alpha synuclein and tau pathology

    h. *Park 9: aka Kufor-Rakeb syndrome; mutation of ATP13A2 on chromosome 1q36; AR;* age of onset in the 30s; vertical gaze palsy, pyramidal signs, facial and finger mini-myoclonus, cognitive impairment

    i. Park 10 and 11: reported but inheritance is still unclear, probably AD, and gene mutation has not yet been identified.

    j. Park 14: mutation of PLA2G6 on chromosome 22q13. AR; parkinsonism asso-ciated with dystonia

4. *Pathology:* many theories on cell death, but no firm conclusions; apoptosis, mi-tochondrial dysfunction, oxidative stress, excitotoxicity, deficient neurotrophic support, immune mechanisms; *loss of pigmentation of the substantia nigra and locus ceruleus with decreased neuromelanin-containing neurons;* affected neurons contain large homogenous eosinophilic cytoplasmic inclusions called *Lewy bodies,* which possess neurofilament, ubiquitin, and crystalline immunoreactivity.

B. **PD** (*cont'd*)

   5. *Pharmacotherapy of PD*

      a. *Amantadine:* N-methyl-D-aspartate antagonist useful for newly diagnosed patients with mild symptoms and in some patients with advanced disease; provides mild to moderate benefit by decreasing tremor, rigidity, and akinesia; rarely effective as monotherapy for more than 1 to 2 years, may be continued as adjunctive agent; effective for levodopa-induced dyskinesias; adverse effects: anticholinergic effects, livedo reticularis, renal disease increases susceptibility to adverse effects, leg edema, neuropsychiatric effects—confusion, hallucinations, nightmares, insomnia

      b. *Anticholinergic agents:* option for young patients (<60 y/o) whose predominant symptoms are resting tremor and hypersalivation (sialorrhea); available agents—trihexyphenidyl and benztropine; adverse effects often limit use—memory impairment, confusion, hallucinations

      c. *Levodopa:* advantages—most efficacious antiparkinsonian drug to date, immediate therapeutic benefits (within 1 week), easily titrated, reduces mortality, lower cost; disadvantages—no effect on disease course, no effect on nondopaminergic symptoms (such as dysautonomia, cognitive disturbances; little or no effect on axial symptoms such as sialorrhea, dysphagia, hypophonia and postural instability), motor fluctuations and dyskinesia develop over time (especially in younger patients, those with more severe disease and those requiring higher doses); acute adverse effects—nausea/vomiting (dopamine decarboxylase inhibitor [carbidopa or benserazide] alleviates by inhibiting amino acid decarboxylase enzyme), confusion, psychosis, dizziness; chronic effects—hallucinations; motor fluctuations—peak dose or diphasic dyskinesias, wearing off (predictable or sudden off), delayed on, yo-yoing; now available in different formulations: short-acting, long-acting, orally dissolving (Parcopa), extended release (Rytary), and in liquid gel form delivered directly to the duodenum through an external pump (Duopa or Duodopa).

      d. *Dopamine agonists*

DRUG	ERGOT DERIVED	D1	D2	D3/D4	HALF-LIFE (HRS)
Bromocriptine	Yes	−	+ +	+	3
*Pergolide**	Yes	+	+ +	+ +	27
Pramipexole	No	−	+ +	+ + +	12
Ropinirole	No	−	+ +	+	4
Rotigotine	No	−	+ +	+ +	5-7**
Cabergoline	Yes	−	+ +	+	65

+, least receptor affinity; +++, greatest receptor affinity.
*Withdrawn from the market due to increased risk of valvulopathy.

**Formulated as a transdermal patch that provides a slow and constant supply of the drug over the course of 24 hours.

        i. Effective for initial monotherapy; also indicated in combination with levodopa to smoothen clinical response in advanced disease; directly stimulate postsynaptic dopamine receptors; effective against key motor symptoms (tremor, bradykinesia, and rigidity); early use shows reduced risk of dyskinesia compared with levodopa therapy, although antiparkinsonian effects consistently inferior to levodopa; adverse effects: slightly higher than levodopa—nausea/vomiting, sedation, orthostatic hypotension, hallucinations, dyskinesia in more advanced disease, leg edema, **NB:** daytime somnolence including sleep attacks; ergot-derived side effects— livedo reticularis, erythromelalgia, cardiac, pulmonary or retroperitoneal fibrosis, valvulopathy; potential to cause impulse control disorders (ICDs), which include pathologic gambling, hypersexuality, compulsive eating.

ii. *Apomorphine:* available in the United States as an injectable (subcutaneous) short-acting dopamine agonist; approved by the U.S. Food and Drug Administration (FDA) as a "rescue therapy" for symptoms of wearing off in advanced PD patients; benefits take effect as early as 5 minutes from the time of injection, but lasts for only 1 to 1.5 hours.

iii. *Rotigotine:* the latest dopamine agonist approved in the United States for monotherapy in early PD and as an adjunct treatment for levodopa in advanced PD; available in transdermal (patch) form; side effects, other than skin reactions, are similar to non-ergot dopamine agonists, including somnolence, sleep attacks, nausea, vomiting, weight gain, hallucinations, and so forth.

iv. Impulse control disorders (e.g., hypersexuality, binge eating, pathological gambling, and compulsive shopping) have been associated with PD medications, especially dopamine agonists. Dopamine agonist withdrawal syndrome (DAWS) has been described to occur in patients when dopamine agonists are withdrawn because of side effects, characterized by agitation, depression, anxiety, and other symptoms similar to that seen with psychostimulant withdrawal.

e. **NB:** *Catechol-O-methyltransferase inhibitors: inhibit levodopa catabolism to 3-O-methyldopa, increasing levodopa bioavailability and transport to brain;* extend duration of levodopa effect; indicated for treatment of patients with PD experiencing end-of-dose wearing off with levodopa; no role as monotherapy; used only in combination with levodopa; two available agents: *entacapone (Comtan®) and tolcapone (Tasmar®);* fatal fulminant hepatitis in four tolcapone-treated patients: requires liver function monitoring and signed patient consent; side effects: dyskinesias, diarrhea (4%–10%), nausea

f. *Monoamine oxidase B (MAO-B) inhibitors*

i. *Selegiline:* selective monoamine oxidase-B inhibitor with doses less than 10 mg/day; Deprenyl and Tocopherol Antioxidative Therapy of Parkinsonism (DATATOP) study showed unlikely neuroprotective effect and mild symptomatic benefit in early PD; with higher doses, avoid tyramine-rich food, meperidine, or selective serotonin reuptake inhibitor, as monoamine oxidase-B selectivity is lost, predisposing to cheese effect

ii. *Rasagiline:* new selective, once-per-day MAO-B inhibitor; FDA approved for monotherapy in early PD, and also for adjunctive treatment to levodopa in moderate to advanced PD; "off time" was decreased by 0.9 hours among PD patients with wearing-off symptoms compared to placebo in the PRESTO trial and LARGO trials; the recently concluded ADAGIO trial showed that early, medication-naïve PD patients placed on rasagiline at 1 mg per day immediately at study entry had a better average total Unified Parkinson Disease Rating Scale (UPDRS) score after 3 years compared to those who received rasagiline 9 months later; unlike selegiline, this new MAO-B inhibitor is not broken down into amphetamine metabolites; however, dietary precaution on tyramine-rich foods is advised.

g. *Management of hallucinations (psychosis) in PD and PD dementia:* eliminate medical causes of delirium (e.g., infection or dehydration); discontinue nonparkinsonian psychotropic medications, if possible; eliminate antiparkinsonian drugs in order of their potential to produce delirium (anticholinergics >

g. *Management of hallucinations (psychosis) in PD and PD dementia (cont'd)*

amantadine > monoamine oxidase-B inhibitors > dopamine agonists > catechol methyltransferase inhibitor > levodopa); use regular levodopa formulation at lowest possible dose; use atypical antipsychotic agents (clozapine > quetiapine > other atypicals). NB: Quetiapine is preferred despite clozapine being the gold standard; risk of agranulocytosis with clozapine necessitates regular white blood cell (WBC) monitoring.

Rivastigmine: for cognitive impairment, *the first FDA-approved medication for Parkinson's disease with dementia (PDD);* available orally and in patch form; may also improve mild hallucinations; most frequent side effects: nausea, vomiting, and tremors (usually mild and transient but can be bothersome to some); no worsening in the UPDRS motor scores in patients who were randomized to rivastigmine compared to placebo in the EXPRESS trial

h. *Surgical management of PD:* lesion versus deep-brain stimulation; *lesion* (thalamotomy—most effective for parkinsonian and essential tremor; pallidotomy—improves bradykinesia, tremor, rigidity, dyskinesia in PD) has the advantage of simplicity, no technology or adjustments required, no indwelling device; however, disadvantages include inability to do bilateral lesions without increased risk of dementia, swallowing dysfunction, and so forth, and side effects could be permanent; *deep-brain stimulation surgery of globus pallidus internus or subthalamic nucleus* may improve most symptoms of PD and has the advantage of minimal to no cell destruction and the ability to perform deep-brain stimulation on both sides and to adjust the stimulation settings as the disease progresses; however, deep-brain stimulation is more expensive, requires technical expertise, and could be prone to hardware malfunctions (e.g., kinks, lead fractures) or infections; the *ideal surgical candidate: clear PD diagnosis with unequivocal and sustained levodopa response, relatively young, nondemented, nondepressed, nonanxious, emotionally and physically stable.*

C. **Multiple system atrophy (MSA) is a neurodegenerative condition characterized by parkinsonism, autonomic dysfunction, and cerebellar dysfunction in variable combination; the term encompasses three overlapping entities: (1) MSA with orthostatic hypotension, previously known as Shy-Drager syndrome; (2) MSA parkinsonism subtype (MSA-P), previously known as striatonigral degeneration; and (3) MSA cerebellar subtype (MSA-C), previously known as olivopontocerebellar atrophy.**

1. *Clinical manifestations*

a. *MSA-P:* a sporadic disorder with an insidious onset of neurologic symptoms in the 4th to 7th decades of life; the mean age at onset is 56.6 years, and there is no sex preference; akinetic rigid syndrome, similar to PD; patients initially present with rigidity, hypokinesia, and sometimes unexplained falling; may be symmetric or asymmetric at onset; the course is relentlessly progressive, with a duration ranging from 2 to 10 years (mean, 4.5–6.0 years); eventually, patients are severely disabled by marked akinesia, rigidity, dysphonia or dysarthria, postural instability, and autonomic dysfunction; mild cognitive and affective changes with difficulties in executive functions, axial dystonia with anterocollis, stimulus-sensitive myoclonus, and pyramidal signs; respiratory stridor due to moderate to severe laryngeal abductor paralysis can sometimes occur; resting tremor is not common; cerebellar signs are typically absent; the majority do not respond to levodopa, except early in the course.

b. *MSA-C:* essentially a progressive degenerative cerebellar-plus syndrome; male-to-female ratio is 1.8:1.0 in familial olivopontocerebellar atrophy and 1:1 in sporadic olivopontocerebellar atrophy; the average age of onset is 28 years for familial and 50 years for sporadic olivopontocerebellar atrophy; the mean duration of the disease is 16 years in familial and 6 years in sporadic olivopontocerebellar atrophy; cerebellar ataxia, especially involving gait, is the presenting symptom in 73% of patients; dysmetria, limb ataxia, and cerebellar dysarthria are characteristic; other initial symptoms include rigidity, hypokinesia, fatigue, disequilibrium, involuntary movements, visual changes, spasticity, and mental deterioration; as the disease progresses, cerebellar disturbances remain the most outstanding clinical features; dementia is the next most common symptom in familial olivopontocerebellar atrophy and is present in 60% of patients; dementia occurs in 35% of sporadic olivopontocerebellar atrophy patients.

2. *Pathology:* MSA is characterized pathologically by cell *loss and gliosis in the striatum and substantia nigra;* macroscopically, the putamen is most affected, with significant atrophy; the substantia nigra exhibits hypopigmentation; microscopically, severe neuronal loss, gliosis, and loss of myelinated fibers are evident in the putamen, less on the caudate; gliosis is found, but Lewy bodies or neurofibrillary tangles are not commonly present; a recent finding in cases of multiple system atrophy is the presence of *argyrophilic cytoplasmic inclusions in oligodendrocytes and neurons;* the inclusions are composed of granule-associated filaments that have immunoreactivity with tubulin, τ protein, and ubiquitin; they seem to be specific for MSA; there is considerable clinical and pathologic overlap among the three MSA syndromes; *in MSA-C, neuronal loss with gross atrophy is concentrated in the pons, medullary olives, and cerebellum; in MSA with orthostatic hypotension, the intermediolateral cell columns of the spinal cord are affected as well.*

3. *Differential diagnosis:* MSA is most frequently misdiagnosed as *PD;* features suggestive of MSA include unexplained falls early in disease, early appearance of autonomic symptoms, rapid progression of parkinsonian disability, lack of or unsustained significant response to levodopa therapy, symmetric presentation, and minimal or no resting tremors; PD is different from MSA-C because of the absence of prominent cerebellar symptoms and from MSA syndrome because of a lack of pronounced orthostatic hypotension; MSA's relatively symmetric presentation will not be confused with *cortical-basal ganglionic degeneration,* and its intact oculomotor function distinguishes it from *progressive supranuclear palsy;* mentation is relatively preserved in MSA-P (less so in MSA-C) and is helpful in differentiating from dementing diseases, such as AD with parkinsonian features, *diffuse Lewy body disease, or Creutzfeldt-Jakob disease;* finally, MSA should be distinguished from *acquired parkinsonism* by ruling out infectious, toxic, drug-induced, vascular, traumatic, and metabolic causes.

> **NB:** Orthostatic hypotension may be treated with fludrocortisone, midodrine, or droxidopa.

D. **Progressive supranuclear palsy: previously known as Steele-Richardson-Olszewski syndrome; clinical: classic PSP (also known as Richardson's syndrome)— supranuclear ophthalmoparesis (especially downgaze) and falls within the first year of onset of parkinsonism are mandatory criteria for probable progressive supranuclear palsy; 60% to 80% with subcortical form of dementia; pathology: widespread diencephalic and mesencephalic (leading to a Mickey Mouse midbrain), brainstem and cerebellar nuclear neuronal loss; with globose neurofibrillary tangles (exhibit paired helical filament, τ protein and ubiquitin immunoreactivity); marked midbrain atrophy.**

> **NB:** Falls and aspiration cause the most frequent complications.

E. Corticobasal ganglionic degeneration: an asymmetric form of parkinsonism presenting with unilateral dystonia, myoclonus, alien limb phenomena plus parkinsonism; dementia is common; pathologically with achromatic neuronal inclusions but no classic Pick bodies; asymmetric findings on MRI or functional imaging

> **NB:** Synucleinopathies: multiple-system atrophy, PD, Lewy body dementia

> **NB:** Tauopathies: AD, Pick's disease, frontotemporal dementia with parkinsonism, progressive supranuclear palsy, corticobasal ganglionic degeneration.

F. Postencephalitic parkinsonism: von Economo's encephalitis; this disease is now almost nonexistent but nevertheless an extremely important disease after the 1914–1918 influenza pandemics; some individuals developed encephalitis, and in the months to years after recovery from the acute illness, they developed parkinsonism with prominent oculogyric symptoms; condition was generally nonprogressive; pathology: depigmentation of the substantia nigra and locus ceruleus, no classic Lewy bodies, with neurofibrillary tangles.

G. Dementia-parkinsonism-amyotrophic lateral sclerosis complex of Guam: exhibits gross atrophy of the frontotemporal regions, depigmentation of the substantia nigra, and loss of anterior roots; histologically, there are neurofibrillary tangles in the cortical neurons, loss of pigmented neurons in the substantia nigra without Lewy bodies, and loss of anterior horn cells with neurofibrillary tangles.

H. Acute parkinsonism: etiology: infectious, postinfectious, autoimmune (e.g. systemic lupus erythematosus), medication (typical side effects of antidopamine drugs, idiosyncratic effects—neuroleptic malignant syndrome, serotonin syndrome, chemotherapeutic drugs), toxic (carbon monoxide, cadmium, MPTP, ethanol withdrawal, ethylene oxide, methanol, disulfiram, bone marrow transplantation), structural (stroke, subdural hematoma, central and extra pontine myelinolysis, tumor, hydrocephalus), psychiatric (catatonia, conversion, malingering)

1. *Structural lesions:* obstructive hydrocephalus is a well-known cause of parkinsonism; may occur in adults and children, either due to shunt obstruction or at presentation of the hydrocephalus; obstructive hydrocephalus after meningitis or subarachnoid hemorrhage may also cause parkinsonism.

   NB: Normal-pressure hydrocephalus often mimics neurodegenerative parkinsonism.

2. *Vascular parkinsonism:* previously called *atherosclerotic parkinsonism;* usually results from tiny lacunes in the basal ganglia; generally insidious in onset and slowly progressive, although sudden worsening may occur with new strokes; *frontal, cingulated gyrus, supplementary motor area strokes* have also caused acute parkinsonism; of interest, strokes in the lenticular nuclei do not cause parkinsonism; acute hemorrhage is a less common cause of acute parkinsonism.

3. *Toxic/metabolic:* some, like *manganese,* develop subacutely or over long periods; parkinsonism may follow *carbon monoxide* poisoning following an acute, life-threatening poisoning after recovery from the coma; carbon monoxide poisoning is a persistent problem in some countries, notably Korea, where faulty oil-burning heaters are used; the globus pallidus is typically involved, but recent data suggest that white-matter deterioration must also be present for parkinsonism to develop; *cadmium and ethylene oxide, disulfiram* (used to prevent alcoholics from imbibing), and *cyanide poisoning* are other uncommon causes.

4. *MPTP:* severe, acute parkinsonism in intravenous drug abusers in the San Francisco Bay area; the drug is taken up by glial cells and converted to MPP+, which is secreted and taken up by dopaminergic cells in the pars compacta of the substantia nigra; the first systemically administered drug that selectively targets these cells and, because it has a similar effect in other primates, it has been widely used to create animal models of PD; the onset of parkinsonism occurs after the first few doses.

5. *Neuroleptic malignant syndrome* is variably defined but generally requires *fever, alteration of mental status, and rigidity; many patients have extreme elevations of creatine phosphokinase* due to rhabdomyolysis; neuroleptic malignant syndrome may occur at any point once a patient is treated with neuroleptics, but it usually occurs relatively shortly after drug initiation and dose increase; the onset of neuroleptic malignant syndrome may be fulminant, progressing to coma over hours, but it usually develops over days; patients develop fever, stiffness, and mental impairment with delirium and obtundation; treatment: requires excluding infection, stopping the suspected offending drug, close monitoring of autonomic and respiratory parameters, and treatment with dopaminergic replacement (either levodopa or dopamine agonists).

6. *Dopamine D2 receptor-blocking drugs* routinely cause parkinsonism; may also occur with *lithium or valproic acid;* syndrome usually develops over the course of weeks, but may occasionally develop over days; in patients with a primary parkinsonian syndrome, a low-potency neuroleptic or even an atypical antipsychotic can induce acute parkinsonism; this is not uncommon when a patient with PD is treated with an antiemetic, such as prochlorperazine or metoclopramide.

III. Chorea: Irregular, rapid, unsustained, purposeless, jerky involuntary movement that flows randomly from one body part to another

A. Etiology

Primary	Essential chorea/senile chorea
Hereditary	Benign familial chorea *Neurodegenerative* Huntington's disease Neuroacanthocytosis syndrome Huntington-disease-like disorders (HDL1,2,3) Wilson's disease *Neurometabolic disorders* Lesch-Nyhan syndrome Lysosomal storage disorders Leigh disease
Secondary	*Infectious:* subacute bacterial endocarditis, subacute sclerosing panencephalitis, AIDS, Lyme disease, tuberculosis, syphilis, Creutzfeldt-Jakob disease, encephalitides *Post-infectious:* Sydenham's chorea Immunological: systemic lupus erythematosus, antiphospholipid antibody syndrome, Henoch-Schönlein purpura Toxins/chemicals: CO, Hg, lithium

(continued)

A. **Etiology** (*cont'd*)

Secondary (cont'd)	Paraneoplastic Postvaccinal Vascular: stroke, venous thrombosis, polycythemia vera *Drugs:* neuroleptics, levodopa, oral contraceptives, anticholinergics, antihistamines, phenytoin, methylphenidate (Ritalin®), pemoline, methadone, cocaine, etc. Pregnancy (chorea gravidarum) *Metabolic and endocrine etiologies:* hypoparathyroidism, hypomagnesemia, Addison's disease, hypernatremia, thyrotoxicosis, hypoglycemia, hyperosmolar hyperglycemic state Mitochondrial myopathies Tumors including metastasis Other: multiple sclerosis, anoxia, kernicterus/ethyl alcohol

> **NB:** The primary treatment of any tardive syndrome (late-onset chorea, dystonia, akathisia, after sustained exposure to dopamine-receptor blocking agents such as antipsychotics and anti-emetics) is elimination of the precipitating medication.

B. **Huntington's disease: AD disorder (with 100% penetrance); caused by CAG repeat in the Huntingtin gene chromosome 4p16**

1. *Clinical:* combines *cognitive (subcortical dementia), movement disorders (chorea, dystonia, motor impersistence, incoordination, gait instability, and, in the young, parkinsonism and seizures, also known as Westphal variant), and psychiatric disorders (depression with a tendency to suicide, anxiety, impulsivity, apathy, obsessive compulsive disorders, etc.);* commonly manifest by age 20 to 40 years; usually progresses relentlessly to death in 10 to 15 years

2. *Pathology:* the brain is atrophic, with striking atrophy of the caudate nucleus, and, to a lesser degree, the putamen; compensatory hydrocephalus may be seen *(box-car-shaped ventricles);* microscopically: preferential *loss of the medium spiny striatal neurons accompanied by gliosis;* biochemically: decreased γ-aminobutyric acid, enkephalins, and substance P.

3. Genetics: HD belongs to a group of disorders known as the trinucleotide repeat diseases; *anticipation:* the age of onset occurs earlier with succeeding generations due to increase in trinucleotide repeat, and, because repeats may amplify between generations, anticipation may be seen.

4. *Trinucleotide-repeat diseases*

DISEASE	INHERITANCE	REPEATS	CHROMOSOME	PROTEIN
Huntington's disease	AD	CAG	4p16	Huntingtin
Fragile X	AD	CGG	X	FMR-1
Myotonic dystrophy	AD	CTG	19	Myotonin

(continued)

DISEASE	INHERITANCE	REPEATS	CHROMOSOME	PROTEIN
SCA type 1	AD	CAG	6p23	Ataxin-1
SCA type 2	AD	CAG	12q24	Ataxin-2
SCA type 3 (Machado-Joseph disease)	AD	CAG	14q32	Ataxin-3
SCA type 6	AD	CAG	19p13	Voltage-dependent calcium channel
SCA type 7	AD	CAG	13p12	Ataxin-7
SCA type 12	AD	CAG	5q31-33	Regulatory subunit of protein phosphatase (PP2A)
SCA type 17	AD	CAG	6q27	TATA-binding protein
Spinobulbar muscular atrophy (Kennedy's)	X-linked recessive	CAG	Xq13	Androgen receptor
Dentatorubropal lidoluysian atrophy	AD	CAG	12p13	Atrophin-1
Friedreich's ataxia	AR	GAA	9q13-21.1	Frataxin

Abbreviation: SCA, spinocerebellar ataxia.

5. *Hereditary causes of chorea*

DISORDER	INHERITANCE	CHROMOSOME	GENE	FINDINGS
Huntington's disease	AD	4p16.3	Huntingtin	See Section III.B
Huntington's disease-like 1 (HDL1)	AD	20p	Prion protein gene (PRNP)	Almost like Huntington's disease; with seizures
HDL2	AD	16q23	Junctophilin 3 (JPH3)	Onset in the 4th decade, like HDL1, but no seizures; seen exclusively in populations with African ancestry
HDL3	AR	4p15.3		Onset at 3–4 years with chorea, dystonia, ataxia, gait disorder, spasticity, seizures, mutism, mental decline

(continued)

5. *Hereditary causes of chorea (cont'd)*

DISORDER	INHERITANCE	CHROMOSOME	GENE	FINDINGS
Neuroacanthocytosis	AR X-linked AD has also been reported	9q21 Xp21	CHAC gene XK gene	Behavioral and personality disorders, chorea, dystonia, dysphagia, dysarthria, seizures, motor axonopathy, high creatine phosphokinase
Neurodegeneration with brain iron accumulation type 1 (formerly known as Hallervorden-Spatz disease)	AR	20p12.3-p13	PANK-2	Childhood onset, progressive rigidity, dystonia, choreoathetosis, spasticity, optic nerve atrophy, dementia with acanthocytosis
Benign hereditary chorea	AD	14q13.1-q21.1		Slight motor delay with chorea, ataxia, usually self-limiting after adolescence
Dentatorubropal-lidoluysian atrophy (DRPLA)	AD	12 (CAG repeat)	Jun NH(2)-terminal kinase (JNK)	Onset typically 4th decade; myoclonus, epilepsy, mental retardation (early onset); ataxia, choreoathetosis, dystonia, rest and postural tremor, parkinsonism, dementia (late onset)
				Others: SCA 2, 3, and 17; Wilson's disease

6. *Treatment: chorea:* dopamine-receptor-blocking agents (e.g., haloperidol, risper-idone, clozapine, quetiapine, reserpine, tetrabenazine), antiseizure medications such as valproic acid and carbamazepine (which also have the benefit of being mood stabilizers), clonazepam, amantadine; *tetrabenazine now available in the United States for the treatment of chorea in HD (monitor patient carefully for development of depression and parkinsonism); gait instability:* reassess if dopamine-blocking agents are causing parkinsonism, physical and occupational therapy; *depression and anxiety:* selective serotonin reuptake inhibitors, clonazepam; *speech and swallowing therapy; genetic counseling; family counseling; multidisciplinary approach for any neurodegenerative cause*

C. Neuroacanthocytosis: second most common cause of hereditary chorea after HD; it is a multisystemic neurodegenerative disorder with a heterogenous presentation consisting of both hyperkinetic and hypokinetic movement disorders as well as other neurological and laboratory abnormalities. Although these disorders have been defined by the presence of red blood cell acanthocytes (deformed erythrocytes with spike-like protrusions), they are not always present and can appear variably during the course of the illness in the same patient, and diagnosis does not require demonstration in peripheral blood smear.

1. *Clinical:* mean age of onset is 32 years (range, 8–62 years), and the clinical course is progressive, but with marked phenotypic variation.

   a. *Psychiatric:* behavioral disorders, emotional disorders, and psychiatric manifestations are common; depression, paranoia, and obsessive-compulsive disorder, self-mutilation behavior; compulsive head banging or biting of tongue, lips, and fingers can lead to severe injury; dementia is often reported.

   b. *Epilepsy:* a considerable proportion of patients have seizures, which may precede onset of movement disorders by many years.

   c. *Involuntary movement disorders:* jerky movements of the limbs; sucking, chewing, and smacking movements of the mouth; shoulder shrugs, flinging movements of the arms and legs, and thrusting movements of the trunk and pelvis; wild lurching truncal and flinging proximal arm movements; oral-facial dyskinesias; tic-like, repetitive, and stereotyped movements; involuntary vocalizations are common; occasional patients have primarily dystonia.

   d. *Disordered voluntary movements:* lack of oral-facial coordination is prominent; dysarthria and dysphagia occur in most cases; many patients have a characteristic eating disorder (feeding dystonia) in which food is propelled out of the mouth by the tongue—patients may learn to swallow with the head tipped back, "facing the ceiling," or place a spoon over the mouth to prevent the food from escaping; bradykinesia in concert with chorea is also common; gait is disordered and features a combination of involuntary movements and poor postural reflexes.

   e. *Neuromuscular weakness:* elevated creatine phosphokinase (in the absence of myopathy); peripheral neuropathy with distal sensory loss and hyporeflexia is common; electrophysiologic studies show increased duration and amplitude of motor unit potentials, indicative of chronic denervation.

2. Classification: two broad groups: (a) core neuroacanthocytosis syndromes—chorea-acanthocytosis, McLeod syndrome, pantothenate-kinase-associated neurodegeneration (PKAN); (b) neuroacanthocytosis with lipoprotein disorders—abetalipoproteinemia, familial hypobetalipoproteinemia, Anderson disease.

> **NB:** HDL-2 is sometimes included among the core neuroacanthocytosis syndromes because of the presence of acanthocytosis in ~10% of cases.

3. *Genetics:* considered to have a genetic basis, but the gene defect is unknown in most patients; some cases are *AD*, others are *AR (chromosome 9q21);* in a subset of patients with a similar but *X-linked* clinical syndrome, the *lack of a common red blood cell antigen, Kx,* has been described; it is caused by mutations in the XK gene encoding the Kx protein, a putative membrane transport protein of yet unknown function; this X-linked illness, known as *McLeod syndrome,* is characterized by *hemolysis, myopathy, cardiomyopathy, areflexia, chorea, elevated creatine phosphokinase, liver disease, and chorea.*

> **NB:** Gene product: chorein.

D. Dentatorubropallidoluysian atrophy (DRPLA): rare disorder, more common in Japan or people with Japanese ancestry (also presents as the Haw River syndrome in African Americans); characterized by the presence of progressive myoclonic epilepsy, ataxia, choreoathetosis, and dementia; age of onset is broad, mostly in the 3rd or 4th decade, but juvenile form occurs in childhood, which is accompanied by mental retardation; two forms—early onset (<20 years) and late onset (>20 years); pathology: degeneration of the dentate nucleus, red nucleus, globus pallidus, and subthalamic nucleus; a trinucleotide CAG repeat mapped to chromosome 12p, producing the protein atrophin-1.

E. Pantothenate-kinase-associated neurodegeneration (PKAN) (formerly Hallervorden-Spatz syndrome): belongs to a group of disorders known as neurodegeneration with brain iron accumulation; regarded as NBIA type I; rare AR disorder pathologically associated with iron deposition and high concentration of lipofuscin and neuromelanin in the substantia nigra pars reticulata and the internal segment of the globus pallidus; mapped to chromosome 20p12.3-13; due to a mutation in the gene for pantothenate kinase gene (PANK2); three presentations: early onset (<10 y/o), late onset (10–18 y/o), and adult variant, although typical presentation is during childhood; characterized by progressive personality changes, cognitive decline, dysarthria, motor difficulties, spasticity; dystonia is common but choreoathetosis tremor may be present; retinitis pigmentosa, optic atrophy, and seizures may also occur; MRI: decreased T2-weighted signal in the globus pallidus and substantia nigra; some have a hyperintense area within the hypodense areas ("eye of the tiger" sign); another neuroacanthocytosis syndrome now considered part of the PKAN spectrum is hyperprebetalipoproteinemia, acanthocytosis, retinitis pigmentosa, and pallidal degeneration (HARP) syndrome.

F. Sydenham's chorea: this is regarded as the classic autoimmune chorea; initial manifestation: usually disturbance in school function, daydreaming, fidgety, inattentiveness, irritability, and increased emotional lability; onset of chorea is rather sudden, lag time between streptococcal infection and chorea averages 6 months; serologic evidence (increase in antistreptolysin-O and anti-DNase B) is absent in one-third of patients; risk of developing carditis with Sydenham's chorea is 30% to 50%; recurrent episodes of chorea are most common at the time of pregnancy in female patients; lab findings: elevated erythrocyte sedimentation rate or C-reactive protein, prolonged PR interval; treatment for chorea: dopamine-receptor-blocking agents, such as haloperidol, pimozide, phenothiazines, or amantadine; for acute rheumatic fever: penicillin V, 400,000 U (250 mg) tid for 10 days, followed by prophylaxis (benzathine penicillin G, 1.2 million U intramuscularly every 3–4 weeks, or penicillin V, 250 mg by mouth bid, or sulfisoxazole, 0.5–1.0 g by mouth qd).

G. Lesch-Nyhan syndrome: rare X-linked disease; uricemia in association with spasticity and choreoathetosis in early childhood with self-mutilation; normal at birth up to 6 to 9 months; self-mutilation (mainly lips) occurs early; spasticity, athetosis, and tremor later; mental retardation moderately severe; gouty tophi appear on ears, risk for gouty nephropathy; lab: serum uric acid, 7 to 10 mg/dL; deficiency in hypoxanthine-guanine-phosphoribosyl transferase that lies on X chromosome by DNA analysis; treatment: allopurinol (xanthine oxidase inhibitor) but no effect on central nervous system; transitory success with 5-hydroxytryptophan with L-dopa; fluphenazine/haloperidol for self-mutilation; behavior modification.

H. Paroxysmal dyskinesias: a heterogeneous group of disorders that have in common sudden abnormal involuntary movements out of a background of normal motor behavior with complete resolution of symptoms in between episodes; may be choreic, ballistic, dystonic, or a combination of these.

FEATURES	PAROXYSMAL KINESIGENIC DYSKINESIA	PAROXYSMAL NONKINESIGENIC DYSKINESIA	PAROXYSMAL EXERTION-INDUCED DYSKINESIA	PAROXYSMAL HYPNOGENIC DYSKINESIA
Inheritance	AD or sporadic	AD or sporadic	AD	AD or sporadic
Male-to-female ratio	4:1	1.5:1.0	1:2	—
Age at onset	<1–40 yrs	<1–30 yrs	2–20 yrs	0–40 yrs
Attacks				
Duration	<5 mins	2 mins–4 hrs	5–30 mins	Seconds to minutes
Frequency	100/day–1/mo	2/day–2/yr	1/day–2/mo	5/night–2/yr
Trigger	Sudden movement/startle, hyperventilation	None	Prolonged exercise, vibration, passive movement, cold	Non-REM sleep
Precipitant	Stress	Alcohol, stress, caffeine, fatigue	Stress	Stress, menses
Treatment	Anticonvulsants, acetazolamide	Clonazepam, oxazepam	L-Dopa	Anticonvulsants, acetazolamide

IV. **Myoclonus:** Sudden, brief, shock-like involuntary movements caused by muscular contraction (*positive myoclonus*) or inhibitions (*negative myoclonus*), usually arising from the central nervous system. Can be classified according to clinical characteristics (body distribution, pattern of movements and relationship to activity), etiology, and area of anatomic origin within the nervous system

A. Clinical characteristics: according to relationship to activity, myoclonus is spontaneous when it develops at rest, action (or intention) myoclonus when it is action-sensitive, and stimulus-sensitive myoclonus is termed reflex myoclonus; classification according to body distribution is as follows: focal or segmental (confined to one particular region of the body), multifocal (different parts of the body affected, not necessarily at the same time), or generalized (whole body part affected in a single jerk), pattern of movements may be rhythmic, in which case it is referred to by some as tremor (will usually have a jerky quality), but more typically, it is arrhythmic.

B. Etiology: physiologic (hiccups), essential (idiopathic or hereditary), epileptic, and symptomatic/secondary myoclonus

> NB: Hypnic jerks (also known as nocturnal myoclonus) used to be regarded as a type of physiologic myoclonus but has now been reclassified as periodic limb movements of sleep.

C. **Area of anatomic origin within the CNS:** most clinically relevant classification system as it has implications for choice of pharmacologic agent

1. **Cortical myoclonus** (frequently multifocal, rather than focal): the jerks are usually more distal than proximal and more flexor than extensor; usually affects the face and hands; typically, stimulus-sensitive and may be precipitated by sudden loud noise or a visual stimulus; *etiology:* any type of focal cortical lesion, including tumors, angiomas, and encephalitis, may be associated with focal cortical myoclonus. Could be caused by dementias (spongiform encephalopathies, especially CJD, CBD, DLB, AD), neurodegenerative disorders (e.g., MSA, PKAN, some of the SCAs, and, rarely, Huntington's disease [Westphal variant]; infectious causes include Whipple disease, postinfectious encephalitis, HSV encephalitis), epileptic syndromes such as progressive myoclonic encephalopathies, and *epilepsia partialis continua* (which refers to repetitive focal cortical myoclonus with some rhythmicity), Angelman syndrome; etiology could also be metabolic in nature—renal/hepatic failure, hyponatremia, Hashimoto encephalopathy. Hereditary cortical myoclonus is usually rhythmic and can be mistaken as a tremor.

2. **Progressive myoclonic epilepsies:** a combination of severe myoclonus, generalized tonic-clonic or other seizures, and progressive neurologic decline, particularly dementia and ataxia; in the *adult, DRPLA* is a consideration; *in the young, the following five conditions* may cause progressive myoclonic epilepsy:

   a. *Lafora body disease:* characterized by polyglucosan–Schiff-positive inclusion bodies in the brain, liver, muscle, or skin (eccrine sweat gland)

   b. *Neuronal ceroid lipofuscinosis (Batten disease):* presents with seizures, myoclonus, and dementia, along with blindness (in the childhood forms); characterized by curvilinear inclusion bodies in the brain, eccrine glands, muscle, and gut

   c. *Unverricht-Lundborg disease:* characterized by stimulus-sensitive myoclonus, tonic-clonic seizures, a characteristic electroencephalography (paroxysmal generalized spike-wave activity and photosensitivity), ataxia, and mild dementia with an onset at around age 5 to 15 years

   d. *Myoclonic epilepsy with ragged red fibers:* maternally inherited, diagnosed by increased serum and CSF lactate and ragged red fibers on muscle biopsy

   e. *Sialidosis:* a lysosomal storage disorder associated with a cherry-red spot by funduscopy and dysmorphic facial features

3. **Subcortical myoclonus:** typically arises from the brainstem or thalamus; most common example of myoclonus arising from the brainstem is reticular myoclonus (also known as brainstem reflex myoclonus); usually proximal and also stimulus-sensitive

> **NB:** *Exaggerated startle disease/hyperekplexia is a rare autosomal dominant inherited startle reflex disorder secondary to mutations in the glycine receptor (GLRA1) in which the startle reflexes are nonhabituating. Note that there are a number of startle syndromes in certain cultures that are not genetically related to hyperekplexia but also exhibit excessive startle—Jumping Frenchmen of Maine, Latah in Indonesia, and Raging Cajuns of Louisiana.*

   a. Other causes of subcortical myoclonus include postanoxic myoclonus (also known as Lance-Adams syndrome), myoclonus-dystonia, Friedrich's ataxia; could also be iatrogenic—medications such as amantadine, levodopa, verapamil, monoamine oxidase inhibitors and heavy metal poisoning.

> **NB:** Myoclonus-dystonia is an autosomal dominant inherited alcohol-responsive disorder secondary to mutations in the epsilon sarcoglycan gene (*SCGE*) on chromosome 7. Classified as one of the genetically inherited dystonias (DYT 11) it has complete paternal inheritance and presents with young-onset disease consisting of lightning-like myoclonic in the arms or trunk, with the lower body (limbs) mostly spared, alone or in combination with a focal dystonia.

> **NB:** Post-anoxic myoclonus is also regarded as a form of subcortical myoclonus and as a posthypercapnic myoclonus. It occurs weeks to months after recovery from cardiac arrest and is commonly seen when respiratory dysfunction precedes cardiac arrest. The most common trigger is severe asthma attack complicated by hypercapnia. It presents as generalized action-induced and intention myoclonus.

4. **Palatal myoclonus (now palatal tremor):** used to be classified as a subcortical myoclonus; on account of its rhythmic nature has been reclassified as palatal tremor and is discussed in the section on tremors.

5. **Spinal myoclonus:** can either be segmental or propriospinal myoclonus

   a. *Spinal segmental myoclonus:* affects a restricted body part, usually contiguous muscle groups; is spontaneous, unilateral rhythmic or arrhythmic in nature, and connotes an underlying structural lesion; etiology: inflammatory myelopathy, cervical spondylosis, tumors, trauma, ischemic myelopathy, and a variety of other causes

   b. *Propriospinal myoclonus involves the trunk and abdomen, is mostly rhythmic, and is worse in the supine position; recently has been found to be psychogenic in a subset of patients.*

> **NB:** **Progressive myoclonic ataxias:** also known as *Ramsay-Hunt syndrome;* seizures and dementia are mild to absent, with myoclonus and ataxia as the major problems; has a much wider span of presentation, ranging from the 1st through 7th decade; may be due either to recognizable etiology or to neurodegenerative disease; *etiology:* mitochondrial encephalomyopathy, celiac disease, late-onset neuronal ceroid lipofuscinosis, biotin-responsive encephalopathy, adult Gaucher's disease, action myoclonus renal failure syndrome, May-White syndrome, and Ekbom syndrome, neurodegenerative diseases (pure spinocerebellar degeneration, spinocerebellar plus dentatorubral degeneration, olivopontocerebellar atrophy, or DRPLA).

5. Spinal myoclonus (*cont'd*)

> **NB:** **Opsoclonus-myoclonus syndrome:** results in random chaotic saccadic eye movements in association with multifocal and generalized myoclonus; *in adults: idiopathic in approximately 50% of cases; second most common cause is paraneoplastic,* usually from ovarian cancer, melanoma, renal cell carcinoma, and lymphoma; in younger patients, can be idiopathic, associated with viral infections, such as Epstein-Barr virus; *neuroblastoma is a major consideration in children,* mainly in tumors with diffuse and extensive lymphocytic infiltration and lymphoid follicles; other causes include drugs, toxins, and nonketotic hyperglycemia.

V. **Dystonia:** Involuntary movement characterized by sustained or intermittent contractions of agonist and antagonist muscles, frequently causing twisting and repetitive movements, abnormal postures, or both; classification now along two axes:

A. Axis I: involves identifying the clinical characteristics and allows the dystonia syndrome to be identified—(i) body distribution: *focal* (involving a single body part, e.g., writer's cramp, blepharospasm, torticollis, spasmodic dysphonia), *segmental* (involving contiguous areas of the body, e.g., Meige's syndrome), *multifocal (involving two or more noncontiguous body regions), generalized (leg, trunk, and another body part or the whole body);* (ii) age of onset: traditionally early onset (< 26 years) and late onset (>26 years); more recently, infancy (birth–2 years), childhood (3–12 years), adolescence (13–20 years), early adulthood (21–40 years), and late adulthood (>40 years); (iii) temporal pattern (progressive disease course or static); and (iv) isolated or combined dystonia and the presence or absence of other neurological or systemic features

> **NB:** *Early onset usually starts in the leg or arm and frequently progresses to involve the other limbs or the trunk; late onset usually starts in the neck, cranial muscles, or arm and tends to remain localized, with restricted spread to adjacent muscles.*

B. Axis II: etiology—inherited (i.e., genetic, acquired, idiopathic, which could be sporadic or familial, and nervous system pathology—degeneration, structural, or neither); acquired causes of dystonia include drugs (some calcium channel blockers, tardive dyskinesias from neuroleptics, levodopa-induced dyskinesias), infections, neoplasms, toxins, primary antiphospholipid syndrome, peripheral nerve injury, perinatal brain injury

C. Based on the two axes, dystonias are now classified as either isolated (dystonia is the only feature) or combined (dystonia with other movement disorders); combined dystonias could either be persistent or paroxysmal. When dystonias are associated with neurologic or systemic features, they are referred to as complex dystonias.

D. Dystonia syndromes: (i) early-onset generalized dystonia (DYT 1, DYT 6), (ii) adult-onset focal or segmental dystonia (Meige's syndrome, task-specific dystonia, e.g., writer's cramp), (iii) myoclonus dystonia (DYT 11), (iv) dystonia parkinsonism (DYT 3, also known as Lubag's; DYT 12; PD; PINK1-, parkin-, and DJ-1- associated parkinsonism; Wilson's disease; NBIA, especially due to PANK2 and PLA2G6 mutations)

> **NB:** **Wilson's disease:** can present with any movement disorder; *AR, mutation in the copper-transporting P-type ATP7B gene on chromosome 13;* diagnosis: decreased serum ceruloplasmin, increased 24-hour urine copper excretion, liver biopsy, slit-lamp examination reveals *Kayser-Fleischer* rings (yellow-brown copper deposits in the cornea); affects mostly young patients (median age 8–20 years); half with liver disease; neurological manifestations: resting and intention tremors, spasticity, rigidity, dystonia, chorea; psychiatric disturbances are present in the majority of patients; penicillamine is the drug of choice (symptoms may worsen in the first months of treatment); trientine and zinc are alternatives.

> **NB:** **Dopa-responsive dystonia: DYT 5** example of a combined dystonia; usually presents as a dystonia-parkinsonism syndrome; usually seen in children with normal neurocognitive development. AD: point mutation in GCH1; starts with gait abnormalities and initially foot dystonia that later progresses to generalized dystonia; unique characteristic is diurnal fluctuation (symptoms worse later in the day). Should not be missed because the condition is treatable (sensitive to levodopa and effect is sustained). Phenotype can also be seen in other biopterin-deficient states (tyrosine hydroxylase mutations, dopamine-agonist-responsive dystonia due to decarboxylase deficiency).

E. Neurodegenerative disorders that can present with dystonia include Huntington's disease, spinocerebellar ataxia type 3, spinocerebellar ataxia type 1, DRPLA, neurodegeneration with brain iron accumulation (NBIA), and neuroacanthocytosis

F. Monogenetic forms of dystonia

DYSTONIA DESIGNATION	PHENOMENOLOGY	INHERITANCE PATTERN	CHROMOSOME	GENE
DYT 1	Early-onset generalized isolated dystonia	AD	9q	TOR1A
DYT 2	Early-onset generalized isolated dystonia	AR	Unknown	Unknown
DYT 3	Dystonia parkinsonism (Lubag)	X-linked	Xq	?TAF1
DYT 4	Whispering dysphonia	AD	19p	TUBB4
DYT 5	Dopa-responsive dystonia; Segawa syndrome	AD	14q	GCH1
DYT 6	Adolescent and early adult-onset isolated dystonia of mixed phenotype	AD	8p	THAP1
DYT 7	Adult-onset focal dystonia	AD	18p	Unknown

(continued)

F.   Monogenetic forms of dystonia (*cont'd*)

DYSTONIA DESIGNATION	PHENOMENOLOGY	INHERITANCE PATTERN	CHROMOSOME	GENE
DYT 8	Paroxysmal nonkinesigenic dyskinesia	AD	2q	MR-1
DYT 10	Paroxysmal kinesigenic dyskinesia	AD	16p	PRRT2
DYT 11	Myoclonus dystonia	AD	7q	SCGE
DYT 12	Rapid-onset dystonia parkinsonism	AD	19q	ATP1A3
DYT 13	Adolescent-onset segmental (cranio-cervical) dystonia	AD	1p	Unknown
DYT 15	Myoclonus dystonia	AD	18p	Unknown
DYT 16	Early-onset generalized dystonia with parkinsonism	AR	2p	PRKRA
DYT 17	Adolescent-onset isolated dystonia	AR	20p	Unknown
DYT 18	Paroxysmal exertion-induced dyskinesia	AD	1p	SLC2A1 (GLUT1)
DYT 19	Paroxysmal kinesigenic dyskinesia 2	AD	16q	Unknown
DYT 20	Paroxysmal nonkinesigenic dyskinesia	AD	2q	Unknown
DYT 21	Adult-onset generalized/ multifocal isolated dystonia	AD	2q	Unknown
DYT 23	Adult-onset cervical dystonia	AD	9q	CIZ1
DYT 24	Adult-onset segmental (cranio-cervical) dystonia	AD	11p	ANO3
DYT 25	Adult-onset cervical dystonia	AD	18p	GNAL

VI. **Ataxia:** Imbalance or incoordination, usually due to disease of the cerebellum and its connections (can also be afferent in nature from severe proprioceptive dysfunction); acquired (usually acute or subacute in nature) or inherited (insidious onset and usually progressive but could also be paroxysmal)

A. Acquired ataxia: stroke, tumors, paraneoplastic, multiple sclerosis, autoimmune (anti-GAD, gluten ataxia), toxins (chronic alcohol intake, heavy metals), drugs (chronic phenytoin, chemotherapy)

> NB: MSA is the most common cause of nonhereditary degenerative ataxia.

B.   Inherited/hereditary ataxias: autosomal dominant (SCA, DRPLA), autosomal recessive (Friedrich's ataxia, ataxia with isolated vitamin E deficiency AVED, ataxia telangiectasia, ataxia with oculomotor apraxia), X-linked (FXTAS)

1. **Friedreich's ataxia:** classic phenotype: *progressive gait disturbance, gait ataxia, loss of proprioception in the lower limbs, areflexia, dysarthria, and extensor plantar responses* with an age of onset younger than 25 years; electrocardiography: early repolarization; echocardiograms: hypertrophic cardiomyopathy; diabetes mellitus in fewer than one-half of patients; skeletal deformities, such as scoliosis and pes cavus; mutation is an *unstable expansion of a GAA repeat in the first intron of the gene X25 on chromosome 9q12-21.1, leading to deficiency of the protein frataxin;* treatment: coenzyme Q10 and vitamin E may improve cardiac and skeletal muscle bioenergetics, idebenone (a coenzyme Q10 analog) may have benefit for cardiomyopathy.

> **NB:** The clinical findings are secondary to involvement of the spinocerebellar and corticospinal tracts, dorsal columns, and a peripheral neuropathy.

2. **Ataxia-telangiectasia** *(Louis-Bar syndrome):* AR; chromosome 11q22-23; characterized by progressive cerebellar ataxia, oculocutaneous telangiectasia, abnormalities in cellular and humoral immunity, and recurrent viral and bacterial infections; neurologic manifestations: cerebellar ataxia, nystagmus, chorea, athetosis, dystonia, oculomotor apraxia, impassive facies, decreased deep tendon reflexes and distal muscular atrophy, progressive deterioration of intelligence, polyneuropathy; other manifestations: immunodeficiency (thymic hypoplasia); patients lack helper T cells, but suppressor T cells are normal; immunoglobulin A is absent in 75% of patients, immunoglobulin E in 85%, immunoglobulin G is low; α-fetoprotein and carcinoembryonic antigen are elevated; ovarian agenesis, testicular hypoplasia, and insulin-resistant diabetes; malignant neoplasms in 10% to 15% of patients; most common are lymphoreticular neoplasm and leukemia; death by 2nd decade from neoplasia or infection.

> **NB:** Recurrent infections are frequently the presenting finding in ataxia-telangiectasia.

3. *AR ataxias with known gene loci*

DISEASE	CHROMOSOME	GENE	MUTATION
Friedreich's ataxia	9q13-21.1	X25/frataxin	GAA expansion
Ataxia-telangiectasia	11q22-23	ATM	Point mutations/deletions
Ataxia with isolated vitamin E deficiency	8q	a TTP	Point mutations
AR ataxia of Charlevoix-Saguenay	13q11	SACS	Point mutations
Ataxia with oculomotor apraxia	9p13	Aprataxin	Point mutations/deletions/insertions
Ataxia, neuropathy, high α fetoprotein	9q33-34	Unknown	Unknown
Infantile onset olivopontocerebellar atrophy	10q24	Unknown	Unknown
Ataxia, deafness, optic atrophy	6p21-23	Unknown	Unknown
Unverricht-Lundborg disease	21q	Cystatin B	Repeat expansion

B. Inherited/hereditary ataxias (*cont'd*)

4. ***AD ataxias:*** present between 3rd and 5th decades of life but with a wide range; many trinucleotide-repeat diseases (1, 2, 3, 6, 7, and 17); large clinical overlap between each type; DRPLA also included sans SCA designation; may be categorized as progressive (SCAs) or episodic (episodic ataxias)

DISEASE	CHROMOSOME	GENE	MUTATION	ADDITIONAL FEATURES
SCA 1	6p23	Ataxin-1	CAG expansion	Young adult; upper motor neuron signs; late chorea
SCA 2	12q23-24.1	Ataxin-2	CAG expansion	Young adult; upper motor neuron signs (rare); parkinsonian; late chorea; very slow saccades; areflexia
SCA 3/ Machado-Joseph disease	14q21	Ataxin-3	CAG expansion	Young adult; upper motor neuron signs; parkinsonian; late chorea
SCA 4	16q24	—	—	Areflexia
SCA 5	11p11-q11	SPTBN2	—	—
SCA 6	19p	CACNA1	CAG expansion	Older adult; benign course; downbeat nystagmus
SCA 7	3p21.2-12	Ataxin-7	CAG expansion	Childhood onset; upper motor neuron signs; very slow saccades; vision loss; seizures
SCA 8	13q21	Ataxin-8	CAG expansion	Upper motor neuron signs
SCA 10	22q13	Ataxin-10	ATTCT repeat expansion	Seizures
SCA 11	15q14-21.3	TTBK2	ATTCT expansion	—
SCA 12	5q31-33	PP2R2B	CAG expansion	Action tremor
SCA 13	10q13.3-13.4	KCNC3	—	—
SCA 14 SCA 15/29	19q13.4 3p26	PRKCG ITPR1	— —	— —
SCA 16	8q23—24.1	ITPR1	—	Action tremor
SCA 17 SCA 19/22	6p21	TBP KCND3	CAG expansion	Parkinsonian Tremor, myoclonus, occasional deafness
SCA 20	11q12	—	Chromosome duplication	Dysphonia, palatal tremor
SCA 21	7p21	—		Hyperreflexia, L-Dopa responsive parkinsonism
SCA 23 SCA 25	PDYN	20p13 2p21	— —	Sensory loss, pyramidal signs Gastrointestinal features, sensory neuropathy
SCA 26 SCA 27	EEF2 FGF14	19p13 13q33	— —	— Tremor, psychiatric features, dyskinesia

(continued)

DISEASE	CHROMOSOME	GENE	MUTATION	ADDITIONAL FEATURES
SCA 28	AFG3L2	18p11	—	upper motor neuron (UMN) signs; ophthalmoparesis; rarely, myoclonic epilepsy
SCA 30	—	4q34	—	—
SCA 31	BEAN	16q21	TGGAA repeat expansion	Late-adult onset
SCA 32	—	7q32	—	Azoospermia, cognitive impairment
SCA 34	—	6p12	—	Infantile skin lesions that resolve by adulthood
SCA 35	TGM6	20p13	—	Spasmodic torticollis, sensory loss, UMN signs
SCA 36	NOP56	20p13	—	Combination of UMN and lower motor neuron (LMN) signs
SCA 37	—	1p32	GGCCTG repeat expansion	—
			—	
Dentatorubropal-lidoluysian atrophy	12p	Atrophin	CAG expansion	Childhood onset; chorea; seizures
Episodic ataxia 1	12p	KCNA 1	Point mutations in ion channels	Short-lived intermittent ataxia; interictally with myokymia
Episodic ataxia 2 Episodic ataxia 3 Episodic ataxia 4 Episodic ataxia 5 Episodic ataxia 6 Episodic ataxia 7	19p 1q42 — 2q23 5p13 —	CACNA 1 — — CACNB4 SLC1A3 —	Point mutations in ion channels	Longer-duration intermittent ataxia; downbeat nystagmus; similar to SCA 6; associated with migraine; *acetazolamide reduces frequency of attacks* *Short episodes of ataxia, vertigo, and tinnitus* *Duration of ataxia and vertigo of several hours* *Duration of ataxia, hemiplegia, and seizures of a couple hours* *Vertigo, weakness, and dysarthria*

> **NB:** SCA 17 is a phenocopy of HD.

5. **Metabolic disorders:** maple syrup urine disease, Hartnup's disease, pyruvate decarboxylase deficiency, argininosuccinic aciduria, hypothyroidism, Leigh disease

VII. Tremor (Rhythmic Oscillation of a Body Part)

TYPE	CHARACTERISTIC	FREQUENCY (HZ)
Parkinsonian tremor	Rest >> posture = action	3–6
Enhanced physiologic tremor	Action = posture	8–12
Essential tremor	Action > posture >> rest	4–10
Cerebellar tremor	Action	2–4
Rubral tremor	Posture = action > rest	2–5
NB: *Orthostatic tremor*	Only when standing still; relieved by walking or sitting	15–18
Dystonic tremor	Posture = action >> rest	4–8
Palatal tremor	Rest	1–6
Neuropathic tremor	Posture >> action	5–9

> **NB:** Palatal tremor (previously palatal myoclonus) can be essential (idiopathic), symptomatic (brainstem disease), or neurodegenerative (adult-onset Alexander disease); movements persist during sleep in symptomatic palatal tremor.

CHEAT SHEET

Dopamine agonists	Assess for hypersexuality, pathological gambling
Corticobasal ganglionic degeneration	Asymmetric parkinsonism, unilateral dystonia, myoclonus, alien limb phenomenon
Huntington's disease	AD 100% penetrance, CAG repeat huntingtin gene chromosome 4p16
Dentatorubropallidoluysian atrophy	Progressive myoclonic epilepsy, ataxia, choreoathetosis, dementia
Pantothenate-kinase-associated neurodegeneration	Priorly known as Hallervorden-Spatz, NBIA type 1
Lesch-Nyhan syndrome	X-linked, uricemia, spasticity, choreoathetosis, self-mutilation
Wilson's disease	AR, mutation in copper-transporting P-type ATP7B gene on chromosome 13

Suggested Readings

Albanese A, Bhatia K, Bressman SB, et al. Phenomenology and classification of dystonia: a consensus update. *Mov. Disord.*2013;28(7):863–873.

Fernandez HH. Updates in the medical management of Parkinson disease. *Clev. Clin. J. Med.*2012;79:28–34.

Gerschlager W, Brown P. Myoclonus. *Curr. Opin. Neurol.*2009;22:414–418.

Klockgether T. Sporadic ataxia with acute onset: classification and diagnostic criteria. *Lancet Neurol.*2010;9:94–104.

Seppi K, Weintraub D, Coelho M, et al. The Movement Disorder Society Evidence-Based Medicine Review update: treatments for the non-motor symptoms of Parkinson's disease. *Mov. Disord.*2011;26(Suppl 3):S42–S80.

Wolf DS, Singer DS. Pediatric movement disorders: An update. *Curr. Opin. Neurol.*2008;21:491–496.

CHAPTER 13

Demyelinating Disorders

I. Overview

A. Commonly accepted pathologic criteria for demyelinating diseases are as follows:

1. Destruction of myelin sheaths or nerve fibers

2. Relative sparing of other elements of nervous tissue, such as axis cylinders (may be incomplete)

3. Infiltration of inflammatory cells in a perivascular distribution

4. Perivenular distribution, primarily in white matter (e.g., Dawson's fingers at callosal septal margin due to perivenular distribution)

5. Lack of Wallerian degeneration or secondary degeneration of fiber tracts (due to integrity of the axis cylinders)

B. Caveat of criteria: Schilder's disease and necrotizing hemorrhagic leukoencephalitis may have massive damage to axis cylinders as well as myelin.

C. Subacute combined degeneration, tropical spastic hemiparesis, progressive multifocal leukoencephalopathy, central pontine myelinolysis, and Marchiafava-Bignami disease were not included because of their known etiology—they are part of either viral or nutritional deficiency; metabolic deficiencies with white-matter involvement are also excluded.

II. Neuroimmunology

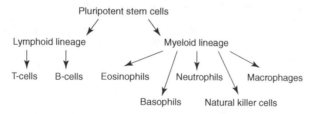

Figure 13.1 Differentiation of stem cells.

A. B-lymphocytes: develop in the bone marrow; acquire immunoglobulin (Ig) receptors that commit them to a specific antigen; express IgM on the surface; after antigen challenge, T-lymphocytes assist B-lymphocytes either directly or indirectly through secretion of helper factors to differentiate and form mature antibody-secreting plasma cells.

B. Igs: glycoproteins; secretory products of plasma cells; the heavy chain on Fc portion determines class: IgM, IgD, IgG, IgA, and IgE; activates complement cascade: IgM, IgG1, and IgG3.

C. T-lymphocytes: thymus derived; CD4: helper cell; CD8: cytotoxic/suppressor cells; specificity of T-cells is to the foreign major histocompatibility complex (MHC) antigens; CD2 and CD3: T-cell activation.

D. Natural killer cells: lymphocytes; lack immunologic memory; have the ability to kill tumor or virus-infected cells without any MHC restriction; role in tumor immunity.

E. MHC and HLA: HLA lies on the short arm of chromosome 6; four major loci: class I (on all nucleated cells; HLA-A, HLA-B, HLA-C) and class II (on macrophages, B-cells, activated T-cells; HLA-DR, -DQ, -DP); class I antigens regulate the specificity of cytotoxic T-cells (CD8) and act on viruses; class II antigens regulate the specificity of helper T-cells (CD4), then CD4 regulates hypersensitivity and antibody response; examples: HLA-DR2 (multiple sclerosis [MS] among white Northern Europeans), HLA-DR3 (young myasthenic without thymoma), HLA-DR2 (narcolepsy).

F. Regulation of immune response

1. Antigen cleared from immune system

2. Formation of antigen-antibody complex, which inhibits B-cell differentiation and proliferation

3. Idiotypic regulation: variable region on Ig molecule expresses proteins that are new and can act as antigens.

4. Suppressor T-cells

G. Lymphokines (cytokines): secreted products of immune cells

1. *Growth factors:* interleukin-1, -2, -3, -4; colony-stimulating factors

2. *Activation factors:* interferons (α, β, and γ)

3. *Lymphotoxins:* tumor necrosis factors

III. Multiple Sclerosis (MS)

A. Also known as disseminated sclerosis, sclerose en plaques: protean clinical manifestations; usually a course of remission and relapse, but occasionally intermittently progressive or steadily progressive (especially in those >40 years old (y/o)) affecting white (more common) and gray matter and spinal cord

B. Pathology: grossly numerous pink-gray (due to myelin loss) lesions scattered surrounding white matter; vary in diameter; do not extend beyond root entry zones of cranial or spinal nerves

1. *Periventricular localization:* characteristic, in which subependymal veins line ventricles

2. Other favored structures: *optic nerves, chiasm, spinal cord;* distributed randomly through brainstem, spinal cord, cerebellar peduncles

3. Astrocytic reaction: *perivascular infiltration with mononuclear cells and lymphocytes; sparing of axis cylinders* prevents Wallerian degeneration.

> NB: Recent reevaluation of pathology shows that gray-matter pathology is common and may not extend into white matter; also, biopsy data show that this may be an early phenomenon due to pial entry of immune cells into the cortical surface.

> NB: Recent pathology studies show significant axon loss even with early demyelinating events, and loss of axons even in normal-appearing white matter.

C. Etiology and epidemiology: prevalence is less than 1 per 100,000 in equatorial areas, 57 to 78 cases per 100,000 in the southern United States, and 110 to 140 cases per 100,000 in the northern United States, with higher rates in Canada and Northern Europe; in southern hemisphere: less well defined; in the United States: blacks at lower risk; few "epidemics" reported.

1. *Migration:* before age 15 years, carries risk from native land; evidence on this is questionable, however.

2. *Familial tendency* also now established: 15% to 20% have an affected relative; *HLA-DR2, DQW1, b1, a1, to a lesser extent -DR3, -B7, and -A3,* on chromosome 6 are overrepresented in MS; low conjugal incidence (supports disease occurring early in life); first-degree relatives have a 10- to 20-fold greater risk. Monozygotic female twin risk is greater than 30%. Both parents having MS confers a 30% risk of MS to children.

3. Low incidence in children, peak at age 30 years, falling sharply in the 6th decade; two-thirds with onset between ages 20 and 40 years; may be greater in rural than urban dwellers; can occur de novo after 60, but may have had subclinical disease prior to clinical onset.

4. Popular view is that initial event is a viral infection of the nervous system with secondary activation by autoimmune reaction; role of *humoral system* is evident by presence of *oligoclonal immune proteins in cerebrospinal fluid (CSF)* that are produced by B-lymphocytes; causation not precisely known. Patients who have never had exposure to mononucleosis do not appear to get MS.

5. *Cellular factor* is demonstrated by abundance of *helper T-cells (CD4$^+$)* in MS plaques; T-cells react to antigens presented by MHC class II on macrophages and astrocytes $\rightarrow$ stimulate T-cell proliferation, activation of B-cells, macrophages $\rightarrow$ secretion of cytokines (e.g., interferon β) $\rightarrow$ breakdown of blood–brain barrier, destruction of oligodendrocytes and myelin.

6. *Physiologic effects of demyelination:* impede saltatory conduction; temporary induction by heat or exercise of symptoms (*Uhthoff phenomenon [visual blurring with exercise]*); rise of 0.5°C can block electrical transmission; smoking, fatigue, and rise in environmental temperature all can cause worsening of symptoms.

D. Clinical manifestations: weakness and numbness, both in one or more limbs, are the initial symptoms in one-half of patients; useful adage that patient with MS presents with symptoms of one leg with signs in both; Lhermitte's phenomenon: passive flexion of the neck induces a tingling, electric-like feeling down one or more of the shoulders, arms, trunk, legs; two particular syndromes are among the most typical modes of onset.

1. **Optic neuritis:** in 25% of all MS patients, this is the initial manifestation; characteristically, rapid evolution over several hours to days of partial or total loss of vision, pain within the orbit, worsened by eye movement and palpation.

    a. *Cecocentral scotoma* (macular area and blind spot) can be demonstrated, as well as other field defects.

    b. Evidence of swelling/edema of nerve head (*papillitis*) in one-half of cases (distinguished from papilledema by severe vision loss).

    c. One-third recover completely, most improve significantly; dyschromatopsia is a frequent persistent finding; one-half or more who present with optic neuritis eventually develop MS; risk is lower in childhood.

    d. *Uveitis and sheathing of retinal veins* (due to T-cell infiltration) are other ophthalmologic findings (e.g., pars planitis) that can occur in MS.

> **NB:** After an episode of optic neuritis, the best predictor of subsequent MS is an abnormal MRI of the brain (presence of one or more demyelinating lesions).

D. **Clinical manifestations** (*cont'd*)

2. **Acute transverse myelitis**: transverse is imprecise: usually asymmetric and incomplete; clinically: *rapidly evolving* (several hours to days) paraparesis, sensory level on the trunk, sphincteric dysfunction, bilateral Babinski signs; cerebrospinal fluid (CSF): may show modest increase in lymphocytes and protein. This term can be used to refer to various disorders:

    a. Idiopathic severe, often following infectious or vaccination myelitis that responds incompletely to treatment with steroids or plasmapheresis, and is often monophasic

    b. Myelitis occurring with neuromyelitis spectrum disorders

    c. Myelitis with other immune conditions, such as Sjögren's, sarcoidosis, lupus

    d. Partial myelitis occurring either before or during the course of MS

> **NB:** Patients with transverse myelitis are at risk for developing MS. However, the presence of partial rather than complete myelitis puts a patient at higher risk for progression to MS! The strongest predictor of subsequent MS is the presence of subclinical lesions on imaging at the time of initial presentation.

3. Other patterns of MS: unsteadiness in walking, brainstem symptoms (diplopia, vertigo, vomiting), disorders of micturition; discrete manifestations: hemiplegia, trigeminal neuralgia, pain syndromes, facial paralysis, deafness, or seizures, or (in the elderly) slowly progressive cervical myelopathy; *Charcot's triad*: nystagmus, scanning speech, intention tremor; *one-and-a-half syndrome*: intranuclear ophthalmoplegia in one direction and horizontal gaze paresis in the other.

> **NB:** The paramedian pontine reticular formation is usually involved in the one-and-a-half syndrome, in addition to the medial longitudinal fasciculus.

4. *Symptoms and signs of established stage of disease*: one-half manifest with a mix of generalized type (involvement of optic nerves, brainstem, cerebellum, and spinal cord); 30% to 40% with spinal form; 5% each have predominantly cerebellar or pontobulbar-cerebellar form; some have euphoria (stupid indifference, morbid optimism), but larger group has depression; global dementia (more subcortical, with prominent frontal lobe syndrome and abulia) or confusional-psychotic state in advanced stage; 2% to 3% have seizures.

5. *Clinical course*

TYPE	PERCENT
Relapsing remitting	80% of patients at diagnosis
Secondary progressive	50% of relapsing remitting progress to this at some time
Primary progressive	10% to 15% from onset progression
Fulminant	3% to 5% severe relapsing disease from onset

> **NB:** Relapsing remitting MS (RRMS) can be active (new relapses or new MRI lesions in the past year) or inactive. Progressive MS (either type) can be active (new relapses or new MRI lesions in the past year) or inactive, and progressive (gradual clinical worsening past year) or nonprogressive. The progressive relapsing form of MS is no longer recognized as a separate variant.

E. **Variants**

1. *Acute or fulminant MS:* highly *malignant* form; combination of cerebral, brainstem, spinal manifestations evolves over a few weeks to months, rendering the patient stuporous, comatose, or decerebrate; death in a few weeks to months, without remission; lesions are of macroscopic dimensions, typical of acute plaques—only difference: plaques are of the same age and more prominent confluence; CSF: shows a brisk cellular response.

> **NB:** The malignant form of MS is also known as the Marburg's variant.

2. *Neuromyelitis optica (NMO) spectrum disorders:* simultaneous or successive involvement of *optic nerves and spinal cord;* acute or subacute blindness of one or both eyes preceded or followed within days or weeks by transverse or ascending myelitis; sometimes, the spinal cord lesions are necrotizing rather than demyelinating (i.e., more permanent); *corticosteroid or plasma exchange* for active neuromyelitis optica relapses; antiplatelets and anticoagulant should be considered in neuromyelitis optica cases with IgG antiphospholipid antibodies; 70% of NMO patients have NMOIGG antibodies, targeting aquaporin-4 located at astrocytic foot processes. Brain MRI is often normal at onset, but may also have episodes of intractable nausea and vomiting or hypothalamic dysfunction due to involvement of regions rich in aquaporin-4 channels. May also get posterior reversible encephalopathy syndrome (PRES). Treatment of NMOSD B-cell targeted immune therapies. May worsen with use of interferon beta. MRI shows longitudinally extensive (three or more segments) lesions in the spinal cord, optic nerve lesions, and atypical brain lesions.

F. **Lab findings**

1. CSF: One-third of patients with MS with slight to moderate mononuclear pleocytosis (<50); in rapidly progressive, may reach or exceed 100 to 1,000; hyperacute cases may have polymorphonucleocytes; 40% have slight increase in total protein in CSF; proportion of γ globulin (IgG) is increased more than 12% to the total protein in two-thirds; *IgG index:* ratio of greater than 1.7 indicates the probability of MS; IgG index and oligoclonal bands elevated (note that these are elevated in other conditions, and are also increased in syphilis and subacute sclerosing panencephalitis); high concentrations of *myelin basic protein* during acute exacerbations; at present, *measurement of γ globulins and oligoclonal bands are the most reliable chemical tests for MS but are not specific for this condition.*

> **NB:** Neuromyelitis optica usually does not present with oligoclonal bands in CSF.

2. Other tests: *visual-evoked potentials* (80% in clinical features of definite MS, 60% in probable); *somatosensory evoked* (69% in definite and 51% in probable); *brainstem auditory-evoked responses* (47% in definite and 20% in probable)

   a. MRI is currently the most important diagnostic test for MS. Characteristic oval-shaped periventricular, juxtacortical, or infratentorial lesions or spinal cord lesions, may enhance, often with open ring sign. Later lesions may be dark and well circumscribed (t1 black holes). Enhancement is a marker of active lesion formation and is present for only 1 to 2 months. Persistent enhancing lesions suggest alternative diagnoses to MS. Spinal cord lesions are usually single

2. Other tests (*cont'd*)

segment and partial cord, often eccentric. Many patients have multiple lesions. Cortical lesions are not well visualized on MRI and are therefore probably underdiagnosed. Over time, generalized brain atrophy occurs.

G. **Diagnosis of multiple sclerosis:** International criteria for the diagnosis of MS were revised in 2010. These are relatively universally adopted criteria.

DISEASE EPISODES (ATTACK)	OBJECTIVE LESIONS	ADDITIONAL REQUIREMENTS
2 or more	2 or more	None
2 or more	1	Dissemination in space (DIS) demonstrated by: ≥1 T2 lesion in at least two of four MS-typical regions of the central nervous system (CNS) (periventricular, juxtacortical, infratentorial, or spinal cord); or await a further clinical attack implicating a different CNS site
1	2 or more	Dissemination in time by MRI or another clinical attack; may include simultaneous presence of Gd+ and Gd− lesions on first scan
1	1	Dissemination in space AND time by MRI, or another attack
0 (progressive from onset)	1	1 year of disease progression (retrospectively or prospectively determined) plus two or three of the following criteria: 1. Evidence for DIS in the brain based on 1 T2 lesion in the MS-characteristic (periventricular, juxtacortical, or infratentorial) regions 2. Evidence for DIS in the spinal cord based on 2 T2 lesions in the cord 3. Positive CSF (isoelectric focusing evidence of oligoclonal bands and/or elevated IgG index)

H. **Differential diagnosis**

1. Acute disseminated encephalomyelitis
2. Nonspecific microvascular MRI change
3. Vitamin B_{12} deficiency
4. Collagen vascular disease
5. Sarcoid and other defined immune conditions (e.g., Behcet's, Susac's)
6. Human T-cell lymphotropic virus (tropical spastic paraparesis)
7. Adult-onset adrenoleukodystrophy
8. Primary lateral sclerosis
9. NMO spectrum disorders

I. **Treatment**

1. *IV or oral high-dose steroids such as methyl prednisone for few days followed by tapering oral steroids or ACTH (Acthar gel).* There is no strong evidence that steroids alter the ultimate course of MS or prevent relapses; high dose often used initially to be effective; attempt to limit the period of corticosteroid administration to <3 weeks but prolong the taper if neurologic signs return.

2. *For optic neuritis, intravenous methylprednisolone* for 3 days followed by oral prednisone for 11 days speeds the recovery from vision loss (compared to placebo or

14 days of oral prednisone), although there was no significant difference after 6 months as compared with placebo (in the Optic Neuritis Treatment Trial).

3. *There is no well-defined treatment for the progressive component of MS to date. Trials of multiple medicines for MS have been negative when blinded, multicenter, and large.*

4. Interferons: several mechanisms—antiproliferative effect, blocking of T-cell activation, apoptosis of autoreactive T cells, interferon gamma antagonism, cytokine shifts, antiviral effect

    a. **Interferon β-1b (Betaseron®/Extavia®):** reduces the number and severity of exacerbations; reduces lesion load on MRI; for secondary progressive MS, interferon β-1b showed minor effect on delaying disability for a few months despite clear evidence of durable effect on reducing relapses; dosage: *8 million U subcutaneously every other day;* complete blood cell count, liver function tests every 3 months. Side effects: local skin reaction (inflammation, thickening, and necrosis); flu-like symptoms (usually within the first 2 weeks); fatigue; decreased white blood cell count, platelets, and hematocrit; increased γ-glutamyltransferase, serum glutamic-oxaloacetic transaminase; depression.

    b. **Interferon β-1a (Avonex®/Rebif®/Plegridy®):** slows accumulation of physical disability and decreases frequency of exacerbation; dosage: *dosage IM or sq depending on agent;* complete blood cell count, platelets, fluid balance profile at least every 6 months; side effects: flu-like symptoms, injection site reactions, myalgias, fever, chills, headache, depression, bronchospasm, anxiety.

5. **Glatiramer acetate (Copaxone®/copolymer-1)**

    a. Acts by blocking autoimmune T-cells, induction of energy, induction of anti-inflammatory Th2 cells, bystander suppression, possibly neuroprotection

    b. Reduces frequency of relapses, reduced new lesion formation on MRI; dosage: *20 mg subcutaneously daily or 40 mg TIW;* side effects: injection-site reactions, immediate postinjection reaction (10%), transient chest pain (26%), anxiety, arthralgias, asthenia, vasodilatation, hypertonia

6. **Mitoxantrone:** Mitoxantrone in Multiple Sclerosis study led to U.S. Food and Drug Administration (FDA) indication for use in aggressive forms of MS; dosage: *5 mg/m² or 12 mg/m² every 12 weeks for 24 months (eight infusions); rarely used for MS at present time despite FDA approval due to risks of cardiomyopathy and treatment-related leukemia*

7. *Natalizumab:* recombinant monoclonal antibody; first selective immunomodulator in the treatment of MS; blocks the molecular interaction of alpha-4-beta-1 integrin with vascular cell adhesion molecule-1 on vascular endothelial cells, thus preventing adhesion of activated T-cells to endothelium, and prevents transmigration of lymphocytes to the CNS; AFFIRM study demonstrated the rate of clinical relapse was reduced by 68% and number of new MRI lesions was reduced by 83%; SENTINEL trial suggested that combination therapy is nearly as effective as natalizumab alone; however, two reported cases of progressive multifocal leukoencephalopathy (PML) have restricted its use; approximately 1:800 risk of PML with use; risk higher with JC virus antibody positive, prior chemotherapy use, use beyond 2 years; monitoring imaging every 6 to 12 months; usually reserved for more aggressive MS or use when breaking through two other agents

8. *Other immunomodulators: azathioprine, methotrexate, cyclophosphamide* (pulse monthly treatments were associated with a small but significant reduction in progression in >30% of patients), *cyclosporine, linomide* (may cause cardiotoxicity and myocardial infarction), *sulfasalazine, cladribine (Leustatin®); monoclonal antibody therapy using anti-CD11/CD18:* no difference with placebo; *intravenous Ig:* a large phase III trial failed to demonstrate a treatment benefit of intravenous Ig in secondary progressive MS; **generally not used for MS now given well-defined disease-modifying therapies available.**

I. **Treatment** (*cont'd*)

9. Fingolimod (Gilenya®): daily oral agent 0.5 mg; binds to Sphingosine 1 phosphate (SIP) receptors on lymphocytes and internalizes receptors; causes impaired exit of lymphocytes from lymph nodes, results in lower circulating lymphocytes; reduces relapses and MRI new lesion activity in relapsing MS. Risks include first-dose bradycardia; macular edema; viral infections, including herpes encephalitis and disseminated zoster; increased urinary tract infections and bronchitis; elevated liver function tests. Few cases of PML have been reported.

10. Teriflunomide (Aubagio®): once-a-day oral agent, either 7 or 14 mg; reduced relapses and MRI activity; used in RRMS; selectively and reversibly inhibits dihydro-orotate dehydrogenase, a key mitochondrial enzyme in the de novo pyrimidine synthesis pathway, leading to a reduction in proliferation of activated T- and B-lymphocytes without causing cell death; side effects: hair loss, activation of tuberculosis, elevated liver tests; teratogenic and remains in system for up to 2 years; may require activated elimination process for both women and men planning on child bearing; modest efficacy

11. Dimethyl fumarate (Tecfidera®): 240 mg bid with titration; specific mechanism of action unknown, but may work through nuclear-related (erythroid-derived 2) factor pathway affecting lymphocyte function; reduces relapses and MRI activity moderately; side effects: diarrhea, flushing, gastrointestinal (GI) upset; lymphocytes drop in small percentage of patients; few cases of PML reported, usually where prolonged lymphopenia seen; monitoring CBC with diff ever 3 to 6 months.

12. Alemtuzumab (Lemtrada®): FDA approved for patients not responding to two standard agents; IV monoclonal antibody that depletes circulating T- and B-cells for months; IV infusion 12 mg daily × 5 days with prophylaxis for infusion reaction; risk of emergence of autoimmune disorders (Grave's disease, immune thrombocytopenic purpura (ITP), glomerulonephritis) during return of lymphocyte population; careful selection of patients for compliance with ongoing lab testing for up to 5 years after treatment

13. *Plasma exchange:* seven alternate-day plasma exchanges hasten at least a moderate clinical improvement in 40% of steroid-unresponsive patients with *acute catastrophic demyelinating illness;* complications: anemia, sepsis, hypotension, heparin-induced thrombocytopenia with hemorrhage. Not used for ongoing MS treatment. Used in NMO spectrum disorders not responding to IV solumedrol high dose.

14. *General measures:* adequate bed rest, prevention of fatigue, infection, use of all rehabilitative measures to postpone bedridden stage; *fatigue* responds to amantadine, 100 mg morning and noon, or modafinil, 100 mg once or twice daily; *bladder dysfunction:* urinary retention use bethanecol chloride; residual urine up to 100 mL are generally well tolerated; for spastic bladder, propantheline or oxybutynin or multiple other agents may relax detrusor muscle; *spastic paralysis:* intrathecal baclofen; oral Lioresal, tizanidine, clonazepam, botulinum toxin type A; Lioresal pump; *surgical procedures:* rhizotomy, myelotomy, crushing of obturator nerves; *disabling tremor:* ventrolateral thalamotomy; isoniazid, 300 to 1,200 mg with 100 mg of B_6 (for severe postural tremor); limited success with carbamazepine and clonazepam. Dalfampridine extended release (Ampyra®) 10 mg bid FDA approved to improve walking speed in patients with MS. Works in about 38% of patients (responders). Side effects: dizziness; increased spasticity; rarely, seizures. Care needed in patients with prior seizures or renal disease (renally excreted).

15. *Specialized, multidisciplinary team approach* to patient with active treatment issues; outpatient and intensive inpatient programs, combined with postdischarge outpatient services, improve patient outcomes.

IV. Diffuse Cerebral Sclerosis of Schilder (*Schilder's Disease, Encephalitis Periaxialis Diffusa*)

A. Overview: more frequent in children and adolescent life; nonfamilial, runs a progressive course, either steady or punctuated by a series of rapid worsening; dementia, homonymous hemianopia, cerebral blindness, deafness, hemiplegia/quadriplegia, pseudobulbar palsy; CSF: often no oligoclonal bands, but myelin basic protein found in large quantity; lesion: large, sharply outlined, asymmetric focus of demyelination involving the entire lobe or cerebral hemisphere, crosses the corpus callosum

B. Concentric sclerosis of Baló: probably a variant of Schilder's disease; distinguishing feature: alternating bands of destruction and preservation of myelin

C. Adrenoleukodystrophy: may be clinically indistinguishable from Schilder's disease, but sex-linked and adrenal atrophy are unique

V. Acute Disseminated Encephalomyelitis (*Postinfectious, Postexanthem, Postvaccinal Encephalomyelitis*)

A. Overview: acute; demyelination scattered throughout brain and spinal cord, surround small- and medium-sized veins; axons and nerves are intact; perivenular inflammation and meningeal infiltration; may precede respiratory infection (Epstein-Barr, cytomegalovirus, mycoplasma rarely, after influenza and mumps), within a few days of onset of exanthem of measles, rubella, smallpox, chickenpox; after rabies, smallpox, and, rarely, tetanus vaccine

B. Prognosis: significant death rate and persistent deficits to those who survive; acute stage is followed by behavioral problems or mental retardation, epilepsy in children; adults make good recoveries; more benign cerebellitis clears over several months.

C. Pathogenesis: unclear; probably immune-mediated complication rather than direct CNS infection; lab model: experimental allergic encephalomyelitis produces pathology between the 8th and 15th day after sensitization.

D. Clinically: acute onset of confusion, somnolence, convulsions, headache, fever, neck stiffness; sometimes with ataxia, myoclonus, and choreoathetosis; in myelinic form: partial or complete paraplegia, quadriplegia, loss of bladder and bowel control, generally no fever; in postexanthem encephalomyelitis: 2 to 4 days after appearance of rash

E. Treatment: high-potency steroids (1g/d for 5 days followed by oral prednisone taper over 1 to 2 weeks); plasma exchange (daily for 5 days) and intravenous Ig (0.4 g/kg/d for 5 days) has been anecdotally successful in fulminant cases; use of embryonated duck eggs for rabies vaccine is free of neurologic complications; chemotherapy used as a last resort for severe, fulminant ADEM, based on anecdotal evidence

VI. Acute Necrotizing Hemorrhagic Encephalomyelitis (*Acute Hemorrhagic Leukoencephalitis of Weston Hurst*)

A. Overview: most fulminant of demyelinating diseases; affects mostly young adults but also children; almost invariably preceded by respiratory infection; neurologic symptoms appear abruptly with headache, fever, stiff neck, and confusion, followed by seizures, hemiplegia, pseudobulbar paralysis, progressively deepening coma; many cases terminate fatally in 2 to 4 days.

B. Lab: leukocytosis, elevated erythrocyte sedimentation rate; increased CSF pressure, pleocytosis (lymph or poly), increased protein, normal glucose; computed tomography/MRI shows massive lesion in cerebral white matter.

C. Pathology: white matter is destroyed almost to the point of liquefaction; resembles disseminated encephalomyelitis but with widespread necrosis.

D. Treatment: corticosteroids; plasma exchange

CHEAT SHEET

Lhermitte's phenomenon	Tingling electric feelings down body with passive neck flexion
Neuromyelitis optica (Devic's syndrome)	NMOIGG, aquaporin-4 antibodies, demyelination and necrosis optic nerves, spinal cord > brain, B-cell
Uhthoff's phenomenon	Visual blurring with exercise due to prior optic nerve demyelination
Schilder's disease	Progressive, high-myelin basic protein, severe injury hemispheric
Concentric sclerosis of Baló	Alternating bands of destruction and preservation of white matter
ADEM	Following infection/vaccine, monophasic usually encephalomyelitis, children more than adults
Acute hemorrhagic leukoencephalitis of Weston Hurst	Most severe form of demyelination; prodromal infection; abrupt, severe demyelinating event

Suggested Readings

Lublin FD. Defining the clinical course of multiple sclerosis: The 2013 revisions. *Neurology*. 2014;83:278–286.

Miller DH, Weinshenker BG, Filippi M, et al Differential diagnosis of suspected multiple sclerosis: a consensus approach. *Mult. Scler.*2008;14:11571–174.

Polman CH, Reingold SC, Banwell B, et al. Diagnostic criteria for multiple sclerosis: 2010 revision to the McDonald criteria. *Ann. Neurol.*2011;69:292–302.

CHAPTER 14

Infections of the Nervous System

I. Bacterial Meningitis

1. Acute bacterial infection of the leptomeninges, subarachnoid space, and structures passing through the subarachnoid space

2. Routes of infection

   a. Nasopharynx (most common)

   b. Open trauma/surgical procedure

   c. Sinus infection

   d. Communicating congenital defect

3. Epidemiology

   a. More common in winter

   b. Annual incidence: 1 to 2 in 100,000 annually

   c. Immunization against *Haemophilus influenza* with polyvalent pneumococcal and meningococcal vaccines has produced a significant reduction in the incidence in the United States.

4. *Etiology*

NEONATE (<1 MO)	INFANT TO YOUNG CHILD (1 MO–5 YRS)	ADULT (15–60 Y/O)	ELDERLY (>60 Y/O)
Group B Streptococcus	*Streptococcus pneumoniae*	*Streptococcus pneumoniae*	*Streptococcus pneumoniae*
Escherichia coli, other enteric gram-negative bacilli	*Neisseria meningitidis*	*Neisseria meningitidis*	*Neisseria meningitides*
Listeria monocytogenes	*Haemophilus. influenzae* type b		*Listeria monocytogenes*

5. Clinical: presents in hours to days with rapid progression. Most patients will have at least two of the tetrad of fever, neck stiffness, headache, and altered mentation.

   a. Fever—85% of cases

   b. Meningismus (neck stiffness) present in 70% of cases; Kernig's and Brudzinski's signs may be present.

   c. Diminished level of awareness

   d. Headache +/− nausea, vomiting

   e. Seizures—poor prognosis

   f. Focal neurologic deficits

5. Clinical (*cont'd*)

    g. Petechial rash *(N. meningitidis)*

    h. Infant: lethargy, seizures, bulging fontanel

    i. Complications

        i. Cerebral edema

        ii. Hydrocephalus

        iii. Stroke due to infectious vasculitis

        iv. Sinus thrombosis

        v. Cranial nerve (CN) palsies

        vi. Disseminated intravascular coagulation (with *N. meningitidis*)

        vii. Syndrome of inappropriate secretion of antidiuretic hormone

        viii. Abscess/subdural empyema

        ix. Respiratory failure

    j. Prognosis: mortality rate of 10% to 15%, highest in pneumococcal meningitis, increased in immunocompromised host

6. Diagnostic testing

    a. CT brain: no diagnostic utility in meningitis. Only used to rule out other intracranial processes prior to lumbar puncture. Indications for undergoing CT imaging prior to lumbar puncture: adult patients who are >60 years of age; immunocompromised state; presentation with focal neurological deficits, new-onset seizures, papilledema, abnormal mentation, or history of central nervous system (CNS) disease.

    b. Lumbar puncture

        i. Initial cerebrospinal fluid (CSF)

            (A) Elevated opening pressure

            (B) White blood cell count (WBC): 100 to 10,000 cells/mL, predominantly polymorphonuclear cells

            (C) Glucose: <20 mg/dL or <40% of serum glucose

            (D) Protein usually elevated, >100 mg/dL

        ii. Gram stain: yield low to 20% if treated with antibiotics

        iii. Culture: within 48 to 72 hours after institution of antibiotic therapy, the CSF culture is usually negative; blood cultures may be positive in 50% of cases.

CSF	APPEARANCE	OPENING PRESSURE	GLUCOSE	PROTEIN	WBC	CELL TYPE	OTHER
Bacterial meningitis	Cloudy, purulent, or clear	Elevated	Low	Elevated	>100 cells	Neutrophils	
Viral meningitis	Clear	Normal or elevated	Normal	Elevated	10–1,000	Lymphocytes	Red blood cells (RBCs) or xanthochromia in herpes simplex virus (HSV)

(continued)

CSF	APPEARANCE	OPENING PRESSURE	GLUCOSE	PROTEIN	WBC	CELL TYPE	OTHER
Tuberculosis	Cloudy or clear	Elevated	Very low	Elevated	50–500	Lymphocytes	
Fungal meningitis	Cloudy or clear	Elevated	Very low	Elevated	10–500	Lymphocytes	

7. Treatment

   a. Supportive care

   b. Antibiotics

   i. Always administer immediately if cannot readily perform spinal tap; administration may produce sterile cultures but associated changes in CSF (if necessary, may need to follow CSF parameters).

   ii. Empiric treatment

   (A) Typical empiric treatment

   (1) Ceftriaxone: 2 g q12h

   (2) Vancomycin: 30 to 45 mg/kg/day, adjusted to renal function

   (a) If Listeria *suspected (in those <3 months old or >60 years old (y/o); immunosuppressed, alcoholic), add ampicillin 2 g IV q 4 hours.*

   (B) *Prophylaxis with rifampin for contacts if meningococcal or* Hemophilus influenza *meningitis*

   iii. *Antibiotics for specific types of bacterial meningitis*

ORGANISM	ANTIBIOTIC	DURATION
Streptococcus pneumoniae	Ceftriaxone and vancomycin	10–14 days
Group B *streptococcus*	Ampicillin	10–14 days
Neisseria meningitidis	Ceftriaxone or cefotaxime	7 days
Listeria monocytogenes	Ampicillin	21 days
Haemophilus influenzae	Ceftriaxone or cefepime	7 days
Pseudomonas aeruginosa	Ceftazidime or cefepime	21 days

   c. Role of corticosteroids: a large randomized trial showed the beneficial effects of 0.15 mg/kg IV q 6 hours for 4 days, in conjunction with antibiotics, for suspected or proven meningitis due to *S. pneumoniae; in kids: dexamethasone, 0.15 mg/kg/day, q6h for 4 to 7 days, should be used in conjunction with antibiotics for suspected or proven* H. influenzae *type B to reduce hearing loss.*

   d. Droplet precautions need to be undertaken until organism is identified.

8. *Recurrent meningitis*

   a. Evaluate for cranial or spinal defect permitting reentry

   b. Evaluate for immune deficiency (i.e., HIV)

   c. Differential diagnosis

   i. *Behcet's syndrome*

   ii. *Sarcoidosis*

   iii. *Mollaret's meningitis*

II. Viral Infections of the Nervous System

A. General

1. A wide range of neurological manifestations, including meningitis, encephalitis, cerebellitis, CN involvement, myelitis, ganglionitis, and polyradiculitis

2. Most viral infections are mild or asymptomatic.

3. Viral meningitis is more common than bacterial meningitis.

4. Etiologies

    a. Enteroviruses cause 90% of viral meningitis.

    b. Herpesviruses and arboviruses are the most common causes of encephalitis.

5. Clinical features

    a. Malaise, anorexia, myalgia, low-grade fever, vomiting, or headache

    b. Physical examination reveals photophobia, somnolence, or irritability, and meningeal irritation.

    c. Systemic features to assess include rash, pharyngitis, lymphadenopathy, arthritis, parotid gland enlargement, and hepatosplenomegaly.

    d. Seizures and altered mentation in encephalitis

    e. Transverse myelitis with flaccid weakness, reduced/absent reflexes, sensory loss, and bladder dysfunction

    f. Other neurological manifestations include CN involvement, extrapyramidal symptoms, cerebellitis, acute inflammatory demyelinating polyneuropathy (AIDP), and acute flaccid paralysis.

    g. **Reye's syndrome**

        i. Seen in infection with *varicella zoster virus* (*VZV*; chicken pox) *and influenza viruses*

        ii. *Develops between ages 2 and 15 years*

        iii. *Strong correlation with aspirin use*

        iv. Clinical

            (A) *<72 hours after viral illness*

            (B) Begins with continuous vomiting followed by increasing lethargy, hypoglycemia, and hyperammonemia with liver failure (and dysfunction of clotting factors)

            (C) Death and neurologic sequelae are related to increased intracranial pressure (ICP)

        v. Treatment

            (A) Supportive care, with strict control of electrolytes and treatment of clotting dysfunction

            (B) Observation/treatment of increased ICP

        vi. Prognosis depends on severity of increased ICP; mortality is 10% to 30%.

6. Diagnostic procedures

    a. Serology—elevated virus-specific antibodies

    b. Lumbar puncture for CSF

        i. Lymphocytic pleocytosis (10–1,000/mm^3), mildly elevated protein, and normal glucose and normal opening pressure

        ii. Polymerase chain reaction (PCR) available for HSV, HIV, cytomegalovirus (CMV), enteroviruses, adenoviruses, Epstein–Barr virus (EBV), VZV, and flaviviruses

c. Neuroimaging

  i. CT: may be normal in encephalitis

  ii. MRI

    (A) More sensitive than CT

    (B) T2 prolongation or enhancement of cortex in encephalitis; T2 prolongation or cord swelling in myelitis

    (C) Distinguish viral encephalitis from acute disseminated encephalomyelitis

d. Electroencephalography (EEG)

  i. Viral meningitis: normal or nonspecific abnormalities

  ii. Encephalitis: slowing of background rhythms and focal or diffuse epileptiform discharges

    (A) *HSV-1 encephalitis often presents with temporal slowing or periodic lateralizing epileptiform discharges.*

7. Specific *antiviral treatment*

VIRUS	MEDICATION
Herpes simplex virus	Acyclovir
Varicella zoster virus	Acyclovir, valacyclovir, famciclovir
Cytomegalovirus	Ganciclovir, foscarnet, cidofovir
Subacute sclerosing panencephalitis	Isoprinosine
HIV	Highly active antiretroviral therapy regimen (see Section II.B.9)

B. Specific viral infections of the nervous system

1. *Herpes viruses*

  a. **Herpes simplex virus 1 and herpes simplex virus 2**

    i. HSV-1: causes 90% to 95% of HSV encephalitis

      (A) Usually adolescent/adult

      (B) Transmitted via oral mucosa

      (C) Most common nonepidemic encephalitis and fatal sporadic encephalitis in the United States

      (D) Remains latent in the trigeminal ganglia with reactivation and retrograde transmission to the central nervous system (CNS) in two-thirds of cases

      (E) Exhibits propensity for the orbitofrontal cortex and temporal lobes

    ii. HSV-2

      (A) Usually neonate

      (B) Transmitted sexually or via birth canal to infant

      (C) Involves the brain diffusely via hematogenous transmission

      (D) Causes 70% of neonatal HSV infections

      (E) Common cause of aseptic meningitis in adult women; may not have concurrent genital herpetic lesions

    iii. Clinical features

      (A) HSV encephalitis

(A) HSV encephalitis (*cont'd*)

   (1) Prodrome of headache, fever, malaise, or vomiting followed by confusion, personality and behavioral changes, focal or generalized seizures, short-term memory dysfunction, and focal deficits, including weakness and aphasia

   (2) Two presentations

      (a) Can be rapidly progressive, with coma and death within 2 weeks

      (b) Indolent, with hallucinations, headache, memory loss, and behavioral disturbances

(B) Other manifestations

   (1) Bell's palsy

   (2) Acute myelitis

   (3) Rhombencephalitis/brainstem encephalitis

   (4) Aseptic meningitis

   (5) Mollaret's meningitis—recurrent episodes of benign lymphocytic meningitis, common in women; most are caused by HSV-2 infection.

iv. Diagnosis

(A) CSF

   (1) Lymphocytic pleocytosis, moderately elevated opening pressure and protein content with normal glucose. Elevated RBC count and xanthochromia may be seen due to hemorrhagic necrosis.

   (2) HSV PCR: 99% sensitive and 95% specific. False negatives can occur in the first 72 hours of the illness.

(B) Neuroimaging

   (1) MRI brain: restricted diffusion and hyperintensities on T2-weighted sequences in frontal regions, mesial temporal lobe, insular cortex, and cingulate gyrus, with or without gadolinium enhancement. Hemorrhagic changes may be seen. Negative MRI does not rule out HSV encephalitis.

(C) EEG: slowing, periodic lateralizing epileptiform discharges (PLEDs), or frank epileptiform discharges

(D) Pathology

   (1) Hemorrhagic encephalitis with neuronal destruction

   (2) Predilection for frontal and temporal regions

   (3) Cowdry A inclusions

      (a) Intranuclear, solitary large viral inclusions with halo due to margination of chromatin

      (b) Seen in HSV, VZV, CMV, and subacute sclerosing panencephalitis

v. Treatment

(A) HSV-1 encephalitis: acyclovir, 10 mg/kg q8h for minimum of 14 to 21 days

(B) HSV-2 in neonates: acyclovir, 20 mg/kg q8h for 21 days

vi. Prognosis

(A) Mortality of untreated cases is 70%; mortality for acyclovir-treated neonates is 15%.

(B) Survivors usually have permanent neurologic complications.

b. **Varicella zoster virus**

   i. Primary VZV infection—*chicken pox*

   (A) Peak incidence between ages 5 and 9

   (B) Respiratory transmission; typically causes no neurological symptoms.

   (C) Postinfectious encephalitis or cerebellitis can occur. In immunocompromised individuals it can cause meningitis or encephalitis.

   (D) Reye's syndrome can be seen in children who receive aspirin.

   ii. Reactivation of VZV: after primary VZV infection, the virus persists in a latent state in the dorsal root ganglia

   (A) *Shingles (herpes zoster)*

   (1) Virus reactivates and migrates via axon to the skin, producing shingles, erythematous, maculopapular rash that progresses to vesicles associated with radicular pain in a dermatomal distribution

   (2) More common among the elderly or immunocompromised

   (3) T5 to T10 dermatomes most commonly affected; can be disseminated in immunocompromised individuals

   (4) Treatment is acyclovir 800 mg oral 5 times a day for 7 days. Early initiation of treatment reduces pain associated with acute zoster.

   (5) Post-herpetic neuralgia can occur, especially in elderly. Gabapentin, pregabalin, and other anticonvulsants, antidepressants, and topical agents are used for treatment of neuralgic pain.

   (6) Live attenuated varicella vaccine has been approved for adults >50 years of age to prevent shingles and post-herpetic neuralgia.

   (B) *Zoster ophthalmicus*: due to involvement of first division of trigeminal ganglion; can be associated with VZV vasculopathy/vasculitis

   (C) *Ramsay-Hunt syndrome*: lower CN VII palsy with associated vesicular eruption in the auditory canal

   (D) Meningitis and myelitis can occur

   (E) Encephalitis is associated with large-vessel vasculitis and can cause focal infarctions. It is usually associated with ipsilateral zoster ophthalmicus. In immunocompromised individuals, small- and medium-sized vessels are involved, causing deep infarctions.

   (F) AIDP and brachial plexus neuritis

   iii. Diagnosis

   (A) Isolation of VZV from the oropharynx or skin lesions

   (B) VZV-specific antibodies in the CSF

   (C) PCR studies of CSF or vesicular fluid

   iv. Treatment

   (A) Patients with CNS involvement are treated with IV acyclovir 10 mg/kg q 8 hours for 7 to 14 days with pulse steroids for 3 to 5 days.

   (B) Supportive care

c. **Epstein-Barr virus**

   i. Fifty percent of children under age 5 and 90% of adults have had EBV infection.

   ii. Acute illness is usually asymptomatic; can present as nonspecific febrile illness or infectious mononucleosis.

    c. **Epstein-Barr virus** (*cont'd*)

       iii. Neurologic complications in <1%

         (A) Aseptic meningitis—most common acute neurologic complication

         (B) Encephalitis

         (C) Optic neuropathy

         (D) Other cranial neuropathy

         (E) Cerebellitis

         (F) Acute transverse myelitis

         (G) AIDP

         (H) Small-fiber sensory or autonomic neuropathy

         (I) Primary CNS lymphoma in immunocompromised patients

       iv. Diagnostic testing

         (A) In meningoencephalitis, brain MRI may be normal or show T2 prolongation involving the basal ganglia, thalamus, white matter, or cerebral cortex.

         (B) Diagnosis of EBV infection is usually established serologically but can also be detected in the CSF by PCR.

       v. Treatment

         (A) Supportive care

         (B) No controlled treatment trials available

    d. **Cytomegalovirus**

       i. Most adults are seropositive for CMV and are asymptomatic.

       ii. Can cause acute and latent or persistent infection

       iii. Acquired by body fluid transmission, blood transfusion, organ transplant, etc.

       iv. Common in immunocompromised host, including HIV-infected patients and post-transplantation (>40%–90% of transplant recipients)

       v. Clinical manifestations:

         (A) Congenital CMV infection

           (1) Most common congenital infection

           (2) Infection occurs in the first trimester. Infection can also occur perinatally during passage through infected birth canal or breastfeeding.

           (3) Ranges from asymptomatic infection in 90% to disseminated disease.

           (4) Systemic: jaundice, petechial rash, hepatosplenomegaly, or intrauterine growth retardation

           (5) Neurologic: encephalitis, retinitis and optic atrophy, microcephaly, microgyria, seizures, abnormal tone, sensorineural hearing loss (CMV infection is the most common cause of congenital deafness).

           (6) May have disorders of neuronal migration (cortical dysplasia, lissencephaly) or absence of the corpus callosum

           (7) Neuroimaging: intracranial calcification in 50% of infected infants (worse prognosis)

             (a) CT: calcification in the periventricular regions, also+ in basal ganglia (BG), cortical, and subcortical regions

             (b) MRI: disruption of gyral pattern and delayed myelination

    (B) Postnatal CMV infection

        (1) Immunocompetent: mononucleosis syndrome, aseptic meningitis

        (2) Immunocompromised:

           (a) Encephalitis (when CD4 $<$50 in HIV patients), meningitis, ventriculitis, ependymitis

           (b) Retinitis

               (i) Occurs in 5% to 10% of persons with AIDS.

               (ii) Unilateral vision loss followed by bilateral vision loss if untreated

               (iii) Ganciclovir, foscarnet, and cidofovir may reduce extent of vision loss.

           (c) Acute myelitis

           (d) AIDP

               (i) Before onset, 10% to 20% of patients are CMV positive.

               (ii) More commonly also have cranial neuropathies and sensorineural hearing loss

  vi. Diagnosis

    (A) CMV-specific immunoglobulin M (IgM): strongly supports infection, but CMV IgG not useful because of the high prevalence of CMV in the general population

    (B) CSF CMV PCR

    (C) CMV DNA can be isolated from urine, saliva, and CSF in newborns

    (D) Pathology: microglial nodules, especially periventricular, on cortical biopsy/autopsy

  vii. Treatment in immunocompromised host

    (A) Initial antiviral dose: ganciclovir, 5 mg/kg q12h for $>$2 to 4 weeks

    (B) Maintenance therapy: ganciclovir, 5 mg/kg/day for 5 days per week for 4 weeks

    (C) Foscarnet for ganciclovir-resistant CMV

  2. *Arthropod-borne infections—transmitted by mosquitos and ticks*

Vectors and animal hosts

ENCEPHALITIS	VECTOR	ANIMAL HOST
Western equine encephalitis	Culex	Birds
Eastern equine encephalitis	Culex	Birds
Venezuelan equine encephalitis	Culex	Rodents, equine
St. Louis encephalitis	Culex	Birds
West Nile virus	Culex	Birds
Japanese encephalitis	Culex	Birds
California encephalitis	Aedes	Rodents
Powassan	Tick—*Ixodes*	Rodents
Colorado tick fever	Tick—*Dermacenter*	Rodents

2. *Arthropod-borne infections* (*cont'd*)

Geographical locations and seasonal occurrence

ENCEPHALITIS	GEOGRAPHICAL DISTRIBUTION	SEASON/MONTHS
Western encephalitis	Western United States and Canada	June to August
Eastern encephalitis	Atlantic and Gulf coasts, Great Lakes region	June to September
Venezuelan encephalitis	Texas and Florida	May to September
St. Louis encephalitis	Central states, Ohio/ Mississippi River valley	June to August
West Nile virus	United States	June to October
Japanese encephalitis	Asia and Western Pacific	Summer and fall
California encephalitis	Midwestern and northeastern United States, southern Canada	June to September
Powassan	North-central United States, eastern Canada	Spring, summer
Colorado tick fever	United States and Canadian Rocky Mountains	March to September

    a. Transmitted by mosquitos

        i. *Alphaviruses*

            (A) Clinical: headache, myalgias, malaise, vomiting, stiff neck, fever, irritability, coma, or seizure

            (B) Diagnosis: detection of virus-specific antibodies in serum and CSF

            (C) Treatment: supportive care

                (1) Western equine encephalitis (EE) virus

                    (a) Mortality: 5% to 15%

                    (b) Most survivors recover completely.

                (2) Eastern EE virus

                    (a) In human infections, 4% to 5% lead to encephalitis.

                    (b) Highest mortality rate of 50% to 70%

                    (c) Complications: most survivors have neurological deficits.

                (3) Venezuelan EE virus

                    (a) Infection rarely causes encephalitis

                    (b) Prognosis is usually good, with low mortality rate (0.4%) and rarely with significant neurological deficits.

        ii. *Flaviviruses*

            (A) St. Louis encephalitis virus

                (1) Clinical infection in less than 1%

                    (a) Encephalitis (60%)

                    (b) Aseptic meningitis (15%)

                    (c) Influenza-like illness

                    (d) Nonconvulsive status epilepticus may occur more frequently than with other arbovirus infections.

        (e) Almost 90% of elderly patients develop encephalitis and have a higher risk of fatal disease.

    (2) Diagnosis, St. Louis encephalitis: virus-specific IgM in serum or CSF or PCR

    (3) Prognosis: mortality rate is 5% to 15%; 10% of survivors have persistent neurologic dysfunction.

  (B) West Nile virus

    (1) Human-to-human transmission can occur via organ transplantation, blood transfusion, and other body fluid transmission, including breastfeeding.

    (2) Clinical

        (a) Usually asymptomatic; less than 1% develop neurological symptoms.

        (b) Elderly, immunocompromised, and patients with other medical illnesses are at greatest risk for neurological complications.

        (c) Prodrome of fever, malaise, headache, nausea, and vomiting followed by neurological symptoms that can include meningitis, encephalitis (60% of symptomatic cases), myelitis, a polio-like syndrome of acute flaccid paralysis, or extrapyramidal symptoms.

    (3) Diagnosis: virus-specific IgM and IgG antibodies in serum and CSF, or CSF PCR. PCR is less sensitive than serology but more specific; useful in immunocompromised patients with weak serological response.

    (4) Imaging: in encephalitis, MRI brain fluid attenuation inversion recovery (FLAIR) and diffusion-weighted imaging (DWI) show changes in basal ganglia, thalamus, brainstem, and cerebellum. Spinal MRI shows T2 changes in myelitis.

    (5) Electrodiagnostic studies: nerve conduction study and electromyography can demonstrate injury to lower motor neurons in patients with flaccid paralysis.

    (6) Prognosis: mortality rate is 5% to 10%; 30% to 40% of survivors have persistent neurologic dysfunction.

  (C) Japanese encephalitis virus

    (1) Most common arboviral encephalitis worldwide

    (2) Vaccination has reduced incidence.

    (3) Most common encephalitis in eastern Asia

    (4) Affects approximately 50,000 persons annually

    (5) Clinical: less than 1% have clinical illness. Headache; fever; anorexia; malaise; convulsions; extrapyramidal, subcortical, or cerebellar signs; coma; symptoms/signs similar to AIDP have been reported.

    (6) Diagnosis: virus-specific IgM serology or CSF

    (7) MRI: abnormalities within thalamus, brainstem, basal ganglia, and cerebellum

    (8) Treatment: supportive care only

    (9) Prognosis: mortality rate of 20% to 40% among those with encephalitis; 30% of survivors have persistent neurologic dysfunction.

  iii. *Bunyaviruses*

  (A) California (La Crosse) encephalitis virus

    (A) California (La Crosse) encephalitis virus (*cont'd*)

        (1) Clinical: fever, vomiting, headache, and abdominal pain, with CNS signs 2 to 4 days later; neurological illness occurs mostly in children under age 16; 50% have seizures, including status epilepticus; 20% have focal neurological signs; 10% have aseptic meningitis.

        (2) Diagnosis: >4 times increase in virus-specific serology or CSF

        (3) Treatment: supportive care only

        (4) Prognosis: mortality rate is <1%; rate of CNS sequelae is low.

  b. Transmitted by ticks

    i. *Flavivirus*

    (A) Powassan encephalitis virus

        (1) Rare cause of human encephalitis in United States

        (2) Clinical: fever, headache, vomiting, and somnolence followed by cognitive dysfunction, ophthalmoplegia, diffuse or focal weakness, ataxia, and seizures

        (3) Diagnosis: virus-specific IgM in CSF or serum and elevations of the virus-specific IgG in convalescent sera

        (4) Treatment: supportive care

        (5) Prognosis: mortality rate is 10% to 15%; neurological sequelae in 35%.

    ii. *Orbivirus*

    (A) *Colorado tick fever virus*

        (1) Clinical: fever, headache, myalgia, anorexia, nausea, and rash (similar to symptoms of Rocky Mountain spotted fever), followed by aseptic meningitis

        (2) Treatment: supportive care only

        (3) Prognosis: mortality rare

3. **Rabies**

  a. Reservoirs: skunks (most common), dogs, raccoons, and bats

  b. Worldwide, 50,000 to 60,000 die annually (but only 1 to 2 per year in United States)

  c. Pathogenesis: virus enters *peripheral nerves followed by axonal transport of the virus to the cell bodies of neurons, where the virus replicates and disseminates throughout the CNS.*

  d. Clinical features

    i. Incubation: 1 week to years (shortest after infection to the head and neck), usually 1 to 3 months

    ii. Prodrome: headache, malaise, sore throat, nausea/vomiting, and/or abdominal pain

    iii. *Furious = agitated encephalitis*

    (A) 80% of human rabies cases

    (B) Confusion, anxiety, agitation, hallucinations, dysphagia, hydrophobia, hypersalivation, autonomic hyperactivity, and seizures

    (C) Death secondary to muscle spasms involving diaphragm or accessory respiratory muscles that lead to respiratory arrest or coma

    iv. *Dumb = paralytic encephalitis*

    (A) Similar course as AIDP; more common with bat virus strains

    (B) The most frequent initial symptoms are pain and paresthesias at the site of infection followed by flaccid paralysis of the same extremity and progress to quadriplegia.

    (C) Death secondary to respiratory arrest and coma

    e. Diagnosis

        i. Neuroimaging: can be normal or show T2 hyperintensities

        ii. Diagnosis confirmed by

            (A) Isolating the rabies virus from saliva

            (B) Pathology

                (1) Negri bodies: eosinophilic intranuclear inclusions in hippocampus and cerebellar Purkinje cells

                (2) Babès nodules: focal microglial nodules

            (C) Serologic responses

            (D) Rabies virus antigen by immunofluorescent staining of full-thickness skin biopsy specimens from the neck

            (E) Rabies virus-specific antibodies can be detected in serum or CSF by day 15.

            (F) PCR in saliva or brain tissues by day 5

    f. Treatment

        i. Postexposure prophylaxis

            (A) Begin with cleaning of the wound with soap and water.

            (B) If animal suspected of having rabies, immediately vaccinate with human diploid cell rabies vaccine and consult local public health officials.

        ii. Symptomatic

            (A) Supportive care only

            (B) Place in isolation because rabies virus is present in body fluids.

    g. Prognosis: 100% mortality, usually within 2 weeks of onset of symptoms

4. **Progressive multifocal leukoencephalopathy (PML)**

    a. Caused by the John Cunningham (JC) virus

    b. Infection is acquired in childhood. About 55% to 85% of adult population is seropositive.

    c. Opportunistic CNS infection due to reactivation of latent JC virus in tonsil, bone marrow, and spleen

    d. Seen in immunodeficiency (5% of AIDS patients have PML when CD4 <200 cells/microliter), hematologic malignancies, and organ transplantation

    e. Seen in patients on immunomodulatory therapy with natalizumab, rituximab, and efalizumab

    f. Pathogenesis: reactivation of virus, dissemination to CNS, and infection of oligodendrocytes (demyelination) and astrocytes (neuronal dysfunction)

    g. Clinical

        i. Cognitive decline, visual field deficits, cranial neuropathies, sensory deficits, motor deficits, speech disturbances, and ataxia progressing to dementia; headaches, extrapyramidal syndromes, and seizures are rare.

    h. Diagnosis

        i. Confirmed by detecting JC virus particles or antigens in brain tissue, isolating the virus from brain, or PCR

        ii. MRI brain: confluent multifocal white-matter lesions with T2 prolongation, typically within cerebral subcortical white matter and brainstem

        iii. Pathology: *oligodendrocytes contain eosinophilic intranuclear inclusions;* bizarre astrocytes.

4. **Progressive multifocal leukoencephalopathy (PML)** (*cont'd*)

   i. Treatment: supportive care; PML lesions may stabilize with improvement of CD4 count with highly active antiretroviral therapy (HAART).

   j. Prognosis: 80% mortality within 9 months

5. *Picornaviruses*

   a. *Enteroviruses*

      i. Non-polio enteroviruses (coxsackie, echovirus, human enterovirus 68-71) are the most common cause of aseptic viral meningitis.

      ii. Transmission is primarily feco-oral; sometimes through respiratory droplets.

      iii. Usually occur in late summer and fall

      (A) Polioviruses

         (1) Clinical

            (*a*) Usually limited symptoms or asymptomatic

            (*b*) Neurologic manifestations

               (i) *Aseptic meningitis (8%)*

               (ii) *Paralytic poliomyelitis (1%)*

                  [1] Usually due to poliovirus type 1

                  [2] Prodrome of fever, headache, vomiting, myalgia, and meningeal signs

                  [3] Acute flaccid paralysis appears within 1 to 2 days due to involvement of alpha motor neurons in the spinal cord.

               (iii) *Bulbar poliomyelitis*

                  [1] Involves the motor CNs of the medulla or pons (usually CNs IX, X, and XI) with dysphagia, dysphonia, and upper airway compromise

               (iv) *Polioencephalitis*

         (2) Diagnosis

            (*a*) Confirmation of poliovirus requires isolation from feces, CSF, or throat.

            (*b*) Detected in feces or CSF with PCR

         (3) Prophylactic

            (*a*) *Salk vaccine*

               (i) *Inactivated poliovirus vaccine*

            (*b*) *Sabin vaccine*

               (i) *Attenuated, live-virus oral vaccine*

               (ii) *No longer distributed in the United States*

         (4) Acute treatment

            (*a*) Supportive care

            (*b*) Immunocompromised: IV immunoglobulin

         (5) Prognosis

            (*a*) Mortality high (50%)

            (*b*) Paralytic poliomyelitis: patients frequently recover but may have residual fatigue, myalgia, arthralgia, and muscle weakness and atrophy. Post–polio syndrome is a late complication in 25% of patients due to exacerbation of motor weakness 30 to 40 years after infection.

(B) **Non-polio enteroviruses—coxsackievirus and echovirus**

   (1) Clinical features

      (a) Range from mild febrile illnesses to severe disseminated multiple organ infections. *Coxsackievirus B has more complications with involvement of the heart, liver, and CNS.*

      (b) Commonly includes pharyngitis, herpangina, pleurodynia, gastroenteritis, neonatal sepsis, or hand-foot-and-mouth disease

      (c) CNS: aseptic meningitis, encephalitis, poliomyelitis-like illnesses, Guillain-Barré syndrome, acute cerebellar ataxia, or opsoclonus-myoclonus

      (d) Echovirus may also produce disseminated intravascular coagulation; 10% present with maculopapular or petechial rash.

   (2) Diagnosis

      (a) Isolated from feces, CSF, or throat washings

      (b) Feces, serum, or CSF PCR

   (3) Treatment: supportive care only

6. **Measles virus—*paramyxovirus***

  a. Spreads via *respiratory droplets*

  b. Measles vaccination has been linked with acute encephalopathy and permanent neurologic deficits.

  c. Clinical (CNS involvement)

    i. *Acute encephalitis*

      (A) Rare

      (B) Begins 2 to 5 days after the rash appears

    ii. *Postviral encephalomyelitis*

      (A) 1/1,000 cases of measles

      (B) Seen within 2 weeks after rash appears

      (C) Usually <10 y/o

      (D) Headache, irritability, seizures, somnolence, or coma; occasionally paralysis, ataxia, choreoathetosis, or incontinence

      (E) Treatment: supportive care

      (F) Prognosis: mortality = 10% to 15%; neurologic sequelae = *20% to 60%*

    iii. *Measles inclusion body encephalitis*

      (A) Rapidly progressive neurodegeneration

      (B) Develops 1 to 6 months after infection

      (C) Patients usually have deficiency of cell-mediated immunity or are immunocompromised.

      (D) Begins insidiously with dementia, myoclonus, and seizures followed by coma and often death

      (E) Treatment: supportive care, reduction in immunosuppression, passive immunoglobulin therapy

    iv. *Subacute sclerosing panencephalitis*

      (A) Persistent measles infection in the brain

      (B) Rare late complication 2 to 12 years after infection

      (C) Pathogenesis: defective measles virus maturation in the brain

      (D) Affects young (50% have had measles before 2 y/o); more common in boys

iv. *Subacute sclerosing panencephalitis (cont'd)*

    (E) Clinical features

        (1) Stage 1: behavior and personality changes followed by myoclonus (usually focal)

        (2) Stage 2: persistent mental status changes with generalization of myoclonus, followed by ataxia, language difficulties, apraxias, and spasticity and chorioretinitis

        (3) Stage 3: vision loss, worsening myoclonus, ballistic movements, quadriparesis, akinetic mutism

        (4) Stage 4: coma or persistent vegetative state

    (F) Diagnosis

        (1) Virus-specific IgG in CSF and serum

        (2) EEG: *bilateral synchronous high-amplitude spike or slow-wave bursts that correlate with myoclonus; EEG progresses to burst-suppression pattern.*

        (3) Pathology

            (a) Patchy demyelination

            (b) Intranuclear eosinophilic inclusions

    (G) Treatment: supportive care and treatment of clinical symptoms

    (H) Prognosis: usually death within 1 to 3 years

7. **Mumps virus—*paramyxovirus***

    a. Respiratory spread

    b. Mild illness, parotitis, orchitis

    c. Common cause of aseptic meningitis and encephalitis in unimmunized populations

    d. Immunization with live attenuated vaccine

8. **Rubella virus**

    a. Mild illness in childhood and adults; can cause postviral encephalomyelitis

    b. **Congenital rubella syndrome**

        i. Serious if infection acquired in first trimester

        ii. CNS involvement in 80%

    c. Clinical features

        i. Infants: lethargy, irritability, bulging fontanelle

        ii. Sequelae: mental retardation, cataracts, sensorineural hearing loss, abnormal tone and posture, congenital heart disease

        iii. Progressive rubella panencephalitis: follows congenital or childhood rubella, with neurological deterioration progressing to death in the second decade of life

    d. Diagnosis: prenatal diagnosis possible via amniotic fluid or rubella-specific IgM in fetal blood

    e. Vaccination: with live attenuated virus (measles, mumps, and rubella [MMR] vaccine)

9. *Retroviruses*

    a. Contain an RNA-dependent DNA polymerase (reverse transcriptase) and replicate through a DNA intermediary

    b. Lentiviruses (HIV-1 or HIV and HIV-2)

        i. **HIV:** worldwide about 35 million people were living with HIV/AIDS as of 2013; the incidence of AIDS-defining illness has decreased in countries with access to HAART.

ii. HIV infection of nervous system occurs within 2 weeks of acquiring infection. Clinical manifestations occur based on stage of infection.

(A) Early (CD4 >500/mm^3)

(1) Asymptomatic CSF abnormalities

(2) Neurological manifestations occur in 10%.

(3) Seroconversion syndromes: meningitis, meningoencephalitis, seizures, myelopathy, inflammatory demyelinating peripheral neuropathies and cranial neuropathies

(B) Midstage (CD4 200–500/mm^3)

(1) Primary HIV-related disorders: cognitive deficits, meningitis, mononeuritis multiplex, distal sensory polyneuropathy, autonomic neuropathy, inflammatory myopathies

(2) Opportunistic infections: shingles

(C) Advanced (CD4 <200/mm^3)

(1) Dementia, vacuolar myelopathy, distal symmetrical polyneuropathy, autonomic neuropathy, myopathies

(2) Opportunistic infections: cryptococcal meningitis, cerebral toxoplasmosis, PML, primary CNS lymphoma

iii. Neurological manifestations of HIV

(A) Aseptic meningitis

(B) HIV-associated neurocognitive disorder (HAND) or AIDS-dementia complex (ADC) or HIV encephalitis

(1) Most common complication

(2) Occurs in 20% to 75% of patients with advanced HIV.

(3) Short-term memory deficit, decreased concentration, bradykinesia, incoordination, gait disturbance, apathy, personality changes

(4) Can be prevented by early treatment of HIV with HAART

(C) Stroke

(D) Cranial neuropathies

(E) HIV-associated vacuolar myelopathy

(1) 20% of AIDS patients

(2) Subacute onset of spastic paraparesis and posterior column involvement

(3) Spongiform changes with vacuolization of myelin sheath

(F) Acute inflammatory demyelinating polyradiculopathy and chronic inflammatory demyelinating polyradiculopathy: treated with IVIg

(G) HIV-associated lumbosacral polyradiculomyelitis

(H) Distal sensory polyneuropathy: predominantly axonal; due to effects of virus and cytokine upregulation

(I) Mononeuritis multiplex: superimposed infection, lymphomatous infiltration or vasculitis

(J) HIV-associated myopathy: polymyositis

iv. Opportunistic infections and malignancies of the nervous system

(A) Most opportunistic infections are due to reactivation of latent infection.

(B) Reduced incidence since the institution of HAART

(C) Usually CD4 <100/mm^3

iv. Opportunistic infections and malignancies of the nervous system (*cont'd*)

   (D) Treatment involves induction phase followed by maintenance therapy and/or secondary prophylaxis to prevent relapse.

     (1) Toxoplasma meningoencephalitis

       (*a*) Affects 5% to 15% of AIDS patients pre-HAART.

       (*b*) Most common focal infection

       (*c*) Primary prophylaxis with trimethoprim/sulfamethoxazole, atovaquone, or dapsone

       (*d*) See other features in Section IX.

     (2) Cryptococcal meningitis

       (*a*) Affects 10% of AIDS patients pre-HAART.

       (*b*) Primary prophylaxis with fluconazole

       (*c*) See other features in Section VII.

     (3) Progressive multifocal leukoencephalopathy

       (*a*) AIDS patients: 5% have PML when CD4 <200 cells/microliter

     (4) CMV encephalitis and ventriculoencephalitis

       (*a*) Usually only when CD4 <50 cells/microliter

       (*b*) 2% of all neurological complications pre-HAART

       (*c*) Death within weeks to months

       (*d*) Prophylaxis with ganciclovir, foscarnet, or cidofovir if prior CMV retinitis

     (5) CMV polyradiculomyelitis

       (*a*) Presents with lower extremity pain, weakness, sensory symptoms, areflexia, and sphincter dysfunction

       (*b*) Evolves over days

     (6) Neurosyphilis

       (*a*) Recent increase in incidence due to HIV

     (7) CNS tuberculosis

     (8) Other causes of meningitis and meningoencephalitis: *Salmonella typhi*, *Pneumococcus* pneumonia, *Nocardia*, *Listeria*, *Bartonella*, *Histoplasma*, *Coccidioides*, *Candida*, *Blastomyces*, varicella zoster, *Trypanosoma*, and *Acanthamoeba*

     (9) Primary CNS lymphomas (PCNSLs)

       (*a*) 5% of AIDS patients

       (*b*) Second most common focal CNS lesion in AIDS

       (*c*) B-cell type

       (*d*) Associated with Epstein–Barr virus

       (*e*) Clinical: focal neurological symptoms over weeks to months

       (*f*) Diagnosis:

         (i) CSF PCR for EBV, monoclonal B lymphocytes in CSF flow cytometry

         (ii) Imaging characteristics: can be solitary, usually uniform contrast enhancement with surrounding edema and mass effect; more likely to "cross the midline" and involve periventricular and deep white matter (as opposed to toxoplasmosis, in which lesions tend to be multiple, with heterogeneous or ring enhancement); Single-photon emission computed tomography (SPECT) and PET also with greater uptake than toxoplasmosis

> (iii) Brain biopsy for definitive diagnosis

   (g) Treatment:

> > (i) Steroids "melt" away lesions, but without long-term improvement in prognosis, should be given after biopsy. Treatment improves edema and mass effect.
> > (ii) Palliative radiation therapy
> > (iii) Use of HAART improves overall prognosis.

  v. Diagnosis:

    (A) HIV Ag/Ab combination immunoassay; if positive, followed by antibody differentiation tests, HIV nucleic acid tests, Western blot, or immunofluorescence assay

    (B) CD4 count and viral load to monitor response to therapy

  vi. Treatment:

    (A) HAART protocol: two nucleoside reverse transcriptase inhibitors in combination with a third active antiretroviral drug from one of three drug classes: an integrase strand transfer inhibitor, a nonnucleoside reverse transcriptase inhibitor, or a protease inhibitor with a pharmacokinetic enhancer (cobicistat or ritonavir)

    (B) *Neurological complications of HAART*

> > (1) Nucleoside analog–associated toxic neuropathy
> > > *(a)* Major dose-limiting complication of didanosine, zalcitabine, and stavudine
> > > *(b)* Painful polyneuropathy similar to distal symmetric polyneuropathy
> > > *(c)* Seen in weeks following initiation of therapy, distal sensory polyneuropathy (DSPN) progresses over months
> > > *(d)* Stopping the offending agent stops progression or causes regression of symptoms.
> > > *(e)* Preexisting DSPN increases risk.
> > (2) Zidovudine myopathy
> > > *(a)* Proximal muscle weakness and myalgia similar to HIV myopathy
> > > *(b)* Due to mitochondrial toxicity from zidovudine
> > > *(c)* Develops after about 6 months of therapy
> > > *(d)* Symptoms improve with discontinuing medication.

Summary of Neurologic Complications of HIV

MUSCLE	HIV myopathy
	Zidovudine myopathy
NERVE AND NERVE ROOTS	HIV distal sensory polyneuropathy
	Antiretroviral drug toxic polyneuropathy
	CMV polyradiculopathy
	CIDP
	HIV or HZV cranial neuropathy
	HIV or CMV mononeuropathy multiplex
SPINAL CORD	HIV vacuolar myelopathy
	Myelitis due to VZV, HSV, CMV, *Toxoplasma*

(continued)

Summary of Neurologic Complications of HIV (*cont'd*)

MENINGES	HIV meningitis
	Neurosyphilis
	Tuberculous meningitis
	Cryptococcal meningitis
BRAIN—FOCAL	Bacterial abscess from atypical organisms
	HIV-associated stroke
	Toxoplasmic encephalitis
	Primary CNC lymphoma
	PML
BRAIN—DIFFUSE	HIV-associated dementia
	Postinfectious encephalomyelitis
	CMV encephalitis
	VZV encephalitis

9. *Retroviruses* (*cont'd*)

 c. Oncoviruses

  i. **Human T-cell leukemia virus type 1**

   (A) Clinical features

    (1) Neurological: progressive myelopathy of lower thoracic segments (only 0.25% of human T-cell leukemia virus type 1 infections)

     (a) Progressive spastic paraparesis

     (b) Urinary incontinence

     (c) Variable sensory loss

    (2) Nonneurological: uveitis, infective dermatitis, T-cell lymphoma and leukemia

    (3) Female-to-male ratio of 3:1

   (B) Diagnosis

    (1) Human T-cell leukemia virus type 1–specific IgG in serum or CSF

    (2) PCR (666)

   (C) Transmission via contact with body fluids, sexual transmission, IV drug use, and vertical transmission

   (D) Treatment: symptomatic treatment; corticosteroids may produce some improvement.

III. Encephalitis

 A. Viral encephalitis (See Section II for specific infections.)

 B. Encephalitis due to Rickettsial disease

  1. Infection acquired by the bite or inoculation of infected vector feces into the skin or mucous membranes

  2. Clinical: initial fever, headache, and malaise followed by rash and neurological symptoms

  3. Diagnosis: serology, PCR and immunohistochemical analysis may be helpful.

4. Treatment: immediate empiric treatment with doxycycline

RICKETTSIAL DISEASE	ORGANISM	VECTOR	ANIMAL RESERVOIR
Epidemic typhus	*Rickettsia prowazekii*	Body louse, tick	Humans
Endemic typhus	*Rickettsia typhi*	Flea	Rodents
Rocky Mountain spotted fever	*Rickettsia rickettsii*	Wood tick, *D. andersoni*	Rodents

    a. Typhus group: epidemic typhus, endemic typhus

       i. Neurological symptoms: agitated delirium associated with pyramidal tract signs and neck stiffness followed by seizures and brainstem dysfunction

       ii. May die in week 2 due to peripheral vascular collapse

    b. Spotted fever group: Rocky Mountain spotted fever

       i. Neurologic: headache with agitation followed by progressive lethargy, stupor, and coma; may also develop transverse myelitis, sensory neuropathy, or AIDP-like syndromes

       ii. Other systems: thrombocytopenia, hyponatremia, increased liver function tests and creatinine, myocarditis

    c. Other Rickettsial diseases—Q fever

       i. Caused by *Coxiella burnetii*

       ii. Spreads from animals to humans by inhalation of the infected dust or by handling infected animals; primarily an occupational disease, mainly affecting shepherds and farmers

       iii. Neurologic: rare but may cause severe encephalitis similar to HSV; optic neuritis, CN palsies, AIDP, and *aseptic* meningitis

       iv. Other systems: *lungs*, liver (hepatitis), heart (myocarditis or endocarditis)

IV. Abscess

A. Brain abscess

  1. **Pathophysiology**

    a. Source of infection

       i. Direct extension of sinusitis (40%); otitis, facial infection, or dental infection (5%)

       ii. Generalized septicemia (30%): usually multiple abscesses; seen in pulmonary infections, bacterial endocarditis

       iii. Cryptogenic (20%–25%)

       iv. Penetrating trauma, post-craniotomy

       v. Meningitis

    b. Common organisms: aerobic and anaerobic streptococci, staphylococci, *Bacteroides*, *Enterobacteriaceae*, and anaerobic organisms

    c. Initial cerebritis followed by central necrosis with surrounding vasogenic edema followed by capsule formation

  2. Clinical features

    a. Onset of subacute cases within 1 month of initial manifestation

    b. Fever, headaches, neck stiffness, focal neurological signs (two-thirds of cases), seizures (one-third of cases), altered mentation

2. Clinical features (*cont'd*)

    c. Complications usually arise from increased ICP or abscess rupture, particularly into the ventricles, causing an empyema

    d. Immunocompromised patients and patients with congenital heart disease more susceptible

3. Diagnostic procedures

    a. CT/MRI: ring-enhancing lesion with surrounding edema

    b. Lumbar puncture not done due to risk of herniation and/or rupture of abscess

4. Treatment

    a. Antibiotics: third-generation cephalosporin with metronidazole and vancomycin if *Staphylococcus* suspected

    b. CT-guided stereotactic aspiration or surgical excision

5. *Other types of brain abscess—toxoplasmosis, candida, and aspergillus*

B. Cranial epidural abscess

1. Source of infection: local spread from cranial infection or after trauma or surgery

2. Common organisms: *S. aureus*, aerobes, anaerobes, and gram-negative bacteria

3. Clinical: fever, headache, unilateral focal neurological signs and symptoms

4. Diagnosis: epidural collection on CT and MRI; increased T1 and T2 signal and dural enhancement

5. Treatment: surgical drainage and antibiotics

C. Subdural empyema

1. Source of infection: local spread from cranial infection

2. Common organisms: microaerophilic, aerobic, and anaerobic streptococci

3. Clinical: fever, headache, unilateral signs, encephalopathy due to raised ICP, seizures

4. Diagnosis: crescent-shaped collection on CT and MRI; increased T1 and T2 signal

5. Treatment: surgical drainage and antibiotics

D. Spinal epidural abscess

1. Source of infection: local spread from cranial infection or after trauma or surgery

2. Common organisms: *S. aureus*, aerobes, anaerobes, and gram-negative bacteria

3. Clinical: fever, headache, unilateral focal neurological signs and symptoms

4. Diagnosis: epidural collection on CT and MRI; increased T1 and T2 signal with marked dural enhancement

5. Treatment: surgical drainage and antibiotics

V. Other Bacterial Infections of the Nervous System

A. **Botulism**

1. Pathophysiology

    a. Caused by the neurotoxins of gram-positive spore-forming anaerobes Clostridium botulinum *and, in rare cases,* Clostridium butyricum *and* Clostridium baratii

    b. Eight distinct type of botulism toxins; neurotoxins types A, B, and E are most frequently responsible for disease in humans, whereas types F and G have been reported only occasionally.

  c. Mechanism:

      i. Irreversible binding to the presynaptic membrane of cholinergic nerve endings in the neuromuscular junction, parasympathetic and sympathetic ganglia

      ii. Toxin is internalized.

      iii. Cleaves SNAP-25 (A, C, E), synaptobrevin (B, D, F, G) and syntaxin (C) required for neuroexocytosis of acetylcholine

  d. Three forms

      i. Food-borne botulism—associated with home-canned vegetables

      ii. Wound botulism—injection drug use and trauma

      iii. Infant botulism—most common type, ages 1 week to 11 months; type A and B

2. Clinical features

  a. Adult botulism:

      i. Symptoms 12 to 38 hours after ingestion of food due to ingestion of pre-formed toxin

      ii. Descending weakness from cranial nerves (ptosis, diplopia, blurred vision, dysphagia, and dysarthria) to proximal muscles, including respiratory muscles

      iii. Autonomic symptoms: dilated pupils, dry mouth, urinary retention, ileus, vomiting, abdominal cramping, constipation

  b. Infant botulism:

      i. Ingestion of pathogenic spores with slow production of toxins in the gastrointestinal (GI) tract

      ii. Constipation, lethargy, hypotonia, poor sucking, weak cry, poorly reactive pupils, respiratory distress

      iii. Most patients recover completely within 6 months.

3. Diagnosis

  a. Clinical exam

  b. Electrodiagnostic tests

      i. Nerve conduction study: normal to mildly reduced compound muscle action potential (CMAP)

      ii. Repetitive stimulation: abnormal incremental response

      iii. Single-fiber electromyography (EMG): jitter and blocking

  c. Tensilon® (edrophonium chloride) test: false positive in 30% cases

4. Treatment

  a. Supportive care

  b. Antitoxin: human-derived botulinum immunoglobulin for infants and equine serum botulism antitoxin for children older than 1 year and adults

  c. Antibiotics: penicillin G or metronidazole may be helpful in eradicating *C. botulinum* in wound botulism, after antitoxin has been administered.

B. Brucellosis (Malta fever)

1. Pathophysiology and epidemiology

  a. Facultative intracellular bacilli of the genus *Brucella* (*B. melitensis*, *B. abortus*, *B. suis*, and *B. canis*)

  b. Disease of domestic animals transmitted to humans by close contact with infected animals (through skin abrasions), by contaminated aerosols, or by consumption

B. **Brucellosis (Malta fever)** (*cont'd*)

  2. Pathology

    a. Systemic: primary involvement of lymph nodes, spleen, and bone marrow, but almost every organ may be involved.

    b. Neuropathology: granulomas, demyelination, thickening of leptomeninges, angiitis, mycotic aneurysms, and degeneration of anterior horn cells

  3. Clinical features

    a. Systemic: chills, fever, headache, generalized weakness, muscle pain, and arthralgias with lymphadenopathy

    b. Neurologic: 5% of patients

      i. Usually acute encephalitis with drowsiness, seizures, and signs and symptoms of increased ICP

      ii. Mononeuritis, acute inflammatory polyradiculoneuritis

  4. Diagnosis: brucella microagglutination test; identification in blood or CSF

  5. Prevention: avoid consumption of undercooked meat and unpasteurized dairy products.

  6. Treatment: doxycycline (200 mg/day) plus rifampin (600–900 mg/day); longer duration for neurological involvement

C. **Leprosy (Hansen's disease)**

  1. Pathophysiology and epidemiology

    a. Caused by *Mycobacterium leprae (obligate intracellular acid-fast bacillus)*

    b. Transmitted by *skin-to-skin contact or through nasal secretions of infected individuals*

    c. *M. leprae* only replicates in body areas where the temperature is low (i.e., skin, distal peripheral nerves).

  2. Clinical: differences in the host's susceptibility to infection result in marked differences in the severity of disease.

    a. *Tuberculoid*

      i. Intense cell-mediated immune reaction at the portal of entry reduces organism proliferation but causes circumscribed acute peripheral nerve and skin damage.

      ii. Skin lesions: well demarcated hypopigmented anesthetic lesions on face, arm, chest

      iii. Thickened nerves and asymmetric neuropathy: ulnar = claw-hand, radial = wristdrop, peroneal = footdrop, and/or facial nerves

    b. *Borderline forms*: borderline tuberculoid, borderline intermediate and borderline lepromatous

    c. *Lepromatous*

      i. Do not mount an adequate immune reaction and more generalized

      ii. Skin lesions poorly demarcated

      iii. Thickened nerves and peripheral neuropathy with symmetric loss of pain and temperature sensations in the distal portions of the extremities and relative preservation of deep sensation

      iv. Anesthetic hands are prone to repeated trauma and infection, leading to ulcerated skin lesions, bone destruction, finger loss, and deformities.

      v. Trigeminal nerve involvement leads to facial hypoalgesia with associated corneal ulcerations and blindness.

  3. Diagnosis: identification of *M. leprae* in skin smears, full-thickness edge biopsy of active skin lesions, nasal smear or peripheral nerve biopsy

4. Treatment: multidrug therapy (MDT)

    a. Paucibacillary: rifampin (600 mg/day) and dapsone (100 mg/day) for 6 months

    b. Multibacillary: clofazimine (50–300 mg/day), rifampin (600 mg/day), and dapsone (100 mg/day) for 2 years

D. Tuberculosis

1. Pathophysiology and epidemiology

    a. Causative organism: gram-positive aerobic bacterium *Mycobacterium tuberculosis*

    b. Transmission: droplet infection, hematogenous spread to extrapyramidal sites

    c. Increased incidence due to HIV

2. Neurological manifestations

    a. Subacute to chronic meningitis:

        i. Most common CNS presentation

        ii. Usually basilar meningitis causing fever, headache, neck stiffness, cranial neuropathies, and altered mentation; seizures can also occur.

        iii. Complications: hydrocephalus and strokes due to vascular involvement of leptomeningeal inflammation.

    b. Parenchymal tuberculosis:

        i. Tuberculoma (central caseating necrosis with collagenous capsule of mononuclear inflammatory cells) or tuberculoid abscess (liquefactive necrosis with neutrophilic infiltrate)

        ii. Cerebral or cerebellar parenchyma and deep gray matter

        iii. Causes headaches, focal neurological deficits, seizures, papilledema, increased ICP

        iv. Very rarely causes tuberculous encephalopathy with diffuse edema and extensive demyelination

    c. Spinal tuberculous meningitis

        i. Rare, causes subacute or chronic radiculomyelitis

    d. Spinal tuberculomas—intramedullary lesions causing myelopathy

    e. Vertebral disease (Pott's disease) <1%

        i. Tuberculous infection of lower thoracic and lumbar vertebral bodies and intervertebral discs, causing collapse of vertebrae

        ii. Causes marked spondylosis with neural foramen and spinal canal stenosis

        iii. Fever, weight loss, progressive back pain, paraspinal muscle spasms

        iv. Involvement of paravertebral tissues can cause abscess; retropharyngeal abscess in cervical spine involvement.

3. Diagnosis:

    a. Tuberculin skin test followed by further testing if positive; blood tests—interferon gamma release assays (QuantiFERON® TB Gold In-Tube test or T-SPOT®).

    b. CSF in tuberculous meningitis:

        i. Lymphocytic pleocytosis, decreased glucose and increased protein

        ii. CSF PCR: sensitivity = 54% to 100%; specificity = 94% to 100%

        iii. CSF amplified *M. tuberculosis* direct test—nucleic acid test, rapidly available

        iv. CSF tests may be negative in only parenchymal disease.

    c. Neuroimaging

        i. Meningitis: meningeal enhancement of the basal cisterns

        ii. Tuberculomas: isointense on T1, central hyperintensity on T2 with ring enhancement and surrounding edema; calcifications in mature lesions

    c. Neuroimaging (*cont'd*)

        iii. Radiculomyelitis: meningeal enhancement; clumping and enhancement of nerve roots

        iv. Pott's disease: hypointense marrow on T1 with hyperintensity on T2, enhancement of dura, discs; epidural or paraspinal fluid collection; may have evidence of cord compression

  4. Treatment:

    a. Antituberculous therapy

        i. Intensive phase for 2 months with isoniazid, rifampin, pyrazinamide, and either fluoroquinolone or injectable aminoglycoside

        ii. Continuation phase for 9 to 12 months with isoniazid and rifampin

    b. *Glucocorticoids*: controversial in treatment of tuberculous meningitis

    c. Surgical treatment:

        i. Surgical decompression in hydrocephalus

        ii. Surgical resection of tuberculoma if diagnosis uncertain or if poor response to medical management

        iii. Spine surgery if progressive symptoms, instability, or poor response to medical management

E. Rheumatic fever

  1. Causative organism: *Group A β-hemolytic streptococci*

  2. Clinical features

    a. Systemic: 1 to 5 weeks after an acute episode of streptococcal pharyngitis; acute migratory polyarthritis, subacute/chronic carditis, subcutaneous nodules and erythema marginatum, congestive heart failure, and valvular heart disease

    b. Neurologic complications

        i. Delirium, seizures

        ii. Embolic stroke due to valvular disease

        iii. Sydenham's chorea:

            (A) Occurs in children, female-to-male ratio of 2:1.

            (B) Usually months after initial infection

            (C) Symptoms: chorea, ballismus, hypotonia, and dysarthria; psychiatric symptoms of irritability, emotional lability, obsessive-compulsive symptoms

            (D) Treatment: oral corticosteroids; valproate and carbamazepine; pimozide or haloperidol if refractory

F. Whipple's disease

  1. Pathophysiology

    a. Caused by *Tropheryma whippelii*

    b. Impaired cell-mediated immunity

    c. Pathology: *infiltration of tissues with foamy macrophages containing periodic acid–Schiff-positive bacilli in the cytoplasm (rectal or jejunal biopsy)*

  2. Clinical features

    a. Systemic: chronic migratory arthralgias; GI tract involvement—abdominal pain, diarrhea with steatorrhea, weight loss; cutaneous hypopigmentation; adrenal insufficiency

    b. Neurological manifestations in 10% to 15% (can present with isolated CNS symptoms)

      i. Triad

        (A) Slowly progressive dementia

        (B) Supranuclear vertical-gaze palsy

        (C) Myoclonic jerks

     ii. Other manifestations

        (A) Oculomasticatory myorhythmia (OMM) and oculofacial-skeletal myorhythmia (OFSM): seen in 20% of cases, pathognomonic of Whipple's disease

           (1) Due to hypothalamic involvement

           (2) Pendular vergence oscillations of the eyes with synchronous rhythmic contractions of the masticatory muscles; can involve proximal and distal skeletal muscles

        (B) Meningitis

        (C) Dysarthria, ataxia

        (D) Deafness, tinnitus

        (E) Seizures

        (F) Visual field loss, motor deficits

        (G) Neuropathy

        (H) Myopathy

3. Diagnosis:

   a. Periodic acid–Schiff-positive macrophage inclusions in biopsy of gastrointestinal (GI) tract

   b. CSF PCR for *T. whippelii* DNA if suspected

4. Treatment

   a. Antibiotics: penicillin G (12–24 million u/day) and ceftriaxone (50–100 mg/kg/day) for 2 to 4 weeks in the initial phase followed by trimethoprim (320 mg) and sulfamethoxazole (1,600 mg) for 1 year in the maintenance phase

   b. Symptomatic treatment of myoclonus, OMM, OFSM: valproate and benzodiazepines

VI. Spirochete Infections of the Nervous System

A. Lyme disease

  1. Pathophysiology

    a. Caused by *Borrelia burgdorferi*

    b. Vector: deer tick *Ixodes dammini*

    c. Early summer most common

  2. Clinical features

    a. Primary stage (within 4 weeks of tick bite): erythema chronicum migrans, constitutional symptoms

    b. Secondary stage (weeks after rash): systemic with cardiac arrhythmias, arthralgia, lymphadenopathy; neurological manifestations:

      i. Aseptic meningitis

      ii. Encephalitis

      iii. Cranial neuropathy—most commonly lower motor neuron (LMN) facial nerve palsy, unilateral or bilateral

      iv. Mononeuritis multiplex, peripheral neuropathy, polyradiculopathy, AIDP

    c. Tertiary stage (months after secondary): neuropathy, encephalomyelitis, dementia

A. **Lyme disease** (*cont'd*)

   3. Diagnosis: enzyme immunoassay or immunofluorescence assay, if equivocal or positive test for serum antibodies; CSF antibodies for neuroborreliosis; MRI may show leptomeningeal enhancement.

   4. Treatment of neuroborreliosis: IV ceftriaxone or penicillin G for 2 to 4 weeks

B. **Syphilis**

   1. Pathophysiology

     a. Caused by *Treponema pallidum*

     b. Transmitted by sexual contact and vertical transmission

   2. Clinical

     a. Primary syphilis: painless genital chancre with asymptomatic systemic spread

     b. Secondary syphilis:

       i. 2 to 12 weeks after exposure

       ii. Systemic dissemination with constitutional symptoms, lymphadenopathy, and rash

       iii. Syphilitic meningitis and cranial neuropathies

     c. Latent phase: asymptomatic

     d. Tertiary syphilis: cardiovascular and delayed neurological complications of tabes dorsalis or dementia

   3. Neurological manifestations <10%

     a. Meningeal and meningovascular syphilis

       i. Meningeal invasion with endarteritis obliterans and vasculitis, causing strokes

       ii. Usually occurs in 4 to 7 years

     b. Tabes dorsalis

       i. Myelopathy symptoms: areflexia, loss of pain and temperature, sensory ataxia, and Charcot's joints

     c. Parenchymatous syphilis

       i. Encephalitic form with progressive dementia, psychiatric disorders, speech disturbance, pupillary abnormalities (Argyll–Robertson pupils—accommodation present; light reflex absent)

   4. Diagnosis

     a. Use both serum nontreponemal and treponemal tests to avoid false positives.

     b. Non-treponemal tests: Venereal Disease Research Laboratory (VDRL) or rapid plasma reagin (RPR)

     c. Treponemal tests: fluorescent treponemal antibody absorbed (FTA-ABS), *Treponema pallidum* particle agglutination assay (TP-PA), syphilis enzyme immunoassay (EIA), immunoblot, or rapid assays

     d. If serum test is positive and neurosyphilis suspected, CSF VDRL should be done.

     e. CSF lymphocytic pleocytosis and/or elevated protein should be treated as neurosyphilis even when CSF VDRL is negative if serum tests are positive.

   5. Treatment of neurosyphilis

     a. IV penicillin G 4 million units q 4 hours for 14 days

     b. Repeat CSF analysis to assess response to therapy.

VII. Fungal Infections of the Nervous System

A. Cryptococcosis

1. Pathophysiology

   a. Caused by *Cryptococcus neoformans*

   b. Spread by respiratory droplet; found in soil and bird feces

   c. Opportunistic infections of cell-mediated immunity (AIDS, lymphoreticular malignancy, chronic steroids)

   d. Most common CNS fungal infection

2. Clinical

   a. Chronic basilar meningitis

      i. Fever, headache, neck stiffness, encephalopathy, behavioral changes, seizures, cranial neuropathies due to basilar meningitis

      ii. Complications: infarctions, hydrocephalus

   b. Cryptococcomas, gelatinous pseudocysts: focal neurological deficits

3. Diagnosis:

   a. CSF

      i. Elevated CSF opening pressure, lymphocytic pleocytosis, increased protein and low glucose

      ii. CSF and serum cryptococcal capsular polysaccharide antigen, CSF fungal cultures (high sensitivity and specificity)

   b. MRI brain:

      i. Leptomeningeal enhancement in meningitis

      ii. "Soap bubble" appearance of gelatinous pseudocysts with hypointense/indeterminate on T1 and FLAIR, hyperintense on T2

      iii. Cryptococcomas: hypointense on T1, hyperintense on T2 and FLAIR with variable enhancement

4. Treatment

   a. Antibiotics

      i. Amphotericin B (0.7 mg/kg/day) plus flucytosine (100 mg/kg/day) for 2 weeks, followed by fluconazole (400 mg/day) or itraconazole (400 mg/day) for 8 weeks

      ii. Long-term maintenance therapy with fluconazole to prevent recurrence

   b. Surgical management for hydrocephalus

B. Aspergillosis

1. Pathophysiology

   a. Aspergillus fumigatus *(85%–90% of cases): septated hyphae*

   b. Acquired by inhalation of airborne spores

   c. CNS infection by hematogenous spread or through contiguous structures

   d. May occur in immunocompetent hosts but usually opportunistic infection

   e. Pathology: angioinvasive hyphae in blood vessels, causing inflammation and necrosis

2. Clinical

   a. *Aspergillus meningitis* with cranial neuropathies (rare)

   b. Vasculitis due to angioinvasion, causing strokes and parenchymal and subarachnoid hemorrhages

2. Clinical (*cont'd*)

   c. Parenchymal disease, causing granulomas and abscesses

   d. Multiple organs involved

   e. Mortality: 80% to 90%

3. Imaging: CT/MRI—mass lesions with minimal mass effect or contrast enhancement

4. Treatment:

   a. IV voriconazole with liposomal amphotericin or posaconazole for secondary therapy

   b. Consider resection for diagnosis and/or treatment.

C. Candidiasis

1. Pathophysiology

   a. Various species of *Candida*

   b. Typically opportunistic infection

   c. Most cases of CNS candidiasis are caused by *Candida albicans.*

2. Neurologic

   a. Meningitis

   b. Parenchymal microabscesses

   c. Granulomas

   d. Angioinvasive, causing infarcts and subarachnoid and parenchymal hemorrhages

3. Treatment: induction of IV lipid-formulation amphotericin with or without flucytosine intravenously for several weeks followed by maintenance with fluconazole until resolution of imaging and CSF abnormalities

D. Coccidioidomycosis

1. Pathophysiology

   a. Caused by *Coccidioides immitis*

   b. Inhabits dry acidic soil endemic in southwestern United States

   c. Inhalation of arthroconidia that is transformed into nonbudding spherules composed of hundreds of endospores

   d. Elicits a caseating granulomatous reaction

   e. CNS involvement occurs in <1%.

2. Neurologic: arachnoiditis, chronic basilar meningitis, brain abscesses

3. Diagnosis: serum and CSF enzyme-linked immunosorbent assay (ELISA) and CSF complement fixation

4. Treatment:

   a. Oral fluconazole or itraconazole with or without intrathecal amphotericin B followed by lifelong azole therapy after normalization of CSF

   b. Surgical management for hydrocephalus

E. Mucormycosis (zygomycosis)

1. Pathophysiology

   a. Rhizopus arrhizus (*90% of cases with CNS involvement*)

   b. Inhabits soil, plants, and certain foods in a mold form

   c. Infection acquired by the inhalation of airborne spores or through direct inoculation of fungi into subcutaneous tissue or bloodstream

   d. Risk factors: diabetic ketoacidosis or acidemia from other causes, malignancies, immunosuppression, organ transplant, iron chelation therapy

   e. Pathology: *broad hyphae invade arteries and veins, causing tissue necrosis.*

2. Clinical

    a. Rhinocerebral form usually begins with fever and a painful swelling of the nose and fronto-orbital area, which rapidly progresses to the striking necrotic lesions.

    b. Sinusitis

    c. Orbital cellulitis

    d. Vascular thrombosis with stroke

    e. Venous sinus thrombosis, most frequently cavernous sinus

    f. Focal CNS involvement via direct extension of infection

    g. Usually fatal disease

3. Treatment

    a. Surgical debridement of necrotic tissue

    b. Amphotericin B, 1.5 mg/kg/day intravenously, for a total dose of 1.0 to 1.5 g; renal function and serum potassium levels should be closely monitored.

F. Blastomycosis

1. Pathophysiology

    a. Caused by *Blastomyces dermatitidis*

    b. Infection acquired by inhalation of spores found in soil and vegetation in Midwest United States

    c. Can cause disease readily in immunocompetent host

    d. Pathology: affects lungs, skin, bones, retina, urinary tract, and CNS (25% of patients)

2. Clinical

    a. Systemic: nonspecific fever, malaise

    b. Neurologic in one-third of disseminated disease

        i. Meningitis with neutrophilic pleocytosis

        ii. Blastomycomas/abscess in brain or spine

        iii. Cranial neuropathies due to skull-base lytic lesions; vertebral osteolytic lesions

3. Treatment: induction with IV liposomal or standard amphotericin for 4 to 6 weeks followed by maintenance therapy with oral azole for >12 months and resolution of CSF abnormalities

G. Histoplasmosis

1. Pathophysiology

    a. Caused by *Histoplasma capsulatum*

    b. Acquire the infection by inhalation of aerosolized contaminated soil or bird and bat droppings; endemic in Mississippi and Ohio River valleys

    c. Usually self-limiting

2. Clinical

    a. Systemic: hepatosplenomegaly, lymphadenopathy, diffuse pulmonary infiltrates, mucosal ulcerations

    b. Neurologic: subacute meningitis and abscesses

3. Diagnosis: CSF *Histoplasma* polysaccharide antigen test

4. Treatment: induction with IV lipid-formulation amphotericin for 4 to 6 weeks followed by maintenance therapy with oral azole for >12 months and resolution of CSF abnormalities, including *Histoplasma* antigen

VIII. Prion Infections of the Nervous System

- Incidence of human prion disease (PrD) is 1 to 1.5 per 1,000,000/ year.

- Normal cellular prion protein PrP^C is transformed to PrP^{Sc}

- 85% = sporadic; 10% to 15% = genetic; <1% = acquired

- Sporadic Creutzfeldt–Jakob disease (sCJD)

- Genetic prion disease (gPrD) occurs due to mutation of PRNP gene encoding prion protein PrP.

  o The three clinico-pathological forms are familial CJD (fCJD), Gerstmann–Sträussler–Scheinker syndrome (GSSS), and fatal familial insomnia (FFI).

  o Mostly autosomal dominant

  o Younger age at onset

  o Insidious course

- Iatrogenic form: cadaver-derived growth hormone, corneal transplants, neurosurgical procedures

- New variant CJD: transmitted from ingestion of cattle products contaminated with agent of bovine spongiform encephalopathy

A. **Creutzfeldt–Jakob disease (CJD)**

  1. Clinical features of sCJD

     a. Usual age at onset is 60s.

     b. Rapidly progressive dementia, neuropsychiatric features, cerebellar ataxia, and myoclonus

     c. >90% mortality within 1 year

  2. Diagnosis

     a. Definitive diagnosis: detecting CJD-specific mutations by prion gene analysis

     b. 14-3-3 protein in CSF: in the appropriate setting, 94% sensitivity and 93% specificity

     c. Pathology: diffuse spongiform encephalopathy with widespread neuronal loss, gliosis, and amyloid plaques

     d. EEG: 80% periodic sharp wave complexes by 12 weeks, which evolve to diffuse slowing

     e. MRI: increased T2 signal in basal ganglia and thalamus; in some CJD variants can see *pulvinar sign*. Hyperintensity in anterior putamen and caudate head is known as the *hockey-stick sign*.

     f. May show cortical ribboning in diffusion-weighted MRI in parietal, occipital, or temporal regions

B. **Gerstmann–Sträussler–Scheinker syndrome**

  1. Clinical features

     a. Begins in third to fourth decade

     b. Slowly progressive over 3 to 8 years

     c. Subacute progressive ataxia/parkinsonian disorder with later-onset cognitive impairment

     d. Mortality within 1 to 10 years

  2. Diagnosis

     a. EEG: diffuse slowing

     b. MRI: cerebellar atrophy or T2 prolongation involving the basal ganglia (iron deposition) *c.* Confirmed by detection of prion gene mutations; P102L is most common

    d. Pathology: spongiform changes are seen; *Kuru-like* plaques in cerebellum and other areas.

C. Fatal familial insomnia

  1. Clinical features

    a. Progressive insomnia, sympathetic hyperactivity, and mental status changes

    b. Typically begins between ages 30 and 60

    c. Death within 6 to 36 months of onset

    d. Loss of circadian rhythm with insomnia to $<$2 hours; behavioral changes, including inattention, poor concentration and memory, hallucinations; dementia is rare. Later, myoclonus, ataxia, spasticity, and parkinsonian features can be seen. Endocrine disturbances are also seen.

    e. Neurophysiologic and polysomnographic features

      i. EEG: diffuse slowing

      ii. Polysomnography: physiologic sleep is absent or decreased to only a few minutes' duration; brief REM sleep may occur but usually has incomplete muscle atonia and may have dream-enacting behavior late in course; myoclonic jerks may accompany periodic slow waves (similar to CJD).

  2. Diagnosis

    a. MRI: normal

    b. Fluorodeoxyglucose (FDG) PET: thalamic and cingulate hypometabolism

    c. Pathology: spongiform degeneration with severe neuronal loss and reactive gliosis in anterior and dorsomedial thalamic nuclei

    d. DNA: single-point mutation of PRNP (prion protein) D178N/129M

D. Kuru

  1. Pathophysiology and epidemiology

    a. Tribes in New Guinea (particularly in women and children) secondary to consumption of brain and/or mucosal and cutaneous contact with neural tissues

    b. Long incubation period ($>$5–20 years)

    c. Genetics: homozygosity for methionine at codon 129 is a risk factor.

  2. Clinical

    a. Dysarthria, gait ataxia, truncal instability, titubation and postural

    b. Emotional lability, psychomotor retardation, and uncontrollable laughter

  3. Diagnosis/pathology: neuronal loss highest in cerebellum, basal ganglia, thalamus, and mesial temporal lobes; PrP^{Sc} reactive plaques called Kuru plaques at highest density in the cerebellum.

  4. Prognosis: death within 1 year

IX. Parasitic Infections of the Nervous System

A. Primary amebic meningoencephalitis

  1. Caused by *Naegleria fowleri* that inhabits soil and water (especially warm climates)

  2. Infections are linked to freshwater swimming between July and August

  3. Enters the nasal cavity and migrates through cribriform plate via olfactory nerves to the frontal lobes

A. **Primary amebic meningoencephalitis** (*cont'd*)

    4. Pathology: purulent meningitis with microabscesses and extensive necrotizing destruction of parenchyma

    5. Clinical:

        a. Severe headache, fever, nausea, vomiting, meningeal signs, seizures, hallucinations, altered consciousness progressing to coma

        b. Rapidly progressive, with mortality >97%

    6. Diagnosis:

        a. CSF shows elevated opening pressure, neutrophilic pleocytosis, increased protein, and decreased glucose.

        b. Motile trophozoites in CSF on wet mount; negative Gram stain

    7. Treatment: supportive only

B. **Cerebral amebiasis**

    1. Caused by *Entamoeba histolytica*

        a. Common intestinal parasite

        b. Infects almost 10% of the world population, causing 100,000 deaths every year

        c. May become aggressive and enter the bloodstream to cause systemic disease and CNS involvement; can cause amebic brain abscess.

    2. Clinical: fever, altered mentation, focal neurological signs, seizures

    3. Diagnosis:

        a. Parasites in fresh-mount preparations of stool

        b. Antibody detection useful in extraintestinal disease—EIA test

    4. Treatment

        a. Metronidazole or tinidazole followed by paromomycin or iodoquinol

        b. Surgical resection of accessible lesions

C. **Toxoplasmosis**

    1. Caused by *Toxoplasma gondii* (intracellular parasite)

    2. Humans are infected by eating undercooked meat or by ingestion of contaminated cat feces.

    3. Seropositive in 30% to 75% of the general population, varies by country

    4. *Congenital toxoplasmosis*

        a. Transmission of the infection from mother to fetus when women acquire the infection during pregnancy

        b. Clinical: hydrocephalus, microcephalus, intracranial calcifications, mental retardation, seizures, deafness, blindness, and hepatomegaly

        c. CT: periventricular or diffuse parenchymal calcification

    5. *Acquired toxoplasmosis*

        a. May occur in immunocompetent (usually asymptomatic and without CNS involvement) or immunocompromised (frequent opportunistic infection)

        b. Clinical: acute mass lesion with focal signs or subacute encephalitis

        c. MRI brain: multiple ring-enhancing lesions with surrounding edema (diffuse focal lesions with predilection for basal ganglia and deep gray matter); differentiate from primary CNS lymphoma (PCNSL).

    6. Pathology: cerebral abscesses consisting of a necrotic center and a periphery in which multiple tachyzoites and cysts are seen together with patchy areas of necrosis, perivascular cuffing of lymphocytes, and glial nodules composed of astrocytes and microglial cells

7. Diagnosis:

   a. Definite diagnosis requires biopsy; not commonly performed.

   b. CSF (contraindicated if mass lesion) lymphocytic pleocytosis, increased protein; PCR very specific (>95%), not sensitive (50%–60%)

8. Treatment

   a. Cerebral toxoplasmosis: pyrimethamine (100–200 mg the first day, followed by 50–75 mg/day) plus sulfadiazine (4–6 g/day) for >2 months

   b. Supplement with folate, 8 to 10 mg/day, to avoid the toxic effects of pyrimethamine.

   c. Clindamycin (2,400 mg/day) is an alternative drug in AIDS patients developing skin reactions to sulfadiazine.

D. Trypanosomiasis

1. *Chagas disease (American trypanosomiasis)*

   a. Caused by *Trypanosoma cruzi*

   b. Found in southern United States, Central and South America

   c. Transmitted by the bite of *Triatoma* (reduviid or kissing bug)

   d. Clinical

      i. Acute stage: meningoencephalitis (more common in children with HIV) with multiple areas of hemorrhagic necrosis, glial proliferation, and perivascular infiltrates of inflammatory cells; myocarditis and hepatosplenomegaly

      ii. Chronic stage: dilated cardiomyopathy, cardioembolic stroke due to heart disease, megacolon, and megaesophagus

   e. Diagnosis: microscopic examination of thin and thick blood smear demonstrate the parasite in the acute phase.

   f. Treatment

      i. Nifurtimox (8–10 mg/kg/day) or benznidazole (5–10 mg/kg/day)

2. *Sleeping sickness (African trypanosomiasis)*

   a. Caused by subspecies of *Trypanosoma brucei* transmitted by *tsetse fly*

   b. Clinical features

      i. Painful erythematous nodules associated with regional lymphadenopathy that disappear spontaneously

      ii. Stage I (lasting months): *Winterbottom's sign*—fever, cervical lymphadenopathy, and hepatosplenomegaly

      iii. Stage II (lasting years): meningoencephalitis—somnolence, apathy, involuntary movements, cerebellar ataxia, delayed hyperesthesia with eventual progression to dementia, stupor, coma, and death if untreated

   c. Diagnosis: clinical signs, parasites in body fluids; CSF exam for Stage II

   d. Treatment

      i. Stage I: pentamidine or suramin

      ii. Stage II: melarsoprol, eflornithine, combination of nifurtimox and eflornithine

E. Cysticercosis

1. Humans are intermediate hosts of the pork tapeworm *Taenia solium.*

2. Acquired by ingesting its eggs from contaminated water/food or by the fecal–oral route

3. After 1 to 3 months, eggs hatch into oncospheres in the human intestine that cross the intestinal wall into the bloodstream and spread mainly to the eye, skeletal muscles, and the CNS, where the larvae (cysticercus) develop.

E. **Cysticercosis** (*cont'd*)

4. Considered the most common helminthic disease of the CNS in the developing world

5. Clinical

   a. Seizures

      i. Most common presentation

      ii. Most common cause of epilepsy in Central America

   b. Focal neurologic deficits from CNS lesions

   c. Vasculitic type: strokes, increased ICP, headaches, hydrocephalus, and (rarely) coma

6. Neuroimaging

   i. Migrating intraventricular cyst is pathognomonic.

   ii. Cystic lesions with or without contrast enhancement and surrounding edema; cysts can be meningobasal, parenchymal, or intraventricular.

   iii. Parenchymal calcification, hydrocephalus, leptomeningeal enhancement

7. Treatment

   a. Calcified lesions: symptomatic treatment only (i.e., antiepileptic drugs)

   b. Viable cysts

      i. Albendazole (10 mg/kg/day divided in 2 doses) for 15 days; better CNS penetration, more effective cyst destruction

      ii. Praziquantel (t3 doses of 25–30 mg/kg given every 2 hours)

      iii. If >50 cysts or with subarachnoid or ventricular involvement, treat for increased ICP/edema prior to initiation of antihelminthics.

   c. Surgical management for hydrocephalus

F. **Trichinosis/Trichinellosis**

1. Intestinal nematode infection due to ingestion of undercooked pork containing encysted larvae of *Trichinella spiralis.*

2. After initial gastroenteritis, may have invasion of skeletal muscle, but weakness is mainly limited to muscles innervated by CNs (e.g., tongue, masseters, extraocular muscle, oropharynx)

3. Rarely, in acute phase may have cerebral symptoms due to emboli from trichinella myocarditis

4. Diagnosis:

   a. Serology positive after 2 to 3 weeks: indirect hemagglutination, indirect immunofluorescence, ELISA

   b. CSF: eosinophilic meningitis may be present, larvae seen in 8% to 24% of patients.

   c. Muscle biopsy: rarely done

5. Neuroimaging: may reveal 3- to 8-mm nodular ring-like lesions

6. Treatment

   a. Prevents systemic invasion when given within 1 week of ingestion

      i. Albendazole, mebendazole, or thiabendazole, 25 mg/kg bid

      ii. Add prednisone, 40 to 60 mg/day, to decrease inflammatory response if hemodynamic instability, CNS, cardiac, or pulmonary involvement.

CHEAT SHEET

Rabies	Negri bodies, Babès nodules
Progressive multifocal leukoencephalopathy	Multifocal confluent T2 subcortical white matter, JC virus
Subacute sclerosing panencephalitis (SSPE)	Persistent measles infection in brain
Adult botulism	Descending weakness from cranial nerves, autonomic symptoms with dilated pupils
Leprosy	Hansen's disease, tuberculoid, borderline, lepromatous
Pott's disease	Tuberculosis (TB) of spine
Whipple's disease	Oculomasticatory myorhythmia and oculofacial-skeletal myorhythmia
Mucormycosis	Cavernous sinus fungal infection in diabetics
Creutzfeldt–Jacob disease	MRI pulvinar sign, hockey-stick sign, cortical ribboning

Suggested Readings

García-Moncó, JC, ed. *CNS Infections: A Clinical Approach*. New York: Springer;2014.

von Geldern G, Nath A. Central nervous system infections. In: Demaerschalk B, ed. *Evidence-Based Neurology: Management of Neurological Disorders*. 2nd ed., London, England: BMJ Books;2015:131.

CHAPTER 15

Neurotoxicology and Nutritional Disorders

I. Heavy Metals

A. Arsenic

1. Pathophysiology: a primary source is pesticides; reacts with sulfhydryl groups of proteins and interferes with several steps of metabolism in the neuron, producing dying-back-type axonal degeneration, particularly in myelinated fibers

2. Clinical

   a. Axonal sensory neuropathy begins within 5 to 10 days.

   b. *Acute gastrointestinal symptoms followed by painful paresthesia with progressive distal weakness*

   c. Central nervous system (CNS) symptoms may develop rapidly in acute poisoning, with drowsiness and confusion progressing to stupor or delirium.

   d. Hyperkeratosis and sloughing of the skin on the palms and soles may occur several weeks after acute poisoning, followed by a chronic state of redness and swelling of the distal extremities.

   e. *Nail changes (Mees' lines)*

   f. Chronic poisoning may develop aplastic anemia.

3. Diagnosis

   a. Acute intoxication: renal excretion greater than 0.1 mg arsenic in 24 hours

   b. Chronic intoxication: hair concentrations greater than 0.1 mg/100 g of hair

4. *Treatment*

   a. *Acute oral ingestion*

      i. *Gastric lavage followed by instillation of 1% sodium thiosulfate*

      ii. *British anti-Lewisite (BAL) given parenterally in a 10% solution*

5. Prognosis

   a. Once neuropathy occurs, treatment is usually ineffective.

   b. Mortality: greater than 50% to 75% in severe cases

B. Gold

1. Pathophysiology: used in the treatment of inflammatory conditions

2. Clinical

   a. Chronic distal axonal sensory neuropathy more common than motor neuropathy

   b. Painful, involving palms or soles

   c. Myokymia

   d. Brachial plexopathy

   e. Acute inflammatory demyelinating polyradiculopathy

B. **Gold** (*cont'd*)

   3. Pathology: loss of myelin as well as active axonal degeneration

   4. Treatment: chelation therapy with BAL has been used but usually is not necessary.

C. **Mercury**

   1. Clinical

      a. Acute: salivation and severe gastrointestinal dysfunction followed by hallucinations and delirium

      b. Chronic

         i. Chronic axonal sensory neuropathy

         ii. Constriction of visual fields, ataxia, dysarthria, decreased hearing, tremor, and dementia

         iii. Parkinsonism

         iv. Children may have acrodynia.

      c. Minamata disease: methylmercury (MeHg) poisoning from ingestion of fish and shellfish contaminated by MeHg discharged in waste water; typical symptoms include sensory disturbances (glove and stocking type), ataxia, dysarthria, constriction of the visual field, auditory disturbances, and tremor

   2. Treatment

      a. Chelating agents (e.g., D-penicillamine, BAL, ethylenediaminetetraacetic acid)

D. **Thallium**

   1. Pathophysiology: found in rat poison; thallium ions act interchangeably with potassium in respect to their transport by the Na/K ATPase system.

   2. Clinical

      a. Hallmark: alopecia; sometimes with cranial nerve and autonomic involvement

      b. Acute

         i. Gastrointestinal symptoms within hours of ingestion

         ii. Moderate doses produce neuropathic symptoms in less than 48 hours consisting of pain and paresthesia, followed by ascending sensory loss and distal weakness.

         iii. May produce acute inflammatory demyelinating polyradiculopathy–like syndrome

         iv. Large doses (>2 g) produce cardiovascular shock, coma, and death within 24 hours.

      c. Chronic: chronic axonal sensorimotor neuropathy

   3. Treatment

      a. Chelating agents

         i. Prussian blue (potassium ferric hexacyanoferrate)

         ii. BAL

         iii. Dithizone

         iv. Diethyldithiocarbamate

      b. If acute, can also perform gastric lavage

E. **Lead**

   1. Pathophysiology

      a. Diminishes cerebral glucose supplies

      b. Intoxication results in inhibition of myelin synthesis with demyelination.

> **NB:** Lead has direct effects on porphyrin metabolism, by inhibiting gamma-aminolevulinic acid dehydrase.

    c. Adults

       i. Use of exterior paints and gasoline

       ii. More likely to present with neuropathy, **predominantly, but not exclusively, the radial nerve**

    d. Children

       i. Pica and eating lead-based paints

       ii. **More likely to present with encephalopathy**

  2. Clinical

    a. Neuropathy

       i. *Chronic axonal motor neuropathy*

       ii. *Classic neurologic presentation: wrist drop (Radial nerve palsy)*

       iii. *Typical clinical triad*

          (A) *Abdominal pain and constipation*

          (B) *Anemia*

          (C) *Neuropathy*

    b. CNS toxicity

       i. Adult

          (A) Prodrome: progressive weakness and loss of weight

          (B) Ashen color of the face

          (C) Mild persistent headache

          (D) Fine tremor of the muscles of the eyes, tongue, and face

          (E) Progression into encephalopathic state

          (F) May have focal motor weakness

       ii. *Children: prodrome usually nonspecific evolving into encephalopathy (50%)*

  3. *Diagnosis*

    a. **Lead lines on gums (also known as Burtonian line)—stippled blue line seen in 50% to 70% of patients with chronic lead poisoning**

    b. **Serum: microcytic anemia and red blood cell basophilic stippling**

    c. **x-rays: may demonstrate lead lines of long bones**

  4. Treatment

    a. Chelating agents (e.g., BAL, ethylenediaminetetraacetic acid, penicillamine)

  5. Prognosis

    a. Mild intoxication: usually complete recovery

    b. Severe encephalopathy: mortality high but lessened by the use of combined chelating agent therapy

    c. Residual neurologic sequelae: blindness or partial visual disturbances, persistent convulsions, personality changes, and mental retardation

    d. Prognosis worse in children than in adults

F. **Manganese**

  1. Pathology: diffuse injury to ganglion cells, *primarily of* **globus pallidus**

  2. Clinical

    a. ***Extrapyramidal signs/symptoms**, including dystonia, bradykinesia, tremor, and gait dysfunction*

2. Clinical (*cont'd*)

    b. Personality changes consisting of irritability, lack of sociability, uncontrollable laughter, tearfulness, and euphoria

3. Treatment: supportive therapy

G. Iron

    1. Acute iron toxicity

        a. Symptoms occur within 30 to 60 minutes.

        b. Initially, bloody vomiting followed by bloody diarrhea

        c. Severe cases: coma or convulsions

        d. Treatment

            i. Supportive care: induction of vomiting, gastric lavage, maintenance of adequate ventilation, correction of acidosis, and control of vital signs

            ii. Chelation: deferoxamine, 5 to 10 g

        e. Mortality: 45%

    2. Iron deficiency can lead to restless leg syndrome.

H. **Tin: Triethyltin exposure acutely results in white-matter vacuolation; with chronic exposure, demyelination and gliosis are seen.**

II. Organic Solvents

A. **Methyl alcohol (e.g., methanol, wood alcohol)**

    1. Pathophysiology

        a. Component of antifreeze and alcoholic drinks

        b. Methanol itself is only mildly toxic, but its oxidation products (formaldehyde and formic acid) induce a severe acidosis.

        c. Methanol may cause bilateral hemorrhagic necrosis of the caudate, putamen, pons, optic nerves, cerebellum, and subcortical white matter.

    2. Clinical

        a. ***Visual disturbance /ocular manifestations***

            i. Amblyopia

            ii. Scotomas

            iii. Total blindness

        b. Extrapyramidal signs (bradykinesia, masked facies, tremor)

    3. Treatment: three-part approach—ethanol, bicarbonate, dialysis (in severe cases)

B. **Ethylene glycol**

    1. Pathophysiology: used as antifreeze, tobacco moistener, and in paint; toxic dose is greater than 100 mL

    2. Clinical

        a. Restless and agitation followed by somnolence, stupor, coma, and even convulsions

        b. Death due to cardiopulmonary failure

        c. Characteristic metabolic findings: **metabolic acidosis with large anion gap,** hypocalcemia, and calcium oxalate crystals in the urine

    3. Treatment

        a. Supportive care

        b. Correct metabolic acidosis and hypocalcemia.

      c. Infuse ethanol at 5 to 10 g/hour.

      d. Dialysis may be necessary to remove ethylene glycol and to treat uremia.

III. Gases

A. Carbon monoxide poisoning

  1. Pathophysiology

     a. Most common cause of death by poisoning in the United States

     b. Damages the brain by three mechanisms:

        i. Production of carboxyhemoglobin that causes hypoxemia

       ii. Decreased release of oxygen to tissues

      iii. Direct mitochondrial toxicity

     c. Pathology

        i. Bilateral necrotic lesions involving the *globus pallidus*

       ii. Hippocampal damage

      iii. Supratentorial demyelination

      iv. Cortical damage (watershed distribution)

  2. Neuroimaging

     a. MRI: lesions usually appear hypointense on T1 and **hyperintense on T2 involving globus pallidus.**

     b. May also involve the thalamus, caudate, putamen, and cerebellum

     c. Differential diagnosis of bilateral basal ganglia lesions

        i. Carbon monoxide

       ii. Cyanide

      iii. Ethylene glycol

      iv. Methanol (more putamen)

       v. Aminoacidopathies

      vi. Infarction

     vii. Pantothenate-kinase-associated neurodegeneration (PKAN; formerly Hallervorden-Spatz disease)

    viii. Leigh disease

      ix. Wilson's disease

       x. Mitochondrial disorders

      xi. Neoplasm

     xii. Multiple system atrophy

  3. Clinical

     a. Hypoxia without cyanosis (cherry-red appearance)

     b. ± Myocardial infarction

     c. Retinal hemorrhages

     d. Neurologic: lethargy that progresses to coma followed by brainstem dysfunction and movement disorders

  4. Treatment

     a. Oxygen 100%

     b. Hyperbaric chamber (if severe)

  5. Prognosis: residual movement disorders are common.

IV. Organophosphates

A. **Pathophysiology**

 1. Irreversible acetylcholinesterase inhibitors

 2. Organophosphates are found in insecticides (e.g., parathion, malathion), pesticides, and chemical warfare agents (e.g., tabun, sarin, soman).

 3. Highly lipid soluble

 4. May be absorbed through the skin, mucous membranes, gastrointestinal tract, and lungs

B. **Clinical**

 1. Symptoms occur within a few hours of exposure.

 2. Neuromuscular blockade; autonomic and CNS dysfunction, including headache, miosis, fasciculations, and diffuse muscle cramping; weakness; excessive secretions; nausea, vomiting, and diarrhea

 3. Excessive exposure: seizures and coma

 4. Delayed neuropathy or myelopathy beginning 1 to 3 weeks after acute exposure

 5. Electrophysiology

   a. Increased spontaneous firing rate and amplitude of the miniature end-plate potentials

   b. Depolarization block

C. **Treatment**

 1. Supportive care: clean patient completely.

 2. Lavage

 3. Atropine, 1 to 2 mg

 4. Pralidoxime, 1 g intravenously

   a. Cholinesterase reactivator

   b. Reversal of peripheral acetylcholinesterase for proportion of enzyme that has not irreversibly bound the inhibitor

V. Other Industrial Toxins

A. **Cyanide intoxication**

 1. Pathophysiology: inhibition of ferric-ion-containing enzymes, including cytochrome oxidase (produces tissue hypoxia by inhibiting the action of respiratory enzymes)

 2. Clinical

   a. Acute: excessive dose: loud cry with generalized convulsions and death within 2 to 5 minutes

   b. Chronic: agitation, salivation, anxiety, confusion, and nausea, followed by vertigo, headache, and ataxia followed by sudden loss of consciousness and seizures ± opisthotonos

 3. Treatment

   a. Supportive care with respiratory assistance, if needed

   b. Sodium and amyl nitrite

   c. Methylene blue: for excessive methemoglobinemia

   d. Commercially available cyanide antidote kit

B. **Acrylamide: impairs axonal transport, causing accumulation of neurofilaments and paranodal swelling, mostly in large myelinated axons, producing a dying-back axonopathy, affecting both peripheral nerves and central tracts (e.g., dorsal spinocerebellar and gracile tract)**

VI. Animal Toxins

A. Snake venoms

1. Pathophysiology

   a. In the United States, estimated 50,000 snakebites annually

   b. Individuals are often drunk

   c. Families

      i. Viperidae

         (A) True vipers, pit vipers, rattlesnakes, moccasins, cottonmouths, and copperheads

         (B) 95% of the annual snakebites in the United States

      ii. Elapidae

         (A) Cobras, kraits, mambas, and coral snakes

      iii. Hydrophiidae

         (A) Sea snakes in Asian and Australian waters

   d. Potent toxins to cardiac muscle, coagulant pathways, and neurologic system

   e. Neurotoxicity

      i. Associated with action on neuromuscular junction, either presynaptically or postsynaptically

      ii. Presynaptic toxins

         (A) *α-Bungarotoxin, notexin, and taipoxin*

         (B) *Act to inhibit the normal release of acetylcholine (ACh) from the presynaptic cell of the neuromuscular junction*

      iii. *Postsynaptic neurotoxins: produce variable degrees of nondepolarizing neuromuscular block*

2. Clinical

   a. Local evidence of envenomation: bite site pain and swelling

   b. Preparalytic signs and symptoms: headache, vomiting, loss of consciousness, paresthesia, ptosis, and external ophthalmoplegia

   c. Paralytic signs and symptoms

      i. Paralysis develops within 1 to 10 hours.

      ii. Facial and jaw paresis compromises swallowing

      iii. Progressive diaphragmatic, oropharyngeal, intercostal, and limb weakness followed by loss of consciousness and seizures

      iv. Death due to circulatory arrest if not stabilized

   d. Other systemic effects: relate to coagulation deficits, including cerebral and subarachnoid hemorrhage

3. Treatment: supportive care, antivenoms

B. Ciguatoxin toxin

1. Found in the Pacific and Caribbean

2. Produced by a marine dinoflagellate (*Gambierdiscus toxicus*) that attaches to algae and is passed up the food chain

3. Carried by numerous fish, but only humans are adversely affected

4. Mechanism: tetrodotoxin-sensitive sodium channel resulting in membrane depolarization

B. **Ciguatoxin toxin** (*cont'd*)

    5. Clinical: begins more than 3 to 5 hours after ingestion, with perioral and distal paresthesia followed by weakness, myalgia, dizziness, and dry mouth; may also have ptosis, dilated pupils, photophobia, transient blindness

    6. Treatment: supportive care

C. **Saxitoxin**

    1. Similar in action and structure to the sodium channel blockers (i.e., tetrodotoxin found in puffer fish and sunfish)

    2. Found in clams and mussels

    3. Produced by dinoflagellates of the genus *Gonyaulax*

    4. Clinical: acute paralysis within 30 to 60 minutes; may have paresthesia and cerebellar ataxia

    5. Mortality: 1% to 10%

    6. Treatment: supportive care

D. **Latrodectism**

    1. Clinical syndrome that follows black widow spider bite

    2. More potent than pit viper venom, but lower volume

    3. Mechanism: forced release of ACh from the presynaptic neuromuscular junction and also stimulation of sympathetic and parasympathetic cholinergic systems

    4. Clinical

       a. Acute: pain with severe local muscle spasm occurs immediately

       b. Subacute: headache, fatigue, weakness

    5. Mortality: less than 1% (fatal if cardiovascular complications)

    6. Treatment: usually supportive care only; antivenom is available but usually not used due to higher risk of adverse effects of sera.

VII. Plant Toxins

A. **Mushrooms**

    1. Most often abundant in summer and fall, resulting in higher rates of intoxication during those seasons

SCIENTIFIC NAME	TOXIN	CLINICAL PRESENTATION	TREATMENT
Amanita muscaria	Cyclic polypeptides	Strong anticholinergic effects, including agitation, muscle spasms, ataxia, mydriasis, convulsions, and hallucinations	No treatment Atropine of minimal benefit
Amanita pantherina	Atropine-like toxins	Strong anticholinergic effects, including agitation, muscle spasms, ataxia, mydriasis, convulsions, and hallucinations Mortality: 10%	No treatment Atropine of minimal benefit

B. **Lathyrism**

    1. *Consumption of the chickpea,* Lathyrus: associated with toxic neurologic signs when *Lathyrus* accounts for more than one-third of calories

2. Three neurotoxins

   a. Amino-β-oxalyl aminopropionic acid

   b. Amino-oxalyl aminobutyric acid

   c. β-N-oxalyl amino-L-alanine: responsible for corticospinal dysfunction by inducing neurodegeneration through excitotoxic actions at the alpha-amino-3-hydroxy-5-methyl-4-isoxazolepropionic acid (AMPA) receptor

3. Pathology: anterolateral sclerosis in the thoracolumbar cord with loss of axons and myelin

4. Clinical: spastic paraplegia

5. Treatment: supportive care only

VIII. Bacterial Toxins

A. Diphtheria

1. Caused by *Corynebacterium diphtheriae*

2. Rare in the United States but may occur with travel, particularly to Eastern Europe

3. Pathology: *noninflammatory demyelinating, primarily affecting muscle and myelin*

4. Clinical

   a. Two clinical forms

      i. Oropharyngeal

      ii. Cutaneous

   b. Often begins with cranial neuropathies, particularly involving oropharyngeal and eye muscles

   c. Over weeks, may develop predominantly sensory polyneuropathy or a proximal motor neuropathy

   d. May be misdiagnosed as acute inflammatory demyelinating polyradiculopathy, but diphtheria has more prominent visual blurring and palatal dysfunction

5. Treatment

   a. Supportive care

   b. Antitoxin administration

6. Mortality

   a. Without antitoxin: 50%

   b. With antitoxin: less than 10%

B. Tetanus

1. *Produced by* Clostridium tetani *under anaerobic conditions of wounds*

2. Mechanism: retrograde axonal transport to nervous system and blocks exocytosis via interaction with synaptobrevin

3. Clinical

   a. Rapidly progressive axonal peripheral neuropathy

   b. Asymmetric sensory and motor responses

   c. May also have CNS involvement

   d. Death in less than 1 week of symptoms

4. Treatment

   a. Removal of the toxin source

   b. Supportive care

   c. Neutralization of circulating toxin via human tetanus immune globulin

C. **Botulism**

1. *Pathophysiology*

    a. *Caused primarily by* Clostridium botulinum, *which is a gram-positive anaerobe*

    b. Three forms

        i. *Food-borne botulism*

            (A) 1,000 cases per year worldwide

            (B) Usually home-canned vegetables

            (C) Most associated with type A spores

        ii. *Wound botulism*

            (A) Injection drug use

            (B) Posttraumatic

        iii. *Infant botulism*

            (A) Most common in children aged 1 week to 11 months

            (B) Usually neurotoxins types A and B

            (C) Death in less than 2% of cases in the United States, but higher worldwide

    c. The most common form now is wound botulism resulting from illicit drug use.

    d. Type A, B, and E neurotoxins are the usual cause, but, rarely, types F and G can also be symptomatic.

    e. *Irreversible binding to the presynaptic membrane of peripheral cholinergic nerves blocking ACh release at the neuromuscular junction*

        i. Three-step process:

            (A) Toxin binds to receptors on the nerve ending.

            (B) Toxin molecule is then internalized.

            (C) Within the nerve cell, the toxin interferes with the release of Ach.

        ii. Cleavage of one of the soluble N-ethylmaleimide-sensitive factor attachment protein receptor (SNARE) proteins (synaptosomal-associated protein [SNAP]-25, synaptobrevin, syntaxin) by botulinum neurotoxin inhibits the exocytosis of ACh from the synaptic terminal

2. Clinical

    a. Blurred vision, dysphagia, dysarthria, dilated/poorly reactive pupillary response to light, dry mouth, constipation, and urinary retention

    b. Tensilon (edrophonium chloride) test: positive in 30% of cases

    c. Infant botulism: constipation, lethargy, poor sucking, weak cry

    d. *Electrophysiologic criteria for botulism*

        i. *↓Compound muscle action potential amplitude in at least two muscles*

        ii. *20% facilitation of compound muscle action potential amplitude*

        iii. *Persistent facilitation for 2 minutes after activation*

        iv. No postactivation exhaustion

        v. Single-fiber electromyography—↑ jitter and blocking

    e. Prognosis

        i. Most patients recover completely in 6 months.

3. Treatment

    a. Supportive care

    b. Antibiotics

        i. Wound botulism: penicillin G or metronidazole

       ii. Antibiotics are not recommended for infant botulism because cell death and lysis may result in the release of more toxin.

    c. Horse serum antitoxin

       i. Types A, B, and E

       ii. Side effects of serum sickness and anaphylaxis

IX. Miscellaneous

  A. **Marchiafava-Bignami disease**

    1. Clinical—seen with chronic alcohol abuse

      a. Insidious cerebral dysfunction

      b. Dementia

      c. Depression

      d. Apathy

      e. Delusions

      f. Slow progression, with death in 3 to 6 years

    2. Pathology: necrosis of corpus callosum; no evidence of inflammation

  B. **Tryptophan: may cause eosinophilic myalgic syndrome**

  C. **Drugs/toxins causing peripheral neuropathy**

    1. Nitrofurantoin

    2. Vincristine

    3. N-hexane

    4. Methyl butyl ketone

    5. Disulfiram (Antabuse®)

    6. Arsenic

    7. Lead

    8. Mercury

    9. Thallium

  D. **Medications/agents associated with myopathy**

    1. Alcohol

    2. Colchicine

    3. Statins

    4. Zidovudine (AZT)

    5. Diazacholesterol

    6. Clofibrate

    7. Steroids

    8. Rifampin

    9. Kaluretics

    10. Chloroquine

  E. **Toxins that cause neuropathy/neuronopathy**

    1. Vitamin B6 (excess > deficiency)

    2. Vitamin E (deficiency)

    3. Taxanes (chemotherapy)

F. Toxins that cause neuropathy and myopathy

   1. Chloroquine

   2. Amiodarone

   3. Colchicine

G. Toxins that cause seizures

   1. Alcohol toxicity or withdrawal

   2. Barbiturate toxicity or withdrawal

   3. Benzodiazepine toxicity or withdrawal

   4. Cocaine

   5. Phencyclidine

   6. Amphetamines

   7. Bupropion

   8. Common medications that may lower the seizure threshold

      a. Antidepressants (tricyclic antidepressants, bupropion)

      b. Antipsychotics (chlorpromazine, thioridazine, trifluoperazine, perphenazine, haloperidol)

      c. Analgesics (fentanyl, meperidine, pentazocine, propoxyphene, tramadol)

      d. Local anesthetics (lidocaine, procaine)

      e. Sympathomimetics (terbutaline, ephedrine, phenylpropanolamine)

      f. Antibiotics (imipenem > penicillin, ampicillin, cephalosporins, metronidazole, isoniazid, pyrimethamine)

      g. Antineoplastic agents (vincristine, chlorambucil, methotrexate, bis-chloronitrosourea, cytosine arabinoside)

      h. Bronchodilators (aminophylline, theophylline)

         i. Immunosuppressants

         ii. Cyclosporine

         iii. Muromonab-CD3 (Orthoclone OKT3®)

      i. Others (insulin, antihistamines, atenolol, baclofen, cyclosporine)

H. Specific action of toxins/agents

   1. *α-Bungarotoxin: irreversible postsynaptic receptor blockade*

   2. *Curare and vecuronium: competitive postsynaptic nicotine receptor blockade*

   3. *Succinylcholine: postsynaptic receptor blockade causing depolarization*

I. Ethanol

   1. **Acute alcohol intoxication features are related to the blood level dose of the toxin.**

      a. 0.05 to 0.1 mg/dL: disinhibited

      b. 0.1 to 0.3 mg/dL: inebriated, ataxic

      c. 0.3 to 0.35 mg/dL: very intoxicated

      d. More than 0.35 mg/dL: potentially lethal (especially when drinking takes on a competitive quality, such as chugging contests, etc.)

   2. Effects of chronic alcohol use

      a. *Wernicke's encephalopathy* (arising from nutritional deficiency of vitamin B_1)

         i. Spongy degeneration

         ii. Petechiae hemorrhage involving mamillary bodies, hypothalamus, thalamus (dorsal and anterior medial nuclei, pulvinar), periaqueductal gray matter, floor of the fourth ventricle, dorsal nuclei, vestibular nuclei

iii. Characterized by confusion, ataxia, ophthalmoplegia

iv. Mortality up to 10% to 20%

v. Treatment: thiamine; dosage may need to be high (300–500 mg IV) for the first few days.

b. *Korsakoff Syndrome*

   i. Chronic phase of Wernicke's syndrome

   ii. Atrophy of the mamillary bodies, dorsomedial nucleus of the thalamus

   iii. Presents with retrograde and anterograde amnesia; confabulation common

c. *Nutritional polyneuropathy*: typically a sensorimotor neuropathy

d. *Hepatic failure* (hepatic encephalopathy or non-Wilsonian hepatocerebral degeneration)

   i. Asterixis with altered level of consciousness

   ii. Alzheimer's type 2 cells ("watery cells")

   iii. Pseudolaminar necrosis, microcavitation of the lenticular nuclei

   iv. Electroencephalogram: general slowing, **triphasic waves**

   v. Serum NH3 may not correspond to symptoms.

e. *Central pontine myelinolysis*

   i. From rapid correction of hyponatremia

   ii. Characterized by progressive paresis, cranial nerve paresis, preserved mental responsiveness

   iii. The demyelination is often M- or W-shaped in the pons.

f. *Anterior superior vermal cerebellar degeneration*

   i. Predominantly in alcoholic men, presenting with truncal ataxia

   ii. Loss of Purkinje cells more common than granule cells

g. *Marchiafava-Bignami disease*: central necrosis of the corpus callosum presenting with a disconnection syndrome

J. **Neurologic complications associated with select chemotherapy agents**

DRUG	NEUROLOGIC COMPLICATION
Busulfan	Seizures
Carboplatin	Peripheral neuropathy / sensory neuronopathy, Ototoxicity (hearing loss > high frequency; tinnitus)
Cladribine	Peripheral neuropathy
Cisplatin	Peripheral neuropathy
Isotretinoin	Pseudotumor cerebri
Methotrexate	Leukoencephalopathy
Paclitaxel (Taxol®)	Peripheral neuropathy
Vinblastine	Peripheral neuropathy
Suramin	Peripheral neuropathy
Vincristine	Peripheral neuropathy

Other side effects of commonly used immunosuppressive medications for neurological conditions:

METHOTREXATE:	HEPATOTOXICITY, PULMONARY FIBROSIS, LEUKOPENIA, ALOPECIA
Azathioprine:	hepatotoxicity, pancreatitis, leukopenia
Cyclophosphamide:	bone marrow suppression, hemorrhagic cystitis, alopecia
Cyclosporine:	nephrotoxicity, hypertension, hepatotoxicity, gum hyperplasia, tremor, hirsutism
Tacrolimus:	tremor, hypertension, hyperglycemia, multifocal demyelinating polyneuropathy
Mycophenolate:	bone marrow suppression, hypertension, tremor, diarrhea
IVIG:	hypotension, aseptic meningitis, nephrotoxicity, flu like syndrome

K. Neurological conditions and associated vitamin deficiencies

DISEASE	VITAMIN DEFICIENCY	CLINICAL FEATURES
Alcoholism	Thiamine (vitamin B_1)	Wernicke-Korsakoff syndrome
Subacute combined degeneration of the spinal cord	B_{12}; also reported in folate deficiency	Peripheral neuropathy, sensory loss, ataxia, anemia; pathology: spongy degeneration of dorsal and lateral columns; peripheral neuropathy—axonal loss; occasional ± demyelination; with or without pernicious anemia
Methylmalonic aciduria	B_{12}	Recurrent lethargy, Reye-like disease, aciduria
Not applicable	Biotin	Alopecia, thrush, recurrent encephalopathy
Multiple carboxylase deficiency	Biotin	Recurrent encephalopathy with aciduria
Pellagra	Niacin	3 Ds = diarrhea, dementia, dermatitis; peripheral neuropathy; pathology: central chromatolysis; if severe, with degeneration of the dorsal and lateral columns of the spinal cord but without the spongy appearance that is characteristic of B_{12} deficiency
Hartnup's disease	Niacin	Recurrent ataxia and aminoaciduria
Mitochondriopathies	Riboflavin	Recurrent encephalopathy, muscle disease
Bassen-Kornzweig disease (Abetalipoproteinemia)	Vitamin E	Neuropathy, ataxia, acanthocytosis
Cholestatic liver disease	Vitamin E	Neuropathy, ataxia
Friedreich-like ataxia	Vitamin E	Ataxia, sensory neuropathy

> **NB:** Nitrous oxide abuse can produce myeloneuropathy that is clinically indistinguishable from vitamin B_{12} deficiency (or copper-deficiency myeloneuropathy): paresthesias of the hands and feet, gait ataxia, and leg weakness, with reverse Lhermitte's sign (shock-like sensation from feet upward with neck flexion). Serum B_{12} and Schilling test are usually normal.

CHEAT SHEET

Lead poisoning
"Fans bleed blue"
f: facial pallor, flaccid paralysis, fertility, and menstrual symptoms
a: anemia, abortion
n: neuropathy, nephropathy
bl: Burtonian line, basophilic stippling
e: eosinophilia
e: encephalopathy
d: dry belly ache (constipation and colic), wrist drop and footdrop
blue: blue stippled line

Mercury poisoning
"SMELL BLACK TEA"
S: salivation
ME: membranous colitis, MGN, Minamata disease
LL: lens deposition
BLACK: black line on gums
T: tremors intentional
E: erethism (excessive sensitivity or rapid reaction to stimulation)
A: acrodynia

Organophosphate (cholinergic) poisoning
"DUMBBELLSS": diarrhea, urination, miosis, bradycardia, bronchospasm, emesis, lacrimation, lethargy, salivation, and seizures

Suggested Readings

Dobbs MR, Rusyniak DE, Evans RW. *Frontiers in Clinical Neurotoxicology*. Philadelphia, PA: Saunders/Elsevier;2011.

Hammond N, Wang Y, Dimachkie MM, Barohn RJ. Nutritional neuropathies. *Neurol.* 2013;31(2): 477–489.

Holstege CP, Borek HA. Toxidromes. *Crit. Care Clin.*2012;28(4):479–498.

Verstappen CC, Heimans JJ, Hoekman K, Postma TJ. Neurotoxic complications of chemotherapy in patients with cancer: clinical signs and optimal management. 2003;63(15):1549–1563.

CHAPTER 16

Sleep and Sleep Disorders

I. Wakefulness and Sleep Overview

A. **Arousal system has two main ascending pathways:**

1. Cholinergic neurons in the pedunculopontine and laterodorsal tegmentum → ventroposterior and mediodorsal nuclei of thalamus ← self-inhibits gamma-aminobutyric acid (GABA) in reticular nucleus (as GABA mediates sleep)

2. Monoamine neurons

   a. Noradrenaline in locus ceruleus

   b. Serotonin in dorsal and medial raphe nuclei

   c. Glutamate in parabrachial nucleus

   d. Dopamine in periaqueductal gray nucleus

   e. Histamine in tuberomamillary nucleus → lateral thalamus (picking up orexin and glutamate) → basal forebrain and cerebral cortex

B. **Sleep-promoting pathway:**

1. GABA and galanin from ventrolateral preoptic (VLPO) nucleus and GABA from median preoptic nucleus → inhibit arousal systems.

2. VLPO important in sleep promotion

3. Two separate systems are necessary to be able to switch completely from wakefulness to sleep (rather than have in-between states). Orexin stabilizes the flip-flop switch.

II. Basics of Sleep Stages

A. **Sleep makeup: N1 = 5% to 10%, N2 = about 50%, N3 = 15% to 20%, rapid eye movement (REM) = 20%**

B. **Wake**

1. Mediated by arousal pathways

2. Electroencephalogram (EEG) will show prominent rhythmic alpha in occipital channels with eyes closed and low-amplitude mixed-frequency (LAMF) with eyes open.

C. **Non-REM (NREM) sleep (N1, N2, N3)**

1. VLPO and basal forebrain critical in initiating sleep

2. In N1, alpha is replaced by LAMF; in N2, sleep spindles and K-complexes; in N3, delta.

D. **REM**

1. Driven by the pons

2. Pontine cholinergic neurons induce REM.

3. Serotoninergic neurons suppress REM.

4. Glutaminergic neurons in sublaterodorsal area induce atonia during REM.

5. EEG: LAMF with sawtooth waves

D. REM (*cont'd*)

6. Polysomnography (PSG) findings in early life key points:

   a. At 26 weeks: will see trace discontinuans—independent activity over each hemisphere or hemispheric asynchrony

   b. At 37 weeks: will see trace alternans—short bursts of high-voltage mixed-frequency activity alternating with low-voltage mixed-frequency activity

   c. At 30 weeks: REMs

   d. At 2 months: sleep spindles

   e. At 4 to 6 months: K complexes

7. Clinical correlates

   a. REM sleep behavior disorder can be caused by lesion of sublaterodorsal nucleus (REM atonia is lost). Remember that REM sleep behavior disorder (RBD) is associated with parkinsonian syndromes (often a precursor).

   b. Loss of orexin causes narcolepsy and incomplete switching of sleep states.

III. Circadian Rhythm Overview

A. The circadian system has three main components: a circadian pacemaker (the suprachiasmatic nucleus [SCN] in the anterior hypothalamus), input pathways (receive light and other stimuli), and output signals regulated by the SCN.

B. Light is the most important and powerful stimulus for regulating sleep cycles.

IV. Sleep Disorders

A. Insomnia

1. Most common sleep disorder

2. Defined as difficulty initiating, maintaining, or staying asleep despite adequate opportunity and environment for sleep; must also have at least one form of daytime impairment (fatigue, sleepiness, mood disorder, lack of concentration, etc.)

3. Disorder of the wake system resulting in round-the-clock hyperarousal

4. Increases risk of comorbid chronic health conditions

5. Diagnosis: sleep history and sleep log; PSG not necessary unless insomnia is felt to be secondary to another sleep disorder (such as obstructive sleep apnea or periodic limb movements)

6. Treatment (of primary insomnia): cognitive behavioral therapy +/– medications (benzodiazepine [BZD], non-BZD hypnotics, melatonin receptor agonist, or selective histamine receptor antagonist)

B. Circadian rhythm disorders

1. Delayed sleep phase syndrome

   a. Go to bed late, wake up late

   b. Most common in teens and young adults

   c. Diagnosis by sleep history and sleep log +/– actigraphy

   d. Triggers: light exposure and stimulating activity in evening

   e. Treatment: first line is morning light exposure with evening melatonin. Light should be used shortly after core body temp nadir, which occurs 2 to 3 hours before natural wake time. Melatonin should be given 5 to 6 hours prior to dim-light melatonin onset (DLMO). DLMO is 13 to 14 hours after natural wake time.

2. Advanced sleep phase disorder

   a. Go to sleep early, wake up early

   b. Linked to hPer2 gene; less common than delayed phase; occurs in middle-aged adults

   c. Diagnosis: sleep history and sleep log+/– actigraphy

   d. Treatment: early-evening light therapy (7–9 p.m.) or chronotherapy (advance bedtime by 3 hours every few days)

3. Non-24-hour sleep wake disorder

   a. Sleep occurs later and later each day and then the cycle repeats itself.

   b. Mostly seen in the blind (no light to regulate cycle)

   c. Diagnosis: sleep history and sleep log; complaint has to be present for at least 2 months; actigraphy can be helpful.

   d. Treatment: melatonin (3–10 mg) 1 hour before bedtime and structured bedtime routines

4. Irregular sleep–wake cycle

   a. Disorganized: intermittent periods of sleep and wake throughout 24-hour period

   b. Common in older adults with dementia

   c. Diagnosis: sleep history and sleep log +/– actigraphy

   d. Treatment: morning light exposure, structured daytime activities, and sleep-conducive nocturnal environment

5. Jet lag

   a. Recurrent insomnia and daytime somnolence due to rapid travel across two or more time zones

   b. Non-sleep symptoms can include malaise, impaired daytime alertness, poor appetite, gastrointestinal (GI) disturbances, menstrual irregularities, decreased cognitive processing, depression, anxiety, and irritability

   c. Eastward travelers may be more at risk.

   d. Diagnosis: sleep history +/– sleep log

   e. Treatment: if the expected stay in the destination is going to be 2 days or less, adapting to the destination's time zone is not needed. Appropriately timed light exposure is a key component: if traveling eastward, light exposure in the mornings to advance circadian clock; if traveling westward, light exposure in evening to delay circadian rhythm.

   f. Melatonin can be used (best if used with appropriate light exposure). If traveling east, take melatonin in the evening for 2 weeks prior to travel and then at bedtime once in destination.

6. Shift-work sleep disorder

   a. Sleepiness during work hours and insomnia during designated sleep periods for at least 1 month

   b. Overnight shift most susceptible

   c. Can result in chronic sleep deprivation and lead to fatigue, mood disorder, GI disturbance, decreased libido; increased risk for polysubstance abuse, weight gain, hypertension, and coronary artery disease

   d. Diagnosis: sleep history and at least 2 weeks of sleep log

   e. Treatment: aimed at increasing alertness during work hours and facilitating sleep during designated sleep hours. For night-shift workers, bright light exposure up to 2 hours before end of shift can increase alertness. Minimize light exposure on commute home (sunglasses) and have dark, quiet environment to help fall asleep.

6. Shift-work sleep disorder (*cont'd*)

   f. Melatonin can be taken at time of sleep, which may help to improve daytime sleep, but does not help with work-hour alertness. Modafinil and armodafinil are treatments approved by the U.S. Food and Drug Administration (FDA) to improve work-hour performance/alertness.

C. Sleep-disordered breathing

1. Key definitions

   a. Obstructive apnea: cessation of airflow with continued respiratory effort, due to complete upper airway occlusion.

   b. Hypopnea: significant decrease in airflow with associated EEG arousal or oxygen desaturation due to partial upper airway collapse

   c. Central apnea: cessation of airflow without respiratory effort

   d. Mixed apnea: components of central and obstructive apneas

   e. Upper airway resistance syndrome: flow limitation, not meeting criteria for apnea or hypopnea; due to narrowed upper airway

   f. Primary snoring: snoring without respiratory compromise

2. Obstructive sleep apnea (OSA): 1.5 to 4 times more common in men, prevalence increases with age

   a. Anatomical risk factors: high arched palate, narrow airway, retrognathia, adenotonsillar hypertrophy, elongated/edematous uvula, enlarged tongue, increased neck circumference, obesity

   b. STOP BANG screening tool; high risk is yes to 5 or more questions

      i. Snoring, tired, observed apneas, pressure (elevated blood pressure), body mass index (BMI) (greater than 35), age (over 50), neck circumference (greater than 40 cm), gender (male)

      (A) Snoring most common symptom

      (B) Diagnosis: by PSG (apnea hypopnea index [AHI] of 5–15 with daytime symptoms or AHI greater than 16)

         (1) AHI: mild = 5 to 14, moderate = 15 to 30, severe = greater than 30

      (C) Treatment: conservative therapies include weight loss, sleep repositioning therapy (if OSA was more prominent during supine position sleep in nonsupine position), maintaining patency of nasal airway, and avoiding sedatives, narcotics, opioids, and alcohol (ETOH).

      (D) First-line therapy is positive airway pressure (PAP) [Continuous PAP (CPAP), Bilevel PAP (BIPAP), Automatic PAP (APAP)]—pressurized air in oronasal cavity to act as a stent to maintain patency of airway.

      (E) If intolerant to PAP or mild to moderate OSA, can use dental appliance (tongue retaining device or mandibular advancement device) or nasal Expiratory PAP (EPAP)

      (F) If severe OSA and unable to use PAP, surgical intervention can be considered (uvulopalatopharyngoplasty most common, but variety of procedures, including septoplasty or turbinate reduction, tonsillectomy, hyoid suspension, and mandibular advancement)

      (G) If patient is morbidly obese, bariatric surgery may help to improve sleep-disordered breathing.

      (H) The main heath risk associated with untreated OSA is cardiovascular, including hypertension, atrial fibrillation, myocardial infarction, congestive heart failure, and stroke.

      (I) OSA also linked to increased risk of metabolic syndrome and autonomic alterations

3. Central sleep apnea (CSA)

    a. Normally, when CO_2 levels rise, there is a certain point at which central sensors in the medulla are stimulated and peripheral sensors in the carotid body are activated to initiate a breath.

    b. Central sleep apnea can occur in association with chronic hypocapnic states (such as congestive heart failure (CHF) or high altitude) in which the body becomes accustomed to lower CO_2 states and the set point to trigger a breath is reduced, leading to apneas.

    c. Other conditions in which CSA is common: with reduced respiratory drive (with opiates/narcotics) or in association with diaphragmatic weakness as can be seen in neuromuscular disorders such as Amyotrophic Lateral Sclerosis (ALS)

    d. Diagnosis: PSG with same AHI criteria as OSA

    e. Treatment: PAP therapy; sometimes triggered respirations are required. Acetazolamide can be used.

    f. Appropriate cardiopulmonary and neurologic workup

4. Sleep-related hypoventilation

    a. Most commonly seen with obesity hypoventilation syndrome (OHS)

    b. OHS diagnosis: BMI greater than 30, waking $PaCO_2$ level of 45 mmHg or greater, hypoxemia PaO_2 of 70 mmHg or less

    c. Higher risk of pulmonary hypertension

D. Hypersomnia

1. Narcolepsy with cataplexy

    a. Excessive daytime sleepiness (EDS) for at least 3 months

    b. Cataplexy (loss of muscle tone triggered by strong emotions)

    c. Diagnosis: Multiple Sleep Latency Test (MSLT) with mean sleep-onset latency (MSOL) 8 minutes or less and two or more sleep-onset REM periods (SOREMPs) **or** a decreased cerebrospinal fluid (CSF) hypocretin level (less than 110 pg/mL)

2. Narcolepsy without cataplexy

    a. EDS for at least 3 months

    b. No cataplexy

    c. Diagnosis: MSLT criteria only (MSOL of 8 minutes or less and two or more SOREMPs)

    d. Narcolepsy key points:

        i. Narcolepsy with cataplexy associated with HLA-DQB1-0602 and low hypocretin levels

        ii. Bimodal peak at 15 years of age and near 35 years of age

        iii. Clinical features aside from EDS and cataplexy include sleep hallucinations, sleep paralysis, and nonconsolidated sleep.

3. Idiopathic hypersomnia (IH)

    a. EDS for 3 months or more

    b. Diagnosis: MSLT with MSOL 8 minutes or less and less than two SOREMPs

    c. Can be further classified as IH with long sleep time (patient getting 10 or more hours of sleep per sleep period) or without long sleep time (6–10 hours of sleep)

4. Kleine-Levin syndrome and menstrual-related hypersomnia

    a. Recurrent episodes of EDS for 2 days to 4 weeks

    b. Episodes occur at least yearly

    c. Baseline (normal) function between attacks

4. Kleine-Levin syndrome and menstrual-related hypersomnia (*cont'd*)

    d. Often accompanied by mood and cognitive alterations, increased appetite, aggressive or hypersexual behavior

5. Treatment

    a. Traditional stimulants (amphetamines, methamphetamine, methylphenidate) or wake-promoting agents that act primarily on norepinephrine and dopamine (modafinil, armodafinil); sodium oxybate acting on GABA-b receptors consolidates sleep and can increase slow-wave sleep—better sleep may allow for more alertness during the day.

    b. Cataplexy is treated with tricyclic antidepressants, selective serotonin reuptake inhibitors (SSRIs), or serotonin-norepinephrine reuptake inhibitors (SNRIs).

E. **Parasomnias: undesirable behaviors that occur during sleep, characterized by complex, seemingly purposeful behaviors, usually longer than 2 minutes, with no conscious recollection of event**

  1. The first distinction to make is NREM versus REM parasomnias:

    a. NREM parasomnias: usually arise from slow-wave sleep during the first half of the night

      i. Confusional arousal: mental confusion or confusional behavior that occurs from waking during nocturnal sleep or a nap; episodes usually last a few minutes; generally no recollection of the event; abnormal sexual behavior (sexsomnia) is a type of confusional arousal.

        (A) Treatment: episodes starting in childhood usually spontaneously remit.

      ii. Sleepwalking or somnambulism: walking or more complex behaviors with eyes generally open

        (A) Peak prevalence ages 8 to 12 years; usually remits spontaneously in teens/early adulthood

      iii. Sleep terrors or parvor nocturnus: sudden arousal, sitting up with cry/vocalization and look of fear; associated with tachycardia, tachypnea, diaphoresis, mydriasis, and facial flushing; episodes usually last a few minutes and then patient returns to normal sleep, with no recollection of event upon waking

        (A) Peak prevalence is early school age, with remission usually by teens.

    b. REM parasomnias—occur during second half of night (when REM periods are longer)

  2. Nightmares: although similar to night terrors in that patient appears to have a sudden arousal with fear/panic, the patient is cognizant that he or she is waking up because of a nightmare and is often able to recall the dream with detail. Most often, there is recollection of the event in the morning.

  3. REM sleep behavior disorder (RBD)

    a. Dream reenactment behavior with motor activity and vocalization

    b. Usually occurring about once per week

    c. This is the only parasomnia that has a definitive PSG diagnosis: there is REM sleep without atonia (RSWA), which is demonstrated by persistent chin EMG activity during REM sleep.

    d. Can be due to bilateral pontine tegmental lesions

    e. Associated with alpha synucleinopathies (Parkinson's disease, dementia with Lewy bodies), with RBD often preceding the neurodegenerative disorder

    f. RBD can also be secondary (induced by medications, including SSRIs, SNRIs, alcohol withdrawal, caffeine) *g.* Pseudo RBD: occurs with untreated OSA; subsides with appropriate treatment of OSA

    h. Treatment: safe sleep environment and clonazepam

F. Nocturnal epilepsies

  1. Two main types: frontal lobe and temporal lobe epilepsy

  2. Autosomal dominant nocturnal frontal lobe epilepsy (ADNFLE): brief, motor seizures; associated with nicotinic acetylcholine receptor gene (CHRNA4/CHRNB2 subunits)

  3. Frontal lobe seizures associated with clonic activity, dystonic posturing, vocalization, and tendency toward secondary generalization; awareness can be preserved; minimal post-episode confusion

  4. Temporal lobe seizures are usually longer episodes associated with automatisms. Awareness is usually preserved, but post-episode confusion is more common. Less likely to generalize.

G. Periodic limb movement disorder/restless leg syndrome (RLS)

  1. Periodic limb movement disorder (PLMD): PSG diagnosis with increased PLMs (significant if PLM index is greater than 15); generally no treatment unless clinical complaints (poor sleep with increased nocturnal waking, EDS) with no other explanation

  2. RLS

    a. Clinical diagnosis often associated with increased PLMs (but not a requirement)

    b. RLS can be secondary to other medical conditions, including iron deficiency, diabetes mellitus, renal failure, and pregnancy.

    c. Prevalence of RLS is 5% to 10% in general population, but 10% to 26% in pregnancy, with peak in the third trimester.

    d. Diagnosis of RLS (four key features)

      i. An urge to move legs; can be accompanied by uncomfortable and unpleasant leg sensations

      ii. The symptoms begin or worsen during times of rest.

      iii. The symptoms improve with movement.

      iv. The symptoms are worse during evening/night.

    e. Workup: check ferritin level (can be associated with low ferritin) and peripheral neuropathy labs (B_{12}, TSH, HgbA1c).

    f. Treatment: if serum ferritin levels less than 50 u/L, treat with iron supplementation +/− medical workup for anemia. Other treatments include dopaminergic agents (dopamine agonists and dopamine replacement—first line), GABA agents, BZDs, and opioids (last line).

    g. Monitor for compulsive behaviors with dopaminergic agents.

    h. Augmentation (where symptoms occur earlier in the day, are more severe, or involve more body parts) can occur with dopaminergic agents; initially can increase frequency of doses, but eventually may require discontinuation of medication.

V. Pharmacology Overview

A. Medications for insomnia

  1. BZDs act as GABA agonists. However, because they have nonspecific GABA attachment sites, BZDs may have a more widespread brain effect (versus just sleep effects).

A. **Medications for insomnia** (*cont'd*)

2. FDA-approved BZDs include flurazepam and quazepam (long half-lives), temazepam and estazolam (medium half-lives), and triazolam (short half-life)

3. BZDs are most commonly used for short-term treatment of insomnia.

4. The most common side effects are drowsiness, dizziness, and headache.

5. There is habit-forming potential.

6. Use with caution in patients with untreated OSA or respiratory disease, as these medications can potentially lower respiratory drive.

7. Non-BZD receptor agonists are modulators of GABA-a receptor complex.

8. FDA-approved non-BZDs include eszopiclone (long half-life), zolpidem (medium half-life), and zaleplon (short half-life)

9. Can be used for short-term or, if needed, longer-term treatment of insomnia

10. Remember that eszopiclone is associated with metallic taste and smell.

11. All non-BZDs have the potential to increase parasomnias (abnormal nighttime behaviors).

12. There are extended-release formulations as well as oral spray and sublingual forms of zolpidem.

13. Selective melatonin receptor agonist

    a. Ramelteon: used mostly for sleep-onset insomnia

14. Selective histamine H1 receptor antagonist

    a. Doxepin: long half-life, used for sleep maintenance insomnia; can have side effect of upper respiratory tract infection

B. **Medications for hypersomnia**

1. Stimulants include amphetamine, methamphetamine, and methylphenidate.

2. Side effects include palpitations, tachycardia, hypertension, anorexia, psychosis, insomnia, and high abuse potential.

3. Wake-promoting agents

    a. Modafinil and armodafinil (act on dopamine receptors) to enhance wakefulness state; common side effect is headache/nausea

4. Sodium oxybate

    a. Activates GABA-b receptors

    b. Consolidates sleep; increases slow-wave sleep; by providing improved sleep quality, enhances daytime alertness

C. **Medications for cataplexy**

1. Tricyclic antidepressants (imipramine, protriptyline, clomipramine)

    a. SSRIs (fluoxetine and fluvoxamine)

    b. SNRI (venlafaxine)

    c. Sodium oxybate

D. **Medications for RLS**

1. Dopamine agonists (generally first-line treatment)

    a. Include pramipexole, ropinirole, rotigotine patch, carbidopa/levodopa

    b. These medications are most often efficacious for RLS.

    c. Side effects include risk of augmentations (making RLS symptoms worse during the daytime), impulse control disorders, and daytime sleepiness.

    d. Impulse control disorders can occur in 6% to 17% of people taking dopaminergic agents and can manifest months after starting treatment.

2. Calcium channel alpha 2 delta ligands (generally first- or second-line agents)
   a. Gabapentin, gabapentin enacarbil, pregabalin
   b. Especially helpful if patients also have neuropathic symptoms
   c. BZDs and opioids are useful as third-line agents for RLS treatment.

CHEAT SHEET

Light	Most powerful zeitgeber
Sleep promoting	VLPO (ventrolateral pontine nucleus)
Flip-flop switch	Stabilized by orexin
Sleep onset	DLMO (dim-light melatonin onset)
Advanced phase sleep disorder	hPER2 gene
K complexes and sleep spindles	Stage II sleep
Delta waves	Stage III sleep
Sawtooth waves	REM sleep
REM behavior disorder	Loss of muscle atonia
REM behavior disorder	Alpha synucleinopathy association
Narcolepsy	HLA-DQB1-0602
Narcolepsy	Low hypocretin level
Restless leg syndrome	Low ferritin level
Obstructive sleep apnea	Airway obstruction with respiratory effort
Central sleep apnea	No respiratory effort
Nightmares	Later in night, REM sleep, memory
Night terrors	Later in night, REM sleep, memory
Sleep seizures	ADNFLE, associated with CHRNA gene
Eszopiclone/Lunesta	Metallic taste and smell
Dopamine agonists	Augmentation, impulse control disorders

Suggested Readings

Kryger MH, Roth T, Dement WC. *Principles and Practice of Sleep Medicine*. 6th ed., Boston, MA: Elsevier;2015.

Westerman DE. *The Concise Sleep Medicine Handbook*. 3rd ed. CreateSpace independent publishing platform;2015.

Neurophysiology

CHAPTER 17

Nerve Conduction Studies (NCS) and Electromyography (EMG)

I. NCS and EMG

A. Basic neurophysiology

1. *Action potential (AP) generation*
   a. Definition: a self-propagating regenerative change in membrane potential
   b. Originally found to be the result of sodium/potassium channels via voltage clamp experiments on axons of the giant squid; involves maintaining membrane potential at a fixed value and then using channel blockers to test current changes
      i. *Tetrodotoxin blocks Na^+ channels*
      ii. *Tetraethylammonium blocks K^+ channels*
   c. *Three phases: resting, depolarizing, repolarizing*
   d. Myelinated are faster than unmyelinated nerves
      i. Myelin decreases membrane capacitance and conductance and the time constant.
      ii. Increases the space constant of the segment of axon between the nodes of Ranvier

> **NB:** AP propagation in myelinated fibers is known as saltatory conduction.

      iii. Velocity is proportional to axon radius.
2. *Neuromuscular junction*
   a. Presynaptic components
      i. Motor neuron body (soma)

a. Presynaptic components (*cont'd*)

　　ii. Axon

　　iii. Terminal bouton: synaptic vesicles contain 5,000 to 10,000 molecules (1 quanta) of acetylcholine; release based on voltage-gated calcium channels.

b. Synaptic cleft: 200 to 500 μm

c. Positive-synaptic components

　　i. Motor end plate

　　ii. Acetylcholine receptors

　　iii. Voltage-gated sodium channels

3. *Volume conduction*

a. Definition: spread of current from the potential source through a conducting medium

b. May cause considerable differences in waveforms when a potential travels from one medium to a different medium

c. The interstitial fluid and body tissues possess a finite resistance capable of attenuating the magnitude of a potential at a distance from the current source. This diminution in potential magnitude is directly proportional to the square of the distance from the current source and falls approximately 20% in 6.25 cell diameters in neural tissue.

d. *The amplitude of the recorded potential is dependent on the following:*

　　i. Membrane's charge density

　　ii. Orientation of the recording electrode and active portion of the membrane

　　iii. Distance between the membrane and recording electrode

　　iv. Type of recording electrode used

e. *The amplitude is also directly proportional to a defined portion of the membrane's surface area and indirectly proportional to the square of the distance between the membrane and the electrode.*

　　i. The amplitude increases if the membrane's surface area increases or the distance to the membrane decreases.

　　ii. *The amplitude of sensory nerve AP (SNAP) or compound muscle AP (CMAP) is the composite of the amplitudes of the individual nerve fibers, some faster or slower than others, resulting in a final amplitude that is less than would be seen if all were summated together in phase.*

f. The triphasic waveform results from the cathode (negative lead) receiving a wave of depolarization that changes in polarity as it passes and subsequent repolarization occurring later.

4. *Far-field recording:* recording electrical activity of biologic origin generated at a considerable distance from the recording electrodes

a. Usually implies stationary rather than propagating signals recorded at a distance

b. Tissue of different density can distort the potential into a complex waveform, with latencies that are different from the actual latencies measured near the generator.

c. Changes in extracellular resistance caused by anatomic "inhomogeneities" and/or by conductivity changes give rise to far-field components.

5. Filters and gain

a. High and low frequencies

　　i. High-frequency (low pass) filters (HFFs) exclude high frequencies.

　　ii. Low-frequency (high pass) filters (LFFs) exclude low frequencies.

b. *Gain:* recorded in microvolts per centimeter

6. *Artifacts*

   a. *Physiologic*

      i. *Temperature: most negative factor; conduction velocity slows 1.5 to 2.5 m per second for every 1°C drop in temperature, and distal latency prolongs by approximately 0.2 millisecond per degree.*

      ii. *Age: newborns have 50% of normal adult nerve conduction velocity (NCV); age 1 year: 75% of normal adult NCV; normal velocities by age 3 to 5 years when complete myelination occurs; upper limb SNAP amplitude drops by up to 50% by age 70 years (lower limb SNAP amplitude may be severely reduced or unevokable by age 60 years); motor unit AP duration is longer in older patients.*

      iii. *Height:* taller individuals have slower NCVs due to longer (and less thickly myelinated) nerves (adjust to normative data).

      iv. *Proximal versus distal nerve segments: distal segments have slower NCVs due to smaller nerve diameter (including reduced myelin thickness).*

   b. *Nonphysiologic:* electrode impedance mismatch and 60-Hz interference

      i. Electrode impedance: minimize by using same electrodes, cleaning skin, using conducting jelly/paste

      ii. 60 Hz (power-line artifact): if problematic, may be faulty ground; reduced by using a 60-Hz notch filter

   c. *Stimulus artifact*

      i. Cathode position: may not stimulate directly over the nerve (producing submaximal stimulation); may also inadvertently stimulate other nerves

      ii. Supramaximal stimulation: all nerve fibers must be depolarized (suboptimal stimulation will give lower amplitude)

      iii. Co-stimulation of adjacent nerves brings in other nerves as artifacts superimposed on desired nerve response

      iv. Electrode placement: if too distant, may result in distortion from far-field effect

      v. *Antidromic versus orthodromic: antidromic* advantage is higher-amplitude potentials; disadvantage is potential for volume-conducting motor potential after the SNAP

      vi. The distance between recording and referencing electrodes must be greater than 4 cm.

      vii. Verify accurate distance.

B. **Equipment**

   1. Principle

     a. The clinical EMG is recorded extracellularly from muscle fibers embedded in tissue (conducting medium).

     b. *The ratio of muscle fibers per motor neuron (innervation ratio) is variable—3:1 in extraocular muscles, 1,000+:1 in limb muscles (e.g. 1,000:1 to 2,000:1 for the gastrocnemius).*

   2. *Sources of generators*

     a. *Fibrillation and positive sharp waves are from the spontaneous depolarization of a muscle **fiber**.*

     b. *Fasciculation, doublets, multiplets, cramps, and myokymic discharges are from the motor neuron and its axon.*

     c. *Complex repetitive discharges (CRDs): result from depolarization of a single muscle fiber followed by nonsynaptic spread to nearby denervated fibers; the depolarization spreads in a "circus" movement back to the original pacemaker muscle fiber (this may be seen with denervation).*

B. **Equipment** (*cont'd*)

3. Technique of needle EMG

    a. Four steps: insertional and spontaneous activity evaluation, minimal contraction to assess different motor unit potentials (MUPs), and maximal contraction to assess recruitment and interference pattern

    b. Sensitivity: 50 to 100 µV/cm for insertional and spontaneous activity; 200 µV/cm to 1 mV/cm to assess voluntary activity

    c. Filter: low, 10 to 20 Hz; high, 10 kHz

    d. Muscles typically assessed in upper and lower extremities

        i. Upper extremities

            (A) First dorsal interosseus (ulnar nerve, C8–T1)

            (B) Abductor pollicis brevis (median nerve, T1 > C8)

            (C) Extensor indicis proprius (radial nerve, mostly C8)

            (D) Flexor pollicis longus (median nerve, C8 > T1)

            (E) Pronator teres (median nerve, C6–C7)

            (F) Biceps brachii (musculocutaneous nerve, C5–C6)

            (G) Triceps (radial nerve, mostly C7)

            (H) Deltoid (axillary nerve, C5 > C6)

            (I) Cervical paraspinal muscles

        ii. Lower extremities

            (A) Abductor hallucis (tibial nerve, mostly S1)

            (B) Extensor digiti brevis (deep peroneal nerve, L5 > S1)

            (C) Tibialis anterior (deep peroneal nerve, mostly L5) and tibialis posterior (tibial nerve, mostly L5)

            (D) Vastus lateralis or rectus femoris (femoral nerve, mostly L3–L4)

            (E) Gluteus maximus (inferior gluteal nerve, S1 > L5) and gluteus medius (superior gluteal nerve, L5 > S1)

            (F) Lumbar and sacral paraspinals

4. *Single-fiber EMG*

    a. *To determine fiber density and jitter*

    b. Records 300-µm radius

    c. Amplifier: higher impedance greater than or equal to 100 megaohms

    d. Sweep faster, higher gain, high-frequency allowed filter

C. **Needle EMG of normal muscle**

1. *EMG of normal muscle*

    a. *Insertional activity*

        i. Produced by mechanic stimulation of the muscle fibers by the penetrating electrode with muscle at rest

        ii. Persists for a few hundred milliseconds (typically, <300 ms)

        iii. Duration slightly exceeds the movement of the electrode.

        iv. Divided into normal, increased, and decreased insertional activity

        v. An isolated positive wave may be present at the end of insertional activity in normal muscle.

        vi. *Prolonged insertional activity occurs in two types of normal variants and in denervated muscle and myotonic discharges.*

(A) *Normal variants:* short trains of regularly firing positive waves—may be familial or subclinical myotonia; short recurrent bursts of irregularly firing potentials—most often seen in muscular individuals, especially in calf muscles

(B) *Reduced insertional activity:* occurs in *periodic paralysis* (during paralysis) and with replacement of muscle by connective tissue or fat in myopathies and neurogenic disorders

(C) *Increased insertional activity:* needle movement resulting in any waveform that lasts longer than 300 ms; needle movement may provoke positive waves; *may be seen in neuropathic and myopathic conditions: denervated muscle, myotonic disorders, inflammatory myopathies*

b. Motor end-plate activity

   i. The end-plate region is the usual place normal resting muscle shows electrical activity when the needle is held in a stationary position.

   ii. *Consists of end-plate noise and end-plate spikes*

   (A) *End-plate noise*

      (1) Monophasic, irregular negative potentials with low amplitude (10–50 μV) and 1 to 2 milliseconds in duration.

      (2) "Ocean"/"sea shell" sound due to depolarization caused by spontaneous release of acetylcholine

      (3) Biphasic potentials with a negative onset are also a constituent of end-plate noise and have duration of 3 to 5 milliseconds and amplitude of 100 to 200 μV.

      (4) Biphasic potentials represent muscle fiber APs arising sporadically at the neuromuscular junction or intramuscular nerve fibers.

   (B) *End-plate spikes*

      (1) Amplitude: 100 to 200 μV

      (2) Duration: 3 to 4 milliseconds

      (3) Frequency: 5 to 50 Hz irregularly firing

      (4) Initially negative amplitude (as opposed to fibrillations)

      (5) Possibly originate in intrafusal muscle fibers

c. *MUP*

   i. Waveform

   (A) *Composed of a group of muscle fibers innervated by a single anterior horn cell*

   (B) *The spatial relation between the needle and the individual muscle fibers plays the greatest role in determining the waveform of the MUP.*

   (C) *Composite of the compound potential of the sum of individual APs generated in the few muscle fibers of the unit that are in the range of the EMG needle*

   (D) Cooling of the muscle (from 37°C to 30°C): increase in the duration; decrease in the amplitude; marked increase in the percentage of polyphasic potentials

   (E) The MUP is made up of less than 20 muscle fibers lying within a 1-mm radius from the electrode tip.

   (F) *MUP waveform*

      (1) *Amplitude: typically 200 μV to 3 mV; determined largely by the distance between the recording electrode and the active fibers that are closest to it;* computer simulations have suggested that MUP is determined by less than eight fibers situated within 0.5 mm of the electrode.

(F) *MUP waveform (cont'd)*

(2) *Rise time*

(a) Time lag from the initial positive peak to the subsequent negative peak

(b) Should be less than 500 microseconds

(c) Area of negative spike depends on number and diameter of muscle fibers closest to electrode and their temporal dispersion.

(d) A crisp sound is associated with minimized rise time (optimal needle electrode position).

(e) Distant units have a slower rise time.

(3) Duration

(a) Relates to anatomic scatter of end plates of the muscle fibers in the units studied

(b) Measured from the initial takeoff to the return to the baseline

(c) Indicates the degree of synchrony among many individual muscle fibers

(d) Varies from 2 to 15 milliseconds depending on the muscle, temperature, and age: decreased temperature causes increased duration and number of polyphasic potentials; increases with age due to increased width of territory of end plates that are scattered

(e) Duration is a more reliable parameter in assessing MUP size, and it reflects more accurately all the muscle fibers within the motor unit.

(f) Pathologic findings

(i) Long duration: seen in lower motor neuron disorders and chronic myositis

(ii) Short duration: seen in all myopathies; occasionally in neuromuscular junction disorders and early phases of reinnervation

(iii) Polyphasia: five or more phases, seen in myopathic and neurogenic disorders

(4) *Phases*

(a) Determined by counting the negative and positive peaks to and from the baseline

(b) Normal: less than four

(c) More than four suggests desynchronization of discharges or drop out of fibers.

(d) May see polyphasic potential in normal muscles, but should not exceed 5% to 15%

(e) Desynchronization may be suggested by complex or pseudo-polyphasic potentials (potentials that have several turns but do not cross the baseline).

d. *Recruitment patterns of MUPs*

i. *Recruitment pattern:* the relationship between the number of MUPs firing and their firing rate varies between muscles but is constant for a particular muscle.

ii. *Recruitment frequency:* frequency at which a particular unit must fire before another is recruited; 5 to 20 Hz; the ratio of the number of active motor units to the firing frequency of individual units is generally less than 5 and is relatively constant for individual muscles.

iii. *Motor units are activated according to Henneman's size principle: early re-cruited units are usually small type I; larger type 2 fibers are activated later during strong voluntary contractions.*

iv. Increase in muscle force results in recruitment of previously inactive units; increased firing rate of already active units

v. Number of active units less than 10 is indicative of loss of motor unit.

vi. *Interference pattern*

(A) *Simultaneous activation of multiple motor units precludes the identifi-cation of individual motor units—interference pattern.*

(B) The spike density and the average amplitude are determined by sev-eral factors, including descending input, number of motor units ca-pable of firing, firing frequency, waveforms, and phase cancellation.

(C) Provides a simple quantitative means of evaluating the relationship between the number of firing units and the muscle force exerted with maximal effort

(D) *Decreased recruitment (interference) pattern*

(1) *Characterized by a rapid rate of firing of MUPs disproportionate to the number of units firing*

(2) *Caused by any disorder that destroys motor axons or neurons, blocks conduction along motor axons, or devastates (or blocks) a large number of muscle fibers so that many motor units are practically lost*

(3) *Can be seen in acute neuropathic conditions (trauma, infarction, Guillain-Barré syndrome [GBS]), acute demyelinating and axonal loss lesions, Kugelberg-Welander disease; in uncooperative patients, the interference pattern may be reduced during maximal voluntary effort (but CMAPs are normal in configuration).*

e. *Clinical applications*

i. *Denervation*

(A) Conditions: acquired neuropathy, hereditary neuropathy, plexopathy, radiculopathy

(B) *Typically long duration, large amplitude (reinnervation), decreased re-cruitment, ± polyphasia*

ii. *Myopathy*

(A) Conditions: acquired myopathies, hereditary myopathies

(B) *Typically short duration, small amplitude, "early" or normal recruit-ment, polyphasic potentials*

iii. *Spontaneous discharges*

(A) *Fibrillation potentials and positive waves: APs of single muscle fibers that are discharging spontaneously in the absence of innervation*

(1) *Fibrillations*

(a) *Triphasic or biphasic, 1 to 5 milliseconds in duration, and 20 to 200 μV in amplitude; firing rate, 2 to 20 Hz; high pitched, bi- or triphasic; first phase is positive except when recorded in end plate.*

(b) *Muscle fibers that show fibrillation potentials:* denervated muscle fibers 3 to 5 weeks after acute lesions (may persist for months or years until muscle fibers are reinnervated or are degenerated)

(c) *Grading (variable methodologies used)*

(i) Fibrillations that are not persistent

(ii) One or more fibrillations persistent in at least two areas

          (c) Grading (variable methodologies used) *(cont'd)*

             (iii) Two or more persistent fibrillations of moderate numbers in three or more areas

             (iv) Three or more persistent fibrillations of large numbers but not obscuring the baseline

             (v) Four or more persistent fibrillations of large numbers that **obscure the baseline**

    (2) *Positive waves*

        (a) Biphasic: 10 to 30 milliseconds in duration and 20 to 200 μV in amplitude

        (b) Arising from single fibers that are injured

        (c) Same significance as fibrillation potentials

(B) *Myotonia*

    (1) APs of the muscle fibers that are firing spontaneously in a prolonged fashion after external excitation

    (2) Regular in rhythm but vary in frequency between 40 and 100 per second

    (3) *Occur as brief spikes or positive waveforms*

    (4) *Sounds like a dive-bomber*

    (5) *Conditions: myotonic disorders (e.g., myotonic dystrophy), acid maltase deficiency*

(C) *Myokymia*

    (1) *Spontaneous muscle potentials associated with the fine, worm-like motoric movement*

    (2) Appears as normal MUPs that fire with a fixed pattern and rhythm

    (3) Burst of 2 to 10 potentials

    (4) Rate of 40 to 60 Hz

    (5) Bursts that recur at regular intervals of 0.1 to 10.0 seconds

    (6) The firing pattern of one potential is unrelated to other potentials.

    (7) Hyperexcitability of lower motor neuron/peripheral nerve, ephaptic excitation

    (8) Unaffected by voluntary activity

    (9) In tetany, similar findings are seen but under voluntary control.

    (10) *Conditions: radiation-induced plexopathy or myelopathy, multiple sclerosis (MS),* acute inflammatory demyelinating polyradiculopathy, *chronic radiculopathy, entrapment neuropathy, gold intoxication, facial myokymia (MS, brainstem tumor)*

(D) *Complex repetitive discharges*

    (1) *APs of groups of muscle fibers discharging spontaneously in near synchrony*

    (2) *May be the result of ephaptic activation of groups of adjacent muscle fibers*

    (3) *Characterized by abrupt onset and cessation*

    (4) Uniform frequency from 3 to 40 Hz

    (5) Typically polyphasic with 3 to 10 spike components with amplitudes from 50 to 500 μV and durations up to 50 milliseconds

    (6) *Conditions: typically, those with chronic denervation*

(E) *Cramp potentials*

    (1) Distinguished from other potentials by their firing pattern

(2) Fire rapidly from 40 to 60 Hz, usually with abrupt onset and cessation

(3) May fire in a sputtering pattern, but typically appear as increasing numbers of potentials that fire at similar rates as the cramp develops and then drop out as the cramp subsides

(4) Common in normal patients and usually occur when a shortened muscle is strongly activated

(F) *Neuromyotonia*

(1) *Manifestation of peripheral nerve hyperexcitability*

(2) Fire at frequencies of 10 to 300 Hz

(3) May decrease in amplitude because of the inability of muscle fibers to maintain discharges at rates lower than 100 Hz

(4) May be continuous or recur in bursts

(5) Unaffected by voluntary activity and are commonly seen in neurogenic disorders

(6) *Conditions: hereditary and acquired; may be seen with peripheral neuropathies or after radiation treatment; classically caused by an autoimmune etiology (with potassium channel antibodies, e.g., Isaacs' syndrome).*

(G) *Fasciculations*

(1) *APs of a group of muscle fibers innervated by an anterior horn cell that discharges in a random fashion*

(2) *Conditions: normal patient, chronic partial denervation, including motor neuron disease*

D. **Pathologic conditions**

1. **Myopathic disorders**

   a. Similar findings are that of reinnervation after severe axon loss nerve damage (these "nascent" motor units are myopathic-appearing)

   b. Assess proximal muscles (e.g., iliacus, glutei, spinati, and paraspinous muscle) and midlimb muscles (brachioradialis and tibialis anterior)

2. **Muscular dystrophies (MDs)**

   a. Decreased insertional activity when muscle replaced by fatty tissue

   b. Increased insertional activity, positive waves, fibrillations, and complex repetitive discharges may occur as a result of segmental necrosis of muscle fiber or regeneration of fibers.

   c. Conditions: Duchenne's MD, Becker's MD, Limb-girdle MD, fascioscapulohumeral MD, Emery-Dreifuss MD

3. **Inflammatory myopathy**

   a. EMG findings may be patchy.

   b. EMG myopathic findings especially common in proximal limb +/− paraspinal muscles

   c. Conditions: polymyositis, dermatomyositis, inclusion body myositis

4. **Endocrine and metabolic myopathies**

   a. *Hypokalemic periodic paralysis*

   i. Typically normal between attacks

   ii. During attacks: no abnormal spontaneous activity; decreased duration and number of MUPs, decreased interference pattern, complete electrical silence in severe cases

D. **Pathologic conditions** (*cont'd*)

    4. **Endocrine and metabolic myopathies** (*cont'd*)

        b. *Hyperkalemic or normokalemic periodic paralysis*

            i. Increased insertional activity; decreased duration and number of MUPs

            ii. Myotonic discharges +/– CRDs

    5. **Drug-related myopathy**

        a. Both myopathic and neuropathic findings

            i. Cimetidine

            ii. D-Penicillamine

            iii. Colchicine

            iv. Chloroquine

        b. Myopathic findings only

            i. Clofibrate

            ii. Lovastatin

            iii. Gemfibrozil

            iv. Niacin

        c. Acute rhabdomyolysis

            i. Lovastatin

            ii. Gemfibrozil

    6. **Critical illness myopathy**

        a. Classic myopathic-appearing MUPs

        b. ± Fibrillations ("necrotizing" feature)

        c. Decreased CMAP

    7. **Neuropathic disorders**

        a. Immediately after acute nerve injury

            i. Decreased CMAP under voluntary control

            ii. No complete interference pattern

            iii. Increased firing rate of individual units

            iv. No electrical activity in severe cases

        b. Reinnervation

            i. Decreased spontaneous activity and amplitude of CMAP

            ii. Variable in size and configuration of CMAP

            iii. Increased duration of CMAP and polyphasia

RECRUITMENT	MUP APPEARANCE	DISORDERS
Normal or "early"	Short duration, low amplitude, polyphasic	*Primary myopathies* *Severe myasthenia gravis*
Normal	Mixed short duration and long duration	*Chronic myositis* *Inclusion body myositis* *Rapidly progressing neurogenic disorder (e.g., amyotrophic lateral sclerosis)*
Reduced	Normal	*Acute neurogenic lesion*
Reduced	Long duration, polyphasic	*Chronic neurogenic lesion*
Reduced	Short duration, polyphasic	*Severe myopathy (end-stage)*
		Early reinnervation after severe nerve damage (with "nascent" units)

E. **Clinical NCS studies**

  1. Miscellaneous: maximum difference of NCS latencies between right and left

      a. Motor: 0.7 millisecond

      b. Sensory: 0.5 millisecond

  2. *Neuropathy*

      a. Axonal: decreased amplitude; mild slowing; reduced recruitment; giant MUPs; fibrillation $+/-$ positive wave potentials.

Motor NCS	
Amplitude	Decreased
Duration	Normal or increased
Morphology	Normal, may include polyphasia
Velocity	Normal or decreased (>60% normal)
Sensory NCS	
Amplitude	Decreased
Duration	Normal
Morphology	Normal
Velocity	Normal or decreased (>60% normal)
H-reflex	Increased (<150% normal) or absent
F-wave	Increased (<150% normal) or absent

      b. Demyelinating: NCV less than 60% of normal; conduction block*; temporal dispersion*; distal latency prolongation (* = seen in acquired causes)

Motor NCS	
Amplitude	Variable
Duration	Dispersion
Shape	Normal or multiphasic
Velocity	Decreased (<60% normal)
Sensory NCS	
Amplitude	Variable
Duration	Increased
Shape	Decreased
Velocity	Decreased (<60% normal)
H-reflex	Increased (>150% normal)
F-wave	Increased (>150% normal)

  3. Reinnervation

      a. May begin as early as 1 to 2 weeks after injury

      b. Reinnervation progresses at 1 mm per day

  4. Motor nerves typically degenerate at faster rates than sensory nerves.

  5. Sensory NCSs are typically better preserved than motor NCVs.

  6. Lesion proximal to dorsal root ganglion will produce sensory loss but preservation of sensory NCS.

F. **H-reflex studies**

1. Technique

    a. Stimulating cathode proximal to avoid anodal block

    b. Stimulus pulse with long duration (1 millisecond)

    c. Submaximal stimulus

    d. Frequency = 0.2 Hz to allow full recovery before next stimulus

    e. Late response must be larger than the preceding direct motor response.

    f. *Lower extremity H-reflex: posterior tibial nerve at popliteal fossa (PF) recorded on soleus muscle*

    g. *Upper extremity H-reflex: flexor carpi radialis muscle via median nerve stimulated at cubital fossa*

2. *Neurophysiologic significance*

    a. *H-reflex involves fast-conducting afferent (Ia) fibers via monosynaptic reflex.*

    b. The tibial H-reflex and Achilles' reflex (ankle jerk) are interchangeable

    c. Uses

        i. It is a standard test available within the routine EMG study to evaluate the preganglionic segment of the sensory fibers of the S1 root.

        ii. Upper limit of normal latency: soleus—35 milliseconds; flexor carpi radialis— 21 milliseconds

        iii. Side-to-side difference of latency: 2 milliseconds between lower extremities; 1.5 milliseconds between upper extremities

        iv. Side-to-side difference of amplitude: less than or equal to 3 milliseconds for both upper and lower extremities

        v. Note: may be normally absent in the elderly

    d. *Disorders of peripheral nervous system: absence early in GBS; important in plexopathies and radiculopathies; important in C6, C7, or S1 radiculopathies; useful in radiculopathies—showing the injury to the anterior rami even when EMG is unrevealing owing to sparing the ventral roots*

    e. *Disorders of central nervous system (CNS): important in CNS lesion with upper motor neuron signs*

    f. *Other uses of H-reflex: decreased in cataplexy and acute spinal cord lesion*

G. **F-response**

1. Physiology: F-waves are produced by *antidromic activation (reflected impulse) of motor neuron; useful to estimate conduction in proximal motor nerves by testing length of entire motor nerve; no synapse is tested.*

2. Technique

    a. Cathodes—proximal

    b. Supramaximal stimulation

    c. No need of long duration

    d. Rate less than 0.5 Hz

    e. Gain amplifier, 200 to 500 μV; sweep, 5 to 10 milliseconds

3. *Clinical application of F-wave*

    a. Normal range

        i. Upper limits of F-wave latency

            (A) Hand: 31 milliseconds

            (B) Calf: 36 milliseconds

            (C) Foot: 61 milliseconds

   ii. Maximal side-to-side difference

      (A) Hand: 2 milliseconds

      (B) Calf: 3 milliseconds

      (C) Foot: 4 milliseconds

   iii. Less than 70% of normal patients do not have peroneal nerve F-wave, but most should have normal tibial nerve F-waves.

   iv. *Disorders of peripheral nervous system*

      (A) Prolonged F-wave latencies

         (1) Polyneuropathies

         (2) Amyotrophic lateral sclerosis

         (3) Myotonic dystrophy

         (4) GBS and chronic inflammatory demyelinating polyradiculoneuropathy: prominent F-wave slowing compared to distal motor NCV

         (5) Syringomyelia

         (6) S1 radiculopathy

   v. *Disorders of CNS*

      (A) Absent in spinal shock, and possibly in other disorders of upper motor neurons

CHEAT SHEET

1. Sources of generators

   a. Fibrillation and positive sharp waves are from the spontaneous depolarization of a muscle **fiber**.

   b. Fasciculation, doublets, multiplets, cramps, and myokymic discharges are from the **motor neuron and its axon.**

   c. Complex repetitive discharges (CRDs) result from depolarization of a **single muscle fiber followed by nonsynaptic spread to nearby denervated fibers.**

2. MUP pathologic findings

   a. Long duration: seen in lower motor neuron disorders and chronic myositis

   b. Short duration: seen in all myopathies; occasionally in neuromuscular junction disorders and early phases of reinnervation

   c. Polyphasia: five or more phases; seen in myopathic and neurogenic disorders

3. Spontaneous discharges

   a. Fibrillation potentials and positive waves

      i. Amplitude; firing rate, 2 to 20 Hz; high pitched, bi- or triphasic; first phase is positive except when recorded in end plate.

      ii. Positive waves

         (A) Biphasic: 10 to 30 milliseconds in duration and 20 to 200 µV in amplitude

(continued)

CHEAT SHEET (continued)

(B) Myotonia: regular in rhythm but vary in frequency between 40 and 100 per second; occurs as brief spikes or positive waveforms; sounds like a dive-bomber

(C) Myokymia: spontaneous potentials associated with fine, worm-like motoric movement; appears as normal MUPs that fire with a fixed pattern and rhythm; burst of 2 to 10 potentials; rate of 40 to 60 Hz; bursts that recur at regular intervals of 0.1 to 10.0 seconds

(D) Complex repetitive discharges: APs of groups of muscle fibers discharging spontaneously in near synchrony; may be the result of ephaptic activation of groups of adjacent muscle fibers; characterized by abrupt onset and cessation; uniform frequency from 3 to 40 Hz; typically polyphasic with 3 to 10 spike components with amplitudes from 50 to 500 µV and durations up to 50 milliseconds

(E) Cramp potentials: fire rapidly from 40 to 60 Hz, usually with abrupt onset and cessation; may fire in a sputtering pattern, but typically appear as increasing numbers of potentials that fire at similar rates as the cramp develops and then drop out as the cramp subsides

(F) Neuromyotonia: fire at frequencies of 10 to 300 Hz; may decrease in amplitude because of the inability of muscle fibers to maintain discharges at rates greater than 100 Hz; may be continuous or recur in bursts

(G) Fasciculations: APs of a group of muscle fibers innervated by an anterior horn cell that discharges in a random fashion

Suggested Readings

Daube JR, Rubin DI. *Clinical Neurophysiology.* Oxford: Oxford University Press;2009.

Daube JR, Rubin DI. Needle electromyography. *Muscle Nerve.*2009;39(2):244–270.

Preston DC, Shapiro EB. *Electromyography and Neuromuscular Disorders: Clinical-Electrophysiologic Correlations.* Philadelphia, PA: Butterworth-Heinemann;2005.

CHAPTER 18

Electroencephalography (EEG)

I. *Physics and Biology of Electricity*

A. Ion fluxes and membrane potentials

1. Most of the charge movement in biologic tissue is attributed to passive properties of the membrane or changes in ion conductance

2. Positive ions/cations: K^+, Na^+, Ca^{2+}

3. Negative ions/anions: Cl^-, protein moieties

4. Resting membrane potential: -70 mV (due to difference in permeability of ions and sodium–potassium pump forcing K^+ in and Na^+ out)

B. Action potential (AP): an AP normally develops if the depolarization reaches the threshold determined by the voltage-dependent properties of the sodium channels. An AP is based on sodium inward currents and potassium outward currents through voltage-dependent channels.

C. Synaptic transmission

1. Intraneuronal negative polarity of 70 mV noted with intracellular recording.

2. Resting membrane potential is based on outward K^+ current through passive leakage channels.

3. If resting membrane potential is diminished and threshold is surpassed, the AP is generated.

4. The AP is conducted along the axons to the terminations.

5. When AP reaches presynaptic region, it causes release of neurotransmitter (NT).

6. NT binds to positive-synaptic receptors, opening positive-synaptic membrane channels.

7. *Depending on the ionic currents flowing through the transmitter (ligand)-operated channels, two types of positive-synaptic potentials are generated.*

   a. *Excitatory positive-synaptic potential (EPSP)*

      i. Occurs when sodium inward current prevails

      ii. Increases the probability that AP will be propagated

   b. *Inhibitory positive-synaptic potential (IPSP)*

      i. Occurs when potassium outward current or chloride inward current prevails

      ii. Causes hyperpolarization of the positive-synaptic membrane, making it more difficult to reach the threshold potential

8. *Summation*

   a. *EPSPs and IPSPs interact to determine whether AP is propagated positive-synaptically.*

   b. *Temporal summation:* EPSPs/IPSPs sequentially summate at a monosynaptic site.

   c. *Spatial summation:* EPSPs/IPSPs simultaneously evoke an end-plate potential polysynaptically.

C. **Synaptic transmission** (*cont'd*)

9. Depolarization of the nerve terminal results in opening of all ionic channels, including those for calcium; calcium entry causes release of NT from the presynaptic terminal that binds to positive-synaptic receptor sites.

10. *Chemical transmission is the main mode of neuronal communication and can be excitatory or inhibitory* (if positive-synaptic binding opens sodium channels and/or calcium channels → EPSP; if opens potassium channels and/or chloride channels → IPSP); most common excitatory NT is glutamate, common inhibitory NTs are γ-aminobutyric acid (GABA) and glycine.

11. Several EPSPs may be necessary to generate depolarization.

12. Summation of EPSPs in the cortex occurs mainly at the vertically oriented large pyramidal cells.

13. EEG waveforms are generated by the summation of EPSPs and IPSPs that are synchronized by the complex interaction of large populations of cortical cells (but, rhythmic cortical activity is believed to arise from subcortical pacemakers, including the thalamus).

D. **Glial cells:**

1. Do not generate AP or postsynaptic potentials

2. Resting membrane potential is based only on potassium outward current through leakage channels.

3. With an increase and a subsequent decrease in extracellular potassium concentration, glial cells depolarize and repolarize, respectively.

E. **Field potentials and volume conduction**

1. Excitatory synapse: the resulting net influx of cations leads to depolarization of the membrane, leading to an EPSP. An intracellular electrode notes the interior becoming more positive than it was at rest, whereas an extracellular electrode sees this as a negative potential.

2. Inhibitory synapse: there is an outflow of cations or an inflow of anions at the synaptic site. Then, the membrane potential is increased at the synaptic site, and a potential gradient develops along the cell membrane EPSPs. The electrode near the synapse "sees" a positivity and the electrode distant from the synapse a negativity.

3. Field potentials are generated by extracellular currents. Negative field potentials at the cortical surface may be based on superficial EPSPs as well as on deep IPSPs, and positive field potentials at the surface may be based on superficial IPSPs as well as on deep EPSPs.

4. The movement of charge from excitable tissue to surrounding tissue is called *volume conduction.*

F. **Generation of EEG rhythms**

1. *Cortical potentials*

   a. Electrical activity in the deep cortical nuclei produces surface potentials of low amplitude.

   b. The largest neurons are involved in efferent outflow and are oriented perpendicular to the cortical surface, producing a vertical columnar orientation of the cortex.

   c. Influx of positive ions into the efferent neurons results in a negative extracellular field potential; electrotonic depolarization of the soma and axon hillock results in a positive field potential; because of the vertical orientation of the large efferent neurons, the negative field potential is usually superficial to the positive field potential, forming a dipole.

   d. *In humans, the thalamus is believed to be the main site of origin of EEG rhythms;* oscillations at the thalamic level activate cortical neurons; EPSPs acting on the dendrites mainly in layer 4 (the main site of depolarization) create a dipole with negativity at layer four and positivity at more superficial layers; scalp electrodes detect a small but perceptible far-field potential that represents the summed potential fluctuations.

2. *Scalp potentials*

   a. It is estimated that 6 to 10 cm^2 of cortex must be synchronously activated for a potential to be recorded at the scalp (note: potentials must be volume conducted through the meninges, skull, and skin before being detected by scalp electrodes).

   b. The source dipole is perpendicular to the surface. Scalp potentials are determined by the vectors of cortical activity; if the superficial layer four of the cortex is a positive field potential and deeper layers are negative, then there is a vertical vector produced, with the positive end pointing toward the scalp electrode; the amplitude of the vector depends on the total area of activated cortex and the degree of synchrony among the neurons.

   c. The source of the electrode is near to the surface. Scalp electrodes can record a few millimeters deep and are not able to detect deep nuclei; scalp EEG, therefore, records approximately one-third of cortical activity.

   d. The head is a uniform and homogeneous volume conductor.

3. At least one recording electrode is essentially over the source and the reference is not contained in the active region.

G. **Generation of epileptiform activity**

1. *Generated when depolarization results in synchronous activation of many neurons*

2. **Spikes and sharp waves**

   a. Duration: spikes, <70 milliseconds

   b. Duration: sharp wave, 70 to 200 milliseconds

   c. Spike potentials are the summation of synchronous EPSPs and APs in the cortex; the foundation for the bursting spike potential is the paroxysmal depolarization shift.

   d. The negative end of the epileptiform dipole points toward the cortical surface, resulting in a negative deflection at the scalp electrode.

   e. The distribution of the epileptiform potential across the cortical surface is called the field.

   f. Occasionally, the surface is positive (and in normal patterns of positives and 14- and 6-Hz–positive spikes).

3. **Paroxysmal depolarization shifts**

   a. Extracellular field potentials characterized by waves of depolarization followed by repolarization

   b. High-amplitude afferent input to the cortex produces depolarization of cortical neurons sufficient to trigger repetitive APs, which in turn contribute to the potentials recorded at the scalp rhythmicity, likely due to a mechanism inherent of neurons to be unable to sustain prolonged high-frequency discharges (termination of the sustained depolarization is likely due to activation of K$^+$ channels and inactivation of Ca^{2+} channels).

   c. Ultimately, termination of epileptiform discharges is due to inhibitory feedback to neurons.

   d. Note: the previous points are for partial seizures $\pm$ secondary generalization; for primary generalized seizures, the generator is likely a loop between the cortex and thalamus (possibly also responsible for sleep spindles).

II. *The EEG Machine, Electrodes, and Their Derivations*

A. Input board: channel—formed by the two selected electrodes, amplifier, and recording unit to form a system to display the potential differences between two electrodes

B. Filters

1. Filters selectively reduce the amplitude of voltage changes or signals of selected frequencies

2. *Types of EEG filters*

   a. Low-frequency filter (LFF; also known as high-pass filter)

      i. Allows frequencies higher than designated

      ii. Typically maintained between 0.5 and 1.0 Hz

   b. High-frequency filter (HFF; also known as low-pass filter)

      i. Should not have HFF <30 Hz on scalp EEG because high-frequency epileptiform discharges may be filtered.

   c. 60-Hz filter (to attenuate artifact caused by electrical power lines)

C. Amplifiers

1. Amplifier sensitivity is typically 7 μV/mm.

2. Two main functions of the amplifier: discrimination and amplification

3. Each amplifier has two inputs connected to the input selector switches.

4. EEG amplifiers are differential amplifiers (increase the difference in voltage between the two input terminals, with identical inputs of the two terminals being rejected); this serves to distinguish cerebral potentials that are likely to have different amplitude, shape, and timing at electrodes in different regions and allows rejection of potentials that will be similar at all electrodes (e.g., 60 Hz) if impedance is equal at all electrodes; failure to reject artifact, such as 60 Hz, may occur if impedance is different at the two input electrodes or there is absence of an effective ground to the patient.

D. Calibration

1. Square-wave calibration: square-wave pulse of 50-μV amplitude is delivered to the inputs of each amplifier at rate of 1-second intervals from square-wave pulse.

2. Biocalibration: assesses the response of the amplifiers, filters, and so forth, to complex biologic signals

E. "Paper" speed: typically 30 mm per second

1. Electrodes

2. Usually made of gold, silver chloride, or other material that does not interact chemically with the scalp; skin is prepared by abrasion to remove excess oils and dead skin containing low levels of electrolytes that may alter impedance; electrode gel (usually NaCl) is used to reduce resistance and improve contact of the electrode to the skin.

3. Impedance between the scalp and electrode must be <1,000 Ω.

4. *Electrode placement*

   a. *Standard 10 to 20 international system*

      i. Measuring the head

         (A) Measure from nasion to inion and mark at 50% point.

         (B) Measure between the two preauricular points and mark at 50%; the intersection with step 1 is CZ.

      b. Intracranial electrodes

         i. Depth electrodes

        ii. Subdural/epidural grids and strips

III. Montage

A. Referential

1. Localizes epileptiform potentials by amplitude and complexity (sharpness) of the waveform.

2. Interelectrode distance alters amplitude; usually CZ or CPz (midline posterior electrodes) are used as reference electrodes or ipsilateral (IL)/contralateral (CL) ear electrodes.

3. Digital EEG allows for average of electrodes as reference.

B. Bipolar: phase reversal—localization based on positive deflection in one channel with negative deflection in adjacent channel (epileptiform potentials on scalp recordings are typically electronegative)

IV. Rhythm and Frequency

A. Frequency categories

1. Δ: *1.0 to 3.9 Hz*

2. θ: *4.0 to 7.9 Hz*

3. α: *8.0 to 12.9 Hz*

4. β: *$\geq$13 Hz*

B. Normal awake rhythm in adult

1. Rhythm and frequency differ in that rhythm is a subcortical generation (likely thalamus) of continuous activity, whereas frequency describes that rate at a given time for recorded activity.

2. α rhythm with attenuation/reactivity with eye opening

V. Artifact

A. Physiologic artifacts: usually due to movement, bioelectric potentials, or skin resistance changes

1. Eye movement: cornea approximately 100-mV positive compared to retina

2. Cardiovascular: often noted in temporal electrodes

3. Perspiration: causes slow waves usually >2 seconds in duration (0.5 Hz) owing to changes in impedance between electrode and skin

4. Muscle: usually $\geq$35 Hz

5. Galvanic skin response: slow waves of 1 to 2 Hz that last for 1 to 2 seconds with two to three prominent phases; represents an autonomic response of sweat glands and changes in skin conductance in response to sensory stimulus or psychic event

B. Nonphysiologic artifacts

1. *Two main sources*

1. *Two main sources* (*cont'd*)

    a. *External electrical signal:* 60-Hz electrical input; factors that reduce 60-Hz artifact:

        i. Proper ground

        ii. Keeping electrode impedance low and approximately equal

        iii. Keeping power lines away from electrodes

        iv. Shielded room to reduce artifact from electricity

    b. *EEG equipment:* electrode pops

        i. Spike-like potentials that occur in random fashion and are caused by sudden changes in junction potentials

        ii. Small movements or alterations of the electrode–gel interface may temporarily short out the junction potential, and the sudden change in junction potential is seen in all channels with that electrode in common.

        iii. Dissimilar metals build up large junction potentials that are discharged into the amplifier.

C. Procedures

1. *Hyperventilation (HV)*

    a. Duration: at least 3 minutes of adequate effort (5 minutes if absence seizure is suspected)

    b. **Useful in primary generalized seizure disorders**; HV will elicit seizure activity in 75% of patients with absence seizures.

    c. HV not performed in elderly or other patients with possible cardiovascular/atherosclerotic disease owing to the risk of vasoconstriction with resultant cardiac or cerebral hypoperfusion.

2. *Photic stimulation*

    a. **Useful in primary generalized seizure disorders**

    b. May demonstrate occipital driving (typically at photic frequency near baseline background cortical frequencies)

3. *Sleep deprivation*

    a. Potential for increased epileptiform activity in light sleep

    b. **Useful in primary generalized seizure disorders and partial seizure disorders**

VI. Normal EEG Findings

A. Normal background cortical activity

1. During the *awake state, the patient demonstrates a well-modulated, well-developed 8- to 10-Hz posterior predominant α rhythm.*

2. *Attenuates with eye opening*

B. Sleep patterns: divided into non-rapid eye movement (NREM) and rapid eye movement (REM)

1. NREM sleep:

    a. *Stage I:*

        i. Drowsiness

        ii. About 5% of sleep time is spent in stage I sleep.

        iii. Slow eye movements (less than 0.5 Hz)

        iv. Attenuation of background and alpha rhythms replaced by theta activity

        v. Enhancement of beta activity in the fronto/central regions.

  b. Stage II:

    i. Light sleep

    ii. About 45% of time is spent in stage II sleep.

    iii. Characterized by **sleep spindles** (11- to 16-Hz, localized in the fronto-central region) **and/or K complexes (vertex waves followed by spindles)**

    iv. Positive occipital sharp transients of sleep (POSTS): triangular waves at irregular intervals (usually $>$1 second)

    v. Vertex (V) waves: negative sharp transients at vertex

  c. Stage III (previously divided into III and IV):

    i. Deep sleep

    ii. 25% of total sleep

    iii. POSTS, sleep spindles, K complexes

    iv. Delta activity

 2. REM sleep

  a. Low-amplitude EEG

  b. **Sawtooth waves** (medium amplitude, theta waves) over central region

  c. Decreased muscle activity

C. μ Rhythm

 1. *7 to 11 Hz*

 2. α *variant, arch-shaped*

 3. Noted with immobility over central regions, generally unilateral

 4. Attenuates with hand movement and/or thinking about moving the limb

> **NB:** μ rhythm attenuates with contralateral hand movement.

D. Normal EEG in premature infant includes:

 1. Occasional sharps in temporal and central regions

 2. Δ brush (which appears between 33 and 35 weeks gestational age [GA])

 3. Tracé-alternant: periods in which there are bursts of high-voltage, slow-wave activity that alternate with periods of low-voltage activity (common between 33 and 35 weeks GA)

 4. Multifocal sharp transients (common between 33 and 35 weeks GA)

 5. **Active sleep (REM sleep):** bursts of REMs, body twitches and face grimace, diffuse low-voltage EEG pattern, absence in chin myogram, irregular cardiorespiratory function

 6. **Quiet sleep (NREM sleep):** no eye movements, reduced body movements, tonic activity of chin myogram, regular cardiorespiratory functions and slow wave EEG and tracé-alternant pattern

E. EEG of neonates and infants

 1. *Preterm*

  a. $<$29 weeks GA

    i. Discontinuous with periodic bursts of moderately high-amplitude activity on suppressed background recurring every 6 seconds ("tracé discontinu"). These periods of EEG activity last less than 5 seconds and are followed by flat background.

  a. <29 weeks GA (*cont'd*)

   ii. Δ brush (which occasionally may also be seen in term infants) at 0.3 to 1.5 Hz in posterior quadrant with overriding faster frequencies

  b. 32 to 34 weeks GA: multifocal sharp transients can be seen as normal variant (and may persist until 44 weeks GA); greater differentiation between quiet and active sleep.

  c. 37 to 42 weeks GA: continuous θ and Δ activity; quiet sleep (QS) with tracé alternant and delta slow; active sleep (AS) with continuous low-amplitude activity or mixed pattern of delta and theta activity

2. *Full term*

  a. Tracé-alternant with mild asynchronies

  b. **Sleep spindles do not occur until 8 weeks postterm.**

  c. **At 3 months postterm, vertex waves present**

CONCEPTUAL AGE	EEG FINDINGS
<29 wks	The discontinuous pattern, or *tracé discontinu*, is accompanied by irregular respiration and occasional eye movement.
27–30 wks	Hemispheric asynchrony and discontinuous EEG are common; temporal sharp waves are common; Δbrush present (Δwith superimposed 14- to 24-Hz activity with posterior prominence); differentiate quiet sleep (QS) (discontinuous EEG and eye movement is rare) from active sleep (AS) (usually continuous △ activity)
30–33 wks	EEG of AS is nearly continuous with low-voltage mixed-frequency patterns; EEG of QS remains discontinuous; Δbrushes and temporal sharp waves remain prominent; amount of indeterminate sleep decreases and NREM–REM cycle becomes more evident, with a duration of 45 mins by week 34 and increases to 60–70 mins by term delivery; state rhythms are more prominent.
	AS demonstrates increased muscle tone compared to QS; QS has more regular cardiac and respiratory rhythms than AS.
33–37 wks	AS develops additional features, including REMs, smiles, grimaces, and other movements; 3rd state develops that is similar to AS but eyes are open; is considered a step toward wake state.
37–40 wks	AS by 37 wks conceptual age is well developed with low- to moderate-voltage continuous EEG, REMs, irregular breathing, muscle atonia, and phasic twitches; QS demonstrates respiration that is regular, extra-ocular movements are sparse/absent, and body movements are few; the discontinuous EEG pattern seen at earlier ages evolves to tracé-alternant (1- to 10-sec bursts of moderate- to high-voltage mixed-frequency activity alternates with 6- to 10-sec bursts of low-voltage mixed-frequency activity); Δbrush becomes less frequent and disappears between 37 and 40 wks conceptual age; periods of continuous slow-wave activity begin to occur during QS at approximately 37 wks conceptual age, becoming more prevalent with increasing age.

3. **By 6 months old, 6-Hz background**

4. **By 3 years old (y/o), typically achieve α background (8-Hz) activity**

VII. Abnormal EEG Findings

A. Slowing: may reflect cerebral dysfunction

B. Polymorphic delta activity: arrhythmic, irregular delta activity associated with white-matter lesions; can be focal or generalized

C. Asymmetry: differences in amplitude between two homologous head regions of at least of 50%; amplitude may be decreased or, less often, increased on abnormal side. A skull defect produces increased amplitudes ("breach rhythm"), whereas subdural hygroma, hematoma, or empyema may cause decrease of amplitudes.

D. Suppression: loss of cerebral activity with less than 20 uV of amplitude

E. Abnormal activity:

1. Spike: sharp ascending and descending (duration <70 msc)

2. Sharp wave (70–200 msc)

3. Slow activity (>200 msc).

4. Excessive fast (beta): seen in fronto-central regions; may be caused by benzodiaze-pines and barbiturates (Figure 18.1)

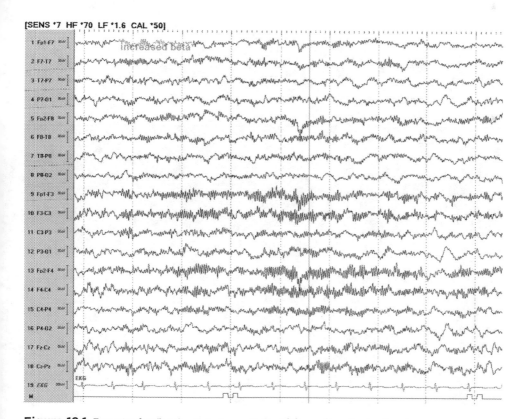

Figure 18.1 Excessive fast (beta) activity in a patient with benzodiazepine treatment.

VIII. Important EEG Findings (for the Boards)

A. EEG of increased intracranial pressure

1. Rhythmic slow activity in Δ-θ range

2. EEG typically not changed by ↑ intracranial pressure until >30 mmHg

B. α coma (8–13 Hz): pattern seen diffusely, predominantly in the frontal regions, monomorphic, nonreactive

1. *Hypoxia*

2. *Drug overdose*

3. *Pontomesencephalic lesion*

> **NB:** α *coma* pattern can be seen in comatose patients with pontine infarctions.

C. **Cerebral death: technical aspects of EEG recording for cerebral death**

1. Interelectrode distance: 10 cm

2. Impedance: 100 to 10,000 Ω

3. Sensitivity: 2 μV/mm

4. Electrocardiography (EKG) monitoring

5. Minimum of eight scalp electrodes

6. LFF <1 Hz

7. HFF >30 Hz

D. **Triphasic waves (Figure 18.2)**

1. *Hepatic/renal encephalopathy*

2. *Generalized frontal maximal discharge with 0.2- to 0.5-second major positive wave preceded and followed by minor negative waves*

3. *Frontal-to-posterior lag in the positive wave*

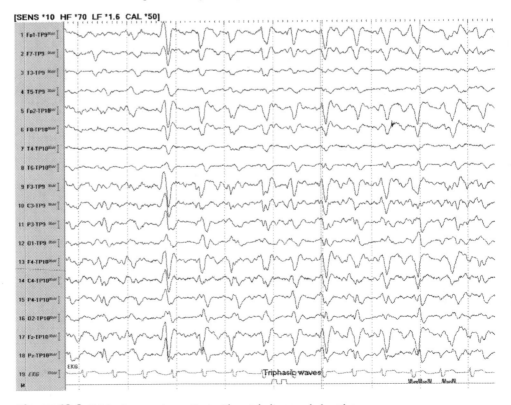

Figure 18.2 Triphasic waves in a patient with metabolic encephalopathy.

E. Periodic lateralizing epileptiform discharges (Figure 18.3): usually positive-anoxic or ischemic state (i.e., stroke) > infection (herpes virus encephalitis) > tumor; frequency, 0.5 to 2.0 Hz. Most common cause is stroke, followed by herpes simplex encephalitis.

F. Epileptiform activity:

1. *3-Hz spike and wave* (see Figure 18.4) *facilitated by*

    a. HV

    b. Alkalosis

    c. Hypoglycemia

    d. Drowsiness

2. Occurrence of 3-Hz spike and wave and other epileptiform discharges is diminished during REM sleep.

3. *Spikes and sharp waves* (see Figure 18.5): duration—spikes <70 milliseconds; sharp wave: 70 to 200 milliseconds

4. *Focal epileptiform potentials:* localization: temporal, 70%; frontal, 20%; occipital/ parietal, 10%

5. *Spike and slow wave:* spike represents excitatory potential; slow wave represents inhibitory potential.

6. In 20% to 30% of patients with epilepsy, no epileptiform potentials may be seen during four separate sleep-deprived EEGs.

7. *Discharges:* associated with infantile spasms/**West syndrome**—EEG with electrodecrement (abrupt attenuation of background)

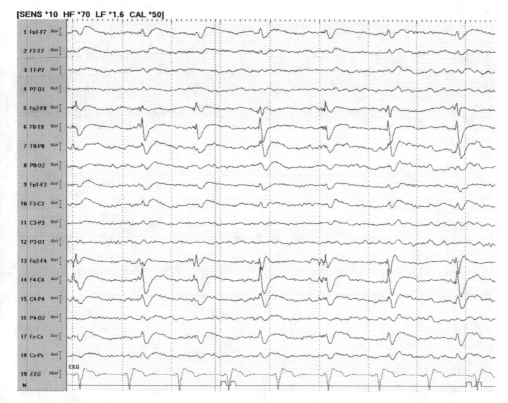

Figure 18.3 Periodic lateralized epileptiform discharges seen in an adult with a right middle cerebral artery (MCA) acute stroke.

7. *Discharges* (*cont'd*)

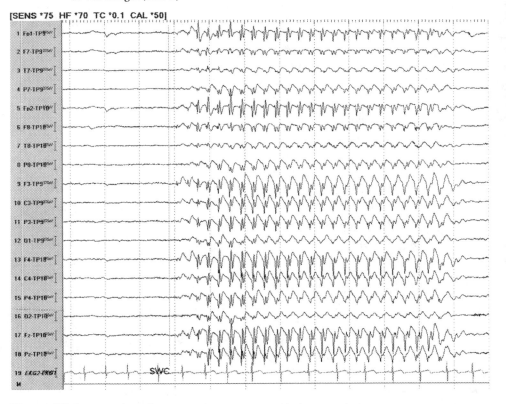

Figure 18.4 3-Hz spike and wave complex in a patient with absences seizures.

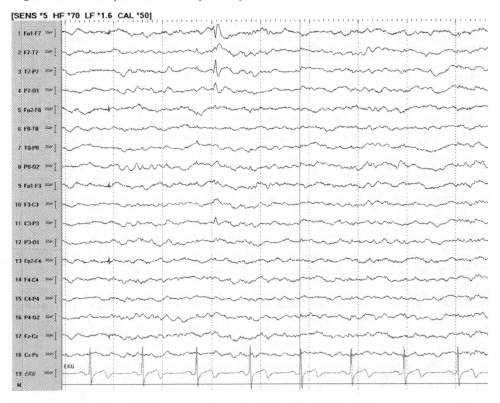

Figure 18.5 Temporal lobe sharp waves in a patient with temporal lobe epilepsy.

8. Slow spike and wave EEG (<2.5 Hz) and generalized seizure => Lennox—Gastaut syndrome

9. Benign rolandic epilepsy or benign childhood epilepsy with centro-temporal spikes (BCECTS): pediatric epilepsy syndrome characterized by centro-temporal spikes

G. **Burst suppression (Figure 18.6)**

1. *Due to anoxic/ischemic injury or medication effect*

2. *Intermittent sharp complexes interspersed with low-amplitude Δ or minimal activity*

H. **Generalized pseudoperiodic sharp waves:** occur in about two-thirds of patients with sporadic Creutzfeldt–Jakob disease (contrasted with periodic sharp waves seen in subacute sclerosing panencephalitis [SSPE], which are bilaterally symmetrical, synchronous, high-voltage [200- to 500-mv] bursts of polyphasic, stereotyped delta wave).

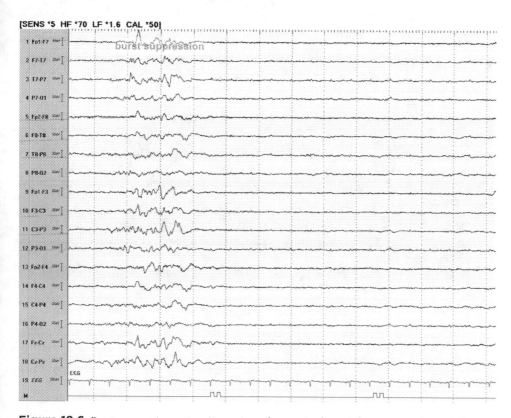

Figure 18.6 Burst suppression pattern in a patient who sustained anoxic brain injury after cardiac arrest.

CHEAT SHEET (see figures)

1. *Beta activity increases (excessive beta) with benzodiazepines and barbiturates.*
2. *Hyperventilation activates abnormal activity in 30% to 50% of patients.*
3. *Photic stimulation => primary generalized epilepsy*
4. *Sleep stage II: spindles and vertex waves; sleep stage III: delta waves*
5. *REM sleep (rapid eye movements): low-amplitude EEG*
6. *Normal EEG in premature infant:* **active sleep (REM sleep)**: *bursts of REMs, body twitches, and face grimace; diffuse low-voltage EEG pattern; absence in chin myogram; irregular cardiorespiratory function.* **Quiet sleep (NREM sleep)**: *no eye movements, reduced body movements, tonic activity of chin myogram, regular cardiorespiratory functions; slow-wave EEG and tracé-alternant pattern.*
7. *3-Hz spike and wave complex seen during absence seizure (pyknolepsy) = increased with* **hyperventilation and hypoglycemia**
8. *Benign* **rolandic** *epilepsy or benign childhood epilepsy with centro-temporal spikes (BCECTS): centro-temporal spikes in children*
9. *Temporal lobe epilepsy: temporal lobe discharges better seen during sleep.*
10. *Hypsarrhythmia: irregular, chaotic, multifocal discharges with a very high amplitude, slow background => epileptic (infantile) spasms, West syndrome*
11. *Generalized* **pseudoperiodic** *sharp waves—***sporadic Creutzfeldt–Jakob disease; periodic** *sharp waves—***subacute sclerosing panencephalitis (SSPE)**
12. *Burst suppression => anoxic brain injury => poor prognosis*
13. *Triphasic waves = hepatic (or renal) encephalopathy*
14. *Brain death => EEG* **sensitivity: 2 μV/mm**
15. *Periodic lateralized epileptiform discharges (PLEDs) =>stroke, herpes encephalitis*

Suggested Readings

Ebersole, JS, Pedley, TA. *Current Practice of Clinical Electroencephalography.* 3rd ed. Philadelphia, PA: Lippincott Williams & Wilkins:2003.

Schomer, DL, Lopes Da Silva, F. *Niedermeyer's Electrocephalography: Basic Principles, Clinical Applications, and Related Fields.* 6th ed. Philadelphia, PA: Lippincott Williams & Wilkins:2011.

Wyllie, E. *The Treatment of Epilepsy: Principles and Practice.* 5th ed. Philadelphia, PA: Lippincott Williams & Wilkins:2011.

CHAPTER 19

Evoked Potentials

I. Evoked Potentials (EPs)

A. Brainstem auditory-evoked responses (BAERs)

Classification of BAERs According to Latency

TYPE	LATENCY (MSECS)	PRESUMED SOURCE
Early (short latency)	<12	
Electrocochleogram	1–4	Auditory nerve compound AP
BAERs	1–12	Wave I = auditory nerve AP
		Waves II–V brainstem
Middle	12–50	Myogenic vs. neurogenic source
Transient		
Steady state		
Slow or late	>50	
Late	50–250	Cortical (N100, P150, N200)
Long	>250	Cortical (P300)

1. *Early auditory-evoked potentials (AEPs)*

   a. *Electrocochleogram*

      i. Sound waves travel via the external auditory canal to the tympanic membrane, in which they produce changes in air pressure and displacement of the tympanic membrane → displacements of the tympanic membrane are transmitted via the ossicular chain (malleus, incus, and stapes) to the oval window of the cochlea.

      ii. The cochlea contains the cochlear duct, an endolymphatic epithelial tube; the endolymph is suspended within another space, the perilymphatic space, which is a spiral tube enclosed at one end by the footplate of the stapes in the oval window and at the other end by the round window; it is continuous with the vestibular labyrinth and cerebrospinal fluid; within the cochlear duct are the basilar membrane and organ of Corti; vibration or displacement of the stapedial foot plate causes change in perilymphatic pressure; vibrations transmitted at the stapedial foot plate are transmitted into a traveling wave at the basilar membrane; high-frequency vibes produce maximum displacement at the base of the cochlea, whereas low-frequency vibes produce maximum displacement at the apex; organ of Corti contains sensory cells: inner and outer hair cells that carry cilia of graded length, with longest embedded in tectorial membrane; when the basilar membrane vibrates, hair cell cilia bend against the tectorial membrane and are moved by the endolymphatic displacement, which produces electrical depolarization of hair cells (receptor potential); inner hair cells transmit to afferent nerve fibers of spiral ganglion cells (the

1. *Early auditory-evoked potentials (AEPs) (cont'd)*

   first-order afferents of the auditory system) and from there form the cochlear nerve; a separate set of spiral ganglion fibers innervates the outer hair cells.

   iii. Occurs within 2.5 milliseconds of stimulus

2. *BAERs*

   a. Physiology

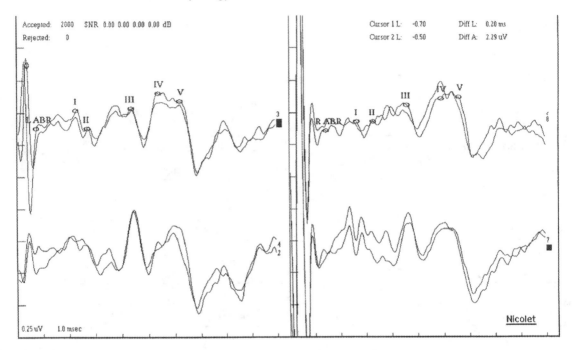

Figure 19.1 Brainstem auditory-evoked potentials. Wave legend: I, acoustic nerve; II, compound AP of the auditory nerve at the entrance into the brainstem, or cochlear nuclei (medulla); III, cochlear nucleus and trapezoid body or superior olivary complex (pons); IV, lateral lemniscus (pons) or superior olivary complex; V, inferior colliculus (midbrain).

Origin of BAER Waves

WAVE	GENERATOR/SOURCE
I	Compound AP recorded from the distal end of the *acoustic nerve* or graded potential of dendritic terminals of the acoustic nerve; approximately 2 msecs positive stimulus
II	Changes in current flow at the acusticus internus, or compound AP of the auditory nerve at the entrance into the brainstem, or graded potentials from *cochlear nucleus*
III	Cochlear nucleus and trapezoid body or *superior olivary complex* and trapezoid body
IV	*Lateral lemniscus*, ventral lemniscus cells, or superior olivary complex or ascending auditory fibers in the pons
V	Generated by projections from the pons to the midbrain, including the ventrolateral *inferior colliculus* and ventrolateral lemniscus; approximately 6 msecs positive stimulus; first wave whose falling edge goes below baseline; last wave to disappear as stimulus intensity is dropped
VI, VII	Higher brainstem structures, including thalamus (medial geniculate body)

    i. All waves used for assessment are negative potentials.

b. *Recording and stimulus parameters*

    i. Earphones must completely envelop the ears to reduce ambient noise; for infants and young children, tubes are placed in the auditory canal because headphones may collapse the external canals.

    ii. Three types of sounds are produced:

        (A) Clicks: most frequently used for routine testing; produced by square wave pulse with the rising phase moving the diaphragm in one direction and the fall of the phase returning it to the origin; condensation = initial movement of diaphragm toward eardrum, refraction = away from eardrum (refraction is used predominantly); duration approximately 100 microseconds (producing a sound complex approximately 2 milliseconds in duration)

        (B) Pure tone: delivers exact frequency; most commonly used for pure-tone audiometry to test hearing

        (C) White noise: composed of all audible frequencies; delivered into non-stimulated ear to mask ambient noise and avoid bone conduction of the click to the contralateral ear

    iii. Stimulus rates: 8 to 10 seconds (waves I, II, VI, and VII have reduced amplitudes at higher frequencies)

    iv. Each acoustic stimulus can be broken down to three components:

        (A) Frequency (Hertz): relates to the location of physical stimulation along the basilar membrane of the cochlea and along the tonotopic representation of the central auditory pathways

        (B) Intensity (decibel): refers to the loudness of the stimulus

        (C) Time: includes duration, rise–fall time, repetition rate, and phase of onset of the stimulus; the phase of onset refers to the initial direction of the basilar membrane displacement.

    v. Intensity of an acoustic stimulus is measured in three ways:

        (A) Hearing level: average threshold in decibels measured in normal adults (0-dB hearing level); ≈30 dB per sound pressure level (SPL)

        (B) Sensation level: subject's individual threshold (decibel sensation level)

        (C) SPL: acoustic stimuli are measured in decibels peak equivalent SPL (dB SPL); SPL uses as a standard reference level of 20 micropascals.

    vi. Recording electrodes should be placed over vertex and bilateral ears and/or bilateral mastoids.

    vii. BAERs are relatively independent of level of consciousness and affected little by sedatives.

    viii. Refraction clicks are recommended because patients with high-frequency hearing loss may have cancellation of out-of-phase responses by condensation and refraction.

    ix. BAER latencies decrease in a quasilinear pattern with increasing stimulus intensities; waves I and V latencies increase as intensity decreases, whereas the I–V interpeak interval remains essentially unchanged; normative values for latency-intensity functions have been derived allowing for comparative analysis.

    x. *Age is another negative variable:*

        (A) In those born prematurely, waves II, IV, and VI are less well defined than I and V, and the I–V interpeak interval is longer than in adults.

        (B) Latencies reach adult level by age 1 year.

    x. *Age is another negative variable* (*cont'd*)

      (C) Latencies also increase as age increases, but the I–V interval usually remains the same; most of the changes are likely related to wave I as a result of associated cochlear dysfunction.

    xi. Gender: females with shorter latencies (presumably attributable to body and brain size)

  c. Clinical applications

    i. *BAERs are useful for:*

      (A) Hearing assessment in infants

      (B) Assessing hearing loss in uncooperative adult

      (C) Evaluating hearing in functional deafness

      (D) Evaluating brainstem function

        (1) Possible multiple sclerosis (MS)

        (2) In central pontine myelinolysis: prolonged waves I–V and III–V latencies (damage to pontine region) with normal wave I (peripheral cochlear nerve/nucleus input)

      (E) Evaluation of neuro-otologic disorders

        (1) Acoustic neuromas

        (2) Cerebellopontine angle tumors

        (3) Brainstem lesions

    ii. Interpretation usually requires measurement of waves I, II, and V and also I–III and I–V interpeak intervals.

    iii. Use of latency-intensity functions allows differentiation of four types of pathology:

      (A) *Latency-intensity functions indicating conductive hearing loss: prolonged waves I and V with latency-intensity curves parallel to the normal curve; I–III and I–V intervals are normal.*

      (B) *Latency-intensity functions indicating cochlear hearing loss: associated with high-frequency hearing loss; recruiting curve for wave I (i.e., normal or mildly prolonged wave I latencies with loud clicks and greater delays decreased intensity, resulting in a steep curve); wave V not markedly affected, and this curve less steep, resulting in a shortened I–V interval.*

      (C) *Latency-intensity functions indicating retrocochlear deficit type I: wave I prolonged with steep latency-intensity function; wave V prolonged; therefore, I–V interval prolonged; associated with lesions of cranial nerve VIII.*

      (D) *Latency-intensity functions indicating retrocochlear deficit type II: wave I latency-intensity curve is normal; wave V and I–V interval is prolonged.*

    iv. Prolonged I–V interpeak interval is most sensitive indicator of brainstem lesion; prolongation of the III–V interval alone suggests at or after the superior olivary complex (in either the high pons or low midbrain).

    v. **NB:** Normal wave V latency practically rules out any peripheral or central lesions in the auditory pathway.

    vi. Most common cause of impaired BAERs is demyelinating disease.

    vii. ↑Age → ↑ hearing loss in high frequency (>1 kHz)

    viii. In brain death, may have complete absence of BAERs or wave I and/or II (wave II noted in 10% of brain-dead patients, which reinforces theory that wave II is generated by intracranial portion of cranial nerve VIII)

ix. Important interpeak intervals may occur in metabolic derangements: vitamin B_{12} deficiency, meningitis, epilepsy, alcoholism, diabetes mellitus; diabetes mellitus and meningitis have findings consistent with damage to acoustic nerve.

x. *Neurologic disorders that cause important transient BAERs*

    (A) *Intramedullary brainstem tumors*

        (1) Wave I: usually preserved because acoustic nerve usually not involved

        (2) Increased interpeak latency (IPL) I–III if pontomedullary

        (3) Increased IPL III–V if pontomesencephalic or midbrain

    (B) *Cerebellopontine angle tumors*

        (1) Absence, increased latency, or increased duration of wave I, and subsequent waves are either distorted or absent but may be present and delayed.

        (2) IPL I–III is often prolonged (if waves I and III are preserved), which is a sensitive indicator for cerebellopontine angle tumors.

    (C) *MS:* no particular BAER impairment is specific for MS.

xi. General interpretation of BAERs

    (A) Absent ipsilateral with contralateral normal: severe unilateral hearing loss due to unilateral cochlear or acoustic nerve lesion

    (B) Absent bilaterally: bilateral acoustic nerve lesions, brain death; rule out technical problems.

    (C) Absent wave I with normal III and V: peripheral hearing disorder with normal central conduction

    (D) Absent peaks after normal wave I: ipsilateral proximal acoustic nerve, ipsilateral pontomedullary lesion

    (E) Absent wave III with normal I and V: normal variant

    (F) Absent wave V with normal I and III: ipsilateral lesion of brainstem (i.e., caudal pons)

    (G) Low amplitude or prolonged latency of entire BAER bilaterally: peripheral hearing loss (especially conductive), distal acoustic nerve lesion; rule out reduced stimulus intensity; in distal acoustic nerve lesions, there may be prolonged latencies of entire BAERs but will have normal IPL I–V.

    (H) Prolonged wave I latency and of all subsequent waves but normal IPL III–V: lesion of distal acoustic nerve, peripheral hearing loss

    (I) Prolonged I–V IPL: most sensitive indicator of brainstem lesion

    (J) Increased I–III IPL (but normal III–V): defect from between proximal acoustic nerve to inferior pons; most common impairment with acoustic neuromas

    (K) Prolonged III–V IPL but normal I–III latencies: if only impaired, suggests lesion at or after the superior olivary complex in caudal pons or midbrain

    (L) Increased I–III and III–V IPLs: IL lesion of lower and upper brainstem

    (M) Increased BAERs threshold: suspect peripheral hearing loss; distal acoustic nerve lesion

    (N) Parallel upward shift of latency-intensity curve: conductive hearing loss

    (O) Shift of latency-intensity curves upward especially at low frequencies: sensorineural hearing loss

   c. Clinical applications (cont'd)

     xii. *Intraoperative BAERs monitoring*

       (A) During surgery in posterior and middle fossa

       (B) Useful for acoustic nerve and brainstem surgery because BAERs are not affected by ordinary anesthetics (e.g., halothane, thiopental; the exceptions are enflurane and imipramine overdose, which increase IPLs)

       (C) During acoustic neuroma surgery, the most common changes are loss of waves II–V or increased I–III IPL.

       (D) Good but not perfect relation between deterioration of intraoperative BAERs and subsequent postoperative hearing deficits

     xiii. *Coma*

       (A) May help differentiate coma due to structural versus metabolic factors (because metabolic/toxic processes usually do not cause important BAERs unless irreversible structural damage is inflicted)

       (B) Body temperature less than 32°C may alter BAERs.

     xiv. *Conditions that may have normal BAERs:* supratentorial lesions, spinocerebellar degeneration, Huntington's chorea, vestibular neuronitis, Meniere's disease, labyrinthitis

     xv. *BAERs in infants and children:*

       (A) All high-risk newborns ($<$1,500 g and infants in neonatal intensive care unit) should have BAERs within first month.

       (B) If normal, nearly 100% will have normal hearing; if impaired, initiate rehabilitation, but be cautious because a small percentage will have significant hearing loss.

     xvi. *BAERs and audiometry*

       (A) Wave V is plotted versus stimulus intensities of 20, 40, 60, and 80 dB greater than hearing threshold, producing a semilog plot with an inverse linear relationship between intensity and latency in normal adults ($\uparrow$ stimulus $\rightarrow$ $\uparrow$latency).

       (B) Effect of hearing loss on threshold and latency

         (1) Hearing loss increases threshold of BAERs, specifically that of wave V if the loss involves the frequencies 1 to 4 kHz, through which click stimuli exert their effect.

         (2) Increases of threshold less than 30 dB above normal hearing threshold cannot be taken as important.

         (3) Increases latency of wave V

       (C) Conductive hearing loss

         (1) Prolongs latency for all intensities, producing an upward shift of the curve but no change in slope

         (2) Interferes with the conduction of sound waves from the ear canal to the cochlea; therefore, acts like a reduction of stimulus intensity that produces a lower amplitude and longer latency of all waves of the BAERs

         (3) At low stimulus intensities, the latency of wave I is more increased than that of other waves in conductive hearing loss, so that IPL I–III and I–V are shortened.

         (4) Does not apply to conductive hearing loss caused by ossicular chain disorders

(5) Impedance audiometry is just as effective as BAERs in assessment of conductive hearing loss.

(6) Latency-intensity curve

(a) Increases the latency of wave V over the range of all intensities, and therefore causes a parallel shift in the curve equivalent to the amount of hearing loss.

(b) The possibility of a central defect must be ruled out by determining that the I–V IPL is normal.

(D) Sensorineural hearing loss

(1) Produces a curve with two slopes; at low intensity, there is decreased responsiveness of end-organs so that for any given intensity → the latency is prolonged; with increased intensity, there is greater than normal recruitment of nerves, so that the curve is steeper; at exceedingly high intensities, there has been sufficient recruitment such that the latency may be normal with the remainder of the slope parallel to the slope of a normal patient (although usually shifted upward).

(2) BAER amplitude is reduced (at least at moderate stimulus intensities).

(3) Amplitude of ratio V to I is usually increased.

(4) Latency of wave V is increased (in keeping with the degree of hearing loss at 4 kHz).

(5) Wave I (if visible) is at least equally increased in latency, causing a normal or importantly short IPL I–V.

(6) Latency-intensity curve

(a) Greatest deviation from normal latency and amplitude at low stimulus intensities (the more the stimulus strength exceeds threshold, the less disparity between the normal and important curve; at high intensities, the latency may be normal, which causes the characteristic steepening of the latency-intensity curve becoming L-shaped)

3. *Middle-latency AEPs*

   a. Occur 12 to 50 milliseconds after stimulation

   b. Middle-latency AEPs uncontaminated by muscle potentials (older theory discusses myogenic etiology as source); probably include components of Heschl's gyrus, thalamocortical projections, posterior temporal gyrus, angular gyrus, and the insula and claustrum

   c. **Lesions of the thalamus or midbrain are more likely to affect the middle-latency AEPs.**

4. Late AEPs

   a. Greater than 50 milliseconds postauditory stimulation

   b. Subdivided into exogenous components N1, P1, and P2 that are primarily dependent on the external stimulus, and into endogenous components P300, N400, cranial nerve V (CNV), and the mismatch negativity (which are more dependent on internal cognitive processes)

   c. Exogenous late AEPs are best elicited by tone bursts and have the highest amplitude over the vertex; N100 may be generated in a posterior-superior temporal plane and adjacent parietal cortex, whereas the later waves may arise from the auditory cortex and frontal association cortex.

   d. N400 is a potential obtained to linguistic stimuli when there is semantic incongruity.

B. **Somatosensory EPs (SSEPs)**

1. *Stimulation parameters*

   a. Unilateral stimulation of a motor/sensory nerve trunk sufficient to produce a moderate motor response is required.

   b. Duration: stimulus artifact is reduced by shorter duration (approximately 100 microseconds); no more than 500 microseconds.

   c. Rate: between 1 and 10 per second (faster than 10 per second is highly painful) and results in low-amplitude somatosensory response; faster rates prolong all absolute and interpeak latencies and suppress cortical amplitudes by 20% to 30% but produce little or no difference on subcortically generated potentials; thus, in short-latency (SSEPs) and AEPs, there is a direct relationship between rate and latency and an inverse relation between rate and amplitude.

   d. Stimulators: either constant voltage or constant current

2. *Recording:* important aspect of recording EPs: replication of waveforms

3. *Generators*

   a. Overview of stimulus and waveform patterns

      i. Near field: cortically generated N20 is a near-field response with maximum voltage between the contralateral central and parietal electrodes on the scalp.

      ii. Far field: in contrast, far-field component is generated by subcortical structures that reach the scalp relatively rapidly via conduction by fluid (e.g., cerebrospinal fluid) mediums (and not via neural paths); typically smaller (microvolts) and faster in frequency and latencies; topographic nonspecificity at scalp.

   b. Most events of SSEPs are from dorsal column–lemniscal system (cuneate neurons not only project to contralateral thalamus, but also to other brainstem structures, including dorsal and medial accessory olives, portions of the inferior and superior colliculi, thalamic nuclei not in the specific projection system, etc.).

4. *General clinical interpretation*

   a. *The undiagnosed patient:* owing to the nonspecific nature of SSEPs, they are of little clinical relevance for the already diagnosed patient, but may have substantial benefit in the undiagnosed patient.

   b. **MS**

      i. *In patients with clinically definite MS, at least one of the EPs is positive in more than 75% to 90%; thus, if all EPs are normal, diagnosis of MS should be questioned.*

      ii. *33% to 50% of SSEPs: clinically silent lesions*

      iii. *Diagnostic yield: visual EPs (VEPs) > SSEPs > BAERs*

      iv. MRI tends to be more sensitive than trimodality EP testing for evaluation of MS.

   c. **Peripheral nerve disorders**

      i. SSEPs are absent with severe peripheral nerve disease or lesion.

      ii. May be useful notably to evaluate proximal nerve pathology (e.g., Guillain-Barré syndrome [GBS])

5. *Median nerve SSEPs*

   a. *Median nerve response components*

      i. *Obligate waveforms*

         (A) *Erb's point potential (EP; N9 [or P9])*

            (1) Near-field triphasic (positive-negative-positive) potential; the prominent negative peak usually occurs at 9 milliseconds (N9) after stimulation at the wrist.

(2) Orthodromic sensory and antidromic motor APs ascending from peripheral nerve stimulation generate EP.

(3) The recording derivation includes negative input potential over the brachial plexus at Erb's point (2 cm superior to the clavicular head of the sternocleidomastoid), and the positive input reference electrode is placed over the contralateral Erb's point or shoulder.

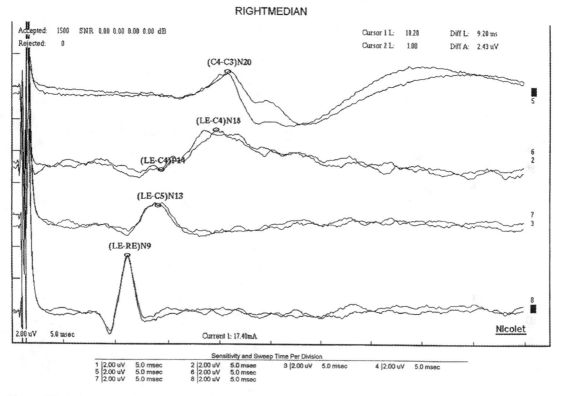

Figure 19.2 Median somatosensory-evoked potential.

(B) *N13*

    (1) Near-field negative potential recorded over the dorsum of the neck (usually at 13 milliseconds after stimulation).

    (2) Can be recorded referentially to any distal point, with Erb's point being a good location because it provides in-phase cancellation of a superimposed slow potential seen at the neck and Erb's point.

    (3) Origin is dorsal horn neurons.

(C) *P14*

    (1) A far-field positive peak present broadly over the scalp (approximately 14 milliseconds after stimulation)

    (2) Subcortically generated and probably reflects activity in the dorsal column nuclei and/or the caudal medial lemniscus within the lower medulla

    (3) In-phase cancellation if recorded scalp-to-scalp, and therefore, should be referenced to Erb's point or torso

(D) *N18*

    (1) Far-field relatively slow potential present broadly over the scalp

    (D) *N18 (cont'd)*

        (2) Subcortically generated, probably from postsynaptic activity from multiple brainstem generators

        (3) Inhalation anesthetics have little effect on N18 (as compared to N20).

    (E) *N20*

        (1) Near-field negative peak

        (2) Generated by the primary cortical somatosensory receiving area

        (3) When recorded referentially, the N20 is preceded by the far-field P9, P11, and P14 and is superimposed on the coincidental N18.

        (4) Origin from thalamocortical radiations

    (F) *Late potentials*

        (1) Include P25, N30, P45

        (2) Largely state dependent

        (3) Typically, these are unsuitable for neuronal evaluation.

        (4) Generators of these are believed to be associated with cortical association areas.

  ii. *Median nerve SSEP interpeak latencies*

    (A) EP-N20, EP-P14, P14-N20, and spinal lumbar potential (LP)-P37 (tibial SSEPs)

    (B) Much more reliable than absolute latencies

    (C) Eliminate most of the peripheral effects, as described earlier

    (D) Not appreciably affected by age/gender in the adult population, but SSEPs of newborns differ substantially from adults because of the immaturity of myelination of the peripheral nervous system and CNS.

        (1) In term neonates, median SSEPs reliably show subcortical potentials but do not demonstrate cortical response (N20) in more than one-third of neonates.

        (2) Cortical response (N20) is not reliably seen until 2 to 3 months of age.

 b. *Clinical interpretation*

N9	N13	P14	N20	N9-P14 INTERVAL	P14-N20 INTERVAL	CLINICAL INTERPRETATION
Normal	—	Normal	Normal	Normal	Normal	Normal; amyotrophic lateral sclerosis; anterior spinal artery syndrome because posterior columns spared; usually normal in cervical radiculopathy but may have delay at N9 and N13; Charcot-Marie-Tooth
↑	—	↑	↑	Normal but may ↑	Normal	Lesion of somatosensory nerves at or distal to brachial plexus (peripheral neuropathy); hypothermia and chronic renal failure should also be considered, particularly if delay noted in all SSEPs

(continued)

N9	N13	P14	N20	N9-P14 INTERVAL	P14-N20 INTERVAL	CLINICAL INTERPRETATION
Normal	—	↑	↑	↑	Normal	Lesion between Erb's point and lower medulla
Normal	—	Normal	↑	Normal	↑	Lesion between lower medulla and cortex
Normal	—	—	Ab or ↑	—	—	Brain death; persistent vegetative state; perinatal asphyxia; hemispherectomy; Minamata disease; parasagittal parietal lesion; thalamic lesion
Ab	—	Ab	Ab	N/A	N/A	Peripheral nerve lesion; rule out technical problem
Ab	—	Normal	Normal	N/I	Normal	Normal
↑	—	↑	↑	↑	Normal	Peripheral nerve lesion
—	↑	—	—	↑	Normal	Brachial plexus lesion
Normal	Ab or ↑	—	↑	—	↑	Cervical cord lesion; cervical spondylitic myelopathy; subacute combined degeneration due to B_{12} deficiency; syringomyelia/hydromyelia; tumor
—	—	—	—	—	↑	Hepatic encephalopathy
—	Ab or ↑	—	—	—	Ab or ↑	Leukodystrophies
Normal	Normal	↑	↑	↑	↑	MS

↑, increased; Ab, absent; N/A, not applicable; N/I, noninterpretable.

   c. **Brachial plexopathy**

     i. Criteria for impairment are decreases of 40% or more in amplitude of N13 or Erb's point potential responses.

     ii. If the N13 were absent or reduced to a greater extent than Erb's point potential, then the lesion is more likely preganglionic.

     iii. If the EP response was reduced to an equal or greater degree than N13, then the lesion is more likely postganglionic.

   d. **Radiculopathy/spondylosis/myelopathy**

     i. *Radiculopathy without myelopathy:* SSEPs are of little clinical benefit.

     ii. *Myelopathy due to cervical spondylosis.*

       (A) Usually seen and are attenuated or absent N13 and N20, a prolonged EP-N13 interval

       (B) Usually little clinical benefit

     iii. An increase in the clavicular-cervical (N9-N13) and the clavicular-scalp (N9-N20) conduction time combined with normal NCVs → is a reliable indicator of root involvement *or cord involvement below the medulla.*

     d. **Radiculopathy/spondylosis/myelopathy** (*cont'd*)

        iv. *Cervical root lesions* are characterized by preservation of the clavicular EP and of sensory nerve action potentials (SNAPs) (unless there is additional involvement of the brachial plexus).

> **NB:** Preganglionic lesions show normal SNAPs because of the integrity of the dorsal root ganglion.

        v. *Postganglionic (but not preganglionic) root damage* is followed by retrograde degeneration of sensory nerve fibers and eventual disappearance of SNAPs.

        vi. Cervical and scalp SSEPs are absent in complete avulsions of the nerve root and delayed or reduced in incomplete lesions (e.g., spondylotic radiculopathy).

    6. *Ulnar nerve SSEPs:* similar to median nerve SSEPs except stimulation of distal ulnar nerve just above wrist

    7. *Tibial nerve SSEPs*

     a. Most normative data are for ankle stimulation.

     b. Responses to femoral stimulation are approximately 20 milliseconds earlier, and popliteal are approximately 10 milliseconds earlier (than ankle stimulation); thus, the tibial P37 is similar to the common peroneal P27 and the femoral P17.

     c. The tibial nerve supplies the gastrocnemius and soleus muscles of the leg, as well as the small intrinsic muscles of the foot.

     d. The proximal stimulus electrode (cathode) is placed at the ankle between the medial malleolus and the Achilles' tendon, and the anode is placed 3 cm distal to the cathode.

     e. Stimulus produces a small amount of plantar flexion of the toes.

        i. Afferent nerve volley recordable at the popliteal fossa (PF)

        ii. LP: potential recorded over lumbar spine

     f. Obligate waveforms

        i. PF potential

          (A) Traveling potential recorded over the midline of the PF

          (B) Near-field potential

          (C) Triphasic with positive-negative-positive waveform; the negative predominates.

          (D) When spinal, cortical, and subcortical responses are absent, it is important to demonstrate this potential to assess preservation of peripheral nerve.

        ii. LP

          (A) Recorded referentially over the broad spinal areas but with highest amplitude at approximately T12 level

          (B) Reflect primarily positive synaptic activity in the lumbar cord with possible origin being dorsal roots and entry zone

        iii. N34

          (A) Subcortically generated far-field potential

          (B) Distribution is broad and can be recorded from several scalp electrode sites.

LEFT TIBIAL

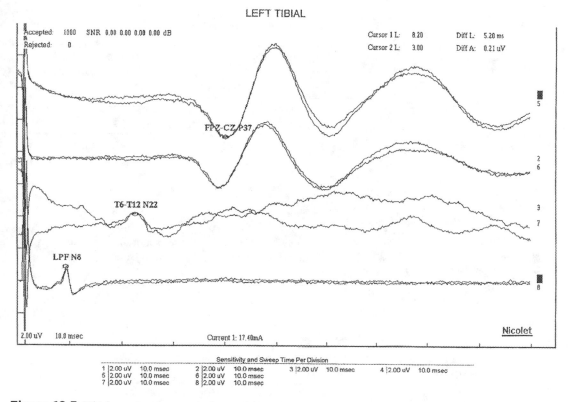

Accepted: 1000   SNR 0.00 0.00 0.00 0.00 dB
Rejected: 0

Cursor 1 L: 8.20   Diff L: 5.20 ms
Cursor 2 L: 3.00   Diff A: 0.21 uV

FPZ-CZ P37

T6-T12 N22

LPF N8

2.00 uV   10.0 msec

Current 1: 17.40mA

Nicolet

Sensitivity and Sweep Time Per Division

1	2.00 uV	10.0 msec	2	2.00 uV	10.0 msec	3	2.00 uV	10.0 msec	4	2.00 uV	10.0 msec
5	2.00 uV	10.0 msec	6	2.00 uV	10.0 msec						
7	2.00 uV	10.0 msec	8	2.00 uV	10.0 msec						

Figure 19.3 Tibial somatosensory-evoked potentials.

    (C) N34 is recorded in isolation referentially from the Fpz electrode and is thought to be analogous to N18 after median nerve stimulation.

    (D) Likely represents postsynaptic activity from multiple generator sources in the brainstem

    (E) N34 is preceded by a small P31 (probably analogous to P14 of median nerve SSEPs).

    (F) Typically not used for clinical assessment

  iv. P37

    (A) Represents primary somatosensory cortex

    (B) Paradoxical lateralization: P37 is maximal at midline and centroparietal scalp ipsilateral to the stimulated leg.

    (C) Major positive wave in the CPi and CPz-Fpz derivations

  g. Clinical interpretation

PF	LP	P37	LP–P37 INTERVAL	CLINICAL INTERPRETATION
↑	↑	↑	Normal	Peripheral nerve lesion; possibly cauda equina; inaccurate measurement; hypothermia
Normal	Normal	↑	↑	Between cauda equina and brain (note: if median SSEPs are normal, this may help localize lesion to spinal cord below the midcervical cord)

(continued)

PF	LP	P37	LP–P37 INTERVAL	CLINICAL INTERPRETATION
↑	↑	↑	↑	Suggests two lesions involving both peripheral nerve and central conduction, or may have single lesion of cauda equina
Normal	Normal	Ab	N/I	Suspected defect above the cauda equina and at or below the somatosensory cortex

↑, increased; Ab, absent; N/A, not applicable; N/I, noninterpretable.

8. *Surgical monitoring using SSEPs*

    a. Loss of median SSEP during surgery is highly predictive of subsequent neurologic deficit.

    b. Anesthetics, such as enflurane, halothane, and isoflurane, may cause a reduction in the amplitude of cortical SSEP (N20); nitrous oxide has little effect.

    c. Subcortical potentials are affected to a lesser extent.

C. VEPs

    1. Anatomy

    a. Retinal function

Properties of Rods and Cones

	RODS	CONES
Operating conditions	Dim (scotopic)	Daylight (photopic)
Visual acuity	Low	High
Sensitivity	High	Low
Pathway	Convergent	Direct
Spatial resolution	Poor	Good
Temporal resolution	Poor	Good
Rate of dark adaption	Slow	Fast
Color vision	Absent	Present

      i. Presume normal optic function to assess retinal function (i.e., cataract alters optic function).

     ii. The opening in the iris diaphragm, the pupil, determines the amount of light reaching photoreceptors.

    iii. Retina has five layers: outer nuclear layer (contains cell bodies of the photoreceptors); outer synaptic layer (aka outer plexiform layer); inner nuclear layer (contains cell bodies of horizontal, amacrine, and bipolar neurons and the cell bodies of the glial cells of Müller); inner synaptic layer; ganglion cell layer

    iv. Visual pigment

      (A) Rhodopsin: visual pigment for the rods

      (B) Iodopsin: visual pigment for the cones

     v. Three subtypes of cones that are sensitive to a particular wavelength of blue, red, or green

    vi. Ganglion cells: three types → (1) Y cells: produce bursts of spikes (APs) in response to stimuli placed in their receptive field and have high conduction velocity and fire preferentially to edge movement; (2) X cells: fire continually in response to visual stimuli and have a small receptive field and are slow conducting and provide fine spatial discrimination; (3) W cells: very slow conducting and are either excited or inhibited by contrast

b. *Function of anterior visual pathways*

   i. Optic nerve: approximately 50 mm long and comprises nerve fibers originating in the ganglion cells; optic nerve fibers are small, myelinated fibers (92% are $<$ 2 µm in diameter).

   ii. Nasal fibers cross to CL cortex and temporal fibers remain IL.

   iii. The functional integrity of the visual pathways, once they enter the optic nerve, can be measured by VEPs recorded from the occipital region; it is presumed these are near-field potentials from the visual cortices.

   iv. It has been determined that full-field stimulation with patterned stimuli is best suited to evaluate anterior pathway function.

c. Anatomy and function of retrochiasmal pathways

   i. From lateral geniculate nucleus, *all* fibers pass to area 17 and then area 18 and 19.

   ii. PET combined with MRI has demonstrated that visual stimulation not only activates areas 17, 18, and 19, but also the lateral temporal cortex.

2. *VEP procedure*

  a. *Pattern-reversal stimulus*

    i. Several parameters influence the response, including:

      (A) Size of checks: affects amplitude and latency of VEP; size is measured in minutes of visual field arc with 60 minutes (60') per degree arc; max response between 15' and 60'; smaller check causes increased latency and reduced amplitude; fovea stimulated better by small checks and the periphery better by large checks; therefore, the recommended size is 28' to 32'.

      (B) Size of the visual field stimulated: should be at least 8 degrees of the visual field arc (because approximately 80% of the response is generated by the central 8 degrees of vision)

      (C) Frequency of pattern reversal

      (D) Luminance: low luminance causes increased latency in P100 and decreased amplitude; pupillary diameter also affects retinal illuminance.

      (E) Contrast between background and foreground: contrast between light and dark squares must be greater than 50% (usually are much larger in routine studies); low contrast may cause increased latency and decreased amplitude P100.

      (F) Fixation: helpful but not essential for reproducible responses; intentionally poor fixation does not affect P100 in most patients but can cause decreased amplitude that may be sufficient to make P100 not identifiable.

  b. *VEP normative data*

    i. *Two most frequent are N70 (negative wave occurring 70 milliseconds after stimulation) and P100 (positive wave at approximately 100 milliseconds $\pm$ 10 milliseconds); often a positive wave P50 (at 50 milliseconds) precedes N70.*

4 CHANNEL OS/OD

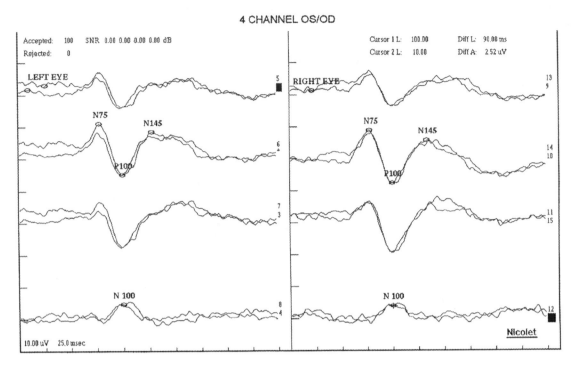

Figure 19.4 Visual-evoked potentials.

b. *VEP normative data (cont'd)*

    ii. N70 and P100 change with age, and delay is most evident after 45 years old (y/o) (likely to ↓ conduction velocities due to defective myelin regeneration or axonal dystrophy, corpora amylacea in optic nerve and chiasm, degeneration of retinal ganglion cells, increased synaptic delay, and/or neuronal loss in the lateral geniculate nucleus or striatal cortex).

    iii. Absolute latency of P100 is important if greater than 117 milliseconds.

    iv. Gender affects latency: women have slightly shorter latency, which may be related to smaller brain size and therefore shorter pathways in women.

    v. P100 also affected by luminance, stimulus field size, acuity, level of alertness

    vi. Pupillary diameter also affects latency, with evidence that small pupils cause delayed latency as a result of decreased retinal illuminance; it is estimated that P100 latency increases by 10 to 15 milliseconds per log unit of decreased retinal illuminance.

3. *Clinical applications*

    a. *General conditions*

       i. *Optic neuritis: in optic neuritis, absent or significantly reduced electroretinograms (ERGs) suggest poor prognosis, likely due to progressive development of optic nerve atrophy.*

       ii. *Papillitis*

       iii. *Ischemic optic neuropathy*

       iv. *Toxic and metabolic optic neuropathy*

       v. *Optic nerve compression*

       vi. *Optic atrophy*

vii. *Early macular disease*

 (A) Funduscopic examination appears normal, and therefore concurrent use of ERG and VEPs helps to elucidate presence of macular component.

  (1) If demyelinating → pattern ERG (P-ERG) is normal.

  (2) If maculopathy → ERG is delayed or severely depressed.

b. *Specific disease processes*

 i. Simultaneous P-ERG and VEPs *in patients with MS detect three abnormalities:*

  (A) Normal ERG/delayed VEP/prolonged retinocortical transient time (RCT) indicate demyelination.

  (B) Normal P-ERG and absent VEP indicate complete block of optic nerve.

  (C) Absent P-ERGs and VEPs, impaired ERGs and delayed VEPs suggest severe axonal damage with retrograde ganglion cell degeneration.

 ii. *VEPs in cortical blindness*

  (A) Surprisingly, VEPs are present in most cases.

  (B) Responses to small checks or gratings may be important but larger often remain constant.

 iii. *Bilateral P100 impairment: bilateral disease of posterior visual pathways*

  (A) Bilateral cataracts

  (B) Bilateral optic nerve disease

  (C) Binocular pathology

 iv. *Reduced P100 on one side is most likely a result of ↓visual acuity.*

4. *ERGs*

a. Flash ERGs

 i. The flash ERG represents the algebraic summation of four basic components: the a-wave, a direct current (DC) potential, the b-wave, and the c-wave.

 ii. The ERG flashes consist of negative-positive deflections labeled a-wave (the photoreceptor potential), b-wave, and c-wave.

 iii. a-wave: negative; results from rising phase of photoreceptor potential

 iv. b-wave: large positive wave; originates in Müller's cells and is related to K^+-mediated current flow; reflects the activity of depolarizing bipolar cells

 v. DC potential: unknown origin

 vi. c-wave: originates in pigmented epithelium

 vii. ERG morphology varies in relation to light and dark, and therefore ERG can differentiate between rod and cone systems.

 viii. Rods can only detect stimuli at less than 20 Hz, and background light less than 8 Lambert can eliminate rod response.

 ix. *Useful in diagnosis of retinal pigmentary degeneration (i.e., retinitis pigmentosa that primarily affects the rods early with impaired night vision [nyctalopia], and normally cones are affected in advanced stages)*

 x. *Congenital nyctalopia:* nonprogressive autosomal dominant disorder characterized by abnormal night vision and normal day vision and normal fundi; ERG → normal cone function but abnormal rod function with absent or severe reduction of b wave in dark-adapted studies.

    a. Flash ERGs (*cont'd*)

       xi. *Oguchi's disease:* night blindness; ERG 26 low-amplitude or absent dark responses of b-wave with diffuse graying of fundus

      xii. *Congenital achromatopsia:* normal dark response but no cone oscillations to red flashes and no light-adapted responses (mediated by cones)

    b. P-ERG

       i. Predominantly a foveal response that originates in the proximal retina

      ii. Dependent on the integrity of the ganglion cells with contribution from amacrine cells

     iii. P-ERGs to transient stimuli consist of a negative a-wave followed by positive b-wave.

     iv. May be used to assess RCT, which, when P-ERG is performed with VEPs, allows assessment of activity outside the retina in the visual pathway; two RCTs have been recorded → RCT (b-N70) and RCT (b-P100).

      v. Delayed P-ERGs occur only in macular diseases: absent or markedly depressed P-ERG in either maculopathies or severe optic nerve disease associated with axonal involvement and retrograde retinal ganglion cell degeneration.

CHEAT SHEET

BAERs—wave origins:
    I = acoustic nerve
    II = compound AP of the auditory nerve at the entrance into the brainstem, or cochlear nuclei (medulla)
    III = cochlear nucleus and trapezoid body or superior olivary complex (pons)
    IV = lateral lemniscus (pons) or superior olivary complex
    V = inferior colliculus (midbrain)
  VI, VII = higher brainstem structures, including thalamus (medial geniculate body)

SSEPs:
Upper limb/median nerve
  Erb's point potential (EP; N9 [or P9])
  N13—recorded over the dorsum of the neck; origin is dorsal horn neurons
  P14—subcortically generated and probably reflects activity in the dorsal column nuclei and/or the caudal medial lemniscus within the lower medulla/caudal medial lemniscus (brainstem)
  N18—subcortically generated probably from postsynaptic activity from multiple brainstem generators.; relatively unaffected by inhalation anesthetics (as compared to N20)
  N20—generated by the primary cortical somatosensory receiving area; origin from thalamocortical radiations

Lower limb/median nerve
  N34—subcortically generated far-field potential; thought to be analogous to N18 after median nerve stimulation; likely represents postsynaptic activity from multiple generator sources in the brainstem; N34 is preceded by a small P31 (probably analogous to P14 of median nerve SSEPs).

(continued)

P37: represents primary somatosensory cortex; paradoxical lateralization: P37 is maximal at midline and centroparietal scalp ipsilateral to the stimulated leg.

VEPs:
The two most frequent are N70 (negative wave occurring 70 ms after stimulation) and P100 (positive wave at approximately 100 ms); often a positive wave P50 (at 50 ms) precedes N70.
Absolute latency of the P100 is important if greater than 117 ms.
P100 also affected by: luminance, stimulus field size, acuity, level of alertness

Suggested Readings

Binnie CD, et al. Osselton JW, ed. *Clinical Neurophysiology: EMG, Nerve Conduction, and Evoked Potentials.* Oxford: Butterworth-Heinemann;1995.

Chiappa KH, ed. *Evoked Potentials in Clinical Medicine.* 3rd [ed]. Philadelphia, PA: Lippincott-Raven;1997.

Kimura J. *Electrodiagnosis in Diseases of Nerve and Muscle: Principles and Practice.* New York, NY: Oxford University Press;2001.

Seyal M, Gabor AJ. Generators of human spinal somatosensory evoked potentials. *J Clin Neurophysiol.* 1987;4(2):177–187.

CHAPTER 20

Sleep Neurology

I. Polysomnography (PSG)

A. Recording

1. To visually stage sleep adequately, the basic monitoring must be at least:
   a. Central and occipital referential (usually to an earlobe or mastoid) electroencephalogram (EEG) linkages
   b. An oculogram for rapid eye movement (REM)
   c. Submental electromyogram (EMG) for axial muscle tone

2. May also place additional EEG electrodes for superficial EMG of upper and lower extremities for evaluation of restless legs syndrome; intercostal EMG for respiratory status; upper airway exchange (thermistors or thermocouplers); monitors of important chest or abdominal patterns, arterial blood gases, or O_2 saturation; EKG; and nocturnal penile tumescence

3. *Standard PSG recording parameters*

PARAMETER	SENSITIVITY (µV)	LFF (Hz)	HFF (Hz)
EEG	5–7	0.3	70
Electro-oculography (EOG)	5–7	0.3	70
EMG	2	10	100
EKG	50	0.3	70
Air-flow with effort	Variable	0.15	0.5
Oximetry	50	DC	15

Abbreviations: LFF, low frequency filter; HFF, high frequency filter.

B. EEG monitoring

1. Colloid provides better contact for long-term monitoring.
2. Resistance/impedance should be kept <5,000 Ω.
3. Basic 10 to 20 international electrode placement.
4. Only C3 and C4 are used to record sleep in adults (with referential to ear); in infants, O1 and O2 are frequently added.
5. A single central channel (either C3-A1 or C4-A2) is necessary to stage sleep, but six or more channels are recommended, including a combo of any of the following electrodes: FP1, FP2, C3, C4, O1, O2, T3, T4; O1 and O2 provide analysis of prominent waking rhythms, whereas central channels are best for V waves, spindles, and/or K complexes.
6. Electrodes to measure eye movement (EOG) are placed at the outer canthus of both eyes; there is a small electrical dipole of the eye with the cornea positive in relation to the retina.

B. **EEG monitoring** (*cont'd*)

7. EMG from chin also recorded

8. Standard paper speed is 10 seconds with 30-second epochs, which results in "compression" of cerebral activity.

C. **EOG**

1. It is commonly recommended to have the referential electrode recording from the lateral canthus to the ipsilateral (IL) ear (provides out-of-phase recording for horizontal eye movements); the disadvantage is marked artifact, especially during slow-wave sleep (SWS) when the EEG reaches max amplitude; this also applies to the referential supra- and infraorbital electrodes for evaluation of vertical eye movements.

2. REMs usually last approximately 50 to 200 milliseconds and have a frequency of >1 Hz.

3. Slow rolling eye movements usually have a frequency between 0.25 and 0.50 Hz, with the duration of the sharpest slope >0.5 seconds.

D. **EMG monitoring**

1. The first electrode is placed submentally on the skin over the mylohyoid muscle, and the second electrode is usually placed 3 cm posterior and lateral (in case first electrode is defective).

2. Tonic EMG activity usually decreases from stage 1 through stage 4 non-REM (NREM) sleep and is absent in REM.

3. A limb EMG is used to evaluate periodic leg movements of sleep (PLMS)/restless legs syndrome, and electrodes are placed over the anterior tibialis muscle (identified by having the patient dorsiflex against resistance); a bipolar derivation is obtained by recording from one electrode on each leg.

4. An intercostal EMG may assist in respiratory monitoring.

E. **Respiratory monitoring**

1. Useful in determining between central, obstructive, and mixed apnea

2. By definition, apnea is a lack of upper airway exchange that must last >10 seconds with >4% oxygen desaturation.

3. All measures of upper airway airflow and of chest/abdominal movement use a band-pass of DC to 0.5 Hz.

4. Monitoring of oxygen saturation/oxygen tension and systemic pulmonary artery or other pressure may also be done, if indicated.

5. *Upper airway breathing:*

   a. *Thermistor*

      i. Thermistor resistor fluctuations are induced by temperature changes in air passing in and out of the mouth/nostrils.

      ii. Useful only for evaluation of respiratory rate

   b. *Thermocouple*

      i. Thermoelectric generators constructed of dissimilar metals (e.g., constantan and copper)

      ii. Generate a potential in response to temperature change

      iii. Usually, two thermocouplers are attached to the nostrils.

   c. *Capnography:* uses carbon dioxide monitor to document CO_2 retention

   d. *Pneumotachography*

      i. Only technique that allows direct quantification of ventilation during sleep

      ii. Can measure flow rate, tidal volume, and other respiratory variables

      iii. Disadvantage: uses uncomfortable airtight mask and is therefore rarely used

6. *Thoracoabdominal movement:*

a. *Strain gauge*

   i. Most consist of a silicone tube filled with a conductor (e.g., mercury or packed graphite), the resistance of which varies with core diameter.

   ii. Inspiration: stretches tube → decreases the core diameter → increases resistance (vice versa for expiration)

   iii. Piezoelectric crystals of quartz or sapphire strain gauges: distortion by inspiration or expiration creates a current; these are more sensitive to movement artifact.

b. *Inductive plethysmography*

   i. It is essentially an improved method of spirometry that separates chest and abdominal movement and adds them together, thus mimicking total spirometric volume.

   ii. The sensors are two wire coils (one placed around the chest and the other around the abdomen).

   iii. A change in mean cross-sectional coil area produces a proportional variation in coil conductance, which is converted into a voltage change by a variable-frequency oscillator.

   iv. Three output channels: rib cage movement, abdominal movement, and total volume

c. *Impedance plethysmography:* rarely used method involving changes in impedance based on abdominal/chest movement

7. *Snoring monitors:*

a. Snoring suggests reduced upper airway diameter and/or hypotonia.

b. Bursts of loud guttural inspiratory snorts after quiescent periods are characteristic of obstructive sleep apnea syndrome.

8. *Arterial oxygen:* transcutaneous oxygen tension for measurement of desaturation with respiratory distress events.

F. EKG

1. Obstructive sleep apnea syndrome patients often may have sinus arrhythmias or extra asystoles, and may have more serious disorders, such as prolonged asystole, atrial fibrillation, or ventricular fibrillation.

G. **Esophageal pH: patients may have insomnia due to esophageal reflux from a hiatal hernia or other conditions.**

H. **Penile tumescence**

1. Strain gauges are placed at the tip and base.

2. Buckling resistance (rigidity) is measured by a technician during the maximal penile circumference during an erection by applying a force gauge to the tip of the penis; force is gradually increased until the penis buckles (or a force of 1,000 g is reached); buckling pressure of >500 g is considered normal (because this has been determined to be the minimal force required to achieve penetration during intercourse).

I. **Technical parameters**

1. Must be performed under conditions conducive to natural sleep

2. A nocturnal sleeper must be tested at night (note that a shift worker must be tested during the period of his or her longest sleep time); for a nocturnal sleeper, daytime testing is not acceptable because there is a circadian distribution of REM and SWS, with REM sleep peaking between 3 a.m. and 6 a.m. and SWS peaking between 11 p.m. and 2 a.m.

I. **Technical parameters** (*cont'd*)

    3. Must avoid prior sleep deprivation (alters arousal threshold) and pharmacologic medications for sleep

J. **Sleep staging**

    1. Basic sleep staging

        a. Most labs use the guidelines set by Rechtschaffen and Kales in 1968.

        b. Usually done at a paper speed of 10 mm per second

        c. Sleep is divided into epochs of 60, 30, or 20 seconds; each epoch is scored as the stage that occupies >50% of the epoch.

        d. A minimum of 6 to 8 recording hours is recommended.

        e. Sleep architecture is commonly altered in patients undergoing initial PSG owing to unusual environment/conditions ("first-night effect"); findings associated with the first-night effect include prolonged sleep latency and REM latency, reduction in sleep efficiency, increased unexplained arousals and awakenings, and reduced or absent stage 3/stage 4 and REM sleep (often accompanied by an increase in stage 1 sleep).

    2. *Sleep parameters and scoring*

Stage 1	May be subdivided into stage 1A (α rhythm diffuses to anterior head regions, often slows by 0.5–1.0 Hz, and then fragments before disappearing) and stage 1B (when EEG contains <20% diffuse slow α [>40 μV] and the EEG consists of medium-amplitude mixed-frequency [mostly θ] activity with occasional vertex waves); scored when >50% of epoch consists of relatively low-voltage mixed frequencies (mainly 2–7 Hz) with relative reduction in EMG activity; other features include slow rolling eye movements and vertex waves (vertex waves may persist into stage 2 and SWS; diphasic sharp transients having initial surface negativity followed by a low-voltage positive phase that is maximum at C3 and/or C4 and with phase reversal over the midline; present by 8 wks postterm)
Stage 2	Characterized by ≥1 sleep spindle, K complexes, and <20% of the epoch containing Δ; spindles are 11.5- to 15.0-Hz central bursts that must last >0.5 secs and have an amplitude >15 μV to be scored, and appear as rhythmic sinusoidal waves of progressively increasing amplitude followed by progressively decreasing amplitude; K complexes are diphasic waves that must contain two of three features (negative vertex sharp wave maximal over central regions, a following negative slow wave maximally frontal, and/or a sleep spindle maximal centrally); K complexes usually occur in trains either spontaneously or after a stimulus; K complexes may appear in infants as early as 5 mos old; may also have vertex waves (see Figure 20.1)
Stage 3	Scored when 20%–50% of epoch contains Δ waves of 0.5–2.5 Hz and >75 μV; sleep spindles may be present but are less frequent than in stage 2 and of lower frequency (10–12 Hz)
Stage 4	Scored when >50% of epoch contains Δ of <2 Hz and amplitude >75 μV; spindles may be present but are rare (note: stages 3 and 4 are collectively also known as SWS; predominates in the first third of night) (see Figure 20.2)

(continued)

REM	Contains medium-amplitude, mixed-frequency (mainly θ and Δ), low-voltage activity associated with REM and relative absence of EMG; bursts of sawtooth waves at 2–6 Hz may appear in frontal or midline regions (generally just before REM bursts); initial REM period may contain some low-voltage spindles, but generally sleep spindles and K complexes are absent; may also demonstrate α frequencies at rate 1–2 Hz slower than patient's waking background rhythm; also may have autonomic instability; although there is relative muscle atonia, bursts of phasic EMG activity may be noted in conjunction with REM; REM stage predominates in the last third of night (see Figure 20.3)
Sleep latency	Time from lights out to the first epoch of sleep (in minutes)
REM latency	Time from sleep onset to the first epoch of REM sleep (in minutes); significantly reduced in certain sleep disorders, sleep deprivation, drug withdrawal; REM latency is usually 60–120 mins
Time in bed	Total time in bed; from time of lights out to lights on
Total sleep	Total time from sleep onset to final awakening (note: some authors do not include stage 1 sleep)
Sleep efficiency	Percentage of time spent in bed asleep (i.e., total sleep time/time in bed)
Arousals	Defined as an abrupt shift in EEG frequency, including θ, α, and/or frequencies >16 Hz (but not spindles) that meet the following criteria: (1) at least 10 secs of sleep of any stage must precede an arousal and must be present between arousals; (2) at least 3 secs of EEG frequency shift must be present; (3) arousals in REM also necessitate a concurrent increase in chin EMG amplitude, because bursts of θ and α are found intrinsically during REM sleep; (4) arousals are not scored based on chin EMG alone; (5) artifacts, K complexes, and Δ are not scored as arousals unless accompanied by EEG frequency shift of >3 secs; (6) pen-blocking artifact is only considered an arousal when contiguous with an arousal pattern and then may be included toward the 3-sec duration criteria; (7) nonconcurrent but contiguous EEG and EMG changes that are <3 secs but together are >3 secs are not scored as arousals; (8) intrusion of α in NREM sleep is scored as arousal only if >3 secs in duration and preceded by >10 secs of α-free sleep; and (9) transitions between sleep stages are not scored as arousals unless they meet the previous criteria; arousals are scored using EEG alone with the exception of REM sleep arousals that also require simultaneous increase in chin EMG amplitude

3. *Sleep onset and sleep cycles*

   a. Sleep onset

      i. No definitive parameters signifying sleep onset

      ii. Three basic PSG assessments

        (A) EMG: gradual diminution but without discrete change

        (B) EOG: slow asynchronous rolling eye movement

        (C) EEG: change from normal background α to low-voltage mixed-frequency pattern (stage 1 sleep), which usually occurs within seconds to minutes of rolling eye movements; patients, if aroused during stage 1 sleep, typically state they were awake, and therefore sleep onset recognized by EEG is taken at stage 2 (presence of K complexes and sleep spindles)

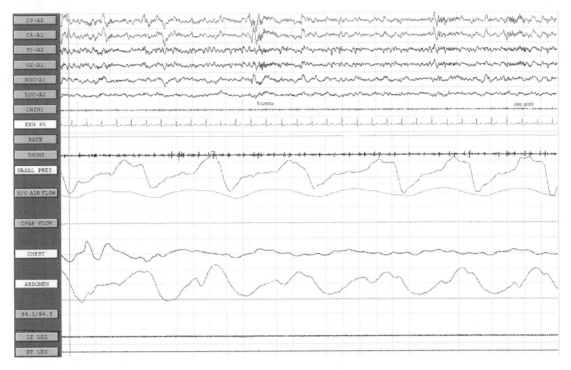

Figure 20.1 Stage 2 sleep.

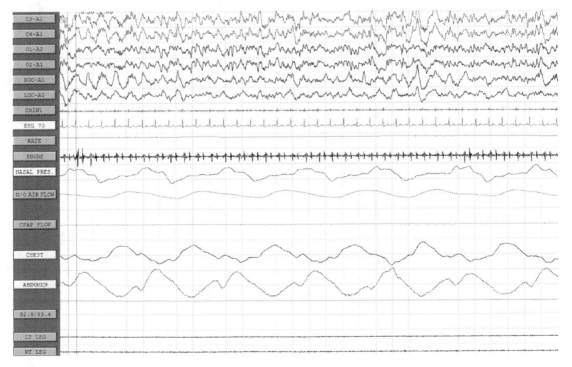

Figure 20.2 Stage 4 slow-wave sleep.

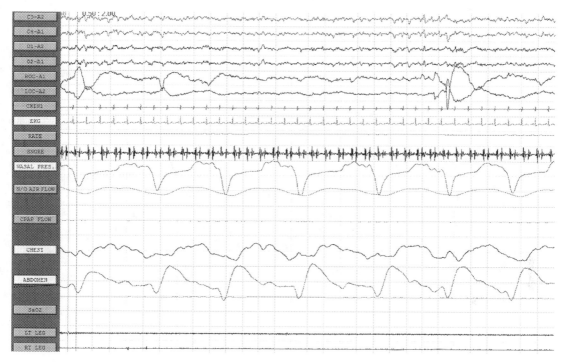

Figure 20.3 REM sleep.

3. *Sleep onset and sleep cycles (cont'd)*
   b. *The first sleep cycle*
      i. Stage 1: in normal adults, the first sleep cycle begins with stage 1 NREM sleep, lasting only a few minutes (1–7 minutes on average).
      ii. Stage 2: follows stage 1 and usually lasts 10–25 minutes; progressive increase in frequency of SWS is appreciated, denoting evolution to stage 3.
      iii. Stage 3: SWS (20–50% of EEG) that usually persists normally for a few minutes and evolves into stage 4
      iv. Stage 4: SWS (>50% of EEG) with higher voltage; lasts 20 to 45 minutes during first cycle; if body movements occur, there is transient return to lighter sleep (stages 1 or 2); often there is transition from stage 4 to stage 2 sleep just before the patient enters REM sleep.
      v. REM: the transition from NREM to REM is not abrupt; REM sleep cannot be identified until the first REM; the REM period during the first cycle is short (between 2 and 6 minutes); REM sleep often ends with a brief body movement, and a new cycle begins.
      vi. The first NREM–REM cycle usually lasts approximately 70 to 100 minutes.
   c. *Later sleep cycles*
      i. The average length for later sleep cycles is 100 to 120 minutes; the last sleep cycle is usually the longest.
      ii. As the night progresses, REM sleep generally becomes longer; stages 3 and 4 occupy less time in the second cycle and may nearly disappear in later cycles, with stage 2 expanding to make up the majority of NREM sleep.

3. *Sleep onset and sleep cycles (cont'd)*

   d. *Dissociated or otherwise atypical sleep patterns*

      i. α-Δ Sleep

        (A) Characterized by presence of α and Δ waves in stages 3 and 4 SWS

        (B) May be induced in healthy individuals without awakening them by using auditory stimuli

        (C) Associated with a number of nonrestorative sleep disorders, especially fibromyalgia

      ii. *REM-spindle sleep*

        (A) Due to breakdown of barriers between NREM and REM sleep

        (B) May occur in up to 8% of normal patients

        (C) Increases in a number of sleep disorders, including increased frequency in the daytime sleep of hypersomniacs and the nocturnal sleep of schizophrenics and narcoleptics

      iii. *REM sleep without atonia*

        (A) Common in patients taking tricyclic antidepressants, monoamine oxidase inhibitors, and phenothiazines

        (B) Disorders include REM behavior disorder.

      iv. *REM burst during NREM sleep*: exhibited by patients being treated with clomipramine (depression, narcolepsy), which is a medication that suppresses REM-based activity

      v. *Isolated REM atonia*

        (A) Cataplexy represents the selective triggering, during wakefulness and by emotional stimuli, of REM sleep atonia.

        (B) Sleep paralysis is the isolated appearance of REM sleep atonia associated with full wakefulness either before entry into REM sleep or during awakenings from REM sleep.

      vi. *Sleep-onset REM periods*

        (A) *The sleep-onset REM period is usually defined as entry into REM sleep within 10 minutes of sleep onset.*

        (B) *Its presence is highly suggestive of diagnosis of narcolepsy-cataplexy and* characterizes approximately 50% of onsets of night sleep in these patients (but sleep deprivation, alcoholism, drug withdrawal, irregular sleep-waking habits, and/or severe depression must be ruled out).

4. *Respiratory parameters and scoring*

   a. Apneas and hypopneas represent decrements in airflow that may or may not be associated with arousals and/or oxygen desaturation.

   b. *Apnea: cessation or >90% reduction of nasal/oral airflow with >4% oxygen desaturation*

   c. Brief central apneas that occur during transitional periods from wakefulness to sleep are believed to have no clinical significance.

   d. *Hypopnea:*

      i. *No consensus agreement of what constitutes a hypopnea*

      ii. *Defined as >50% reduction of airflow lasting >10 seconds and also reductions of airflow between 30% and 50%, which are associated with arousal or desaturation of at least 4%*

   e. Hypopneas and apneas have the same clinical significance as apneas (i.e., apneas and hypopneas are combined to give a total number divided by number of hours of sleep = apnea-hypopnea index or respiratory distress index).

5. *Leg movement (LM) parameters and scoring*

   a. LMs can be periodic (PLMS) or aperiodic/random (after arousals, respiratory events, snoring, etc.).

   b. An *LM* is defined as a burst of anterior tibialis muscle activity with a duration from onset to resolution of 0.5 to 5.0 seconds, and an amplitude of >25% of the bursts recorded during calibration.

      i. LMs do not include hypnic jerks that occur on transition from wake to sleep, aperiodic activity during REM, phasic EMG during REM sleep, other forms of myoclonus, or restless legs.

   c. When scoring LMs, must document whether there are arousals, awakenings, or respiratory events; arousals attributed to LMs should occur no >3 seconds after termination of LM.

   d. PLMS:

      i. Characterized by rhythmic extension of the great toe and dorsiflexion of the ankle with occasional flexion of the knee and hip (similar to triple flexor response).

      ii. Lasting from 0.5 to 5.0 seconds

      iii. Occur at intervals of 20 to 40 seconds

      iv. Occur intermittently in clusters lasting minutes to hours throughout the night

      v. Typically, the total number of LMs is reported with a breakdown of the number associated with arousals or awakenings and respiratory events.

      vi. PLMS arousal index of >5 is important in middle-aged adults (but a cutoff of 10–15 should be used in elderly patients).

      vii. If associated with arousals, patient may present with hypersomnia/excessive daytime sleepiness.

      viii. Patients also commonly will have restless legs syndrome (may be associated with anemia due to iron deficiency, renal failure, and a variety of neurologic disorders).

      ix. A PLMS sequence or epoch is a sequence of four or more LMs separated by at least 5 seconds and not by >90 seconds (measured from LM onset to LM offset).

      x. *PLMS are more abundant in stages 1 and 2 and less frequent in stages 3 and 4 and REM sleep.*

II. The Epworth Sleepiness Scale (ESS)

The ESS: self-administered questionnaire with 8 items; it provides an index of the general level of daytime sleepiness, or the average sleep propensity in daily life. The ESS requests respondents to rate, on a 4-point scale (0–3), their usual chances of dozing off or falling asleep in eight different situations or activities that most people engage in as part of their daily lives, although not necessarily every day.

Interpretation:

   0 to 7: It is unlikely that you are abnormally sleepy.

   8 to 9: You have an average amount of daytime sleepiness.

   10 to 15: You may be excessively sleepy depending on the situation. You may want to consider seeking medical attention.

16 to 24: You are excessively sleepy and should consider seeking medical attention.

III. Multiple Sleep Latency Test (MSLT) and Maintenance of Wakefulness Test

A. MSLT

1. Use

   a. Developed by Carskadon and Dement (1977) and first tested on excessive daytime sleepiness patients by Richardson (1978)

   b. *Used to evaluate*

      i. *Excessive daytime sleepiness (by quantifying the time required to fall asleep)*

      ii. *REM latency (to evaluate specific disorders, e.g., narcolepsy)*

   c. Must perform urine toxicology screen for narcotics, psychotropics, stimulants, hypnotics, and so forth

2. General procedures

   a. Standard montage using the Rechtschaffen and Kales (1968) guidelines

   b. Monitored for five 20-minute nap periods with 2 hours between each period; the first is standard setup for between 9:30 a.m. and 10:00 a.m.; first nap is performed at least 90 minutes after wake-up time.

   c. MSLT is usually performed on the night after PSG so that sleep disorders that might artifactually produce short daytime sleep latencies are ruled out (*important note*: nocturnal PSG will negate the usefulness of MSLT); patient must have at least 360 minutes of sleep on night before MSLT.

   d. General considerations for MSLT

      i. 2 weeks of sleep diaries preceding MSLT

      ii. PSG on night before MSLT to evaluate habitual sleep and quantitate possible sleep-confounding deprivation before MSLT

      iii. Consideration of drug schedule (both prescribed and illicit drugs) with stable regimen for at least 2 weeks before testing (especially benzodiazepines, barbiturates, etc.)

      iv. Minimum of four tests at 2-hour intervals beginning 1.5 to 3.0 hours after waking

      v. Quiet, dark, controlled-temperature room

      vi. No alcohol or caffeine for at least 2 weeks before MSLT

3. Scoring

   a. *Sleep onset* is defined by any of the following parameters:

      i. The first three consecutive epochs of stage 1 NREM sleep

      ii. A single epoch of stage 2, 3, or 4 NREM sleep

      iii. REM sleep

   b. *Sleep offset* is defined as two consecutive epochs of wakefulness after sleep onset

   c. A nap is terminated after one of the following:

      i. No sleep has occurred after 20 minutes

      ii. After 10 minutes of continuous sleep as long as sleep criteria are met (if sleep onset is at 20 minutes, the sleep is allowed to continue until 30 minutes, etc.)

      iii. After 20 minutes or any point thereafter if the patient is awake

d. Sleep latency is measured from the time of lights out to first sleep epoch; usually an average sleep latency of four or five naps is calculated.

e. REM latency: time of sleep onset to first epoch of REM sleep

4. Interpretation of MSLT

   a. *Normal sleep latency on MSLT*

AGE	SLEEP LATENCY
Young adult (21–35 y/o)	10 mins
Middle-aged adult (30–49 y/o)	11–12 mins
Older adults (50–59 y/o)	9 mins

   b. *Decreased REM-onset latencies during MSLTs can occur with:*

      i. *Sleep pathology (e.g., narcolepsy, severe obstructive sleep apnea)*

      ii. Sleep deprivation

   c. *MSLT interpretation of sleep-onset latency*

SEVERITY OF SLEEPINESS	SLEEP LATENCY ON MSLT	CLINICAL CORRELATION
Severe	<5 mins	Presence of pathologic or significant sleepiness; sleep episodes are present daily during times that require moderate attentiveness, such as eating, driving, and so forth, resulting in impairment of normal daily function
Moderate	5–10 mins	Excessively sleepy; sleep episodes occur daily during times that require moderate attentiveness, such as watching a movie/performance or attending a meeting
Mild	10–15 mins	Sleep episodes occur normally during times of relaxation, requiring little attentiveness, such as a passenger in a car or watching television

   d. Eighty-five percent of narcoleptics have a mean sleep latency of <5 minutes.

   e. Patients with mild to moderate obstructive sleep apnea syndrome or sleep deprivation may have borderline sleep latency between 5 and 10 minutes.

   f. Sleep latency may be affected by several factors, including:

      i. Sleep deprivation: causing a shortened sleep-onset latency

      ii. Sleep–wake schedule: must assess during patients' normal sleep schedule (e.g., shift worker)

      iii. Medications

      iv. Environment: environmental factors (e.g., noise) may cause prolonged sleep latency.

B. **Maintenance of wakefulness test**

   1. An alternative to MSLT

   2. Requires subject to sit in dark room with eyes closed reclining at a 45-degree angle

   3. Required to attempt to stay awake for 20 minutes

   4. Three to four testing periods every 2 hours

CHEAT SHEET

A. Stages of Sleep:
Stage 1:
1A (α rhythm diffuses to anterior head regions, often slows by 0.5–1.0 Hz, and then fragments before disappearing)
1B (when EEG contains <20% diffuse slow α; scored when >50% of epoch consists of relatively low-voltage mixed frequencies [mainly 2–7 Hz] with relative reduction in EMG activity)
Stage 2:
≥1 sleep spindle, K complexes, and <20% of the epoch containing Δ
Stage 3:
20% to 50% of epoch contains Δ waves of 0.5 to 2.5 Hz and >75 μV; sleep spindles may be present but are less frequent than in stage 2 and of lower frequency (10–12 Hz)
Stage 4:
>50% of epoch contains Δ of <2 Hz and amplitude >75 μV; spindles may be present but are rare (note: stages 3 and 4 are collectively also known as slow-wave sleep [SWS])
B.
Apnea: cessation or >90% reduction of nasal/oral airflow with >4% oxygen desaturation
Hypopnea: defined as >50% reduction of airflow lasting >10 seconds and also reductions of airflow between 30% and 50%, which are associated with arousal or desaturation of at least 4%
C:
The ESS: self-administered questionnaire with 8 items; it provides an index of the general level of daytime sleepiness, or the average sleep propensity in daily life. Interpretation: 0 to 7: unlikely for patient to be abnormally sleepy; 8 to 9: average amount of daytime sleepiness; 10 to 15: excessively sleepy depending on the situation and might consider seeking medical attention; 16 to 24: excessively sleepy and should consider seeking medical attention.
D:
Severity of sleepiness on MSLT:
Severe = <5 mins; moderate = 5 to 10 mins; mild = 10 to 15 mins.

Suggested Readings

Shelgikar, AV, Chervin, R. Approach to and evaluation of sleep disorders. *Continuum (Minneap Minn)*.2013;*19*(1):32–49.

Rechtschaffen, A, Kales, A. A manual of standardized terminology, techniques and scoring system for sleep stages of human subjects. Bethesda, MD: U.S. Department of Health, Education, and Welfare, 1968.

Voderholzer, U, Guilleminault, C. Sleep disorders. In: Sclaepfer, TE, Nemeroff, CB. eds. *Neurobiology of Psychiatric Disorders*. Amsterdam, Netherlands: Elsevier;2012:527–540.

Watson, NF, Viola-Saltzman, M. Sleep and comorbid neurologic disorders. *Continuum (Minneap Minn)*.2013;*19*(1):148–169.

Pediatric Neurology

CHAPTER 21

Pediatric Neurology

I. Embryology and Development

A. Embryology of nervous system and corresponding disorders (*high-yield items*)

DEVELOPMENTAL PROCESS	TIME OF OCCURRENCE	DISORDER	ETIOLOGY (EXAMPLES)	ADDITIONAL INFORMATION
Primary neurulation	1st month of gestation	Craniorachischisis totalis	Failure of neural tube formation	Notochord
		Anencephaly	Failure of anterior neural tube closure	
		Myeloschisis	Failure of posterior neural tube closure	
		Encephalocele	Restricted failure of anterior neural tube closure	*Usually occipital*, part of Chiari III malformation
		Myelomeningocele	Restricted failure of posterior neural tube closure	Can be associated with *hydrocephalus and Chiari II*

(continued)

DEVELOPMENTAL PROCESS	TIME OF OCCURRENCE	DISORDER	ETIOLOGY (EXAMPLES)	ADDITIONAL INFORMATION
Prosencephalic development	2nd month of gestation	*Holoprosencephaly*	Failure of prosencephalic cleavage	Can be associated with *trisomy 13*
		Agenesis of corpus callosum	Disorder of midline prosencephalic development	Associated with *Aicardi syndrome*
		Septo-optic dysplasia		Optic atrophy and endocrine abnormalities
Neuronal proliferation	3rd month of gestation	Microcephaly (<3rd percentile head circumference)	Syndromic (trisomy 13/18) Infection (TORCH) Metabolic—toxic (fetal alcohol, maternal phenylketonuria [PKU])	
		Macrocephaly (>95th percentile head circumference)	Familial Genetic (fragile X, tuberous sclerosis, Sotos)	
Neuronal migration	4th month of gestation	Schizencephaly	Cleft in the brain from agenesis of germinative zones	MRI diagnosis, cleft lined by gray matter
		Lissencephaly	Smooth brain—few to no gyri due to defect in pace of migration	Type 1: smooth, *LIS1 gene (Miller-Dieker) or X-linked lissencephaly/DCX gene in males*
			Failure of neurons to terminate radial migration in cerebral cortex	Type 2: cobblestone (Fukuyama muscle dystrophy and Walker-Warburg syndrome)

(continued)

DEVELOPMENTAL PROCESS	TIME OF OCCURRENCE	DISORDER	ETIOLOGY (EXAMPLES)	ADDITIONAL INFORMATION
		Polymicrogyria	Multiple small gyri from fusion of molecular layers	Common in *Zellweger syndrome*
		Neuronal heterotopia	Collections of nerve cells arrested in radial migration	Periventricular heterotopia: filamin gene *Subcortical band heterotopia DCX/doublecortin gene in females*
Organization	5th month to postnatal	Multiple disorders causing intellectual disability		
myelination	Birth to postnatal	Multiple disorders, including periventricular leukomalacia and organic acidopathies, affecting myelination		

1. **Risk factors for neural tube defects:** *maternal diabetes (caudal regression syndrome),* folate deficiency and use of antiepileptics during pregnancy (especially valproic acid)
2. **Occult dysraphic states:** High suspicion with abnormal tuft of hair, skin dimples or tracts
   a. Myelocystocele—localized cystic dilation of caudal spinal cord
   b. Diastematomyelia—bifid spinal cord
   c. Meningocele—no spinal cord tissue in sac, usually contiguous with tumors; lipoma, teratoma
   d. Tethered cord—caudal end of the spinal cord fixed with fibrous bands

B. **Normal developmental milestones**

AGE	FINE MOTOR	GROSS MOTOR	SOCIAL/VERBAL
1 mo	Hands fisted near face		Follows face
2 mo	Hands unfisted ~50%		Social smile Visual tracking to 180 degrees; coos
3 mo		Head control; chin up when prone; rolls over	Babbling and cooing
4 mo	Reaches for objects consistently		Laughs out loud
5 mo		Will hold up head and straighten back with horizontal suspension	

(continued)

AGE	FINE MOTOR	GROSS MOTOR	SOCIAL/VERBAL
6 mo	Transfers objects between hands	Sits with support; turns over	
8 mo	Thumb finger grasp	Sits unsupported	Separation anxiety
9 mo	Transfers objects	Stands; creeps, crawls	Says "mama," "dada" (nonspecific)
10 mo		Crawls; walks with support	
11 mo			Plays peek-a-boo
12 mo	Pincer grasp; tower of two cubes; hand-edness develops	Walks alone or holding hand/furniture	Two words (besides "mama," "dada")
15 mo		Should walk by self	Points to what is wanted
18 mo	Cube in box; builds tower of three blocks	Walks forward and back; stoops and recovers; climbs steps	Six words
2 yrs	Tower of eight cubes	Runs; climbs	Combines two to three words
2.5 yrs			Says name; asks questions; says "I"; points to body parts
3 yrs	Copies circle; knows left and right	Throws, catches, kicks ball; pedals tricycle; stands on one foot	Talks constantly; nursery rhymes; knows name; speaks in sentences; follows two commands
4 yrs	Copies square	Hops	Tells a story; uses syntax; writes name
5 yrs	Writes name	Skips	Begins to read
6 yrs			Reads and writes

II. Neonatal Neurology

A. The neonate nervous system functions essentially at a brainstem–spinal level; examination should be directed to diencephalic–midbrain, cerebellar–lower brainstem, and spinal functions; control of respiration and body temperature, regulation of thirst, fluid-balance appetite (hypothalamus and brainstem); automatisms, sucking, rooting, swallowing, grasping (brainstem–cerebellum); movements and postures of neck, extension of neck, trunk, flexion movement, steppage (reticulospinal, cerebellar, spinal); muscle tone of limbs and trunk; reflex eye movements (tegmental midbrain, pons); state of alertness (diencephalon); reflexes: Moro.

B. Intraventricular hemorrhage (IVH): common in preterm infants, especially very-low-birth-weight infants (<1,500 g); originates from rupture of germinal matrix vessels; screening and monitoring done with serial cranial ultrasound; increased incidence of hydrocephalus with Grade III to IV IVH

IVH GRADING SYSTEM	
I	Germinal matrix hemorrhage
II	Intraventricular hemorrhage with NO ventricular dilatation or hemorrhage <50% of ventricles
III	Intraventricular hemorrhage WITH ventricular dilatation or hemorrhage >50% of ventricles
IV	Intraventricular hemorrhage with hemorrhagic infarction into the parenchyma

C. Periventricular leukomalacia (PVL): white-matter injury with cystic changes usually associated with high-grade IVH or decreased cerebral blood flow in watershed areas

D. Hypoxic-ischemic encephalopathy (HIE): "neonatal encephalopathy"; may be due to prenatal (maternal/placental disease), perinatal (difficult delivery), or postnatal factors (trauma), usually presents as neonatal seizures

   1. Two patterns: (1) acute severe asphyxia leads to damage in deep gray-matter areas; (2) partial prolonged asphyxia (more common) leads to cortical involvement with edema and watershed injuries.

   2. Can be mild, moderate, or severe and be associated with multiple-organ involvement. Moderate to severe HIE can be treated with hypothermia (whole-body or head cooling) within the first 6 hours.

E. Cerebral palsy (perinatal encephalopathy): defined as a fixed, nonprogressive neurologic motor deficit of multiple etiologies; not necessarily cognitive impairment

SUBTYPE	MAIN INJURY	CLINICAL FEATURES
Spastic diplegia (most common)	Preterm: PVL	Spasticity in lower extremities Can have normal intelligence
Spastic quadriplegia	Preterm: PVL Term: HIE and central nervous system (CNS) infections	Bilateral spasticity Epilepsy and cognitive impairment common
Spastic hemiplegia	Preterm and term: congenital malformations, perinatal stroke	Early handedness Epilepsy common 1/3 with normal intelligence
Dyskinetic (extrapyramidal or athetoid)	Usually term infants: basal ganglia injury—kernicterus	Dystonic movements Normal to borderline intelligence
Ataxic, mixed types (less common)	Varied, may be genetic syndromes or congenital malformations	

F. **Floppy infant**

1. *Cerebral lesion:* atonic cerebral palsy, Prader-Willi, Down syndrome, storage/amino acid disorders

2. *Cord lesion:* transection during breech delivery, myelopathy from umbilical artery catheters, spina bifida, dysraphism

3. *Anterior horn cell:* spinal muscular atrophy (Werdnig-Hoffman, Kugelberger-Welander) Pompe's, poliomyelitis

4. *Peripheral nerves:* rare, congenital peripheral neuropathies

5. *Neuromuscular junction:* botulism, aminoglycosides, hypermagnesemia (from maternal treatment of eclampsia)

6. *Muscle:* nemaline rod, central core, myotubular myopathy, congenital muscular dystrophy

7. *Systemic:* hypercalcemia, hypothyroidism, renal acidosis, celiac, cystic fibrosis, Marfan, Ehlers-Danlos

8. *Benign:* Amyotonia congenita (diagnosis of exclusion)

III. Inherited Metabolic Disease of the Nervous System: The nervous system is the most frequently affected system by genetic abnormality; one-third of all inherited diseases are neurologic.

A. **Modes of inheritance**

1. *Autosomal dominant (AD):* manifest disease as heterozygotes, but variation in the size of the gene abnormality; may produce *several phenotypes; variable degree of penetrance and expressivity are characteristic;* tendency to *appear long after birth*

2. *Autosomal recessive (AR):* more *uniform phenotypic expression,* onset soon after birth, usually an *enzyme deficiency*

3. *X-linked:* mutant gene affects *mainly one sex; Lyon hypothesis:* female will experience same fate as the male if one X chromosome is inactivated in most cells during embryonic development; biochemical abnormality more often a basic protein.

4. *Multifactorial* genetic disease: may present as constitutional disorders with gene abnormalities located on several chromosomes (polygenic); relative contributions of "risk genes" and environmental influences are highly variable.

5. *Mitochondrial* disease: *mitochondrial DNA:* double-stranded circular molecule that encodes protein subunits required; essential feature: inherited maternally; genetic error is most often single-point mutation; may also be deletions or duplications that do not conform with maternal inheritance (sporadic, e.g., Kearns-Sayre); some enzymes of respiratory chain are coded by nuclear DNA, which is imported to the mitochondria, resulting in a Mendelian pattern of inheritance.

(*text continued on page 479*)

B. Metabolic disorders

DISORDERS INVOLVING ORGANELLES

LYSOSOMAL DISORDERS: lysosomes hydrolyze complex molecules, specific enzyme deficiency leads to accumulation of products and manifestation of disease

DISEASE NAME OR EPONYM	ENZYME DEFICIENCY	CLINICAL FEATURES	MODE OF INHERITANCE	ADDITIONAL INFORMATION
1) **Tay Sachs disease** (GM2 gangliosidosis)	**Hexosaminidase A**	***Excessive startle*** Psychomotor delay and regression Hypotonia → spasticity Seizures **Cherry red spot** and optic atrophy Death by age 3	AR (usually Jewish infants)	None
2) Sandhoff disease	Hexosaminidase A and B	Same as Tay-Sachs but with hepatosplenomegaly	AR	None
3) Landing disease (GM1 gangliosidosis type 1)	Beta-galactosidase	Pseudo-Hurler (coarse features, macroglossia, hirsutism) Hypotonia, psychomotor delay Cherry red spot	AR	None
4) **Gaucher disease**	**Glucocerebrosidase**	*Type 1:* no CNS involvement, hepatosplenomegaly, hypersplenism, and bone involvement *Type 2: **neuronopathic type in infants**:* hypotonia → spasticity, bulbar signs, seizures, death *Type 3:* juvenile type: ataxia, seizures, cognitive decline, myoclonic epilepsy, ***supranuclear horizontal ophthalmoplegia***	AR	***Gaucher cell:*** histiocyte with lacy, striated cytoplasm ("tissue paper") found in bone marrow and liver biopsy Enzyme replacement available but does not treat neurologic manifestations

(continued)

LYSOSOMAL DISORDERS: lysosomes hydrolyze complex molecules, specific enzyme deficiency leads to accumulation of products and manifestation of disease (continued)

DISEASE NAME OR EPONYM	ENZYME DEFICIENCY	CLINICAL FEATURES	MODE OF INHERITANCE	ADDITIONAL INFORMATION
5) **Niemann-Pick disease A and B**	**Sphingomyelinase**	*Type A: neurovisceral* Loss of reactivity to environment Myoclonic seizures, blindness, spasticity; marked enlargement of liver, spleen, lymph nodes	AR (Ashkenazi Jews)	Pathology: ***foam cells*** (vacuolated histiocytes) and balloon ganglion cells
		Cherry red spot in some Occurs in infants *Type B: visceral* Rare neurologic manifestation, occurs in older children		
6) **Fabry disease**	**Alpha-galactosidase**	Skin lesion: ***angiokeratoma corporis diffusum*** in periumbilical area Painful peripheral neuropathy *Cornea verticillata* in slit lamp Associated with renal disease, heart disease and posterior circulation stroke	***X-linked recessive***	Enzyme replacement treatment available Females may have milder form of disease due to Lyonization
7) Lipogranulomatosis (Farber's disease)	Ceramidase	Irritable infant with hoarse cry and multiple erythematous swelling over joints, death by 2–3 years of age	AR	None
8) **Metachromatic leukodystrophy**	**Arylsulfatase A**	Progressive impairment of motor function with cognitive decline, onset usually in early childhood Also with nystagmus, dysarthria, areflexia May have cherry red spot	AR	***MRI pattern shows bilateral symmetric periventricular white matter involvement with sparing of U fibers***

(continued)

LYSOSOMAL DISORDERS: lysosomes hydrolyze complex molecules, specific enzyme deficiency leads to accumulation of products and manifestation of disease (continued)

DISEASE NAME OR EPONYM	ENZYME DEFICIENCY	CLINICAL FEATURES	MODE OF INHERITANCE	ADDITIONAL INFORMATION
9) Krabbe disease (globoid cell leukodystrophy)	**Galactocerebrosidase**	Hypertonia then generalized rigidity, opisthotonic posturing, seizures Onset usually in infancy High cerebrospinal fluid (CSF) protein Death by 2–3 years of age	AR	Multinucleated globoid cells on pathology MRI pattern shows bilateral symmetric periventricular white matter involvement with sparing of U fibers
10) Mucopolysaccharidosis *Enzyme defects cause accumulation of glycosaminoglycans (GAGs)*				
A. Type IH Hurler	L-iduronidase	Coarse features, hepatosplenomegaly, can have hydrocephalus, corneal clouding, cognitive impairment	AR	Diagnosed by urine excretion of GAGs Enzyme replacement and bone marrow transplant available
B. Type IS Scheie	L-iduronidase	Similar to Hurler, carpal tunnel syndrome common, normal IQ	AR	
C. *Type II Hunter*	Iduronate-2—sulfatase	Sensorineural deafness, retinitis pigmentosa, *nerve entrapment syndromes*	*X-linked recessive*	Bone marrow transplant available
D. Type III Sanfilippo	Multiple: Heparan-N-sulfamidase (most common)	Progressive mental deterioration and seizures	AR	
E. Types IV–VII (less common with rare neurologic manifestation)				

(continued)

LYSOSOMAL DISORDERS: lysosomes hydrolyze complex molecules, specific enzyme deficiency leads to accumulation of products and manifestation of disease (continued)

DISEASE NAME OR EPONYM	ENZYME DEFICIENCY	CLINICAL FEATURES	MODE OF INHERITANCE	ADDITIONAL INFORMATION
11) Mucolipidosis and sialidosis		Action and intention *myoclonus*		
A. Sialidosis I	Sialidase	*Retinal cherry red spot* Normal intelligence		
B. Mucolipidosis II (I-cell disease)	N-acetylglucosamine phosphotransferase	Resembles Hurler phenotype, hyperplastic gums, rapid neurological deterioration in infants	AR AR	Looks like Hurler but no urine excretion of GAGs
C. Mannosidosis	Mannosidase	Rare, Hurler-like appearance, intellectual disability	AR	
D. Fucosidosis	Fucosidase	Rare, onset in infancy with vertebral beaking, hepatosplenomegaly, dystonia	AR	
12) Neuronal ceroid lipofuscinosis (Batten disease)				
A. Infantile CLN (CLN1)	Palmitoyl protein thioesterase (PPT1)	Hand-knitting movements Psychomotor regression Microcephaly		EEG with response to photic stimulation at low frequency
B. Late infantile CLN (CLN2)	Tripeptyl peptidase-1	Same as CLN1		
C. Juvenile CLN (CLN3)		*Myoclonic epilepsy,* macular degeneration, psychiatric disturbance		
D. Adult CLN (Kufs disease or CLN 4)		Similar to CLN3		

(continued)

PEROXISOMAL DISORDERS: ubiquitous organelles that are more numerous in cells that metabolize complex lipids				
DISEASE NAME OR EPONYM	ENZYME DEFICIENCY GENETIC MUTATION	CLINICAL FEATURES	MODE OF INHERITANCE	ADDITIONAL INFORMATION
1) *Zellweger spectrum disorder* includes: *Zellweger syndrome (cerebrohepatorenal syndrome, most severe)* *Neonatal adrenoleukodystrophy (intermediate)* *Infantile Refsum (least severe, can reach adulthood)*	Multiple enzymes involved Mutation in PEX genes, most commonly PEX1	Dysmorphic—high forehead, wide fontanelle, broad nasal ridge Severe hypotonia Epilepsy Hepatomegaly and liver dysfunction Polycystic kidneys Hearing and vision loss Death in the 1st year of age	AR	MRI shows multiple malformations usually polymicrogyria or pachygyria, vermian hypoplasia Increased very long chain fatty acid (VLCFA)
2) *X-linked adrenoleukodystrophy*	ALDP deficiency, which transports VLCFA into peroxisomes Mutation in ABCD1 gene	*Cerebral childhood form:* rapidly progressive decline in school performance, gait disturbance, dementia, seizures, death *Adolescent form:* slower progression *Adult form (amyeloneuropathy):* spastic paraparesis and psychiatric symptoms *Addison disease only*	***X-linked recessive***	***MRI shows symmetric white-matter involvement in parieto-occipital area with sparing of U fibers***
3) Classical Refsum	Phytanic acid oxidase Mutation in PEX7	Retinitis pigmentosa Anosmia Bony abnormalities Demyelinating hypertrophic neuropathy Usually in adults	AR	Dietary restriction of phytanic acid

DISORDERS INVOLVING ENDOPLASMIC RETICULUM AND GOLGI BODY

DISEASE NAME	ENZYME DEFICIENCY GENETIC MUTATION	CLINICAL FEATURES	MODE OF INHERITANCE	ADDITIONAL INFORMATION
Congenital disorders of glycosylation (CDG)	Multiple	Poor feeding, hypotonia, psychomotor delay, ataxia, epilepsy Acquired microcephaly ***Dysmorphic with inverted nipples, abnormal fat pads above buttocks*** Stroke-like episodes Wide spectrum of disease	AR	
Oligosaccharide + Protein = glycosylated protein Elongation process occurs in endoplasmic reticulum (CDG type 1)	Most common is 1a: phosphomannomutase	Severe developmental delay, hypotonia, seizures	AR	***MRI shows olivopontocerebellar atrophy***
Trimming process occurs in Golgi body (CDG type II)	Multiple	Stereotypic handwashing movements, head banging		

Disorders of Amino Acids and Organic Acids

AMINOACIDOPATHIES: ½ present with neurologic manifestation, usually psychomotor delay

DISEASE NAME OR EPONYM	ENZYME DEFICIENCY	CLINICAL FEATURES	MODE OF INHERITANCE	ADDITIONAL INFORMATION
1) Phenylketonuria (PKU) or hyperphenylalanemia (HPA)	***Phenylalanine hydroxylase*** (most common)	Psychomotor regression Intellectual disability Behavioral disturbance Poor coordination Microcephaly in 2/3 Fair rough skin, blue eyes	AR	Treatment with phenylalanine-restricted diet ***Maternal PKU results in babies born with microcephaly, low birth weight, dysmorphism, and congenital defects***
2) Tyrosinemia (HT-1)	Fumarylacetoacetase	Intellectual disability Self-mutilation Porphyria-like crisis with ascending peripheral neuropathy	AR	

(continued)

AMINOACIDOPATHIES: ½ present with neurologic manifestation, usually psychomotor delay (continued)

3) Disorders of branched-chain amino acids A. Maple syrup urine disease (MSUD) B. Methylmalonic aciduria C. Propionic aciduria D. Isovaleric aciduria	Multiple enzymes involved in branched-chain amino acid catabolism	Severe neonatal forms: initial symptom-free period then deterioration after feeds initiated, progressive coma, severe acidosis, dystonic posturing, seizures Late-onset forms: recurrent attacks of coma or lethargy during enhanced protein catabolism (infection, etc.)	AR	Dietary restriction of branched-chain amino acids ***MSUD: musty odor*** ***Isovaleric aciduria: "sweaty socks" odor*** ***Labs may show ketotic hyperglycinemia***
4) *Glutaric aciduria (GA-1)*	Glutaryl–COA dehydrogenase (GDH–riboflavin cofactor)	Dystonia Choreoathetosis Macrocephaly Encephalopathic crisis before age 2 (hypotonia, seizures, regression)	AR	***MRI shows widening of Sylvian fissure, chronic subdural collections***
5) *Canavan disease*	*Aspartoacyclase*	***Macrocephaly*** Hypotonia → spasticity Irritability Death by age 3	AR	Neuropathology: status spongiosus MRI shows diffuse demyelination involving U fibers Increased N-acetylaspartate (NAA) level in magnetic resonance spectroscopy (MRS)
6) *Homocystinuria*	*Cystathionine beta-synthase (vitamin B₆ cofactor)*	*Marfanoid habitus* *Lens dislocation* Intellectual disability (Marfan's syndrome has normal intelligence) Coronal, renal, and cerebral vasculopathy "Charlie Chaplin" gait	AR	Treatment includes low-methionine diet, pyridoxine supplementation, and antiplatelet medication
7) Hartnup disease	Transport error of neutral amino acids	Pellagra-like rash Developmental delay Episodic cerebellar ataxia Psychosis	AR	Treatment with nicotinamide

(continued)

Disorders of Neurotransmitter Metabolism

DISEASE NAME OR EPONYM	ENZYME DEFICIENCY	CLINICAL FEATURES	MODE OF INHERITANCE	ADDITIONAL INFORMATION
1) Tetrahydrobiopterin (THB) deficiency THB is cofactor of phenylalanine, tyrosine, and tryptophan hydrolases	Multiple dihydropteridine deficiency (DHPR) most common	Malignant HPA with progressive neurologic deterioration despite low-phenylalanine diet Hypotonia Developmental delay Abnormal movements Hyperthermia Grand mal and myoclonic seizures	AR	Treatment with low-phenylalanine diet and supplementation with folinic acid, neurotransmitter replacement therapy with L-dopa
2) Nonketotic hyperglycinemia or glycine encephalopathy	Defect in P protein (GLDC gene) in glycine cleavage system most common	Lethargy and apnea in neonates Spastic cerebral palsy if they survive neonatal period	AR	EEG shows burst suppression MRI usually shows agenesis of corpus callosum Treatment with sodium benzoate

Disorders of Vitamin Metabolism

DISEASE NAME OR EPONYM	ENZYME DEFICIENCY	CLINICAL FEATURES	MODE OF INHERITANCE	ADDITIONAL INFORMATION
1) Biotin deficiency	Holocarboxylase deficiency (neonates) Biotinidase deficiency (late onset)	Episodic coma Ataxia Basal ganglia necrosis Deafness Skin rashes, alopecia, and conjunctivitis	AR	Ketoacidosis and lactic acidosis on labs Treat with biotin replacement
2) Pyridoxine dependency (vitamin B₆)	Antiquitin	***Intractable seizures in neonates*** Encephalopathy	AR	***IV pyridoxine immediately effective***

(continued)

Disorders of Vitamin Metabolism (continued)

DISEASE NAME OR EPONYM	ENZYME DEFICIENCY	CLINICAL FEATURES	MODE OF INHERITANCE	ADDITIONAL INFORMATION
3) Pyridoxine 5' phosphate oxidase (PNPO) deficiency	PNPO (converts pyridoxine to active form)	Pyridoxine resistant epileptic encephalopathy	AR	Low pyridoxal phosphate in CSF Treatment with pyridoxine and oral pyridoxal phosphate
4) Vitamin B$_{12}$ A. Absorption or transported defects B. Intracellular metabolism	Multiple enzymes	Developmental delay, subacute combined degeneration, anemia Developmental delay, seizures, microcephaly	AR	Labs show methylmalonic aciduria, homocystinuria, and high methionine

Other Metabolic and Heredodegenerative Disorders

DISEASE NAME OR EPONYM	ENZYME DEFICIENCY GENE MUTATION	CLINICAL FEATURES	MODE OF INHERITANCE	ADDITIONAL INFORMATION
1) Urea cycle disorders	Carbamoyl phosphate synthetase deficiency (type 1) ***Ornithine transcarbamylase deficiency (type 2)***	Neonate with initial symptom-free period then progressive vomiting, hypotonia, lethargy, coma, seizures	AR ***X-linked recessive***	Labs show high ammonia but no acidosis Treat with protein restriction
2) Fatty acid beta-oxidation defects	Multiple enzymes including medium chain acyl dehydrogenase **(MCAD)**	Muscle weakness ***Recurrent rhabdomyolysis*** ***Dilated or hypertrophic cardiomyopathy*** Reye-like episodes	AR	Avoid fasting and catabolic states

(continued)

Other Metabolic and Heredodegenerative Disorders (continued)

DISEASE NAME OR EPONYM	ENZYME DEFICIENCY GENE MUTATION	CLINICAL FEATURES	MODE OF INHERITANCE	ADDITIONAL INFORMATION
3) Cholesterol disorders A. Smith-Lemli-Opitz	7-Dehydrocholesterol reductase	Brain malformations Dysmorphisms Autism	AR	
B. Niemann-Pick type C	NPC1/NPC2 gene—codes for transport of cholesterol along cell membranes	Intellectual disability Hepatosplenomegaly Cataplexy Intellectual disability *Vertical supranuclear ophthalmoplegia*	AR	
4) Abetalipoproteinemia	MTTP gene mutation	Peripheral neuropathy Vitamin A, D, E, K deficiency Steatorrhea Retinitis pigmentosa Ataxia	AR	Peripheral blood smear shows *acanthocytes*
5) Wilson's disease (hepatolenticular degeneration)	Defect in copper excretion Mutation in gene ATP7B	Movement disorders Intellectual deterioration Psychosis Kayser-Fleischer ring	AR	High urinary copper Low serum ceruloplasmin Chelation therapy
6) Menkes disease (kinky hair disease)	Deficiency in copper transporter ATPase (unable to absorb copper) Mutation in MNK gene	Failure to thrive Seizures Hypothermia Steel wool hair	*X-linked recessive*	
7) Lesch-Nyhan disease	*Hypoxanthine guanine phosphoribosyl transferase (HGPRT) deficiency*	Spasticity Choreoathetosis Self-mutilation Gouty nephropathy	*X-linked recessive*	Labs show *hyperuricemia*, treat with allopurinol

(continued)

Other Metabolic and Heredodegenerative Disorders (continued)

DISEASE NAME OR EPONYM	ENZYME DEFICIENCY GENE MUTATION	CLINICAL FEATURES	MODE OF INHERITANCE	ADDITIONAL INFORMATION
8) Pelizaeus- Merzbacher disease	Defective synthesis of proteolipid protein (PLP)	**Pendular nystagmus** Optic atrophy Spasticity Choreoathetosis Developmental delay	**X-linked recessive**	**MRI shows hypomyelination (T2 hyperintensity of unmyelinated periventricular white matter, tigroid pattern)**
9) Alexander disease	Mutation in GFAP gene	**Macrocephaly** Spasticity Seizures Episodes of regression with mild head trauma Bulbar symptoms in older patients		**Rosenthal fibres on pathology** MRI shows extensive signal enhancement of white matter with **anterior predominance,** involves U fibers

MITOCHONDRIAL DISORDERS

Huge diversity in clinical presentation and age of onset; many but not all show elevations in lactate

DISEASE NAME OR EPONYM	ENZYME DEFICIENCY GENE MUTATION	CLINICAL FEATURES	MODE OF INHERITANCE	ADDITIONAL INFORMATION
1) Leigh syndrome (subacute necrotizing encephalopathy)	Multiple different gene mutations usually nuclear DNA Most common is disruption of complex IV (COX deficiency with mutation in SURF1 gene)	Hypotonia Seizures Ataxia **Hyperventilation during infections**	Usually AR, 20%-25% maternal inheritance	Neuropathology shows spongionecrosis of thalamus, basal ganglia, brainstem, spinal cord

(continued)

MITOCHONDRIAL DISORDERS (continued)

Huge diversity in clinical presentation and age of onset; many but not all show elevations in lactate

DISEASE NAME OR EPONYM	ENZYME DEFICIENCY GENE MUTATION	CLINICAL FEATURES	MODE OF INHERITANCE	ADDITIONAL INFORMATION
2) **Kearns-Sayre syndrome**	Deletion in mtDNA	***Retinitis pigmentosa*** ***Ophthalmoplegia and Ptosis*** ***Ataxia*** ***Deafness*** ***Heart block***	Mostly sporadic	None
3) Chronic progressive external ophthalmo-plegia (CPEO)	Deletions in mtDNA Deletions in nuclear DNA	Progressive ptosis and ophthalmoplegia Muscle weakness with exercise	Maternal AD	None
4) **Myoclonic epilepsy with ragged red fiber myopathy (MERRF)**	Point mutation in mtDNA	***Myoclonic epilepsy*** Muscle weakness Ataxia Deafness	Maternal	None
5) **Mitochondrial myop-athy, encephalopa-thy, lactic acidosis, and stroke-like epi-sodes (MELAS)**	Mutations in mtDNA	***Stroke in nonvascular distribution*** ***Recurrent vomiting*** ***Migraines*** Focal seizures Short stature Diabetes mellitus Deafness	Maternal	***Arginine supplementation for strokes***
6) **Leber's hereditary optic neuropathy (LHON)**	Mutations in mtDNA	***Optic atrophy*** ***Cardiac conduction abnormalities***	Maternal	None
7) Alpers-Huttenlocher disease (hepatocere-bral syndrome)	POLG mutations	Progressive cerebral poliodystrophy with intractable seizures Ataxia, blindness Progressive spasticity Liver failure after valproic acid administration	AR	"Walnut brain" on MRI

C. Metabolic diseases by age of presentation

NEONATAL	EARLY INFANCY	LATE INFANCY AND EARLY CHILDHOOD	LATE CHILDHOOD AND ADOLESCENCE
Aminoacidopathies	Tay-Sachs	Same disease in early infancy	X-linked adrenoleu-kodystrophy
Urea cycle defects	Infantile Gaucher	Metachromatic leukodystrophy	Wilson's disease Lesch-Nyhan
Pyridoxine dependency	Infantile Niemann-Pick	Neuronal ceroid lipofuscinosis	Homocystinuria Fabry's disease
Nonketotic hyperglycinemia	Krabbe disease Pelizaeus-Merzbacher Canavan disease Alexander disease Alpers disease Zellweger disease	Mucopolysaccharidoses Mucolipidosis and sialidosis	Juvenile Gaucher's Mitochondrial disorders (CPEO, MELAS, LHON)

IV. Neuromuscular Disorders

A. Neuropathies

1. **Hereditary motor and sensory neuropathies (HMSN) type 1:** *Charcot-Marie-Tooth, peroneal muscular atrophy;* all types generally have insidious clinical onset and slow progression from adolescence; rarely, they can present in infancy; **pes cavus and hammer toes** often cause initial complaints; segmental *demyelination* and remyelination occur, resulting in distal muscle atrophy and weakness and tremor and ataxia in some (39%); *autosomal dominant;* multiple genetic subtypes; in older patients, nerve biopsy shows a hypertrophic onion bulb appearance; may have elevated CSF protein; life expectancy is normal; *duplication of PMP22.*

2. **HMSN type 2a:** autosomal *dominant;* map to chromosome 1; *axonal* neuropathy; milder course compared to type 1; *HMSN type 2b: childhood onset; autosomal recessive*

3. **HMSN type 3** *(Dejerine Sottas):* autosomal *recessive;* presents at birth; may be a homozygous form due to a sporadic point mutation; hypotonia and slow motor development are common in the first year; sensory ataxia develops; clubfoot and scoliosis are seen; usually with elevated CSF protein.

4. **HMSN type 4** *(Refsum's):* autosomal recessive deficiency of phytanic acid oxidase affects lipid metabolism; onset is 1st to 3rd decade with cerebellar ataxia, chronic hypertonic neuropathy, and retinitis pigmentosa; other findings: night blindness, deafness, ichthyosis, cardiac myopathy, hepatosplenomegaly, and increased CSF protein; dietary restriction of phytanic acid (avoiding nuts, spinach, and coffee) is beneficial, as phytanic acid is not produced endogenously; infant and adult forms are seen.

5. **Hereditary neuropathy with liability to pressure palsies** *(tomaculous neuropathy):* 10% have *deletion of PMP-22 protein.*

B. Anterior horn cell/muscle disorders

1. **Infantile spinal muscular atrophy:** three types, all related to *chromosome 5;* frequency of carriers is 1 in 60; prenatal screening available.

    a. *Werdnig-Hoffman: infantile form; autosomal recessive;* presents at birth with proximal hypotonia and respiratory insufficiency; reduced fetal movement,

1. **Infantile spinal muscular atrophy** (*cont'd*)

    hypotonia, areflexia, quivering tongue; progressive feeding difficulty and death can occur by age 6 months; muscle biopsy is also diagnostic.

    b. *Kugelberg-Welander: chronic form; autosomal recessive or sporadic;* presents after 3 months with pelvic girdle weakness and runs a variable course; mean survival is 30 years.

    c. Third form affects primarily the neck and respiratory muscles; presenting with head droop; survival to age 3 years.

2. **Neurogenic arthrogryposis:** *sporadic* disease; affects fetus, causing *contractures* by the time of birth; electromyography (EMG) is normal but shows a neuropathic process.

3. **Fazio-Londe:** onset in early childhood; *progressive bulbar paralysis, with anterior horn cell involvement*

4. *Glycogen storage diseases:* autosomal *recessive*

    a. **Type 2 (Pompe's):** *deficient acid maltase activity (1,4 glycosidase)* results in glycogen deposition in the anterior horn cells; infantile form presents as *floppy infant with congestive heart failure, macroglossia, hepatomegaly;* muscle biopsy shows periodic acid–Schiff-positive deposits and vacuolation.

    b. **Type 3 (Forbes-Cori):** *debrancher enzyme (1,6 glucosidase) deficiency* associated with hypotonia, hypoglycemia, hepato-/cardiomegaly; prognosis is variable; skeletal and cardiac muscles affected.

    c. **Type 5 (McArdle's):** results from *inactive myophosphorylase;* childhood and adult forms seen; exercise induces painful cramps; *ischemic exercise test shows no lactate production;* biopsy shows periodic acid–Schiff-positive subsarcolemmal blebs or crescents.

    d. **Tarui's (type 7):** *phosphofructokinase deficiency* results in cramping and fatigue.

> **NB:** **McArdle's disease and Tarui's disease do not produce lactate in the exercise ischemic test.**

    e. *Nonmyopathic types:* **type 1** (*von Gierke; deficient glucose-6-phosphate causes neonatal seizures*); **type 4** (*Anderson's; deficiency of 1,4 debrancher enzyme results in failure to thrive*); **type 6** (*Hers'; liver phosphorylase deficiency* results in growth retardation)

5. *Muscular dystrophies*

    a. **Paramyotonia congenita:** autosomal *dominant;* defect on *chromosome 17q23.1* affects voltage-gated **Na$^+$ channels;** causes myotonia on exposure to cold; electrolytes are normal; compare to: **myotonia congenita** (*Thomsen's disease*)— autosomal *dominant on chromosome 7; mutation of the* **chloride channel;** seen at birth, muscle hypertrophy (mini-Hercules); EMG: myotonic discharges

    b. **Duchenne's muscular dystrophy:** the *most common* dystrophy, affects boys by age 5 years; incidence is 1 in 3,500; 30% mutation rate; *localized to Xp21;* defects in the gene for *dystrophin* results in variable amounts of this essential muscle structural protein; weakness, *pseudohypertrophy of the calf muscles and tendon shortening* are classic; mild MR and cardiac involvement are also present; treatment: prednisone may improve strength and function; creatine phosphokinase (CPK) is elevated; death usually by age 20 years; biopsy: atrophy and hypertrophy, central nuclei, fiber splitting, necrosis, fibrosis, fatty changes, and hyaline fibers; EMG: myopathic units denervation, fibrillation and sharp waves.

    c. **Becker's dystrophy:** also *X-linked;* but *milder* defect, slower progression

d. **Limb-girdle dystrophy:** autosomal *recessive (chromosome 15), autosomal dominant (chromosome 5), severe childhood autosomal recessive muscular dystrophy (chromosome 13);* slowly progressive proximal weakness: iliopsoas, quadriceps, hamstrings, deltoids, biceps, triceps; facial and extraocular muscles spared; slightly elevated CPK; EMG: myopathic changes; pathology: fiber size variations; fiber splitting; degeneration/regeneration

e. **Fascioscapulohumeral dystrophy:** autosomal *dominant;* on *chromosome 4;* onset at end of the 1st decade; slowly progressive *weakness of facial musculature (Bell's phenomenon);* **serratus anterior (winging of the scapula) and biceps;** deltoid and forearm muscles preserved (giving *Popeye appearance*); scapuloperoneal form: on chromosome 5; CPK slightly elevated; EMG and pathology: myopathic changes.

f. **Congenital muscular dystrophy:** rare; onset at age 2 to 3 years

g. **Emery-Dreifuss** *(humeroperoneal):* X-linked recessive (most common) but also has other inheritance patterns; weakness over biceps, triceps, distal leg; **contractures early, cardiac conduction block**

h. **Oculopharyngeal dystrophy:** common in French Canadians or Spanish Americans; autosomal *dominant;* onset in 5th decade, slowly progressive; ptosis first, pharyngeal weakness later; CPK slightly elevated; pathology: myopathic changes, rimmed vacuoles, and intranuclear tubulofilamentous inclusions

i. **Myotonic dystrophy:** autosomal *dominant;* **cytosine-thymine-guanine (CTG) triplet repeat** (>50 copies on *chromosome 19q*); related to defective protein kinase and membrane instability; it is a multisystem disease that usually presents in adults (20–40 years old [y/o]), not in children; results in facial weakness (ptosis, *fish mouth*), *hatchet face, some MR, posterior capsule cataracts, cardiac disease, diabetes, testicular or ovarian atrophy;* congenital form is severe at birth but improves in 4 to 6 weeks; *EMG: spontaneous bursts of high frequency amplitude discharges;* pathology: type 1 fiber hypertrophy and *ring fibers;* congenital myotonic dystrophy in children of mothers with myotonic dystrophy.

6. *Myopathies*

a. **Nemaline:** autosomal *recessive on chromosome 1; occasionally autosomal dominant;* non-progressive; also high-arched palate, small jaw and thin face; Marfanoid features, cardiomyopathy; CPK is normal; type 1 fiber predominance with Z-line rods.

b. **Central core:** autosomal *recessive on chromosome 19;* floppy baby, motor delay, spine abnormalities, proximal, nonprogressive; CPK is normal; type 1 fibers have *central pallor; on electron microscopy: core lacks mitochondria.*

c. **Myotubular** *(centronuclear):* X-linked recessive; age of onset is 5 to 30 years; involvement of ocular, facial, and distal muscle; variable progression; CPK is normal or mildly increased; biopsy: central nuclei with halos and type 1 fiber atrophy.

d. **Dermatomyositis:** affects *females more than males; skin lesions: diffuse erythema, maculopapular eruption, heliotrope rash, eczematoid dermatitis of extensor surface joints;* carcinoma in 15% (affects more adults than children); lab: CPK high, aldolase high, IgG and IgA levels may be elevated; myoglobinuria; inflammatory muscle changes; sometimes tissue calcification.

e. **Hypokalemic periodic paralysis:** may be autosomal *dominant or associated with thyrotoxicosis;* age between 10 and 20 years; attacks are frequent and usually severe, lasting for hours to days; trigger: rest, cold, stress; low serum K^+; *calcium channelopathy;* treatment: acetazolamide, K^+ replacement.

f. **Hyperkalemic periodic paralysis:** autosomal *dominant;* age between 10 and 20 years; attacks are frequent with moderate severity lasting minutes to hours;

6. *Myopathies* (*cont'd*)

triggers: rest, cold, hunger; high serum K^+, occasional myotonia, *Na^+ channelopathy;* treatment: acetazolamide, low potassium.

C. **Neuromuscular junction disorders**

1. **Neonatal (transient) myasthenia:** *transient disorder seen in 15% of infants born to mothers with myasthenia gravis; due to placental transfer of acetylcholine receptor (AChR) antibodies;* symptoms: intrauterine hypotonia; may be born with arthrogryposis; usually evident within 24 hours of life, lasting for 18 days (range, 5 days to 2 months); may need exchange transfusion and/or neostigmine, 0.1 mg intramuscularly before feeding.

2. **Congenital myasthenia:** heterogeneous disorder due to *genetic defects in the presynaptic (mostly autosomal recessive) and postsynaptic (mostly autosomal recessive, some autosomal dominant [slow channel syndrome]) neuromuscular junction;* not associated with antibodies to AChR; symptoms: usually begin in the neonatal period, ocular, bulbar, respiratory weakness, worse with crying or activity; ptosis, ophthalmoplegia, or ophthalmoparesis; diagnosis: positive family history in some, Tensilon® (edrophonium chloride) test negative in most, *AChR is negative,* EMG: decremental response and increased jitter.

> **NB:** *In contrast to neonatal myasthenia, congenital myasthenia is not an autoimmune disorder.*

3. **Juvenile myasthenia:** *sporadic, autoimmune; due to antibodies to AChR; similar to adult myasthenia gravis;* special characteristics: less often have detectable AChR antibodies, have other autoimmune disorders such as diabetes mellitus/rheumatoid arthritis/asthma/thyroid disease, also have nonautoimmune disease such as epilepsy/neoplasm; thymectomy recommended for moderate to severe cases; *little to no correlation with thymus pathology and response to surgery (77% with hyperplasia, 16% normal, and 3% thymoma).*

V. Neuro Phakomatoses

A. **Neurofibromatosis type 1 (NF1): autosomal dominant; chromosome band 17q11.2; spontaneous mutations occur in approximately 50% of patients; the most common genetic disorder of the nervous system: 1 in 3,000 people; chromosome 17 encodes the tumor suppressor neurofibromin; the loss of neurofibromin may contribute to tumor progression.**

1. *National Institutes of Health criteria for NF1*

   a. *Café au lait macules: six or more*

   b. *Two or more neurofibromas or one plexiform neurofibroma (neurofibromas often multiple, nonpainful, intermingled with nerves, and can become malignant)*

   c. *Axillary or inguinal freckling*

   d. *Optic glioma*

   e. *Lisch nodules (iris hamartomas)*

   f. *Dysplasia or thinning of long bone cortex*

   g. *First-degree relative with NF1*

2. Neurologic complications of NF1: *optic gliomas are the most common,* occur in approximately 15% of patients; other associated CNS neoplasms are *astrocytomas, vestibular schwannomas (acoustic neuroma), and, less often, ependymomas and meningiomas;* hydrocephalus, seizures, learning disabilities; bilateral optic nerve

gliomas; congenital *glaucoma; pheochromocytoma (0.1%–5.7%) or renal artery stenosis;* growth hormone deficiency, short stature, and precocious puberty have been reported in patients with NF1.

B. **Neurofibromatosis type 2 (NF2) (central type): autosomal dominant; chromosome 22q11-13.1; this gene codes for schwannomin/merlin proteins, which may affect tumor suppressor activity at the cell membrane level; spontaneous mutations exist in 50% to 70% of patients; NF2 is less common than NF1, occurring in 1 in 35,000; paucity of cutaneous lesions.**

   1. *Diagnostic criteria for NF2*

      a. Bilateral vestibular schwannomas (visualized with CT scan or MRI)

      b. A first-degree relative with the disease plus a unilateral vestibular schwannoma before 30 y/o

      c. Any two of the following: neurofibroma, meningioma, glioma, schwannoma, or juvenile posterior subcapsular opacity

   2. Complications of NF2: ocular manifestations include *juvenile posterior subcapsular lenticular opacity, retinal hamartomas, optic disc glioma, and optic nerve meningioma; intracranial and spinal meningiomas, astrocytomas, and ependymomas;* subcutaneous schwannomas are superficial-raised papules with overlying pigment and hair.

C. **Tuberous sclerosis (TS): autosomal dominant; two gene loci have been identified: chromosome 9q34, which codes for a protein (termed hamartin) and is a probable tumor suppressor gene, and chromosome 16q13.3, which codes for an amino acid protein (termed tuberin): triad of MR, epilepsy, and adenoma sebaceum is characteristic.**

   1. Neurologic complications of TS

      a. Infantile spasms (EEG may show *hypsarrhythmia*): generalized tonic-clonic, complex partial, and myoclonic seizures are the most common forms; of children with infantile spasms, 10% have TS.

      b. Cortical tubers: potato-like nodules of glial proliferation occurring in the cortex, ganglia, or ventricle walls; often calcified

      c. Other CNS findings include *subependymal hamartomas, paraventricular calcifications, or "candle gutterings," and giant-cell astrocytomas.*

   2. Cutaneous presentation of TS

      a. Congenital *ash-leaf hypopigmented macules:* in 87% of patients

      b. Confetti macules: 1 to 3 mm, hypopigmented, on the pretibial area

      c. Shagreen patch (subepidermal fibrous patches): 1- to 10-cm, flat, flesh-colored plaque, most often in the lumbosacral region; orange-peel appearance

      d. Facial angiofibromas (adenoma sebaceum): diagnostic of TS, usually appear in children aged 4 to 10 years

      e. Koenen tumors: on nail plates *(ungual fibroma)* appear at puberty

   3. Other complications of TS: retinal hamartomas (phacomata); gingival fibromas; renal cysts; phalangeal cysts and periosteal thickening; lung cysts, pulmonary lymphangiomyomatosis; rhabdomyomas occur in 50% of patients; angiomyolipomas; *renal failure* most common cause of death

> **NB:** *Giant-cell astrocytomas are nonmalignant and are treatable with rapamycin but may cause obstruction of the foramen of Monroe.*

D. **Sturge-Weber syndrome: trigeminocranial angiomatosis with cerebral calcification; congenital facial port-wine stains and leptomeningeal angiomatosis; present clinically as epilepsy, MR, and hemiplegia; complications: ocular complications in 30% to 60%**

D. Sturge-Weber syndrome (*cont'd*)

of patients; glaucoma can begin at age 2 years; the most common ocular manifestation is diffuse choroidal angioma; parenchymal calcifications (train tracks on radiographs by age 2 years) are classic; caused by mosaic mutations in the GNAQ gene.

E. Ataxia-telangiectasia (Louis-Bar syndrome): autosomal recessive; chromosome 11q22-23; mutation in ATM gene, which is involved in the detection of DNA damage; 1 in 80,000 live births; characterized by progressive cerebellar ataxia, oculocutaneous telangiectasia, abnormalities in cellular and humoral immunity and recurrent viral and bacterial infections; increased risk of cancers

1. Neurologic manifestations: cerebellar ataxia at 2 y/o, nystagmus; chorea, athetosis, dystonia, oculomotor apraxia, impassive facies; decreased deep tendon reflexes, and distal muscular atrophy; intelligence progressively deteriorates; polyneuropathy

2. Other manifestations: immunodeficiency (thymic hypoplasia); patients *lack helper T cells, but suppressor T cells are normal; IgA is absent in 75% of patients, IgE in 85%, IgG is low;* α-*fetoprotein and carcinoembryonic antigen are elevated;* ovarian agenesis, testicular hypoplasia, and insulin-resistant diabetes.

3. Increased risk of malignant neoplasms in 10% to 15% of patients due to defect in DNA repair; most common are lymphoreticular neoplasm and leukemia; death by 2nd decade from neoplasia or infection

4. Cutaneous manifestations: telangiectasias develop at age 3 to 6 years: first on the bulbar conjunctiva (red eyes) and ears and later on the flexor surface of the arms, eyelids, malar area of the face, and upper chest; granulomas, café au lait macules, graying hair, and progeria can occur.

F. Incontinentia pigmenti: X-linked dominant disorder; lethal to male patients; few affected males have been documented, and most had Klinefelter syndrome (47,XXY); skin lesions arranged in a linear pattern (begin as linear bullous lesions and progress to hyperkeratosis and hyperpigmentation with linear streaks and whorls), slate-gray pigmentation, alopecia, ocular defects, dental, and neurologic abnormalities; more than 700 cases have been reported; pathology: atrophy, microgyria, focal necrosis in white matter; lab: eosinophilia.

1. Complications: characterized by seizures, MR, and generalized spasticity, cortical blindness in 15% to 30% of patients; the findings include cerebral ischemia, cerebral edema, brain atrophy, and gyral dysplasia.

2. Ocular manifestations include *strabismus, cataracts, retinal detachments, optic atrophy, and vitreous hemorrhage.*

G. Osler-Weber-Rendu disease (hereditary hemorrhagic telangiectasia; familiar telangiectasia): autosomal dominant; chromosome 9q33-q34 (endoglin gene); 1 in 100,000 births; neurologic complications include vascular lesions, including telangiectasias, arteriovenous malformations, and aneurysms of the brain and/or spinal cord, cerebellar ataxia, varying degrees of MR, and possible hearing loss; multiple telangiectasias on the face, hands, a white forelock, and depigmented patches with spots of hyperpigmentation, epistaxis.

H. von Hippel-Lindau syndrome (hemangioblastoma of the cerebellum): autosomal dominant; chromosome 3; cerebellar hemangioblastomas (obstructive hydrocephalus); retinal hemangioblastomas; renal cell carcinoma; hepatic, pancreatic cysts; polycythemia (increased erythropoietin); pheochromocytomas; usually presents in adults

I. Sneddon syndrome: characterized by livedo reticularis and multiple strokes resulting in dementia; antiphospholipid antibodies and anti–β_2-glycoprotein antibodies also have been detected in some patients with this disorder; not usually a pediatric disorder but a neurocutaneous syndrome.

J. Chediak-Higashi syndrome: autosomal recessive; defective pigmentation and peripheral neuropathy

VI. Infections and Toxins

A. **Perinatal infections (TORCH [toxoplasmosis, other infections, rubella, cytomegalovirus infection, and herpes simplex])**

1. **Toxoplasmosis:** protozoan comes from *cat feces or uncooked meat;* transmission *is least likely in the first trimester; hydrocephalus, chorioretinitis, granulomatous meningoencephalitis, late periventricular and cortical calcification,* seizures, MR, hepatosplenomegaly, thrombocytopenia; diagnosis by enzyme-linked immunosorbent assay; CT for congenital toxoplasmosis: periventricular calcifications; treatment: sulfadiazine, pyrimethamine and folate.

2. **Rubella:** fetus is most susceptible in the first trimester; clinical findings: *MR, heart disease, cataracts, deafness, microgyria/microcephaly, seizures, spasticity.*

3. **Cytomegalovirus:** infection occurs transplacentally in the second to third trimester, and reinfection can occur at the time of birth; multifocal necrosis, periventricular calcification, and hydrocephalus are seen; clinical findings: MR, microcephaly, rash, hepatosplenomegaly, jaundice, and chorioretinitis; treatment: acyclovir/ganciclovir.

> **NB:** *The most common sequela after congenital cytomegalovirus infection is deafness.*

4. **Herpes simplex virus (type 2;** *adult encephalitides are usually type 1*): infection is usually due to exposure at birth and may not be recognized by age 1 to 3 weeks; there is a high risk (35%–50%) with primary (active) maternal infection and lower risk (3%–5%) with recurrent maternal infection; predilection is for the temporal lobes, insula, cingulate gyrus; clinically: *cyanosis/respiratory distress, jaundice, fever, microcephaly, periventricular calcification;* treatment: acyclovir or vidarabine; pathology: *Cowdry type A inclusions.*

5. **Congenital syphilis:** etiology: *Treponema pallidum;* meningovascular form may present as hydrocephalus; general paresis can occur by age 10 years; tabes dorsalis is rare in the young.

B. **Other viruses**

1. **Coxsackie A:** encephalitis, herpangina, rash (usually ages 5–9 years during summer)

2. **Coxsackie B:** pleurodynia and encephalitis

3. **Echovirus:** meningitis, morbilliform rash (summer and fall months)

4. **HIV:** CNS signs (motor and cognitive) occur in 50% to 90% of infected children; 10% develop opportunistic infection; 30% develop bacterial infections; seizures are common, stroke in 10%; mothers treated with zidovudine (AZT) have a lower transmission rate.

5. **Measles:** encephalitis can occur in children less than 10 y/o with low mortality; pathology: multinucleated giant cells, intranuclear and intracytoplasmic inclusions are present.

6. **Subacute sclerosing panencephalitis:** rare but often *fatal complication of measles (rubeola);* onset occurs at age 5 to 15 years in children with previous rubeola infection; personality changes, poor school performance, macular changes, progress to myoclonus, ataxia, spasticity, dementia; treatment is with γ-globulin or intrathecal interferon-α; pathology: *rod cells and Cowdry type A nuclear inclusions,* patchy demyelination and gliosis, CSF increased IgG and measles antibodies, + oligoclonal bands; *EEG: periodic sharp wave complexes (like burst suppression).*

7. **Mumps:** encephalitis presents 2 to 10 days *after parotitis and orchitis;* note: parotitis and encephalitis can also occur with coxsackie A, cytomegalovirus, Epstein-Barr virus, and lymphocytic choriomeningitis.

B. **Other viruses** (*cont'd*)

8. **Poliomyelitis:** etiology: *enterovirus (picornavirus), coxsackie, echovirus;* rare in the United States with widespread use of vaccine; transmission: feco-oral; clinical: *mild flu-like illness in 95% with no CNS involvement;* nonparalytic: flu-like illness, muscle pains, aseptic meningitis; paralytic: rapid limb and bulbar weakness, fasciculations, most patients recover completely, some with residual weakness (atrophied limb); pathology: *neuronophagia; immune response in thalamus, hypothalamus, cranial nerve motor nuclei, anterior horn and cerebellar nuclei, Cowdry B inclusions in the anterior horn cells*

9. **Reye syndrome:** *after varicella or influenza B infection and use of salicylates,* acute encephalopathy develops; results in hypoglycemia, hyperammonemia, increased intracranial pressure, cerebral edema and seizures; treatment: glucose, hyperventilation, fluid restriction, and mannitol; mortality is high unless caught early.

C. **Bacterial**

1. Meningitis risk increases with prematurity, maternal infection, complicated delivery; subdural effusion is a common complication of purulent meningitis; etiology: *newborns up to 1 year* (Enterobacter coli, *group B streptococcus*), *6 months to 1 year* (Haemophilus influenzae, pneumococcus, meningococcus), *post-traumatic (pneumococcus), abscess (staphylococcus, streptococcus, pneumococcus).*

> **NB:** *Frontal lobe abscesses are more likely contaminated with streptococcus; in the temporal lobe, it is more likely polymicrobial.*

2. **Sydenham's chorea:** initial manifestation: usually disturbance in school function, daydreaming, fidgety, inattentiveness, and increased emotional lability; onset of chorea is rather sudden, *lag time between streptococcal infection and chorea averages 6 months;* serologic evidence is absent in one-third of patients; risk of developing carditis with Sydenham's chorea is 30% to 50%; *recurrent episodes of chorea are most common at the time of pregnancy in patients;* lab: elevated erythrocyte sedimentation rate or C-reactive protein, prolonged PR interval; treatment for chorea: dopamine receptor blocking agents such as *haloperidol, pimozide, phenothiazines, or amantadine;* for acute rheumatic fever: *penicillin V, 400,000 U (250 mg) tid for 10 days followed by prophylaxis (benzathine penicillin G, 1.2 million U intramuscularly every 3–4 weeks or penicillin V, 250 mg orally bid or sulfisoxazole, 0.5–1.0 g orally qd).*

   a. Differential diagnosis: phenothiazine reactions, tics, Huntington's disease, Wilson's disease, benign paroxysmal choreoathetosis, lupus, polyarteritis and other vasculopathies, hyperparathyroidism, neoplastic lesions of the basal ganglia, and ataxia telangiectasia

   b. *Jones criteria for acute rheumatic fever:* diagnosis—*two major manifestations or one major and two minor manifestations* plus evidence of streptococcal infection

      i. Major manifestations: *carditis, polyarthritis, chorea, erythema marginatum, subcutaneous nodules*

      ii. Minor manifestations: arthralgia, fever, increased erythrocyte sedimentation rate, increased C-reactive protein, increased PR interval

      iii. Supporting evidence of streptococcus group A infection: throat culture or rapid streptococcus antigen screen, high or rising streptococcus antibody titer

D. **Toxins**

1. **Kernicterus:** *(bilirubinemia) is usually from ABO and Rh incompatibility,* especially in premature, hypoxic, acidotic, or septic newborns; it can affect the pallidum,

substantia nigra, cranial nerves III, VIII, and XII selectively or be diffuse, staining neurons yellow.

2. **Fetal alcohol syndrome:** growth delay, small face, MR, abnormal cortical lamination, small cerebrum and brainstem; alcohol is also associated with stillbirth, prematurity, and low birth weight.

3. **Thallium:** axonal neuropathy, vomiting, diarrhea, headache, and confusion

4. **NB: Lead:** irritability, motor regression and encephalopathy; testing shows *positive urine coproporphyrin III and basophilic stippling of red blood cells;* treatment: oral chelation with dimercaptosuccinic acid; lead paint may have been used in homes until 1973.

5. **Arsenic:** *Mees' lines* are seen in the nail bed.

6. **Mercury (organic):** in utero exposure at Minamata resulted in severe MR, cerebral > cerebellar atrophy.

7. **Botulism:** spores can be found in honey; results in hypotonia, mydriasis, and apnea.

VII. Learning Disorders

A. **Attention deficit disorder:** onset is before age 7 years; affects males more than females; duration is greater than 6 months; problems occur in two or more settings; at least three types of inattentions, three impulsivities, and two hyperactivities must be present; treatment: behavior modification, methylphenidate, amphetamine, guanfacine.

B. **Autism:** onset is before age 3 years; male-to-female ratio is 4 to 1; without clear etiology; failure to develop normal language, lack of imagination, abnormal response to contact, repetitive behavior, and fear of change are key features; treatment: early intervention with behavior modification. *Diagnostic and Statistical Manual of Mental Disorders,* fifth edition (*DSM-5*) incorporates Pervasive Developmental Disorder and Asperger's Syndrome under Autism Spectrum Disorder.

CHEAT SHEET

Key Words	High-Yield Information
Abetalipoproteinemia	Acanthocytosis, progressive ataxia, deficient in vitamin A, D, E, K
Acquired microcephaly	Rett's syndrome, Angelman syndrome
Adrenoleukodystrophy	X-linked recessive, spastic gait, decline in school function, high VLCFA
Aicardi syndrome	X-linked dominant, agenesis of corpus callosum, chorioretinal lacunae, infantile spasms
Alexander disease	Macrocephaly, GFAP mutation, Rosenthal fibers
Alpers disease	Progressive gray-matter disease, walnut brain, epilepsy—do not use valproic acid (VPA), causes liver failure; POLG mutation
Anencephaly	Failure of anterior neural tube closure

(continued)

CHEAT SHEET (continued)

Key Words	High-Yield Information
Angelman syndrome	"Happy puppet," seizures, microcephaly, paternal transmission of 15q deletion
Ataxia-telangiectasia syndrome	Choreoathetosis, oculomotor apraxia, conjunctival telangiectasia, immunodeficient, DNA repair mechanism defect
Becker's muscular dystrophy	Milder than Duchenne, not wheelchair bound at 16 years old
Canavan disease	Macrocephaly, aspartoacylase deficiency, increased NAA on MRS
Congenital myopathies	All AR except, myotubular/centronuclear which is X-linked; malignant hyperthermia risk
Congenital myotonia	Chloride channel, mini-Hercules
Cornelia de Lange syndrome	Duplication of 3q, synophrys "unibrow," short stature, dystonia,
Cri du chat syndrome	Deletion of 5p, "cat's cry," microcephaly
Duane syndrome	Congenital nonprogressive horizontal ophthalmoplegia, usually difficulty with abduction
Duchenne muscular dystrophy	Gower's maneuver, calf pseudohypertrophy, X-linked, dystrophin gene
Fabry's disease	X-linked recessive, alpha-galactosidase deficiency, angiokeratomas, renal disease, painful neuropathy, posterior strokes
Fazio-Londe disease	Progressive bulbar palsy in early childhood
Fetal alcohol syndrome	Flat philtrum, short stature, microcephaly, small eyes
Fragile X	Trinucleotide repeat disorder—CGG (giant gonads), autism
Friedrich's ataxia	Trinucleotide repeat disorder GAA, ataxia, peripheral neuropathy, hypertrophic cardiomyopathy, diabetes mellitus
Galactosemia	Newborn with failure to thrive, hepatomegaly, jaundice, cataracts, intellectual disability, deficiency of galactose-1-UDP
GLUT-1 disorder	Low CSF glucose, neonatal seizures, atypical absence, dystonias, treat with ketogenic diet
Hallervorden-Spatz disease	Pantothenate-kinase-associated neurodegeneration (PKAN), choreoathetosis, spasticity, iron deposits in basal ganglia, "eye of the tiger" on MRI

(continued)

CHEAT SHEET (continued)

Key Words	High-Yield Information
Homocystinuria	Marfanoid, increased stroke, cystathionine synthetase deficiency
Hydranencephaly	Brain replaced by CSF, usually only brainstem and cerebellum intact
Incontinentia pigmenti	X-linked dominant, linear vesicular or bullous lesions that become hyperpigmented, seizures, spasticity, intellectual disability
Isovaleric acidemia	Smells like "sweaty socks"
Joubert syndrome	"Molar tooth sign" on MRI, oculomotor apraxia, hyperpnea with central apnea, cerebellar vermis agenesis
Kearns-Sayre syndrome	MtDNA deletion, retinitis pigmentosa, deafness, cardiac arrhythmias, ophthalmoplegia
Klinefelter syndrome	47 chromosomes: XXY, gynecomastia, small testes, learning disability
Krabbe disease	Rigidity; galactocerebrosidase deficiency
Lafora body disease	Lafora body—basophilic cytoplasmic inclusions; progressive myoclonic epilepsy ataxia, optic atrophy
Leigh disease	Encephalopathy during infections, ataxia, seizures, necrosis of basal ganglia, nuclear DNA mutation
Lesch-Nyhan syndrome	Self-mutilation, X-linked, deficiency in HGPRT enzyme causing hyperuricemia
Lissencephaly	Type 1: smooth brain (Miller Dieker syndrome) Type 2: cobblestone brain (Walker Warburg syndrome, Fukuyama muscular dystrophy)
Lowe syndrome	Oculocerebrorenal symptoms: cataracts, glaucoma, buphthalmos, renal tubular acidosis, renal failure, X-linked recessive
Macrocephaly	Alexander disease, Canavan disease, PTEN mutation, fragile X
Maple syrup urine disease	Urine smells like maple syrup
MELAS	Migraine, stroke not following vascular distribution, mtDNA mutation
Menkes disease	Hair like steel wool (pili torti), hypothermia, seizures, profound copper deficiency
MERRF	Myoclonic epilepsy, deafness, optic atrophy, ophthalmoplegia

(continued)

CHEAT SHEET (continued)

Key Words	High-Yield Information
Metachromatic leukodystrophy	Arylsulfatase deficiency, spasticity in early childhood
Migraine variants in children	Benign paroxysmal torticollis: episodes of head tilt, age of onset 2–8 months Benign paroxysmal vertigo: episodes of vertigo—may be unexplained fright or refusal to walk, age of onset 2–4 y/o Cyclic vomiting: episodes of intense vomiting, age of onset 3–5 years
Miller-Dieker syndrome	LIS 1 gene, lissencephaly, intractable seizures
Mobius syndrome	Congenital facial diplegia—agenesis of cranial nerve nuclei, usually 6 and 7
Mucopolysaccharidoses	Coarse facies, carpal tunnel in a child, AR except Hunter's (X-linked)
Myelomeningocele	Restricted failure of posterior neural tube closure, associated with hydrocephalus and Chiari II
Neuroaxonal dystrophy	Psychomotor retardation, blindness, EEG shows high-amplitude fast rhythms
Neurofibromatosis 1	Chromosome 17, neurofibromin, café au lait macules, neurofibromas, optic glioma, Lisch nodules, pseudoarthrosis
Neurofibromatosis 2	Chromosome 22, merlin protein, bilateral acoustic schwannoma, meningiomas
Neuronal ceroid lipofuscinosis	Retinitis pigmentosa, myoclonic epilepsy
Niemann-Pick A and B	May have cherry red spot, hepatosplenomegaly, sphingomyelinase deficiency; lysosomal storage disorder
Niemann-Pick c	Cholesterol disorder, vertical supranuclear ophthalmoplegia
Nonaccidental trauma (NAT)	Child abuse, retinal hemorrhage, subdural or parenchymal hemorrhage, multiple healing fractures, seizures
Nonketotic hyperglycinemia	Seizures in utero = fetal hiccups
Opsoclonus myoclonus ataxia syndrome	"Dancing eyes" syndrome, associated with neuroblastoma
Osler-Weber-Rendu syndrome	AD, arterio-venous malformation (AVM), and aneurysms in brain; multiple skin telangiectasias

(continued)

CHEAT SHEET (continued)

Key Words	High-Yield Information
Paramyotonia congenita	Sodium channel, cold trigger
Pelizaeus-Merzbacher disease	Pendular nystagmus; X-linked; hypomyelination syndrome
Phenylketonuria	Musty body odor, cataracts, hyperactive, aggressive, low IQ
Pompe's disease	Glycogen storage disease type 2, floppy infant, cardiomyopathy
Posterior fossa tumors	Medulloblastoma and pilocytic astrocytoma most common Can also be ependymoma, hemangioblastoma, brainstem glioma When resected, children can develop cerebellar mutism
Prader-Willi syndrome	Triple H—hyperphagia, hypotonia, hypogonadism; paternal transmission of 15q deletion
Rett's syndrome	X-linked dominant, acquired microcephaly, autism, regression, "hand wringing," MECP2 gene
Schizencephaly	Cleft in brain lined by gray matter
Septo-optic dysplasia	Absence of septum pellucidum, panhypopituitarism, optic atrophy
Sialidosis	"Cherry red spot myoclonus syndrome," neuraminidase deficiency
Spasmus nutans	Head tilt, Nystagmus, Torticollis in healthy infant, benign
Spinal muscular atrophy (SMA)	Floppy but alert infant, SMN gene 1 and 2
Sturge-Weber syndrome	Facial port wine stain, glaucoma, leptomeningeal angiomatosis
Tay-Sachs disease	Cherry red spot, regression, hexosaminidase A deficiency
Tourette's syndrome	AD, combination of motor and vocal tics, associated with attention deficit disorder and obsessive-compulsive disorder
Trisomy 13—Patau syndrome	Holoprosencephaly, cardiac defects, cleft lip and palate

(continued)

CHEAT SHEET (continued)

Key Words	High-Yield Information
Tuberous sclerosis complex 1 and 2	TSC 1—chromosome 9, hamartin TSC 2—chromosome 16, tuberin Infantile spasms—treat with vigabatrin Cortical tubers, giant-cell astrocytoma Skin: ash leaf spots, Shagreen patch, facial angiofibroma
Turner syndrome	45 chromosomes: XO, webbed neck, short stature, coarctation of aorta
Unverricht-Lundborg disease	Progressive myoclonic epilepsy, preserved cognition, EPM1 gene
Von Hippel Landau syndrome	AD, cerebellar hemangioblastoma, multiple tumors
X-linked OTC (ornithine transcarbamoylase) deficiency	Most common urea cycle defect, neonatal encephalopathy, high ammonia, respiratory alkalosis
Zellweger disease	Peroxisomal disorder, dysmorphic, floppy infant, seizures, hepatic and renal involvement

Suggested Readings

Aicardi J. *Diseases of the Nervous System in Childhood.* 3rd ed. London: Mac Keith Press;2009.

Bradley WG, Daroff RB, Fenichel GM, et al. *Neurology in Clinical Practice.* 5th ed. Philadelphia, PA: Elsevier;2008.

Fenichel GM. *Clinical Pediatric Neurology: A Signs and Symptoms Approach.* 6th ed. Philadelphia, PA: Saunders Elsevier;2009.

Swaiman KF, Ashwal S, Ferriero DM. *Pediatric Neurology Principles and Practice.* 5th ed. Philadelphia, PA: Mosby Elsevier;2012.

Volpe JJ. *Neurology of the Newborn.* 5th ed. Philadelphia, PA: Saunders;2008.

Subspecialties

CHAPTER 22

Neurourology

I. Micturition

A. Involves coordination of central nervous system (CNS) and peripheral nervous system (PNS)

B. Initiated by cerebral cortex

C. First step is relaxation of striated external urethral sphincter (EUS) by inhibition of somatic efferents

D. Inhibition of sympathetic efferents

E. Activation of parasympathetic efferents causing bladder contraction and urethral smooth muscle relaxation

1. *CNS*

   a. Pontine micturition center (PMC) or Barrington nucleus mediates normal micturition reflex by coordinating activity of detrusor and urethral sphincter.

   b. Afferent signals from the lower urinary tract are received in the periaqueductal grey matter (PAG) and relayed to insula.

   c. Anterior cingulate gyrus controls micturition reflexes.

   d. Prefrontal cortex makes voluntary voiding decisions.

2. *PNS*

   a. Somatic nervous system S2 to S4, pudendal nerve

      i. Striated external urinary sphincter

         (A) Striated sphincter contraction via nicotinic cholinergic receptors

         (B) Preganglionic **efferent** nerves exit from **S2 to S4.**

         (C) Nerve bodies are located in **Onuf's nucleus.**

         (D) Nerve fibers travel with **pudendal nerve** to EUS, where they modulate voluntary sphincteric control.

         (E) Release of acetylcholine stimulates nicotinic cholinergic receptors in EUS, causing contraction (storage).

2. *PNS* (*cont'd*)

   b. Autonomic nervous system

      i. Parasympathetic pathways S2 to S4, pelvic nerve

         (A) Detrusor contraction via muscarinic receptors

         (B) Preganglionic **efferent** nerves exit from **S2 to S4.**

         (C) Travel in **pelvic nerve** to **inferior pelvic plexus** located adjacent to the bladder to modulate bladder contractions

         (D) Release of acetylcholine stimulates muscarinic acetylcholine receptors (M3) in bladder, causing contraction (emptying).

      ii. Sympathetic pathways T11 to L2, hypogastric nerve

         (A) Smooth muscle relaxation via B-adrenergic receptors

         (B) Preganglionic **efferent** nerves exit from **T10 to L2.**

         (C) Ganglia are paraganglia (next to vertebrae), preganglia (between vertebrae and end organ), or peripheral ganglia (in end organ).

         (D) Nerves travel within **hypogastric nerve to the inferior pelvic plexus,** where they modulate urethral smooth muscle contraction and inhibit parasympathetic activity.

         (E) Release of norepinephrine stimulates beta-3 adrenergic receptor in bladder, causing relaxation (storage).

         (F) Release of norepinephrine stimulates alpha-1 adrenergic receptors in involuntary sphincter, causing sphincter contraction (storage).

II. Voiding Dysfunction Classification System

A. Failure to store

1. Bladder: overactivity (idiopathic, neurogenic), decreased compliance, increased sensation

2. Outlet: stress urinary incontinence, intrinsic sphincteric deficiency

3. Both

B. Failure to empty

1. Bladder: underactive, acontractile

2. Outlet: anatomic (tumor, detrusor sphincter dyssynergia, stricture), functional (dysfunctional voiding, Fowler's syndrome [failure of urethral sphincter relaxation in young women], primary bladder neck obstruction)

3. Both

III. Location of the Neurologic Lesion and Effect on Bladder (Figure 22.1)

A. Suprapontine (including cerebral cortex): detrusor overactivity with bladder and sphincter synergy, normal bladder sensation, usually adequate emptying

B. Pons to spinal cord above S2 (upper motor neuron damage): detrusor sphincter dyssynergia and spastic paresis of lower limbs

C. S2 to S4 (lower motor neuron damage): acontractile detrusor, flaccid striated sphincter, flaccid lower limbs

D. Peripheral nerves: acontractile detrusor and absent bladder sensation

IV. Evaluation

A. History

   1. Urinary symptoms

     a. Frequency, volumes of urination, urinary incontinence

     b. Hesitancy, force of urinary stream, incomplete emptying

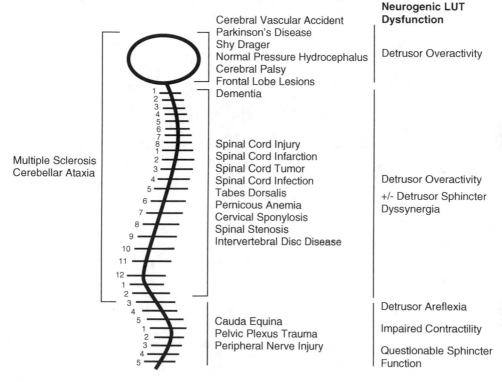

Figure 22.1 Symptoms associated with level of neurologic lesion.

   2. Review of symptoms

     a. Gastrointestinal (GI): frequency and consistency of bowel movements

     b. Need to splint—use fingers to press on the vagina or perineum to aid in obtaining a sense of complete evacuation during defecation, manual disimpaction.

B. Examination

   1. General: appearance, nutritional status, upper extremity dexterity

   2. Abdominal examination: presence of masses, assess for constipation

   3. Neurologic examination: should include assessment of perineal sensation

   4. Pelvic examination in women

     a. Evidence of leakage with cough

     b. Presence of pelvic organ prolapse beyond the hymen

     c. Strength of anal sphincter, presence of hemorrhoids

C. Testing

   1. Voiding diary: record volume voided, fluid consumed, incontinence episodes, pads/diapers for 3 days

   2. Postvoid residual

C. Testing (*cont'd*)

   3. Noninvasive uroflow

   4. Urodynamic study with or without video (video to assess outlet)

     a. In patients with spinal cord injury (SCI), wait until spinal shock resolves (~12 weeks).

   5. Cystoscopy

   6. Upper tract imaging: voiding cystourethrogram (assess for reflux), renal ultrasound (US) (assess for hydronephrosis, stones, renal scarring)

V. Urodynamic Findings Associated With Common Neurologic Disorders (Table 22.1)

A. Detrusor function: normal (N), overactive (O), acontractile (A), detrusor underactivity (D)

B. Detrusor compliance: normal (N), decreased (D), increased (I)

C. Smooth sphincter activity: synergic (S), dyssynergic (D), open (O)

D. Striated sphincter activity: synergic (S), dyssynergic (D), bradykinetic (B), impaired voluntary control (I), fixed tone (F)

VI. Management

A. Upper urinary tract preservation/preservation of renal function

B. Absence of infection

C. Adequate bladder capacity at low intravesical pressure (to prevent upper tract damage)

D. Adequate emptying at low intravesical pressure

E. Urinary control

Table 22.1 Detrusor Function, Sphincteric Function, and Bladder Compliance Associated With Common Neurologic Diseases

DISORDER	DETRUSOR FUNCTION	COMPLIANCE	SMOOTH SPHINCTER	STRIATED SPHINCTER
Cerebral vascular accident	O	N	S	S
Normal-pressure hydrocephalus	O	N	S	S
Cerebral palsy	N, O	N	S	S
Parkinson's	O, D	N	S	S, B
Multiple system atrophy	O, D	N	O	S
Multiple sclerosis	O	N	S	S, D
Myelomeningocele	A	N	O	F
Pernicious anemia	D, A	N	S	S
Diabetes mellitus	O, D, A	N	S	S
Pelvic surgery	D, A	N	O	F
Cauda equina	A	N	O	F
Spinal shock (after suprasacral injury)	A	N	S	F

F. **Failure to store**

1. Bladder: overactive bladder idiopathic
   a. Bladder retraining
   b. Dietary modification
   c. Pelvic floor physical therapy
   d. Pharmacotherapy
      i. Anticholinergics: oxybutynin, tolterodine, trospium chloride, fesoterodine, solifenacin, darifenacin
      ii. β-3 agonists: mirabegron
   e. Refractory treatments (fail pharmacotherapy)
      i. Sacral nerve stimulation (InterStim)
      ii. OnabotulinumtoxinA 100 units
      iii. Posterior tibial nerve stimulation
      iv. Augmentation cystoplasty

2. Bladder: neurogenic detrusor overactivity
   a. Bladder retraining
   b. Dietary modification
   c. Pelvic floor physical therapy
   d. Pharmacotherapy
      i. Anticholinergics: oxybutynin, tolterodine, trospium chloride, fesoterodine, solifenacin, darifenacin
   e. β-3 agonists: mirabegron
   f. Refractory treatments (fail pharmacotherapy)
      i. OnabotulinumtoxinA 200 units
      ii. Posterior tibial nerve stimulation
      iii. Augmentation cystoplasty

3. Outlet: stress urinary incontinence
   a. Pelvic floor physical therapy
   b. Incontinence pessary
   c. Intra-urethral bulking agents
   d. Mid-urethral synthetic sling
   e. Pubovaginal fascial sling

G. **Failure to empty**

1. Bladder: underactive, acontractile
   a. Timed, double voiding
   b. Intermittent self-catheterization (ISC)
   c. Suprapubic tube
   d. Sacral nerve stimulation (only in nonobstructive idiopathic urinary retention)
   e. Catheterizable stoma
   f. Indwelling Foley catheter (last resort)

2. Outlet:
   a. Pelvic floor physical therapy
   b. ISC
   c. OnabotulinumtoxinA 100 units into urinary sphincter (off-label usage)
   d. Sacral nerve stimulation in Fowler's syndrome

CHEAT SHEET

Neurologic lesions above the brainstem that affect micturition generally result in neurogenic detrusor overactivity (NDO) and involuntary bladder contraction, with coordinated smooth and striated sphincter function. Sensation and voluntary striated sphincter function are generally preserved, but sensation may be deficient or delayed.
Complete spinal cord lesions above the sacral spinal cord result in NDO, absent sensation below the level of the lesion, smooth sphincter synergia, and striated sphincter dyssynergia. Lesions at or above the spinal cord level of T7 or T8 may result in smooth sphincter dyssynergia.
For patients with SCI above T6, must rule out autonomic dysreflexia.
SCI or nerve root trauma below spinal cord level S2 typically results in detrusor acontractility. An open smooth sphincter area may result and various types of striated sphincter dysfunction may occur, but commonly the area retains a residual resting sphincter that is not under voluntary control.
Spinal shock typically lasts 12 weeks and is characterized by detrusor acontractility and a closed and competent bladder neck. The smooth sphincter is functional. The striated sphincter is maintained but may be reduced. The normal guarding reflex (striated sphincter response during filling) is absent, and there is no voluntary control. Urodynamic studies should be avoided until resolution of spinal shock.

Suggested Readings

Haylen BT, de Ridder D, Freeman RM, et al. An International Urogynecological Association (IUGA)/International Continence Society (ICS) joint report on the terminology for female pelvic floor dysfunction. *Neurourol Urodyn*.2010;29:4–20.

Jeong SJ, Cho SY, Oh SJ. Spinal cord/brain injury and the neurogenic bladder. *Urol Clin North Am*.2010;37:537–546.

Stohrer M, Blok B, Castro-Diaz, et al. EAU guidelines on neurogenic lower urinary tract dysfunction. *Eur Urol*.2009;56:81–88.

Wein AJ, Kavoussi LR, Novick AC. *Campbell-Walsh Urology*. 10th ed. Philadelphia, PA: Saunders Elsevier;2012.

CHAPTER 23

Neuro-ophthalmology

I. Anatomy and Examination

A. Photoreceptors

1. *Rods:* use *rhodopsin* pigment; mediate *light perception*
2. *Cones:* use *iodopsin* pigment; mediate *color vision*

B. Eyelids

1. *Three muscles control lid position.*
   a. *Levator palpebrae superioris*
      i. Main elevator of the upper lid
      ii. Innervated by the superior division of cranial nerve (CN) III
      iii. Right and left levators originate from the caudal central nucleus
   b. *Müller's muscle:* upper and lower eyelids; innervated by sympathetic fibers
   c. *Orbicularis oculi:* closes eyelids; innervated mainly by ipsilateral CN VII

C. Ocular muscles

1. *Horizontal eye movement*
   a. Lateral rectus—abducts the eye
   b. Medial rectus—adducts the eye
2. *Vertical eye movement*
   a. Superior rectus and inferior oblique—elevate the eye
   b. Inferior rectus and superior oblique—depress the eye
3. *Torsional eye movement:* the superior muscles produce intorsion (superior oblique muscle) and the inferior eye muscles produce extorsion (inferior oblique muscle).

> **NB:** When eye is turned outward, eye depressor is inferior rectus, and when turned inward, is superior oblique.

D. Ocular motor nerves

1. *Oculomotor nerve (CN III)*
   a. Innervates: superior rectus, inferior rectus, medial rectus, inferior oblique, levator palpebrae superioris, iris sphincter, ciliary muscle (required for focusing on near objects)
   b. Controls all adduction, extorsion, and elevation of the eye; controls most depression; and contributes to intorsion through the secondary action of the superior rectus
   c. Edinger-Westphal nucleus: rostral part of CN III, supplies the iris sphincter and ciliary muscle

D. **Ocular motor nerves** (*cont'd*)

    2. *Trochlear nerve (CN IV):* innervates: superior oblique; intorsion, particularly during abduction

    3. *Abducens nerve (CN VI):* innervates: lateral rectus muscle; eye abduction

E. **Oculomotor systems**

    1. *Vestibulo-ocular response system*

        a. Three semicircular canals

            i. Resting firing rate increased by acceleration/rotation of the head.

            ii. Canal function is initiated by head rotation toward it.

            iii. Each canal works in tandem with one on the opposite side.

            iv. Generate compensatory eye movements in the direction opposite the head motion to keep the eye stable during fixation

            v. Project through the vestibular component of CN VIII

        b. Otoliths

            i. Also component of the vestibular system

            ii. *Saccule and utricle consist of maculae embedded in a gelatinous substance with calcium crystals.*

            iii. *Detect linear accelerations of the head*

    2. *Optokinetic response*

        a. Main function is to hold images steady on the retina during sustained head movement

        b. Precise pathways are unknown but likely associated with *pathways for smooth pursuit extending from visual association areas (Brodmann's 18 and 19) to the horizontal pontine gaze center.*

        c. Smooth eye movement generated when large portions of the visual scene move across the retina, which usually happens when the head is moving

        d. Generates a *jerk nystagmus with the slow phase in the direction of stripe motion*

        e. Vestibulo-ocular response works together with optokinetic response: vestibulo-ocular response: rapid head rotation greater than 0.5 Hz; optokinetic response: slower rotations.

        f. Pursuit

            i. *Main function is to hold an object of interest on the fovea*

            ii. *Motion-sensitive regions of the extrastriate cortex, parieto-occipitotemporal junction, and the frontal eye fields supply input into superior colliculi, which control horizontal and vertical pursuit.*

            iii. Involved in horizontal ipsilateral pursuit

        g. Saccades

            i. Main function is to bring objects of interest onto the fovea

            ii. Saccades are quick eye movements that shift gaze from one object to another

            iii. Involve parietal and frontal eye fields

            iv. Mediate saccades toward the opposite side

            v. Superior colliculus involved in triggering saccades

            vi. Parapontine reticular formation and medial longitudinal fasciculus are responsible for horizontal saccades,

F. **Pupillary anatomy**

1. *Parasympathetic pathway*

   a. *Muscles innervated*

      i. *Iris sphincter: for pupillary constriction*

      ii. *Ciliary muscle: for accommodation*

   b. *Edinger-Westphal nucleus*

   c. *CN III*

      i. Innervation of intraocular muscles is located in the inner aspect of CN III.

      ii. Pupillomotor fibers are located on the outside (susceptible to compression).

      iii. Courses within the cavernous sinus, where it bifurcates into an inferior (preganglionic pupillomotor fibers) and superior division

      iv. Within the orbit, the parasympathetic fibers synapse in the ciliary ganglion and postganglionic parasympathetic fibers proceed anteriorly as short ciliary nerves to innervate the iris sphincter and ciliary muscles.

      v. Acetylcholine released at both the preganglionic presynaptic terminal within the ciliary ganglion and the postganglionic neuromuscular junction

2. *Sympathetic pathway*

   a. First-order neurons: originate in the *posterolateral hypothalamus and synapse within the intermediolateral gray-matter column* of the lower cervical and upper thoracic spinal cord

   b. *Second-order (preganglionic) neurons: arise from the ciliospinal center and exit the spinal cord through the ventral roots of C8 to T2 to synapse in the superior cervical ganglion*

> **NB:** Sympathetic pathway exits the spinal cord in the lower trunk of the brachial plexus.

   c. *Third-order (postganglionic) neurons: originate* from the superior cervical ganglion and travel as a plexus along the internal carotid artery. In the cavernous sinus they travel briefly with the 6th cranial nerve before entering the orbit.

> **NB:** These fibers, if lesioned, produce a Horner's syndrome in carotid dissection, sometimes with an associated VI nerve palsy.

II. Clinical Assessment

A. **Localization**

1. Pre-chiasmal: ocular or optic nerve

   a. Loss of vision in one eye

2. Chiasmal

   a. Bitemporal deficits may be incongruous.

3. Retrochiasmal

   a. Hemianopia or quadrantanopia

   b. May be misinterpreted as monocular visual loss

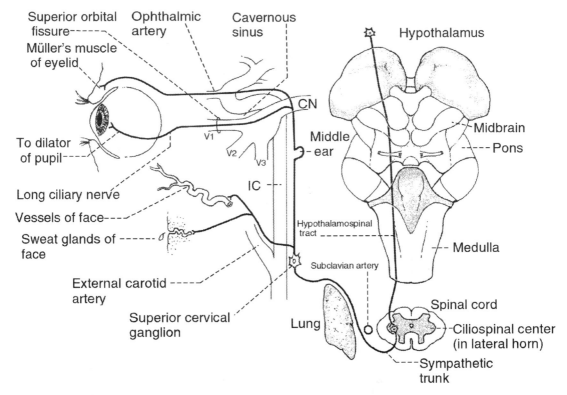

Figure 23.1 The course of the oculosympathetic pathway, where any interruption results in Horner's syndrome. Hypothalamic fibers project to the ipsilateral ciliospinal center of the intermediolateral cell column at T1, which then projects preganglionic sympathetic fibers to the superior cervical ganglion. The superior cervical ganglion projects postganglionic sympathetic fibers through the tympanic cavity, cavernous sinus, and superior orbital fissure. CN, cranial nerve; IC, internal carotid.

A. **Localization** (*cont'd*)

    4. Associated phenomenology

        a. Positive (hallucinations, scotoma, diplopia, etc.)

        b. Negative (vision loss with darkness; complete versus partial)

        c. Associated symptomatology (eye pain, headache, focal weakness)

B. **Examination**

    1. General examination of eye

        a. Eyelids

            i. Periorbital edema, injection, warmth

            ii. Ptosis

            iii. Blepharospasm

            iv. Retraction

        b. Conjunctiva

            i. Transparent with only a few visible blood vessels

            ii. Corkscrew conjunctival vessels—carotid cavernous fistula

            iii. Halo of redness at the limbus—uveitis or acute glaucoma

            iv. Interpalpebral redness—keratopathy or dry eye syndrome

            v. Diffuse eye injection—viral conjunctivitis

        c. Visual acuity: *Snellen visual acuity test*

    i. Ishihara or *Pseudoisochromatic color plates—assessment of color discrimination*

    ii. Visual field testing: confrontation methods—comparisons between hemifields and quadrants; Humphrey or Goldmann perimetry—standardized visual field testing

d. *Visual fields*

    i. *Nasal: 50 degrees*

    ii. *Superior: 60 degrees*

    iii. *Inferior: 70 degrees*

    iv. *Temporal: 80 degrees*

e. Extraocular movement

    i. Supranuclear upgaze palsy: confirmed by an intact Bell's phenomenon

    ii. *Tropias*

      (A) *Both eyes are not aligned, whether the patient is viewing with one eye or both.*

      (B) Patients usually have diplopia (if not, either vision in one eye is poor or the image of one eye is suppressed, which can occur with chronic lesions).

      (C) Differential diagnosis

        (1) Childhood ocular alignment problems (strabismus)

        (2) CN III, IV, VI palsies

        (3) Thyroid ophthalmopathy

        (4) Myasthenia gravis (MG)/neuromuscular junction disorders

        (5) Botulism

        (6) Convergence spasm

        (7) Traumatic ocular muscle entrapment in orbital fracture

        (8) Duane's retraction syndrome

        (9) Posterior fossa tumors

> **NB:** *Monocular diplopia is an ocular, not a neurological, problem.*

    iii. *Phorias*

      (A) *Eyes are misaligned when either eye is viewing alone.*

      (B) When both eyes are viewing, the two eyes are aligned.

    iv. *Fixation*

      (A) Opsoclonus: fixation interrupted by repetitive saccades that immediately reverse direction and randomly directed ("saccad-o-mania").

    v. *Smooth pursuit*: assessed as the patient follows an object; requires attention

    vi. *Saccades*: assessed as patient rapidly moves eyes from one object to another

      (A) Hypometria: nonspecific

      (B) *Hypermetria: cerebellar disturbance, MS—always pathological*

      (C) Saccadic velocity

    vii. *Nystagmus*

      (A) Evaluation

        (1) Waveform: amplitude and velocity

        (2) Direction: horizontal versus vertical versus torsional

        (3) Monocular versus binocular

       vii. *Nystagmus (cont'd)*

         (B) *Pendular nystagmus has a sinusoidal oscillation without fast phases.*

         (C) *Jerk nystagmus* has a slow drift of the eyes in one direction alternating rhythmically with a fast movement in the other.

         (D) *Latent nystagmus (version of infantile nystagmus)*

            (1) Only present when one eye covered

            (2) Fast component away from covered eye

            (3) Decreased visual acuity due to nystagmus

            (4) Usually congenital and often seen in conjunction with esotropia

         (E) *Downbeat nystagmus: lesion at cervicomedullary junction (e.g., Chiari malformation), also paraneoplastic syndrome*

         (F) *Upbeat nystagmus lesions of medulla, cerebellar vermis, and Wernicke's*

         (G) *Seesaw nystagmus: parasellar lesions, septi-optic dysplasia*

         (H) *Torsional nystagmus*

         (I) *Rotary nystagmus:* differential diagnosis/etiologies—thalamic lesion

         (J) *Convergence retraction nystagmus: Parinaud's dorsal midbrain syndrome*

         (K) *Gaze-evoked nystagmus: not present in primary position; beats in direction of gaze, not visually disabling*

       viii. *Oculopalatal myoclonus: vertical pendular nystagmus and tremor of palate and or facial muscles, larynx, diaphragm; lesion of Mollaret triangle (connecting red nucleus, inferior olive, and dentate nucleus)*

       ix. *Ocular bobbing: metabolic encephalopathy or massive pontine lesion*

       x. *Opsoclonus; paraneoplastic encephalitis*

   f. Pupillary reactivity

     i. Direct versus indirect

     ii. Swinging flashlight

   g. Red reflex

     i. Routine step before the fundus is examined

     ii. May be abnormal and detects corneal opacities, cataracts, vitreous blood, and retinal detachments

   h. Ophthalmoscopic examination

     i. Funduscopic examination

       (A) Optic disc: assess for edema, pallor, and cupping.

       (B) Vessels

       (C) Macula

       (D) Retina

       (E) Assess for emboli, edema, and hemorrhage.

III. Disorders

  A. Disorders of the eyelids

    1. *Periorbital edema*

      a. Ocular inflammation, infection, allergy

      b. Cavernous sinus disease

      c. Thyroid ophthalmopathy

2. *Ptosis*

   a. Can originate anywhere from the cortex to the levator aponeurosis

   b. Differential diagnosis

      i. Supranuclear palsy

      ii. CN III palsy

      iii. Horner's syndrome (mild ptosis, 1–2 mm only)

      iv. Neuropathic

      v. Neuromuscular junction (MG, botulism)

      vi. Myopathic

      vii. Congenital

      viii. Progressive external ophthalmoplegia

      ix. Trauma

3. *Blepharospasm*

   a. Involuntary intermittent eyelid closure

   b. Form of focal dystonia, often with transient resolution during sensory input

   c. Orbicularis oculi resulting in eyelid closure may contract in synchrony with lower facial muscles with aberrant regeneration of CN VII after Bell's palsy.

   d. Types and etiologies

      i. Idiopathic, isolated

      ii. Associated with other facial dystonias: Meige's syndrome

      iii. Part of a generalized dystonia

      iv. Occurs with parkinsonian syndromes

      v. Medications (levodopa or the neuroleptics)

      vi. Pontine lesions

      vii. Severe dry eyes

   e. Treatment

      i. Botulinum type A toxin injections of the orbicularis muscles (treatment of choice)

      ii. Medications: anticholinergic agents, baclofen, clonazepam but rarely successful

B. **Disorders of eye movement**

   1. *Myopathic disorders*

     a. Congenital myopathy

       i. Myotubular

       ii. Central core

     b. Muscular dystrophy

       i. Myotonic dystrophy

       ii. Oculopharyngeal dystrophy

     c. Myotonic disorders

       i. Thomsen's disease

       ii. Paramyotonia congenita

       iii. Hyperkalemic and hypokalemic periodic paralyses

     d. Mitochondrial myopathy

       i. Progressive external ophthalmoplegia/Kearns-Sayre syndrome

       ii. *Mitochondrial myopathy, encephalomyopathy, lactic acidosis, and stroke-like episodes (MELAS)*/myoclonus epilepsy with ragged red fiber

1. *Myopathic disorders (cont'd)*
    e. *Metabolic myopathy:* abetalipoproteinemia
    f. *Endocrine myopathy*
        i. *Thyroid (Graves') ophthalmopathy:* characteristic feature is lid retraction; downgaze increases the distance between the cornea and upper lid, transiently resulting in lid lag (von Graefe's sign).
        ii. *Steroid myopathy*
    g. *Traumatic myopathy (muscle entrapment)*
    h. Autoimmune: orbital inflammatory pseudotumor
2. *Neuromuscular disorders*
    a. **MG**
        i. Symptoms more likely as day progresses or with significant motor activity
        ii. Ptosis that increases throughout the day, ptosis that worsens with repeated eye opening or prolonged upgaze, and Cogan's lid twitch
        iii. Lid retraction may also occur.
        iv. Diplopia with extraocular muscle involvement
    b. Lambert-Eaton myasthenic syndrome: ocular signs are rare.
    c. Amyotrophic lateral sclerosis
    d. *Toxins*
        i. Organophosphate insecticides
        ii. Botulism
        iii. Venom (cobras, kraits, coral snakes, and sea snakes)
3. *Neuropathic disorders*
    a. *Etiologies*
        i. Ischemic (diabetes mellitus, hypertension, vasculitis [giant-cell arteritis])
        ii. Hemorrhagic
        iii. Intra-axial tumors
        iv. Compression (tumor, aneurysm)
        v. Trauma
        vi. Acute inflammatory demyelinating polyradiculopathy (Miller-Fisher variant)
            (A) Clinical
                (1) *Ophthalmoplegia: symmetric paresis of upgaze with progressive impairment of horizontal gaze and late involvement or relative sparing of downgaze*
                (2) *Areflexia* ·
                (3) *Ataxia*
            (B) Male-to-female ratio: 2 to 1
            (C) Upper respiratory infection or gastrointestinal (*Campylobacter jejuni*) infection preceding the neurologic symptoms
            (D) Autoantibodies to *GQ1b-ganglioside*
        vii. Demyelinating (multiple sclerosis [MS]) (internuclear ophthalmoplegia, saccadic dysmetria)
        viii. Meningitis (basilar-cryptococcus)
        ix. Increased intracranial pressure (6th nerve palsy)

x. Cavernous sinus

    (A) Compression/metastatic   (meningioma,   pituitary   adenoma, craniopharyngioma)

    (B) Pituitary adenoma

    (C) Chordoma

    (D) Carotid aneurysm

    (E) Inflammation (Tolosa-Hunt)

    (F) Infection (mucormycosis, infiltrating sinus infection)

    (G) Carotid-cavernous fistula

b. *Oculomotor (CN III) palsy*

  i. Pathophysiology

    (A) Etiologies in adults

      (1) Idiopathic (30%–35%) (likely microvascular infarction)

      (2) Aneurysmal compression

      (3) Tumor

      (4) Inflammation (e.g., sarcoidosis)

      (5) Infection (meningitis)

      (6) Trauma

    (B) Etiologies in children

      (1) Congenital

      (2) Trauma

      (3) Posterior fossa tumors

      (4) Meningitis

  ii. *Clinical*

    (A) Symptoms

      (1) Diplopia: usually oblique in primary position

      (2) Ptosis

      (3) Blurred near vision

    (B) Complete CN III palsy

      (1) Eye in primary position is down and out.

      (2) Cannot elevate or adduct

      (3) Full abduction

      (4) Some residual depression accompanied by intorsion

      (5) *Ptosis is severe.*

      (6) Accommodation impaired

      (7) Pupil is large and does not constrict to light or on convergence.

    (C) *Pupil rule*

      (1) *Ischemic: pupil is spared in 75%.*

      (2) *Aneurysm: pupil eventually involved in* more than *90%.*

    (D) *Oculomotor synkinesis, aberrant regeneration*

      (1) Anomalous contraction of muscles

      (2) Most common is lid elevation on adduction

c. *Trochlear (CN IV) palsy*

  i. Pathophysiology

    (A) Etiologies in adults

   (A) Etiologies in adults (*cont'd*)

    (1) Microvascular ischemia

    (2) Trauma

    (3) Idiopathic

    (4) Congenital

    (5) Tumor

  ii. Clinical

   (A) Vertical separation largest in downgaze

   (B) Compensatory lateral head tilt away from the side of the lesion to minimize the diplopia

   (C) Extraocular muscles examination: decreased depression of the adducted eye

   (D) Bilateral CN IV = head trauma

   (E) Differential diagnosis of vertical diplopia

    (1) Ocular MG

    (2) Thyroid ophthalmoplegia

    (3) Orbital lesion (i.e., tumor)

    (4) CN III palsy

    (5) CN IV palsy

    (6) Skew deviation

 d. Abducens (CN VI) palsy

  i. Pathophysiology

   (A) Etiologies in adults

    (1) Microvascular ischemia (25%)

    (2) Tumor (20%)

    (3) Trauma (15%)

    (4) Elevated intracranial pressure (ICP)

  ii. Clinical

   (A) Horizontal diplopia that is uncrossed, meaning that the ipsilateral image belongs to the ipsilateral eye and is more noticeable for distant targets

4. Cavernous sinus syndromes

 a. May also affect CN V-1 or CN V-2

 b. Can produce a Horner's syndrome

 c. Anterior disease may damage the optic nerve.

 d. Etiologies

  i. Tumors (70%)

   (A) Nasopharyngeal carcinoma (most common cause)

   (B) Pituitary

   (C) Adenoma

   (D) Meningioma

   (E) Craniopharyngioma

   (F) Chondroma

   (G) Metastatic (breast, lung, and prostate) carcinoma

ii. Aneurysms (20%)

iii. Infection

iv. Cavernous sinus fistula

e. **Tolosa-Hunt syndrome**

   i. Pathophysiology

     (A) Accounts for only 3% of cavernous sinus syndromes

     (B) Pathology: *idiopathic noncaseating granulomatous inflammation in the cavernous sinus*

     (C) Diagnosis of exclusion

   ii. Clinical

     (A) Acute, painful ophthalmoplegia

     (B) Progression over days to weeks

     (C) Most commonly, CNs III and VI involved

     (D) CN IV and CN V-1 in one-third of cases

     (E) Optic nerve is affected in 20%.

     (F) CN V-2 sensory loss in 10%

     (G) Horner's syndrome, CN V-3 sensory loss, and CN VII palsy are unusual.

     (H) May have elevated erythrocyte sedimentation rate and positive systemic lupus erythematosus preparation

     (I) May have recurring attacks over months to years

   iii. Treatment

     (A) High-dose oral prednisone

5. **Pituitary apoplexy**

   a. Multiple oculomotor palsies

   b. Severe headache

   c. Bilateral vision loss

6. **Wallenberg lateral medullary syndrome**

   a. Infarction in posterior-inferior cerebellar artery, usually due to ipsilateral vertebral arterial occlusion or possibly MS

   b. Clinical

     i. *Imbalance*

     ii. *Vertigo*

     iii. *Numbness of the face or limbs*

     iv. *Dysphagia*

     v. *Headache*

     vi. *Vomiting*

     vii. *Horner's syndrome*

     viii. *Decreased pain and temperature sensation of ipsilateral face and contralateral body*

     ix. *Skew deviation with ipsilateral eye hypotropic, causing diplopia*

     x. *Primary position horizontal or horizontal-torsional nystagmus*

7. *Internuclear ophthalmoplegia*

   a. Lesion of the medial longitudinal fasciculus (MLF) blocks information from the contralateral CN VI to the ipsilateral CN III.

   b. Internuclear ophthalmoplegia named after ipsilateral MLF lesion.

7. *Internuclear ophthalmoplegia (cont'd)*

   c. Clinical

      i. Impaired adduction during conjugate gaze away from the side of the MLF lesion

      ii. Nystagmus of the abducting during conjugate version movements

      iii. Slowed adducting saccades with lag in the adducting eye compared with the abducting eye

   d. Etiologies

      i. Brainstem ischemia (usually unilateral)

      ii. MS, often bilateral

      iii. Brainstem encephalitis

      iv. Behcet's disease

      v. Cryptococcosis

      vi. Guillain-Barré syndrome

8. *One-and-a-half syndrome*

   a. *Combined damage to:*

      i. *MLF plus ipsilateral paramedian pontine reticular formation*

      ii. *MLF and ipsilateral CN VI nucleus*

   b. Clinical

      i. Internuclear ophthalmoplegia on gaze to the contralateral side (the "half")

      ii. Pontine conjugate gaze palsy to the ipsilateral side (the "one")

9. *Mobius syndrome:* heterogeneous group of congenital anomalies consisting of *facial palsies and abnormal horizontal gaze*

C. Nystagmus

1. *Pendular nystagmus: back-and-forth slow phase movements without a fast phase*

   a. Etiologies

      i. MS (most common)

      ii. Strokes

      iii. Encephalitis

      iv. Brainstem vascular

   b. Pathophysiology unclear

   c. Treatment: may improve with gabapentin, memantine, clonazepam

2. *Spasmus nutans*

   a. *Disorder of young children, with age at onset usually 6 to 12 months and resolves by age 3 years*

   b. *Clinical triad (not all three are required)*

      i. *Ocular oscillations*

      ii. *Head nodding*

      iii. *Head turn*

   c. Pathophysiology is uncertain.

3. *Seesaw nystagmus*

   a. Pendular

   b. Present in all gaze positions

   c. Etiologies

      i. Tumor (parasellar lesions)

        (A) Pituitary adenoma

        (B) Craniopharyngioma

   ii. Stroke

    (A) Pontomedullary infarct

    (B) Midbrain/thalamic infarct

   iii. Trauma

   iv. Congenital (septo-optic dysplasia)

   v. Vision loss: retinitis pigmentosa, albinism, optic nerve hypoplasia

   vi. Prognosis variable

 4. *Jerk nystagmus*

  a. *Downbeat nystagmus*

   i. Clinical

    (A) Associated signs/symptoms

     (1) Ataxia

     (2) Blurred vision

     (3) Oscillopsia

   ii. Etiologies

    (A) Arnold-Chiari syndrome (20%–25%)

    (B) Idiopathic (20%)

    (C) Spinocerebellar degeneration (20%)

    (D) Brainstem stroke (10%)

    (E) MS (5%–10%)

    (F) Tumor

    (G) Medication (lithium, antiepileptic drugs)/alcohol

    (H) Trauma

  b. *Upbeat nystagmus*

   i. Associated with:

    (A) Oscillopsia

    (B) Ataxia

   ii. Etiologies

    (A) Spinocerebellar degeneration (20%–25%)

    (B) Brain stem stroke/vascular malformation (20%) (medulla common)

    (C) MS/inflammatory (10%–15%)

    (D) Tumor

    (E) Infection

    (F) Medication/alcohol

    (G) Trauma

  c. *Torsional nystagmus*

   i. Usually attributed to dysfunction of vertical semicircular canal inputs

   ii. Etiologies

    (A) Stroke

    (B) MS

    (C) Vascular malformation

    (D) Arnold-Chiari syndrome

    (E) Tumor

    (F) Encephalitis

    (G) Trauma

C. **Nystagmus** (*cont'd*)

    5. *Gaze-evoked nystagmus*

        a. Most common nystagmus; often age related

        b. Dysfunction of cerebellar flocculus in conjunction with the lateral medulla for horizontal gaze and the midbrain for vertical gaze

        c. Differential diagnosis/etiologies

            i. Medications

                (A) Antiepileptic agents

                (B) Sedative hypnotics

            ii. Bilateral brainstem lesion

            iii. Cerebellar lesion

            iv. MG

    6. *Convergence retraction nystagmus: bilateral adducting saccades, causing convergence of both eyes*

        a. Best seen when testing eyes with a downward moving optokinetic nystagmus tape/drum because this requires upward saccades

        b. Differential diagnosis/etiologies

            i. Differential diagnosis by age

                (A) 10 years old (y/o): pinealoma

                (B) 20 y/o: head trauma

                (C) 30 y/o: brainstem vascular malformation

                (D) 40 y/o: MS

                (E) 50 y/o: basilar stroke

        c. **Parinaud syndrome**

            i. *Dorsal midbrain lesion*

            ii. *Supranuclear upgaze palsy*

            iii. *Lid retraction*

            iv. *Convergence-retraction nystagmus*

            v. *Light-near dissociation of pupil response*

    7. *Treatment of nystagmus*

        a. Acquired pendular nystagmus: gabapentin, memantine

        b. Downbeat and upbeat: aminopyridine

        c. Periodic alternating: Lioresal, clonazepam, valproic acid

D. **Opsoclonus (saccadomania)**

    1. Pathophysiology: *dentate nucleus lesion*

    2. Clinical

        a. Involuntary bursts of spontaneous saccades in all directions

        b. Classic triad

            i. Opsoclonus

            ii. Myoclonus

            iii. Ataxia (trunk and gait)

    3. Etiologies

        a. Neuroblastoma (childhood)

        b. Infection (young adults)

            i. Enterovirus

   ii. Coxsackie virus B3, B2

   iii. Louis encephalitis

   iv. *Rickettsia*

   v. *Salmonella*

   vi. Rubella

   vii. Epstein-Barr virus

   viii. Mumps

  c. Paraneoplastic (older adults), usually anti-Ri antibodies

   i. Breast

   ii. Lung

   iii. Uterine/ovarian

  d. Brainstem stroke or encephalitis

  e. Hyperosmolar coma

  f. MS

  g. Midbrain tumor

  h. Medications/toxins (lithium, phenytoin, cocaine)

E. Ocular bobbing

 1. Clinical: rapid downward jerk with slow return to primary gaze

 2. Etiology

  a. Pontine lesion

  b. Subarachnoid hemorrhage

  c. Head trauma

  d. Leigh disease

  e. Metabolic encephalopathy

F. Ocular myoclonus (see Chapter 27): lesion associated with Mollaret's triangle

G. Oculogyric crisis

 1. Temporary period of frequent spasms of eye deviation, often upward

 2. Lasts seconds to hours

 3. Etiology

  a. Medication

   i. Neuroleptics

   ii. Carbamazepine

   iii. Tetrabenazine

   iv. Lithium toxicity

   v. Metoclopramide (and other antiemetics)

  b. Brainstem encephalitis

  c. Paraneoplastic

  d. Rett's syndrome

  e. Tourette's syndrome

  f. Wilson's disease

H. Disorders of the visual system and pathways

 1. *Optic disc edema*

  a. Optic disc edema results from stasis of axoplasmic flow at the optic disc, with swelling of the axons that cause an elevation of the disc and an increase in the diameter of the disc.

1. *Optic disc edema (cont'd)*

    b. Causes of optic disc edema

        i. Papilledema (elevated intracranial pressure)

        ii. Optic neuritis

        iii. Anterior ischemic optic neuropathy (AION) (either microvascular [non-arteritis] or giant-cell arteritis)

        iv. Diabetic papillitis

        v. Orbital mass

        vi. Infiltration (tumor, lymphoma)

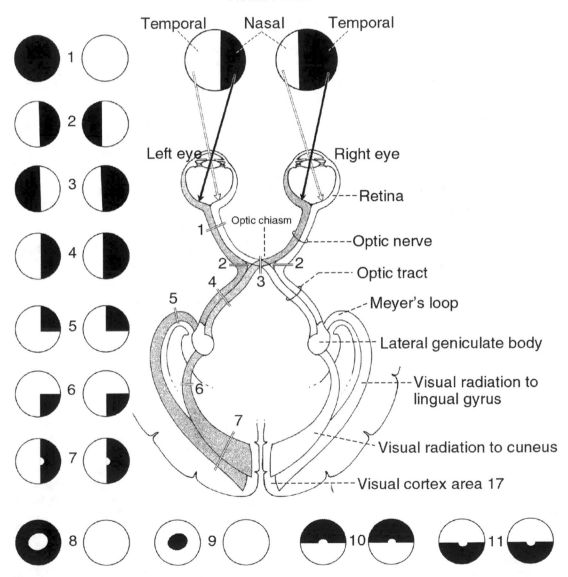

Figure 23.2 The visual pathway from the retina to the cortex illustrating the visual field defects. (1) Ipsilateral blindness. (2) Binasal hemianopia. (3) Bitemporal hemianopia. (4) Right hemianopia. (5) Right upper quadrantanopia. (6) Right lower quadrantanopia. (7) Right hemianopia with macular sparing. (8) Left constricted field as a result of end-stage glaucoma. (9) Left central scotoma seen in optic neuritis. (10) Upper altitudinal hemianopia from destruction of the lingual gyri. (11) Lower altitudinal hemianopia from bilateral destruction of the cunei.

  vii. Retinal vein occlusion

  viii. Venous congestion

  ix. Malignant hypertension

   x. Infection

  xi. Uveitis

2. *Optic neuritis*

 a. Describes any condition that causes inflammation of the optic nerve

 b. Pain in the involved eye worsened with eye movement followed by monocular vision loss

 c. Usually young adults

 d. Female-to-male ratio: 5 to 1

 e. Visual acuity is usually affected, with diffuse field depression as the common finding.

 f. *Relative afferent pupillary defect may persist even after the visual function improves.*

 g. *Visual-evoked potential: prolonged P100*

 h. Treatment

   i. The Optic Neuritis Treatment Trial

   (A) Three groups

    (1) Placebo tablets

    (2) Moderate-dose oral prednisone

    (3) High-dose intravenous (IV) methylprednisolone for 3 days (followed by 11-day therapy with oral prednisone)

   (B) Results

    (1) Oral steroids: higher rate of recurrence of optic neuritis.

    (2) Patients with abnormal brain MRI more likely to develop MS, but the risk of new events was reduced in those patients who received IV methyl prednisone.

    (3) Patients treated with IV steroids improved more quickly, but all patients improved to the same degree within 6 months to 1 year.

3. **Anterior ischemic optic neuropathy (AION)**

 a. Pathophysiology: ischemic infarct of the optic disc due to atherosclerotic disease (nonarteritic AION), or from vasculitis, most commonly giant-cell arteritis (arteritic AION)

 b. Clinical

   i. **NB:** Sudden *painless* vision loss associated with unilateral optic disc swelling

   ii. *Usually* greater than *45 y/o*

  iii. *Arteritic AION*

   (A) Giant-cell arteritis

    (1) Inflammation of small- and medium-sized extracranial arteries

    (2) Usually greater than 60 y/o

    (3) Female-to-male ratio: 3 to 1

    (4) Vision loss most commonly from vasculitic occlusion of the posterior ciliary

    (5) Systemic symptoms include headache, scalp and temple tenderness, myalgias, arthralgias, low-grade fever, anemia, malaise, weight loss, anorexia, and jaw claudication.

(A) Giant-cell arteritis (*cont'd*)

    (6) Associated with polymyalgia rheumatica

    (7) Inflamed temporal arteries can be palpated as a firm "cord" with a poor pulse.

    (8) Labs: elevated erythrocyte sedimentation rate greater than 50 (erythrocyte sedimentation rate may be normal in ~10%); elevated C-reactive protein; platelets greater than 400,000

    (9) Diagnosis via biopsy at least 2 cm long and sectioned serially, because the vasculitis is patchy (skip lesions)

    (10) Treatment

        (a) *High-dose IV steroids (1 g/day) for patients with vision loss (duration variable), followed by maintenance oral prednisone (sometimes for years)*

        (b) *Patients without acute vision loss can be started immediately on oral prednisone, 60 to 80 mg/day.*

4. *Papilledema*

    a. Associated with bilateral optic disc edema due to elevated intracranial pressure

    b. Secondarily, compression of the venous structures within the nerve head that causes venous engorgement and tortuosity, capillary dilation, and splinter hemorrhage

    c. Etiologies

        i. Intracranial mass lesion

        ii. Pseudotumor cerebri

        iii. Hydrocephalus

        iv. Intracranial hemorrhage

        v. Venous thrombosis/obstruction

        vi. Meningitis

        vii. Vitamin A toxicity

5. *Graves' disease*

    a. Autoimmune disorder

    b. Clinical

        i. Diplopia due to enlargement of the extraocular muscles and primarily inferior and medial rectus muscles

        ii. Increase in orbital fat volume

        iii. Proptosis

        iv. Diplopia

        v. Eyelid retraction

        vi. Ocular congestion

6. *Tumors affecting the anterior visual system*

    a. Optic nerve sheath meningiomas

        i. *Classic triad*

            (A) Disc pallor

            (B) Optic disc venous collaterals

            (C) Progressive vision loss

        ii. In children, usually bilateral and often associated with neurofibromatosis type 2

        iii. May extend into the optic canal or may originate from the dura within the optic canal

iv. MRI with contrast and orbital fat suppression shows enhancement of the sheath with optic nerve sparing ("railroad track" on axial images and "bull's eye" on coronal views).

v. Treatment

(A) Surgery if intracranial or complete visual loss

(B) Radiation (most viable) if partial vision remains

b. *Optic nerve gliomas*

i. Usually present in childhood (75% before 20 y/o)

ii. Clinical

(A) Proptosis

(B) Vision loss

(C) Strabismus

(D) Nystagmus

iii. In children: associated with neurofibromatosis type 1 (15%); usually pilocytic astrocytomas

iv. In adults: more malignant; rapidly leads to blindness and death

7. Inflammatory optic neuropathies

8. Infectious optic neuropathies

9. *Toxic/nutritional optic neuropathies*

a. Nutritional deficiencies

i. Pyridoxine

ii. B_{12}

iii. Folate

iv. Niacin

v. Riboflavin

vi. Thiamine

vii. NB: gastric bypass patients

b. Toxic

i. Ethambutol

ii. Ethanol with tobacco

iii. Methanol

iv. Ethylene glycol

v. Amiodarone

vi. Isoniazid

vii. Chloramphenicol

viii. Chemotherapy

c. *Toxic amblyopia*

i. Typically affects heavy drinkers and pipe smokers deficient in B vitamins

ii. Insidious onset of slowly progressive bilateral central visual field impairment associated with loss of color vision

iii. Ophthalmoscopic examination: splinter hemorrhages or minimal disc edema, but most are normal.

10. *Hereditary optic neuropathies*

a. **Leber's optic neuropathy**

i. Pathophysiology: maternal *mitochondrial DNA point mutation*

ii. Clinical

   ii. Clinical (*cont'd*)

    (A) Painless sequential bilateral central scotomata

    (B) *Asymptomatic cardiac anomalies including accessory cardiac atrio-ventricular conduction pathways (Wolff-Parkinson-White and Lown-Ganong-Levine syndromes)*

    (C) Adolescent males

  11. Ophthalmoscopic examination: mild hyperemia and swelling of optic discs with irregular dilation of peripapillary capillaries (telangiectasia microangiopathy) early; mild temporal pallor late

I. Disorders associated with the optic chiasm

 1. Clinical: classic pattern is bitemporal visual field defects, but variable.

 2. Etiologies

  a. Sella tumors

   i. Pituitary macroadenomas (may have associated endocrine abnormalities): pituitary apoplexy—acute enlargement of a pituitary adenoma due to necrotic hemorrhage or postpartum (Sheehan's syndrome)

   ii. Craniopharyngiomas

   iii. Gliomas

   iv. Meningiomas

  b. MS

  c. Aneurysm

  d. Trauma

  e. Sarcoidosis

 3. *Anterior chiasm lesion (Willebrand's knee)*

  a. *Nasal retinal fibers cross anterior in the chiasm before joining the contralateral temporal fibers.*

  b. Signs/symptoms

   i. Ipsilateral monocular central scotoma

   ii. Contralateral upper temporal field cut

> **NB:** This is also known as a junctional scotoma.

J. Retrochiasmal visual pathways

 1. Disorders of the optic tract

  a. Etiologies

   i. Tumors

   ii. Aneurysm

 2. *Disorders involving the lateral geniculate nucleus*

  a. **NB:** Lateral geniculate nucleus is somatotopically arranged.

   i. *Uncrossed fibers = layers 2, 3, 5*

   ii. *Crossed fibers = layers 1, 2, 6*

  b. Etiologies

   i. Stroke

   ii. Tumors

 3. *Optic radiations:* etiologies: stroke, tumors, traumatic brain injury

4. *Occipital lobe*

    a. Etiologies

        i. Stroke: thromboembolism from the heart and vertebrobasilar system

        ii. Tumors

    b. Clinical

        i. Produces highly *congruous homonymous visual field defects,* usually without any other accompanying neurologic symptoms

        ii. *Riddoch phenomenon: patient can detect motion in an otherwise blind hemifield (can be associated with any retrochiasmal visual field defect).*

        iii. Bilateral occipital lobe infarctions

            (A) Bilateral blindness

            (B) Normal pupillary response

            (C) No other neurologic signs

        iv. Closed head injury can cause transient cortical blindness (may be difficult to distinguish from functional vision loss).

K. Disorders of pupillary function

  1. Topical cholinergic agents that influence pupil size

    a. Cholinergic agonists that produce miosis

        i. *Pilocarpine*

        ii. *Carbachol*

        iii. *Methacholine*

        iv. *Physostigmine*

        v. *Organophosphate insecticides*

    b. Cholinergic antagonists that produce mydriasis

        i. *Atropine*

        ii. *Scopolamine*

  2. Topical adrenergic agents that influence pupil size

    a. Adrenergic agonists that produce mydriasis

        i. *Epinephrine*

        ii. *Phenylephrine*

        iii. *Hydroxyamphetamine*

        iv. *Ephedrine*

        v. *Cocaine*

    b. Adrenergic antagonists that produce miosis

        i. *Guanethidine*

        ii. *Reserpine*

        iii. *Thymoxamine*

  3. *Afferent pupillary defect (Marcus Gunn pupil)*

    a. Diagnosis via swinging flashlight test

    b. Etiologies

        i. Diffuse unilateral retinopathies or dense vitreous hemorrhage

        ii. Optic neuropathies

        iii. Optic chiasm lesions

        iv. Optic tract lesions

   b. Etiologies (*cont'd*)

    v. Midbrain lesion involving the pretectal nucleus or the brachium of the superior colliculus

    vi. Lateral geniculate nucleus

4. *Large and poorly reactive pupil*

    a. Differential diagnosis

      i. Unilateral

        (A) Adie's tonic pupil

        (B) Pharmacologic (anticholinergic agent, jimson weed, adrenergic agonist)

        (C) Trauma/surgery

        (D) Ischemia (carotid artery insufficiency, giant-cell arteritis, carotid cavernous fistula)

        (E) Iridocyclitis

        (F) Complication of infection (e.g., herpes zoster)

        (G) CN III palsy

        (H) Tonic pupil associated with peripheral neuropathy or systemic dysautonomia

      ii. Bilateral

        (A) Adie's tonic pupils; usually sequential

        (B) Pharmacologic (anticholinergic agent, jimson weed, adrenergic agonist)

        (C) Parinaud syndrome

        (D) Argyll-Robertson pupils

        (E) CN III palsy

        (F) Carcinomatous meningitis

        (G) Chronic basilar meningitis

        (H) Guillain-Barré syndrome

        (I) Eaton-Lambert syndrome

        (J) Botulism

5. *Argyll-Robertson syndrome*

    a. Clinical

      i. Miotic irregular pupils

      ii. Light-near dissociation

        (A) Absence of light response associated with normal anterior visual pathway function

        (B) Brisk pupillary constriction to near object

      iii. Normal visual acuity

      iv. Diminished pupillary dilatation, particularly in dark

      v. Usually bilateral

    b. Etiology

      i. Neurosyphilis

      ii. Dorsal midbrain damage

      iii. MS

      iv. Chronic alcoholism

      v. Diabetes mellitus

      vi. Bilateral tonic pupils

6. **Horner's syndrome**

   a. Clinical

      i. Miosis

      ii. Ptosis (denervation of Müller's muscle); 1- to 2-mm ptosis

      iii. Anhidrosis (ipsilateral facial)

   b. Etiologies

      i. Central (first-order) neuron

         (A) Brainstem (Wallenberg's) or thalamic stroke

         (B) Intra-axial tumor involving the thalamus, brainstem, or cervical spinal cord

         (C) Demyelination or inflammatory process involving the brainstem or cervical spinal cord

         (D) Syringomyelia

         (E) Neck trauma

      ii. Preganglionic (second-order) neuron

         (A) Tumors involving the pulmonary apex, mediastinum, cervical paravertebral region, or C8 to T2 nerve roots

         (B) Lower brachial plexus injury

         (C) Subclavian or internal jugular vein catheter placement

         (D) Stellate or superior cervical ganglion blocks

         (E) Carotid dissection below the superior cervical ganglion; often unilateral neck or facial pain

         (F) Neck surgery

      iii. Postganglionic (third-order) neuron

         (A) Internal carotid artery dissection

         (B) Cluster headache

         (C) Skull base or orbital trauma or tumors

         (D) Intracavernous carotid artery aneurysm

         (E) Carotid endarterectomy

         (F) Herpes zoster ophthalmicus

         (G) Complicated otitis media

   c. **NB:** Diagnostic procedures

      i. Apraclonidine (0.5%–1.0%) causes dilation of miotic pupil and improvement in ptosis due to denervation supersensitivity, which occurs within 3 to 5 days after onset of Horner's syndrome.

      ii. **Cocaine 4% to 10%**

         (A) *Confirms oculosympathetic denervation by blocking presynaptic reuptake of norepinephrine, allowing norepinephrine to accumulate at the iris and produce mydriasis*

         (B) *If injury occurs anywhere along the oculosympathetic pathway, the amount of tonically released norepinephrine is reduced and the ability of cocaine to dilate the pupil is impaired.*

      iii. **Hydroxyamphetamine 1%**

         (A) *Test third-order neuron*

         (B) Releases stored norepinephrine from the third-order nerve terminal to dilate pupil

        c. **NB:** Diagnostic procedures (*cont'd*)

           iv. Differentiation between pre- and postganglionic Horner's syndrome

              (A) **1% hydroxyamphetamine** → *releases catecholamines from postsynaptic neurons → dilation of the pupil if the lesion is presynaptic*

              (B) **1% phenylephrine** → *dilates supersensitive pupil in postganglionic Horner's syndrome*

    7. *Light-near dissociation*

        a. Better pupillary response to near than to light

        b. Differential diagnosis

           i. Severe retinopathy

           ii. Optic neuropathy

           iii. Adie's tonic pupil

           iv. Argyll-Robertson syndrome

           v. Dorsal midbrain syndrome

           vi. Aberrant CN III regeneration

    8. *Opiate overdose*

        a. Bilateral pinpoint pupils

        b. Also seen in pontine dysfunction

    9. *Barbiturate coma: pupils remain reactive*

L. Other pearls

    1. **Balint's syndrome**

        a. Paralysis of visual fixation

        b. Optic ataxia

        c. Simultanagnosia

    2. *External ophthalmoplegia*

        a. Etiologies

           i. MG

           ii. Kearns-Sayre syndrome

           iii. Oculopharyngeal dystrophy

    3. **De Morsier's syndrome (septo-optic dysplasia)**

        a. Triad

           i. *Short stature*

           ii. *Nystagmus*

           iii. *Optic disc hypoplasia*

        b. Spectrum of midline anomalies, including absent septum pellucidum, agenesis of corpus callosum, dysplasia of anterior third ventricle

        c. 60%: hypopituitarism with decreased growth hormone

    4. **Aicardi's syndrome**

        a. X-linked dominant

        b. Only females because lethal in utero for males

        c. Ophthalmoscopic examination: *chorioretinal atrophy, retinal pigment epithelial changes, large colobomatous disk*

    d. Other ocular features: strabismus, microphthalmos

    e. Associated with infantile spasms, agenesis of corpus callosum, developmental delay

    f. Usually death within first few years of life

5. *Unilateral proptosis*

    a. Etiologies

        i. Intraorbital tumor

        ii. Sphenoid ridge meningioma

        iii. Cavernous sinus/internal carotid artery fistula

        iv. Hyperthyroidism

6. Aberrant regeneration of CN III may cause lid elevation on attempted adduction and infraduction.

7. Cerebellar disease can cause:

    a. Vertical or horizontal nystagmus

    b. Ocular dysmetria

    c. Impaired saccadic pursuit

8. *Differential diagnosis of central scotoma*

    a. Optic neuritis

    b. Macular disease

    c. Ischemic papillitis

    d. Leber's hereditary optic neuropathy

    e. Drug toxicity: ethambutol, Plaquenil

> **NB:** Central scotoma is not seen in papilledema.

9. *Achromatopsia*

    a. *Unable to differentiate colors on Ishihara plates; may be congenital*

    b. Lesion: occipital lobe inferior to calcarine fissure (therefore, also often have superior visual defect)

10. *Devic's disease (neuromyelitis optica)*

    a. Variant of MS

    b. Bilateral optic neuritis with transverse myelitis

11. *Behçet's disease*

    a. Recurrent, painful orogenital ulcers

    b. Uveitis

    c. CN palsies

    d. Seizures

    e. Strokes

    f. Recurrent meningoencephalitis

    g. Joint effusions

    h. Thrombophlebitis

CHEAT SHEET

Aicardi's syndrome	X-dominant, females, chorioretinal atrophy, agenesis corpus callosum
Argyll-Robertson pupils	Miotic irregular pupils, light-near dissociation
Balint's syndrome	Paralysis visual fixation, optic ataxia, simultagnosia
Cogan's lid twitch	Seen in myasthenia gravis
Convergence retraction nystagmus	Parinaud's dorsal midbrain syndrome
De Morsier's syndrome	Short stature, nystagmus, optic disc hypoplasia
Downbeat nystagmus	Lesion cervicomedullary junction (e.g., Chiari)
Edinger-Westphal nucleus	Rostral part of CN III, iris sphincter, and ciliary muscle
Horner's syndrome	Ptosis, miosis, anhidrosis
Meige's syndrome	Blepharospasm and other facial dystonias
Monocular diplopia	Ocular, not neurological, problem
Müller's muscle	Upper and lower eyelids, sympathetic innervation
Oculopalatal myoclonus	Vertical pendular nystagmus, tremor of palate, lesion of Mollaret triangle
One and a half	MLF and ipsilateral parapontine reticular formation (PPRF)
Pituitary apoplexy	Multiple oculomotor palsies, severe headache, bilateral visual loss
Visual association cortex	Brodmann's areas 18 and 19
Wallenberg syndrome	Lateral medullary syndrome

Suggested Readings

Lee AG, Brazis PW. *Clinical Pathways in Neuro-ophthalmology: An Evidence-Based Approach.* New York, NY: Thieme;2011.

Savino PJ, Danesh-Meyer HV, eds. *Color Atlas and Synopsis of Clinical Ophthalmology—Wills Eye Institute—Neuro-Ophthalmology.* Philadelphia, PA: Lippincott Williams & Wilkins;2012.

CHAPTER 24

Neuro-otology

I. Anatomy and Physiology

A. Hair cells

1. Transduce mechanical forces associated with sound and motion into nerve action potentials

2. *Stereocilia:* multiple hair-like protrusions from the surface of the hair cell

3. *Kinocilia:* longest protrusion from the hair cell

4. Modulate the spontaneous afferent nerve-firing rate

    a. Bending stereocilia toward the kinocilium depolarizes the hair cells, increasing their firing rate.

    b. Bending stereocilia away from the kinocilium hyperpolarizes the hair cells, decreasing their firing rate.

B. Receptor organs

1. *Vestibular labyrinth (otolith, anterior, posterior, and lateral semicircular canals)*

    a. Hair cells embed within the macules and cristae.

        i. *Maculae:* sensitive to gravitational forces and linear acceleration

        ii. *Cristae:* sensitive to angular head acceleration

    b. *Cupula:* hair-cell cilia in the cristae of the semicircular canals are embedded in this gelatinous material.

    c. *Otoconia:* comprised of calcium carbonate crystals, a critical component of otolith

2. *Cochlea*

    a. Hair cells mounted on the flexible basilar membrane of the organ of Corti

    b. Tectorial membrane

        i. Covers the organ of Corti

        ii. Relatively rigid structure attached to the wall of the cochlea

        iii. Hair cells vibrate at the frequency of sound, and the hair cells are displaced in relation to the tectorial membrane.

    c. *Hair cells in the cochlea are sensitive and vary from 20 to 20,000 Hz.*

C. Fluids

1. *Perilymph*

    a. Primarily formed by filtration from blood vessels in the ear

    b. Perilymphatic fluid resembles the extracellular fluids (low potassium and high sodium).

2. *Endolymph*

    a. Produced by secretory cells in the stria vascularis of the cochlea and the dark cells of the vestibular labyrinth

    b. Contains intracellular-like fluids (high potassium and low sodium)

D. **Cranial nerve VIII**

1. *Scarpa's ganglion:* afferent bipolar ganglion cells of the vestibular nerve

2. *Superior division*

   a. Cristae of the anterior and lateral canals

   b. Macule of the utricle

   c. Anterosuperior part of the macule of the saccule

3. *Inferior division*

   a. Crista of the posterior canal

   b. Saccule

4. Bipolar cochlear neurons are in the spiral ganglion of the cochlea.

II. Examination of Vestibular and Auditory Dysfunction

A. **Vestibular**

1. Past pointing

2. Romberg's test

3. *Vestibulo-ocular reflex (oculocephalic reflex)*

   a. Compensatory eye movements that are scaled equally to the amplitude, velocity, and direction of the head movements

   b. Critical for the assessment of the semicircular canals

4. *Caloric testing*

   a. *Cold-water caloric testing*

      i. Principle

         (A) Cupula deviates away from utricle, producing nystagmus with fast component directed away from stimulated ear

      ii. Procedure

         (A) Make sure ears are clear.

         (B) The patient is in the supine position with the head tilted 30 degrees forward.

         (C) Ice-cold-water injection of 2 to 3 mL in the external auditory canal induces transient nystagmus lasting for approximately 3 minutes.

      iii. Clinical interpretation

         (A) Comatose patient: only a slow tonic deviation toward the side of stimulation is observed.

         (B) Normal subjects: a decrease greater than 20% in nystagmus duration suggests an ipsilateral lesion.

   b. *Warm-water caloric testing*

      i. Principle

         (A) Cupula deviates toward utricle, producing nystagmus with fast component directed toward stimulated ear

5. Positional testing (*Dix-Hallpike*)

   a. Maneuvering head position from erect (sitting) to the supine, and then right or left ear facing the ground

   b. Aids diagnosis of positional nystagmus—seen in benign paroxysmal positional vertigo or central positional vertigo

B. **Auditory**

  1. **Rinne's test**

    a. Principle

      i. Comparison of hearing from air conduction with bone conduction

    b. Procedure

      i. Tuning fork (512 Hz) first held against the mastoid process until the sound fades and then placed 1 inch away from the external auditory meatus

    c. Interpretation

      i. Healthy subjects can hear the tuning fork approximately twice as long by air conduction as by bone conduction.

      ii. Bone conduction > air conduction = conductive hearing loss

  2. **Weber's test**

    a. Principle

      i. Lateralizes hearing deficit with bone conduction

    b. Procedure

      i. Tuning fork (512 Hz) placed at the center of the forehead and patient asked on which side tone is best heard

    c. Interpretation

      i. Healthy subjects hear sound in the center of the head.

      ii. Unilateral conductive loss: hear sound ipsilateral to lesion

      iii. Unilateral sensorineural loss: hear sound contralateral to lesion

  3. **Audiometry:** quantitative assessment of hearing by precisely controlled auditory stimuli

  4. **Brainstem auditory-evoked responses:** localization of hearing deficit in the central neuraxis (see also Chapter 19)

III. Vestibular Dysfunction

A. **Unilateral**

  1. Acute

    a. Labyrinthitis

    b. Vestibular neuritis

    c. Anterior inferior cerebellar artery infarct

    d. Benign paroxysmal positional vertigo (see details in Section III.B.2)

  2. Chronic

    a. Semicircular canal dehiscence (Tullio phenomenon—sound induced nystagmus, eye movement evoked by vibratory stimulation to bony prominences in severe cases)

    b. Ménière's disease

    c. History of vestibular neuritis

    d. History of labyrinthitis

    e. Acoustic neuroma

    f. Ototoxicity

  3. Phenomenology:

    a. Vertigo (acute and chronic)

    b. Oscillopsia (acute and chronic)

3. Phenomenology (*cont'd*)

    c. Nausea (acute)

    d. Nystagmus (acute)

    e. Gait and standing—leans ipsilesional (acute and chronic)

B. Bilateral

  1. Chronic:

    a. Ototoxicity

    b. Ménière's disease

  2. *Benign paroxysmal positional vertigo (BPPV)*

    a. Brief episodes of vertigo with head position change, head turning, or any movement

    b. Typically follows thrust to head (classic examples: fall and hitting head to ground, prolonged procedure that requires head tilting [barber visit or dentist visit]), or can be idiopathic

    c. Principle: otoconia dislodges and blocks in semicircular canal (thus canal acts as a "gravity sensor")

    d. Bedside diagnosis: Dix-Hallpike test

    e. Most common type: posterior canal BPPV

      i. Treatment: repositioning maneuver (Epley maneuver)

    f. Second common type: horizontal canal BPPV—often sequelae of repositioning maneuver of posterior canal BPPV (canalith dislodges from the posterior canal and lodges in lateral canal)

      i. Treatment: repositioning with log-roll maneuver

IV. Auditory Dysfunction

A. **Conductive hearing loss: results from lesions involving the external or middle ear**

B. **Sensorineural hearing loss**

  1. Results from lesions of the cochlea or the auditory division of cranial nerve VIII

  2. Sound distortion, tinnitus, and hyperacusis can be present.

  3. Causes

    a. Presbycusis

    b. Ménière's disease

    c. Labyrinthitis

    d. Neuritis

    e. Acoustic neuroma

    f. Ototoxicity

C. **Central hearing disorders**

  1. Only happens if the lesion is between the inner ear and cochlear nucleus; lesions between cochlear nucleus and auditory cortex never cause hearing loss.

D. **Tinnitus**

  1. Subjective (heard by patient only)

  2. Objective (heard by examiner)

3. Common causes
    a. Presbycusis
    b. Idiopathic
    c. Conductive hearing loss
    d. Ménière's disease
4. Differential diagnosis
    a. Eustachian tube abnormality
    b. Spontaneous contractions of soft palate muscles (palatal myoclonus)
    c. Normal vascular flow through jugular bulb
    d. Vascular malformation

V. Ototoxic agents

A. Aminoglycosides

1. Auditory and vestibular toxins
2. *Streptomycin and gentamicin are more vestibular toxic.*
3. *Kanamycin, tobramycin, and amikacin are more auditory toxic.*
4. *Likely due to hair-cell damage*
5. Hearing loss at higher frequencies and progresses to 60- to 70-dB loss across all frequencies

B. Salicylates

1. Hearing loss
2. Tinnitus
3. Involves all frequencies
4. Highly concentrated in perilymph and may interfere with enzymatic activity of hair cells, cochlear nuclei
5. Symptoms reversible if medication stopped

VI. Ménière's Syndrome

A. Clinical

1. *Fluctuating hearing loss at low frequencies (shift >10 dB at two frequencies is pathognomonic)*
2. *Tinnitus*
3. *Episodic vertigo*
4. *Sensation of pressure in the ear*
5. *Pathology: distention of the entire endolymphatic system (endolymphatic hydrops)*

B. Etiologies

1. Idiopathic (most cases)
2. Bacterial
3. Viral
4. Syphilitic labyrinthitis

CHEAT SHEET

1. COWS for calorics: *cold—opposite, warm—same*
2. *Posterior semicircular canal BPPV: positional nystagmus—upbeat and torsional beating quick phases; treated with repositioning maneuver*
3. *Cogan syndrome = autoimmune, inner ear deficit, interstitial dermatitis*
4. *Glomus body tumor = most common tumor of middle ear, conductive hearing loss, pulsatile tinnitus, rhinorrhea*
5. *Acoustic neuroma = neurofibromatosis present*
6. *Alport's syndrome = X-linked, sensory neural hearing loss, interstitial nephritis*
7. *Usher's syndrome = autosomal recessive, retinitis pigmentosa, sensorineural hearing loss*
8. *Wernicke's = confusion, extra-ocular motion (EOM) abnormalities, nystagmus, ataxia, decreased reflexes*

Suggested Readings

Goldberg JM, Wilson VJ, Cullen KE, Angelaki DE, Broussard, DM, Buttner-Ennever J, Fukushima K, Minor LB. *The Vestibular System: A Sixth Sense*. New York, NY: Oxford University Press;2012.

Leigh RJ, Zee DS. *The Neurology of Eye Movements* (Contemporary Neurology Series), 5th ed. New York, NY: Oxford University Press;2015.

Wray SH. Eye Movement Disorders in Clinical Practice. New York, NY: Oxford University Press;2014.

CHAPTER 25

Neurorehabilitation

I. **Background and General Principles:** approximately 500 million people worldwide are disabled in some way; prevalence: one in 10 of the world population; three main groups of roughly equal size: developmental, acute, and chronic conditions; four-fifths of disabled live in developing countries; one-third are children.

II. Mechanisms of Functional Recovery

A. Artifact theories: secondary tissue effects, such as inflammation, edema, and vasospasm, may be associated with temporary changes in neurotransmitter pathways and nonspecific inhibition of neural activity (diaschisis); as innervation is regained elsewhere, so does function return to otherwise undamaged structures; examples: spinal shock or the remote effects of a cortical stroke.

B. Regeneration: classically regarded as confined to the peripheral nervous system; potential for regeneration within the central nervous system (CNS) may exist; animal experiments with neural trophic factors or transplantation offer an additional method of artificial tissue regeneration. Human axon growth rates can reach 2 mm/day in small nerves and 5 mm/day in large nerves.

C. Anatomic reorganization: after damage to higher cortical levels of control, certain functions could be taken over by a lower, subcortical level, albeit in a less sophisticated way; rather than strict hierarchical ordering, certain adjacent cortical association areas or even symmetric regions in the contralateral cerebral hemisphere might fulfill equipotential roles, or have the capacity to take over what are termed vicarious functions; greatest potential exists in the immature, developing brain.

D. Behavioral substitution: a person with a right hemiplegia may recover the ability to write by learning how to use the left hand; also called functional adaptation.

E. Pharmacologic intervention: examples: amphetamine, physostigmine, nerve growth factor, corticosteroids, 21-aminosteroids, opiate receptor antagonists, free radical scavengers

III. Aims of Rehabilitation

A. Ethical issues

1. *Respect for autonomy* is paramount: do not ignore the disabled person's responsibility for self-care.

2. *Beneficence:* doing good

3. *Nonmaleficence:* doing no harm

4. *Justice:* ethical duty to ensure that disabled patients receive equally high standards of care and equitable distribution of resources

B. **Management aims**

1. Prevent complications.

2. Promote intrinsic recovery.

3. Teach adaptive strategies.

4. Facilitate environmental interaction.

IV. Management of Specific Neurologic Impairments

A. **Cognitive impairment**

1. *Reception by sense organs:* arousal and alerting techniques (e.g., verbal, tactile, visual, oral stimulation in a patient in a vegetative state)

2. *Perception:* training the patient in obeying commands; miming

3. *Discrimination:* selective attention may be facilitated by performance of matching and selecting tasks.

4. *Organization:* sorting, sequencing, and completion tasks can be practiced.

5. *Memory and retrieval:* psychological techniques (e.g., interactive visual imagery, mental peg systems, etc.), behavioral techniques (e.g., reinforcement with partial cueing), alerting the environment (e.g., checklists, physical cues, etc.), drugs

B. **Language and speech**

1. *Aphasia*

   a. *Traditional aphasia therapy:* rote learning; selective stimulation

   b. *Cues or deblocking techniques*

   c. *Behavioral modification* using operant conditioning: programmed instructions break tasks down into small steps, initially with the use of cues, which is later slowly faded.

   d. *Melodic intonation or rhythm therapy:* based on the belief that musical and tonal abilities are subserved by an intact right hemisphere

2. *Dysarthria:* improving person's awareness of deficit may allow him or her to compensate for it; specific exercises for one or two weak muscle groups; self-monitoring; use of ice or palatal training appliances.

3. *Dyslexia:* prognosis for acquired dyslexia is generally poor; use of right-hemisphere strategies; arrangement of sentences into vertical columns; tactile presentation of material.

C. **Aural impairment: requires full evaluation of communication; visual acuity is relevant to lipreading; hearing aids: cornerstone of therapy, but unable to overcome the common problem of auditory distortions; environmental aids (e.g., amplification devices); sensory substitution aids (for profound or total deafness; e.g., wearing a belt that converts sound into patterns of vibrotactile stimulation); direct nerve stimulation via cochlear implant; communication training.**

D. **Visual impairment**

1. *Vision loss:* magnifying devices; psychological and environmental adjustments (e.g., large-print books, radio, prerecorded "talking books," white stick, guide dog)

2. *Visual agnosia:* intensive visual discrimination training can improve agnosia and neglect.

3. *Diplopia:* alternating covering each eye; prisms; surgery; botulinum toxin injection

4. *Oscillopsia:* resistant to treatment

5. *Swallowing and nutrition:* need direct observation; videofluoroscopy
6. *Dysphagia:* counseling and advice on positioning, exercises, diet modification; ice may reduce bulbar spasticity; treatments: baclofen, preprandial pyridostigmine (for lower motor neuron weakness); appliances; Teflon injection of vocal cords; cricopharyngeal myotomy (controversial).

E. **Motor impairment**

1. *Weakness:* physical therapy; variable loading with springs, fixed loads with weights, self-loading; suspension devices and hydrotherapy (for very weak muscles)
2. *Spasticity:* stretching; drugs: benzodiazepines, baclofen, tizanidine, dantrolene (acts directly on muscle, inhibiting excitation-contraction coupling by depressing calcium release from the sarcoplasmic reticulum); botulinum toxin injection; nerve or motor point blocks; surgery: lengthening or division of soft tissues; rhizotomy, cordectomy (rare); electrical stimulation of dorsal columns
3. *Ataxia:* use of visual, kinesthetic, and conscious voluntary pathways to compensate should be encouraged; repeated practice of exercises of increasing complexity; avoidance of fatigue; redevelopment of self-confidence.

V. General Prognostic Pearls After a Cerebrovascular Accident

Ambulation	95% of recovery occurs in 11 wk
	There is generally no increase in the number of patients able to walk after 2 mo
Arm weakness	Most recovery occurs in 6 wk
	There is some increase in neurologic capacity up to 3 mo
	There is some functional improvement after 1 yr
Sensory recovery	Usually occurs within 2 mo
Visual field defect	Usually recovery occurs within 2 wk
	Some at 3 wk
	No further recovery at 9 wk
Neglect	Most recovery occurs in 10 days
	Some up to 3 mo
Continence	50% of patients recover in 1 wk
	Some can take up to 6 mo
Aphasia	Recovery occurs in weeks to months
	Some recovery can still occur up to 1 yr, especially with comprehension
Apraxia	Recovery can occur up to 3 yrs

> **NB:** After a cerebrovascular accident, tone is usually the first finding to improve.

CHEAT SHEET

• **Autonomy**: to honor patients' right to make their own decisions
• **Beneficence**: to help the patient advance his or her own good
• **Nonmaleficence**: to do no harm
• **Justice**: to be fair and treat like cases alike

Suggested Readings

Bernat J. Challenges to ethics and professionalism facing the contemporary neurologist. *Neurology*. 2014;83(14):1285–1293.

Dromerick A, Wolf SL, Winstein CJ. Arm rehabilitation study after stroke "ICARE." The Internet Stroke Center. http://www.strokecenter.org/trials/clinicalstudies/arm-rehabilitation-study-after-stroke/description.

Takeuchi N, Izumi SI. Rehabilitation with post stroke motor recovery: a review with a focus on neural plasticity. Stroke Res. Treat. 2013.

CHAPTER 26

Neuroendocrinology

I. Hypothalamus

A. Hormones that affect pituitary function

1. *Corticotropin-releasing hormone:* mainly from the paraventricular nucleus; stimulates adrenocorticotropic hormone (ACTH); stimulated by stress, exercise; inhibited by glucocorticoids through negative feedback

2. *Thyrotropin-releasing hormone:* a tripeptide secreted mainly from the paraventricular nucleus; stimulates thyroid-stimulating hormone (TSH) and prolactin; decreased by stress, starvation, and thyroid hormones through negative feedback

3. *Gonadotropin-releasing hormone (GnRH):* secreted mainly from the arcuate nucleus; pulsatile release stimulates follicle-stimulating hormone (FSH) (slower pulse frequency) and luteinizing hormone (LH) (more rapid pulse frequency); continuous exposure to GnRH actually decreases luteinizing hormone and FSH through down-regulation; negatively affected by stress, low body weight, weight loss, excessive exercise (which cause hypothalamic amenorrhea); *clinical application:* treatment of precocious puberty of hypothalamic origin makes use of long-acting GnRH agonists (through down-regulation).

4. *Growth hormone (GH)–releasing hormone:* a peptide secreted from the arcuate nucleus; stimulates GH; *clinical application:* recombinant human GH replacement therapy is given for GH deficiency.

5. *Somatostatin or somatotropin release-inhibiting factor:* a peptide secreted mainly from the periventricular nuclei; also from the gastrointestinal tract; inhibits release of GH; *clinical application:* somatostatin analogues (e.g., octreotide and lanreotide) and GH receptor antagonists (pegvisomant) are used as adjuncts in treatment of acromegaly (GH excess).

6. *Dopamine:* from the arcuate nucleus; inhibits release of prolactin; prolactin inhibitory factor; suppression, not stimulation of prolactin release, is the major hypothalamic effect on prolactin; *clinical applications:* destruction of the hypothalamic-pituitary connection (such as transection of the pituitary stalk) produces a decrease in the release of pituitary hormones, except for prolactin, which is increased because dopamine (prolactin *inhibitory* factor) is the major regulator of this pituitary hormone; dopamine agonists such as bromocriptine and cabergoline are used in the treatment of prolactin-producing tumors.

B. Appetite

1. The hypothalamus has mediators or *receptors* for mediators of food intake.
   a. For increased appetite: ghrelin, neuropeptide Y
   b. For satiety or reduced food intake: leptin, cholecystokinin, serotonin (lorcaserin, a selective serotonin agonist, is an appetite suppressant)

2. Areas of the hypothalamus that control eating
   a. *Lateral nuclei = feeding center;* lesions in this area produce adipsia, aphagia.
   b. *Ventromedial nuclei = satiety center;* lesions in this area produce hyperphagia.

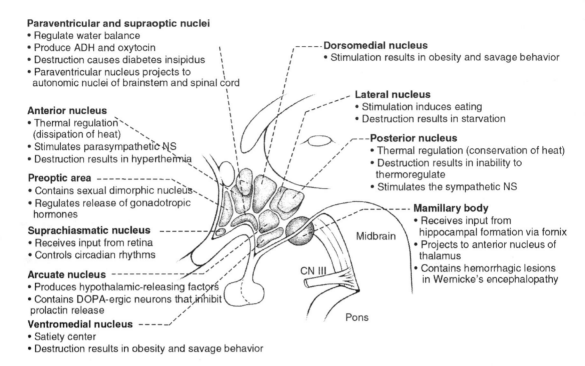

Paraventricular and supraoptic nuclei
• Regulate water balance
• Produce ADH and oxytocin
• Destruction causes diabetes insipidus
• Paraventricular nucleus projects to
  autonomic nuclei of brainstem and spinal cord

Anterior nucleus
• Thermal regulation
  (dissipation of heat)
• Stimulates parasympathetic NS
• Destruction results in hyperthermia

Preoptic area
• Contains sexual dimorphic nucleus
• Regulates release of gonadotropic
  hormones

Suprachiasmatic nucleus
• Receives input from retina
• Controls circadian rhythms

Arcuate nucleus
• Produces hypothalamic-releasing factors
• Contains DOPA-ergic neurons that inhibit
  prolactin release

Ventromedial nucleus
• Satiety center
• Destruction results in obesity and savage behavior

Dorsomedial nucleus
• Stimulation results in obesity and savage behavior

Lateral nucleus
• Stimulation induces eating
• Destruction results in starvation

Posterior nucleus
• Thermal regulation (conservation of heat)
• Destruction results in inability to
  thermoregulate
• Stimulates the sympathetic NS

Mamillary body
• Receives input from
  hippocampal formation via fornix
• Projects to anterior nucleus of
  thalamus
• Contains hemorrhagic lesions
  in Wernicke's encephalopathy

Midbrain

CN III

Pons

Figure 26.1 The hypothalamus with its various nuclei and corresponding functions. ADH, antidiuretic hormone; CN, cranial nerve; NS, nervous system.

C. Emotion/behavior: stimulation of the septal region results in feelings of pleasure and sexual gratification; lesions in the caudal hypothalamus produce attacks of rage; impaired GnRH release causes decreased libido; the opioid peptides enkephalin and dynorphin are involved with sexual behavior.

D. Temperature

1. *Pre-optic anterior hypothalamus:* lesions of this area produce *hyperthermia.*

2. *Posterior hypothalamus:* lesions of this area produce *hypothermia and poikilothermia.*

II. Pituitary

A. Anterior pituitary (adenohypophysis) hormones

PITUITARY HORMONE	EXCESS (ADENOMAS)	DEFICIENCY
ACTH	Cushing's disease	Adrenal insufficiency (glucocorticoid axis)
TSH	Hyperthyroidism	Hypothyroidism
FSH and LH	Usually silent	Infertility, hypogonadism
GH (somatotropin)	Gigantism in children; acromegaly in adults	GH deficiency
Prolactin	Amenorrhea, galactorrhea	Inability to lactate

Abbreviation: LH, luteinizing hormone.

1. *Pituitary tumors:* 30% to 40% are prolactinomas; 20% are somatotropinomas; 10% to 15% are corticotropinomas; 1% are thyrotropinomas; 25% are clinically non-functioning (includes gonadotropinomas)

   a. *Hyperprolactinemia:* produces amenorrhea, galactorrhea, low testosterone levels in males

      i. Causes: prolactinomas: more than *70% are microadenomas* (<10 mm); the rest are macroadenomas (>10 mm);

      ii. Diagnosis: prolactin levels, pituitary MRI

      iii. Treatment of choice: dopamine agonists—bromocriptine, cabergoline

Physiologic	Pregnancy
	Sleep
	Nursing
	Stress
	Nipple stimulation
Drugs	Dopamine receptor blockers
	Antipsychotics, especially first generation
	Opioid analgesics
	Estrogens
	α-Methyldopa
CNS lesions	*Prolactinomas*
	Lesions of the hypothalamus or pituitary stalk, granulomatous disease
Others	Liver cirrhosis
	Chronic renal failure
	Primary hypothyroidism (via TRH stimulation)

Abbreviations: CNS, central nervous system; TRH, thyrotropin-releasing hormone.

   b. *Acromegaly:* causes frontal bossing, coarse facial features, increased shoe and ring size, carpal tunnel syndrome, hyperhidrosis;

      i. Diagnosis: elevated GH and insulin-like growth factor-1; lack of GH suppression after oral glucose tolerance test; pituitary MRI

      ii. Treatment of choice: transsphenoidal surgery; adjuncts: radiation, dopamine agonists such as bromocriptine (because dopamine attenuates GH secretion in one-third of patients), GH receptor antagonist (pegvisomant), somatostatin analogues (octreotide, lanreotide)

   c. *Cushing's disease:* Cushing's syndrome due to a pituitary adenoma (other causes of Cushing's syndrome are exogenous glucocorticoid intake, adrenal tumors, and ectopic ACTH production); presents with moon facies, buffalo hump, purple striae, diabetes, centripetal obesity; diagnosis: screening by 1-mg overnight dexamethasone suppression test, 48-hour low-dose dexamethasone suppression test, midnight salivary cortisol, or by urinary-free cortisol

      i. To differentiate from adrenal causes: ACTH, corticotropin-releasing hormone test; to differentiate from ectopic causes: pituitary MRI, inferior petrosal sinus sampling

c. *Cushing's disease (cont'd)*

  ii. Treatment: transsphenoidal pituitary surgery is the treatment of choice; other treatments: mifepristone (glucocorticoid receptor antagonist for glucose intolerance) and pasireotide (analog of somatostatin receptor subtype 5 which is overexpressed in corticotroph adenoma cells).

d. *Thyrotropinomas:* rare; manifests with hyperthyroidism (symptoms include palpitations, nervousness, weight loss, increased appetite, increased sweatiness), diffuse goiter; diagnosis: TSH levels are normal or high, thyroxine (T_4) and triiodothyronine (T_3) levels are high (as opposed to hyperthyroidism from a thyroid origin such as Graves' disease, in which TSH is low while T_4 and T_3 are high); elevated α subunit levels; pituitary MRI; macroadenoma in 90% of cases.

  i. Treatment: surgery is the treatment of choice; adjuncts are radiation, somatostatin analogs such as octreotide, or treatment targeted toward the thyroid gland itself, such as antithyroid drugs, radioactive iodine ablation, or thyroidectomy.

e. *Gonadotropinomas:* rare, usually clinically silent

2. *Hypopituitarism:* may be inherited or acquired (e.g., from compression, inflammation, invasion, radiation of the hypothalamus or pituitary); for acquired disorders: prolactin deficiency is rare and occurs only when the entire anterior pituitary is destroyed (e.g., pituitary apoplexy) (remember that tonic inhibition by dopamine is the predominant control of prolactin); of the remaining cells, the corticotrophs and thyrotrophs are usually the last to lose function.

a. *Adrenal insufficiency:* affects the glucocorticoid, not the mineralocorticoid, axis (for adrenal insufficiency originating from the adrenals, both glucocorticoid and mineralocorticoid axes are affected); presents acutely with hypotension, shock; chronic adrenal insufficiency presents with nausea, fatigue

  i. Diagnosis: ACTH stimulation test (however, will not differentiate between primary adrenal failure and secondary pituitary failure)—draw baseline cortisol levels, administer synthetic ACTH (e.g., Cortrosyn®), 250 µg intramuscularly or intravenously, then draw cortisol levels again at 30 and 60 minutes; normal if peak cortisol is greater than or equal to 18 to 20 µg/dL; may give false normal results in acute cases because the adrenal glands may still produce cortisol; in the acute setting, do not need to wait for lab values to come back before instituting glucocorticoid treatment if clinically warranted; in acute stressful situations, hydrocortisone has conventionally been given at a total daily dose of 300 mg intravenously, but lower doses are also effective; maintenance treatment is usually with hydrocortisone, 20 mg in the morning and 10 mg at night, or prednisone, 5 mg in the morning and 2.5 mg at night, or less if tolerated.

b. *Hypothyroidism:* not apparent acutely because the half-life of serum T_4 is approximately 7 days

  i. Diagnosis: normal or low TSH, low T_4 and T_3 (as opposed to primary hypothyroidism, in which TSH is high)

  ii. Treatment: glucocorticoids should be replaced before thyroid hormone replacement; replacement is with levothyroxine preparations such as Synthroid®

c. *Hypogonadotropic hypogonadism:* delayed puberty, amenorrhea in females: can be seen in female athletes; low testosterone levels in males (causes sexual dysfunction, decreased libido)

  i. Treatment: delayed puberty: testosterone for boys, estrogen for girls; luteinizing hormone-releasing hormone or FSH and human chorionic gonadotropin to induce ovulation/fertility; treatment with testosterone replacement in adults: intramuscular or topical preparations; monitoring of prostate-specific antigen levels (link with prostatic cancer though causality not yet proven) and complete blood count (can cause polycythemia)

ii. Inherited disorders

(A) **Kallmann's syndrome:** hypogonadotropic hypogonadism, anosmia

(B) **Laurence-Moon-Biedl:** autosomal recessive, hypogonadotropic hypogonadism, mental retardation, obesity, retinitis pigmentosa, syndactyly

(C) **Prader-Willi:** hypogonadotropic hypogonadism, hyperphagia, obesity, mental retardation; caused by loss of function in region of chromosome 15; most cases occur when segment of paternal chromosome 15 is deleted in each cell.

> **NB:** Prader-Willi is produced when the chromosomal defect is inherited from the father; if inherited from the mother, the result is Angelman's syndrome.

d. *GH deficiency:* short stature in children; in adults with pituitary disease, GH is the most frequently deficient of the pituitary hormones; in adults: present with fatigue, increased fat mass, decreased muscle mass, decreased bone density; diagnosis: gold standard is the insulin tolerance test in which GH response to insulin-induced hypoglycemia is measured; treatment: recombinant human GH.

B. **Posterior pituitary (neurohypophysis) hormones: axons from the hypothalamus have direct connections with the posterior lobe of the pituitary.**

1. *Arginine vasopressin or antidiuretic hormone:* from the supraoptic and paraventricular nuclei

a. *Hypothalamic diabetes insipidus (DI):* deficiency of arginine vasopressin

i. Causes: head trauma, neurosurgery, tumors such as craniopharyngioma, CNS infections, CNS vascular disease, pituitary apoplexy *(Sheehan's syndrome)*, autoimmune disorders, familial DI, idiopathic; presents with polyuria and polydipsia; new-onset enuresis in children; presents with hypernatremia if with deficient thirst mechanism or without access to fluids, otherwise normal serum sodium; dilute urine

ii. Differential diagnosis procedure: *water deprivation test* to differentiate hypothalamic from nephrogenic DI

iii. Treatment: fluid replacement then IV or intramuscular DDAVP in acute setting; intranasal or oral desmopressin when more stable

b. *Syndrome of inappropriate antidiuretic hormone secretion:* usually a diagnosis of exclusion; hyponatremia with plasma osmolality less than 275 mOsm/kg H_2O and inappropriate urine osmolality ($>$100 mOsm/kg H_2O); with normal renal function; with euvolemia; without adrenal insufficiency, hypothyroidism, or diuretics

i. Caused: CNS infections, tumors and trauma, pulmonary and mediastinal infection and tumors, drugs—phenothiazines, tricyclic antidepressants, desmopressin, oxytocin, salicylates, nonsteroidal anti-inflammatory drugs

ii. Diagnosis: in difficult cases can be aided by *water loading test* (oral water load of 20 mL per kg body weight in 15–20 minutes, inability to excrete 80%–90% of the oral load in 4–5 hours, and inability to suppress the urine osmolality to $<$100 mOsm/kg H_2O)

b. *Syndrome of inappropriate antidiuretic hormone secretion* (*cont'd*)

    iii. Treatment: 3% NaCl in acute severe symptomatic hyponatremia; restriction of free water intake if chronic with option of vasopressin-2 receptor antagonist if not responding

2. *Oxytocin:* from the supraoptic and paraventricular nuclei; release during suckling results in myoepithelial cell contraction and milk ejection, as well as myometrial contractions

III. Pineal Gland: Secretes melatonin, which is high at night and low during the day; melatonin influences (1) circadian rhythmicity, (2) induction of seasonal responses to changes in day length, and (3) the reproductive axis; melatonin is synthesized from tryptophan; treatment with melatonin has been used for jet lag and to regulate sleep, but controlled clinical trials are lacking

> **NB:** Afferent input to the pineal gland is transmitted from retinal photoreceptors through the suprachiasmatic nucleus and sympathetic nervous system, the supply of which comes from the superior cervical ganglion.

CHEAT SHEET

Anterior pituitary hormones	ACTH, TSH, FSH, LH, GH, prolactin
Kallmann's syndrome	hypogonadotropic hypogonadism, anosmia
Laurence-Moon-Biedl	autosomal recessive, hypogonadotropic hypogonadism, mental retardation, obesity, retinitis pigmentosa, syndactyly
Prader-Willi	hypogonadotropic hypogonadism, hyperphagia, obesity, mental retardation
Posterior pituitary hormones	ADH, oxytocin
Pineal gland hormones	melatonin

Suggested Readings

Barrett EJ. Organization of endocrine control. In *Medical Physiology*, 2nd ed., W Boron and E Boulpaep, eds. Philadelphia, PA: Saunders Elsevier;2012:1011–1027.

Ellison DH, Berl T. Clinical practice: syndrome of inappropriate antidiuresis. *N. Eng. J. Med.* 2007;356(20):2064–2067.

Low MJ. Neuroendocrinology. In *Williams Textbook of Endocrinology*, 12th ed., S Melmed, KS Polonsky, PR Larsen, HM Kronenberg, eds., Philadelphia, PA: Elsevier Saunders;2011:103–174.

CHAPTER 27

Neuro-oncology and Transplant Neurology

I. Central Nervous System (CNS) Tumors

A. Epidemiology

1. Metastatic brain tumors outnumber primary brain tumors 10 to 1.

2. Gliomas are the most common primary brain tumors in adults (70%), whereas primitive neuroectodermal tumors (PNETs) are the most common primary brain tumors in children.

3. Genetics and radiation exposure to the head are important risk factors for gliomas.

4. Young age, high performance status, and low pathological grade are favorable prognostic factors for primary brain tumors.

5. Children less than 1 year old (y/o) have mainly supratentorial tumors; after 1 year, approximately 70% are infratentorial; only 30% of tumors in adults are infratentorial.

6. The most common infratentorial pediatric brain tumors include medulloblastoma, cerebellar astrocytoma, brainstem glioma, and ependymomas.

7. The most common supratentorial pediatric tumors are gliomas and craniopharyngioma.

8. Common differentials for intracranial masses include CNS infections, atypical stroke/vasculitis, tumefactive multiple sclerosis (MS), and radiation necrosis.

B. Oncogenes and chromosomal aberrations in the CNS (see Chapter 2)

C. Neuroepithelial tumors

2007 WORLD HEALTH ORGANIZATION (WHO) CLASSIFICATION FOR DIFFUSE GLIOMAS			
TYPE	GRADE	DESCRIPTION	MEDIAN SURVIVAL
Astrocytomas	II	Found diffusely infiltrating into surrounding neural tissue; increased hypercellularity, no mitosis	6–8
Oligodendroglioma	II	Occur in the white matter and cortex of the cerebral hemispheres, low mitotic activity, no necrosis	12
Oligoastrocytoma	II	Diffuse mixed tumor with mixed glial background	3 to >10
Anaplastic astrocytoma/ oligodendroglioma	III	Highly infiltrating tumors with increased mitotic activity; no necrosis or vascular proliferation	3
Glioblastoma	IV	Infiltrating glial neoplasm with necrosis and microvascular proliferation; high rate of mitosis	1–2

II. Common CNS/Peripheral Nervous System (PNS) Tumors

TUMOR TYPE	COMMENTS/CLINICAL FEATURES	PATHOLOGY
Astrocytic tumors		
Fibrillary	Grade II; age 30–50 years Malignant change after several years occurs frequently; complete resection/cure often not possible Do not enhance on scans	Sparse and fairly regular proliferation of astrocytes without histologic evidence of malignancy, mitotic figures, or vascular endothelial proliferation and without area of necrosis or hemorrhage
Anaplastic	Considered Grade III; poorly responsive to therapy; frequently evolve into glioblastoma	Cellular atypia, mitotic activity and endothelial proliferation is common (but no necrosis)
Glioblastoma	Most malignant grade; also the most common malignant primary tumor in adults (50% of all gliomas); chiefly supratentorial; MRI: enhancing lesion surrounded by edema (may be indistinguishable from abscess); frequently crosses the corpus callosum (butterfly glioma)	Pathologically demonstrate a pseudopalisading pattern (arrangement of nuclei around an area of necrosis)
Juvenile pilocytic astrocytoma (JPA)	More common in children and young adults; *location:* commonly in the cerebellum, optic nerve, hypothalamus; generally discrete and well circumscribed *MRI:* cystic mass with enhancing mural nodule; other differential for intracranial lesions presenting with this imaging include pleomorphic xanthoastrocytoma (PXA) and ganglioglioma. 80% 20-year survival	Cystic structures containing mural nodule, hair-like cells with pleomorphic nuclei, contain *Rosenthal fibers* (opaque, homogeneous, eosinophilic structures), microcystic, endothelial proliferation
Subependymal giant cell astrocytoma (SEGA)	*Grade I astrocytoma;* well demarcated; *location:* lateral ventricles, may cause obstructive hydrocephalus; *associated with tuberous sclerosis;* may produce hydrocephalus if it occurs at the foramen of Monro; *MRI:* well circumscribed, enhance homogenously	Large, round nuclei, few mitoses, few endothelial proliferations; prognosis: good

(continued)

TUMOR TYPE	COMMENTS/CLINICAL FEATURES	PATHOLOGY
Pleomorphic xanthoastrocytoma (PXA)	Common in adolescents and young adults; located in the superficial cortex; frequently in the temporal lobe; thus, often causes seizures Good prognosis	Often cystic, large pleomorphic, hyperchromatic nuclei, minimal mitotic activity, no necrosis Eosinophilic granular bodies usually seen; Rosenthal fibers rare
Gemistocytic astrocytoma	Variant of astrocytoma 80% subsequently transform into glioblastoma	Contains neoplastic astrocytes with abundant cytoplasm
Gliomatosis cerebri	Fairly uncommon; hemispheric or bihemispheric, poor prognosis	Diffuse, neoplastic astrocytic infiltration
Gliosarcoma	Prognosis and treatment are similar to glioblastoma	*Collision tumor;* combination of malignant glial and mesenchymal elements
Ependymal tumors		
Ependymoma	Account for 6% of gliomas; occur at any age but more common in childhood and adolescence; location: more likely infratentorial, with the most frequent site being the 4th ventricle; in the spinal cord, 60% are located in the lumbosacral segments and filum terminale Prognosis has improved, although tumor generally recurs at some point	Gross—reddish nodular and lobulated; microscopic—rudimentary canal and gliovascular (pseudo) rosettes, ciliated cells, but can have *Flexner-Wintersteiner (true) rosettes;* glial fibrillary acidic protein (GFAP positive)
Anaplastic ependymomas	Usually well circumscribed and benign	
Myxopapillary ependymomas	More commonly at the cauda equina or filum terminale; may mimic herniated disc or present with posterior rectal mass; generally benign and well circumscribed Differential for filum terminale tumor is paraganglioma	Contain mucinous structures surrounded by ependymal cells GFAP and S-100 positive
Subependymoma	Usually incidental findings at autopsy in adults; well-circumscribed ventricular lesions; usually asymptomatic (or can cause obstructive hydrocephalus)	Cluster of nuclei separated by acellular areas; GFAP positive

(continued)

TUMOR TYPE	COMMENTS/CLINICAL FEATURES	PATHOLOGY
Choroid plexus tumors		
Choroid plexus papilloma	Account for 2% of intracranial tumors; most frequently in the 1st decade of life; location: 4th ventricle, lateral ventricle (left > right), 3rd ventricle; in children, more commonly supratentorial; in adults, more commonly infratentorial; more common to cause ventricular obstruction than cerebrospinal fluid (CSF) overproduction; *MRI:* well-delineated ventricular lesion with fairly homogeneous enhancement; Curable by surgical resection; does not invade the brain (no recurrence)	Papillary, calcified, single layer of cuboidal or columnar cells with a fibrovascular core
Choroid plexus carcinoma	Also affects young children; location: 4th ventricle, occipital lobe	Less differentiated, increased mitosis, necrosis, invades the parenchyma, may seed CSF
Oligodendroglial tumors		
Oligodendroglioma	Account for approximately 5% of intracranial gliomas; most frequently between ages 30 and 50 years; location: usually cerebral hemispheres, clinical behavior is unpredictable and depends on degree of mitotic rate	Pathology: uniform *fried-egg cells,* delicate vessels, calcification; mitotic figures are rare, GFAP negative; MRI: diffuse wispy white-matter appearance; treatment: radiation and chemosensitive; better prognosis than astrocytic tumors Deletion of 1p19q with better treatment response
Anaplastic oligodendroglioma	Higher grade with propensity to turn into glioblastoma	Larger pleomorphic nuclei; with mitotic activity, endothelial proliferation and necrosis
Mixed oligoastrocytomas	Glioblastoma with presence of oligodendroglial component may have better prognosis (more responsive to chemotherapy)	With oligodendroglial and astrocytic components; low grade or anaplastic
Neuronal and mixed neuronal-glial tumors		
Gangliocytoma	Benign tumor most frequently at the floor of the third ventricle followed by the temporal lobe, cerebellum, parieto-occipital region, frontal lobe, and spinal cord	Tumor of mature-appearing neoplastic neurons only
Ganglioglioma	Mature neoplastic neurons and neoplastic astrocytes; almost always benign; commonly in the temporal lobe of a young adult; may cause long-standing seizure	May appear *cystic with a mural nodule,* microscopic—binucleate, round, GFAP negative, and synaptophysin-positive neoplastic neurons

(continued)

TUMOR TYPE	COMMENTS/CLINICAL FEATURES	PATHOLOGY
Central neurocytoma	Relatively uncommon intra-ventricular tumor in the lateral ventricle; discrete, well circum-scribed; enhance with contrast administration	Microscopically indistinguish-able from oligodendroglioma; small, round, bland nuclei, *Ho-mer-Wright rosettes,* no histologic anaplasia (benign), confirmation comes with immunohistochemical demonstration of neural antigens or electron microscopy showing neuronal features
Dysembryoplastic neuroectodermal tumor	Multiple intracortical lesions mainly in the temporal lobe	Small islands of mature neurons mimicking oligodendrocytes float-ing in a *mucin-like substance*
Dysplastic infan-tile ganglioglioma	Highly characteristic supratento-rial neuroepithelial neoplasms that occur as large cystic masses in early infancy; most frequently in the frontal and parietal region Very favorable clinical course af-ter successful complete or subto-tal resection	Marked fibroblastic and desmo-plastic component but mature neuroepithelial cells of both glial and neuronal lineage; more primi-tive cells are also present
Dysplastic gan-gliocytoma of the cerebellum (Lher-mitte-Duclos)	Slowly evolving lesion that forms a mass in the cerebellum	Composed of granule, Purkinje, and glial cells; lack of growth potential; therefore, favorable prognosis
Paraganglioma (chemodectoma)	Neural crest derived; location: filum terminale, supra-adrenal, carotid body; *glomus jugulare, glomus vagale;* can produce neurotransmitters Treatment: surgery or chemotherapy/radiotherapy	Nodules surrounded by reticulin—Zellballen
Olfactory neuroblastoma (esthesioneuro-blastoma)	Nasal obstruction/epistaxis may be the presenting symptoms; may erode through the cribriform plate	Small blue cell tumor (also a type of primitive neuroectoder-mal tumor [PNET]); treatment: responsive to chemotherapy/radiotherapy; fairly good prognosis
Embryonal tumors		
PNETs	Small blue cell tumors that are named depending on their lo-cation; 50% are calcified; 50% are cystic; propensity to spread along CSF; generally sensitive to radiotherapy (NB: blastomas are PNET tumors except for hemangioblastoma)	They resemble germinal matrix; >90% are nondifferentiated cells (capable of differentiating along astrocytic, ependymal, oligoden-droglial, and neuronal lines)

(continued)

TUMOR TYPE	COMMENTS/CLINICAL FEATURES	PATHOLOGY
Medulloblastoma	The most common intracranial PNET; in children, most commonly located at the cerebellar midline (25% of pediatric brain tumors); 50% have drop metastasis; 50% 10-year survival with multimodality therapy (surgery, radiation, chemotherapy) Suspect medulloblastoma in child presenting with headaches and ataxia; *loss of alleles on chromosome 17p; oncogenes called c-myc and n-myc are known to be amplified in some medulloblastomas*—poor prognostic indicators	*Homer-Wright rosettes,* carrot-shaped nuclei, mitosis, necrosis
Pineoblastoma	PNET of the pineal gland; occurs most commonly in children; contrast-enhancing pineal region mass; Treatment: surgical resection; Prognosis: rapid recurrence with wide dissemination	Resembles medulloblastomas, may form *fleurettes*
Retinoblastoma	Sporadic in 60% of all cases, *autosomal dominant in 40%; emergence of tumor requires inactivation of Rb gene (tumor suppressor gene) on chromosome 13q14;* in the familial form, one gene is inactivated in the cell; thus, only one gene needs inactivation to produce the tumor; in the sporadic form, both need inactivation; trilateral (rare): bilateral retinoblastomas + pineoblastoma Treatment: enucleation, intra-arterial chemotherapy	*Flexner-Wintersteiner rosettes* with mitosis and necrosis
Neuroblastoma	Rare in the CNS; most commonly arise in the sympathetic chain (or in adrenal) in childhood; clinical correlate of dancing eyes and dancing feet syndrome (opsoclonus myoclonus) Anti-Ri (ANNA-2) antibodies reported in children with neuroblastoma Treatment: ACTH	Small blue cell tumors, *Homer-Wright rosettes*

(continued)

TUMOR TYPE	COMMENTS/CLINICAL FEATURES	PATHOLOGY
Tumors of nerve sheath cells		
Neurilemmoma (schwannomas; neurinoma)	Benign tumors arising from Schwann cell; usually *solitary except in neurofibromatosis type 1*, in which they are multiple; *in neurofibromatosis type 2, bilateral acoustic schwannomas* can be found; location: most commonly cranial nerve VIII, also other cranial nerves, spinal roots (thoracic segments > cervical, lumbar, cauda equina); *MRI:* hyperintense on T2; gross total resection usually possible; Schwannomas are strongly positive for S-100 protein	*Antoni type A*—dense fibrillary tissue, narrow elongated bipolar cells with very little cytoplasm and nuclei that are arranged in whorls or palisades *Antoni type B*—loose reticulated type tissue, round nuclei are randomly arranged in a matrix that appears finely honeycombed
Neurofibroma	Differ from schwannomas in that they almost always occur within the context of neurofibromatosis type 1, almost always multiple, may undergo malignant transformation in 0.5%–1.0% of tumors (neurofibrosarcoma); *plexiform neurofibroma:* cord-like enlargement of nerve twigs	Single cells, axons, myxoid background, parent nerve is usually intermingled with tumor
Tumors of the meninges		
Meningioma	Benign tumors originating from arachnoid cells; account for 13%–18% of primary intracranial tumors and 35% of intraspinal tumors (frequently in the thoracic segment in the lateral compartment of the subdural space); most meningiomas have *a partial or complete deletion of chromosome 22;* primarily in adults (20–60 y/o), although it may occur in childhood; female predominance, especially in the spinal epidural space (NB: women with breast cancer have a higher incidence of meningioma) *Radiology:* dural-based tumors cause enhancement of the peripheral rim of the dura surrounding the meningioma, producing *the dural tail*	Gross—spherical, well circumscribed, and firmly attached to the inner surface of the dura; microscopic—*psammoma bodies*(whorls of cells wrapped around each other with a calcified center), xanthomatous changes (presence of fat-filled cells), myxomatous changes (homogeneous stroma separating individual cells), areas of cartilage or bone within the tumor, foci of melanin pigment in the connective tissue trabeculae, rich vascularization; may produce hyperostosis (local osteoblastic proliferation of skull); most are epithelial membrane antigen positive

(continued)

TUMOR TYPE	COMMENTS/CLINICAL FEATURES	PATHOLOGY
	Location: convexity meningiomas (parasagittal, falx, lateral convexity); basal meningiomas (olfactory groove, lesser wing of the sphenoid, pterion, suprasellar meningiomas); posterior fossa meningiomas, meningiomas of the foramen magnum, as well as intraventricular meningiomas, are considerably less common Foster Kennedy syndrome, characterized by contralateral papilledema and ipsilateral optic atrophy and anosmia, can occur when a meningioma directly compresses ipsilateral optic nerve in olfactory groove	
Hemangiopericytoma	Tumors originating from fibroblasts in the dura Considered a variant of solitary fibrous tumor	Irregular, elongated tumor cells with a mesenchymal component Stain strongly for CD34
Melanocytoma	Most commonly posterior fossa tumors arising from meningeal melanocytes, usually slow growing and low grade Important to distinguish from malignant melanomas, which are aggressive with a poor 5-year survival	Melanocytomas are usually spindle shaped or fusiform, looking much like meningiomas If associated necrosis and hemorrhage is seen, consider melanoma.
Lipoma	Low-grade tumors, often inter-hemispheric/pericallosal, with very slow growth Arise from mesenchymal component within meninges May be associated with vascular malformations and present with headaches or seizures	Mature adipose tissue containing engorged blood vessels; often found in subarachnoid space
Tumors of uncertain histogenesis		
Hemangioblastoma	The most common primary cerebellar neoplasm; sporadic or genetic; 20% are associated with von Hippel-Lindau syndrome (hemangioblastoma, retinal angiomatosis, renal cell carcinoma, renal and pancreatic cysts); location: cerebellum > brain stem > spinal cord Gadolinium-enhanced MRI is the best modality for detection	Gross—cystic lesion with mural nodule; microscopic—foamy cells in clusters separated by blood-filled channels, surrounding parenchyma contains Rosenthal fibers

(continued)

TUMOR TYPE	COMMENTS/CLINICAL FEATURES	PATHOLOGY
Lymphomas and hematopoietic neoplasms		
Malignant lymphoma	Most CNS lymphomas *are B cell;* usually non-Hodgkin's (usually a diffuse large cell variety); more common in the immunocompromised population; Epstein-Barr virus may play a role; *ghost tumor:* initially may respond dramatically to steroids and/or radiation but eventually recurs; commonly originate in the basal ganglia or periventricular white matter; may be radiology: homogeneous contrast enhancement located in the deep brain rather than the gray–white interface; Treatment: methotrexate; responds to steroids and radiation but recurs Prognosis: overall survival in HIV is 3 months or less, in non-HIV is 19 months	Multifocal; angiocentric or perivascular distribution
Cysts and tumor-like lesions		
Rathke cleft cyst	Epithelial cyst in the sella	
Epidermoid cyst	*Radiology:* low-density cyst with irregularly enhancing rim, may not enhance with contrast; Treatment: surgical excision preferred Prognosis: recurrence with subtotal excision	Occur due to slow-growing ectodermal inclusion cysts; secondary to ectoderm trapped at the time of closure of neural tube; cyst lined by keratin-producing squamous epithelium; leakage of contents into the CSF produces chemical meningitis; occurs mostly laterally instead of midline
Dermoid cyst	Mostly present in childhood; hydrocephalus common Location: usually midline, related to fontanel, 4th ventricle, spinal cord; Treatment: surgical resection Prognosis: recurrence with subtotal excision	Comprising mesoderm and ectoderm lined with stratified squamous epithelium and filled with hair, sebaceous glands, and sweat glands
Colloid cyst	Account for 2% of intracranial gliomas; mainly in young adults; location: always at the anterior end of the 3rd ventricle, adjacent to the foramen of Monro; *MRI:* increased signal on T1-weighted images (due to the proteinaceous composition of contents); obstructive hydrocephalus is common	

(continued)

TUMOR TYPE	COMMENTS/CLINICAL FEATURES	PATHOLOGY
	Therapy: drainage, surgical resection	
Hypothalamic hamartomas	Rare; associated with gelastic seizures and endocrine abnormalities; location: hypothalamus; radiology: small discrete mass near the floor of the 3rd ventricle Treatment: surgical resection or ablation, if possible Prognosis: cure is possible if resected	Well-differentiated but disorganized neuroglial tissue
Tumors of the sellar region		
Pituitary adenoma	15% of all intracranial neoplasms; women > men; most common neoplasm of the pituitary gland; can present early if they hypersecrete hormones or later owing to compressive effects; microadenoma (<10-mm diameter) tend to be hormone secreting, with hyperprolactinemia as the most common hormonal abnormality; may be due to hypersecretion or stalk effect in which the flow of prolactin inhibitory factor (dopamine) is absent; Treatment: bromocriptine—may induce tumor fibrosis (which may make pathologic diagnosis difficult)	a. *Acidophilic:* growth hormone ± prolactin; rare follicle-stimulating hormone or luteinizing hormone; acromegaly b. *Basophilic:* adrenocorticotropic hormone >> thyroid-stimulating hormone; hyperadrenalism (Cushing's disease) c. *Chromophobic:* prolactin; null; rarely follicle-stimulating hormone/luteinizing hormone; amenorrhea-galactorrhea; men impotent d. *Mixed*
Craniopharyngioma	*Rathke pouch cyst;* origin is uncertain; bimodal age of distribution of childhood and adult life	Calcified and cystic; *crankcase oil;* more commonly adenomatous but can be papillary; benign but locally adherent
Germ cell tumors	Occur in midline, mostly in first three decades; much more common in children; most common germ cell tumor is Germinoma; prognosis is good	Histologically similar to other germ cell tumors such as ovarian or testicular; may be mixed Reactive to alpha fetoprotein, embryonal carcinoma, placental alkaline phosphatase, HCG, CD30
Pineal gland tumors		
Pineocytoma	WHO grade I, symptoms due to local compression of adjacent structures—tectum compression can cause Parinaud's syndrome (up-gaze paralysis and convergence nystagmus)	Well circumscribed, slow-growing tumor composed of pinealocyte-like cells Small, well-differentiated cells with oval nuclei. Normal pineal gland tissue is lobular and contains calcifications

(continued)

TUMOR TYPE	COMMENTS/CLINICAL FEATURES	PATHOLOGY
Pineoblastoma	Aggressive tumor primarily affecting children; WHO grade IV; 40% of all pineal parenchymal tumors; can be associated with retinoblastoma	Densely packed small blue cells; irregular nuclei with necrosis
Metastatic tumors	20–40% of all brain tumors; well defined, round, with surrounding edema*; location:* gray–white junction; most common site of CNS metastasis is cerebellum. 1. *Primary CNS tumors:* can metastasize to extracranial regions (any anaplastic glial tumor, PNET, meningioma), lymph nodes, and/or lung (gliomas, meningiomas) or bone (PNET) 2. *Secondary metastasis to brain:* bronchogenic cancer > breast cancer > melanoma > hypernephroma 3. *Hemorrhagic transformation*—melanoma, bronchogenic cancer, choriocarcinoma (the only pineal region tumor that may bleed spontaneously; increased β-human chorionic gonadotropin), renal cancer, thyroid cancer 4. Metastasis to the skull/dura: prostate, lung, breast, lymphoma 5. Meningeal carcinomatosis: adenocarcinomas (gastrointestinal, breast, lung)	

III. Paraneoplastic Syndromes

A. Group of disorders associated with tumors but not directly caused by tumor invasion. They are likely due to autoimmune mechanism affecting neural and nonneural tissue. Neurologically, these immune phenomena may target:

1. Neuromuscular junction (e.g., myasthenia gravis)
2. Target neurons in central or peripheral nervous system (e.g., anti-Hu Ab)
3. Intracellular proteins (e.g., GAD 65)
4. Surface antibodies (e.g., NMDA-R)

	CLINICAL SYNDROME	ANTIBODY	COMMON ASSOCIATED TUMOR
Brain and cranial nerves	Cerebellar degeneration Opsoclonus/ myoclonus Encephalopathy Cancer-associated retinopathy Stiff-person syndrome	Anti-Yo (PCA-1), ANNA-2, GAD-65, CRMP-5 ANNA-2 (Ri) ANNA 1-3, Ma, Ta, NMDA-R, LGI1, CRMP-5 Recoverin, CRMP-5 GAD-65, GlyR, amphiphysin	Gynecological malignancies, breast Neuroblastoma (kids), lung, breast Germ cell (Ma/Ta), lung (Hu), often not associated with malignancy Small-cell lung cancer None
Spinal cord and dorsal root ganglia	Progressive encephalomyelitis Transverse myelitis	GlyR ANNA 1,2	Possible Hodgkin's lymphoma Small-cell lung cancer

(continued)

	CLINICAL SYNDROME	ANTIBODY	COMMON ASSOCIATED TUMOR
Peripheral nerves and muscle	Peripheral neuropathy associated with paraproteinemia Lambert-Eaton myasthenic syndrome Myasthenia gravis Dermatomyositis Isaac syndrome Sensory neuropathy/neuronopathy Motor neuron disease	Paraproteins VGCC Ach-R, MuSK Jo-1 VGKC ANNA 1 (anti-Hu) ANNA 1	MGUS/POEMS Small-cell lung cancer Thymoma Breast, lung, urinary tract Possibly thymoma Small-cell lung Ca Lymphoma

IV. Common Tumor Classifications

A. Most common tumors by location

SUPRATENTORIAL TUMORS	HEMISPHERIC	SELLAR REGION	PINEAL REGION
	Glioma	Pituitary adenoma	Pineocytoma
		Craniopharyngioma	Pineoblastoma
	Metastasis	Meningioma	Germinoma
	Meningioma	Optic glioma	Astrocytoma
		Germ cell tumor	
		Epidermoid/dermoid	
		Hypothalamic glioma/hamartoma	
INFRATENTORIAL TUMORS	CEREBELLAR MIDLINE	CEREBELLAR HEMISPHERE	
Pediatric	Medulloblastoma	Juvenile astrocytoma	
	Ependymoma		
	Pontine glioma		
Adult	Medulloblastoma	Hemangioblastoma	
	Schwannoma	Astrocytoma	
	Meningioma	Metastasis	
	Choroid plexus papilloma	Medulloblastoma	
	Metastasis		

(continued)

SPINAL CORD TUMORS	EXTRADURAL	INTRADURAL EXTRAMEDULLARY	INTRAMEDULLARY
	Metastases	Meningioma	Astrocytoma
		Schwannoma	Ependymoma
		Neurofibroma	Glioblastoma
Extra-axial CNS tumors	Meningioma		
	Epidermoid cyst		
	Dermoid cyst		
	Arachnoid cyst		
Intraventricular tumors	Ependymoma: frequency—20%; location: 4th ventricle (in pediatrics) or lateral ventricle (in adults); calcified in 20% to 40%		
	Astrocytoma: frequency—18%; location: frontal horn, 3rd ventricle; calcified in 30%		
	Colloid cyst: frequency—12%; location: 3rd ventricle (anterior roof); may be associated with hydrocephalus		
	Meningioma: frequency—11%; location: lateral ventricle (atrium)		
	Choroid plexus papilloma: frequency—7%; location: lateral ventricle (pediatrics), 4th ventricle (adults)		
"Seeding" CNS tumors	Medulloblastoma: >66% have subarachnoid space seeding at the time of first operation		
	Glioblastoma		
	PNET		
	Ependymoma		
	Pineoblastoma		
	Germinoma		
	Plexus papilloma		
Corpus callosum tumors	Glioblastoma		
	Oligodendroglioma		
	Lipoma		
Conus/filum terminale	Ependymoma		
	Lipoma		
	Paraganglioma		
	Meningioma		
	Drop metastasis		
Cystic tumors	Pilocytic astrocytoma		
	Hemangioblastoma		
	Ganglioglioma		
	Pleomorphic xanthoastrocytoma		
	Glioblastoma		

B. Posterior fossa lesions

Extra-axial	**Foramen magnum**	Chordoma (clival)	
		Meningioma (anterior)	
		Neurofibroma (posterior)	
	Cerebello-pontine angle	M	Meningioma
			Metastasis
		E	Epidermoid
			Exophytic brainstem glioma
		A	Acoustic neuroma
			Arachnoid cyst
			Aneurysm
		T	Trigeminal neuroma
		S	Seventh nerve neuroma
Intra-axial	**anterior compartment**	Brainstem glioma (25% of pediatric, 3% of adults)	
		Syringobulbia	
		Cavernous malformations	
	Posterior compartment	Metastasis (most common adult tumor)	
		Hemangioblastoma (most common primary adult tumor)	
		Ependymoma (>70% are posterior fossa; peak ages: 5 and 50 y/o; 0% Ca^{2+})	
		Medulloblastoma (most common pediatric tumor; midline in pediatrics; lateral in adults)	
		Choroid plexus papilloma	
		Oligodendroglioma (rare in the posterior fossa; 90% are calcified)	

> **NB:** Meningioma/epidermoid/acoustic neuroma account for 75% of cerebello-pontine angle lesions.

V. Chemotherapy

A. Nervous system complications of chemotherapy

L-Asparaginase	Cerebral venous thrombosis Stroke Headache Acute encephalopathy
Azathioprine Bleomycin Busulfan	Posterior reversible encephalopathy syndrome (PRES) Raynaud's phenomenon Seizures Venous thrombosis
Bevacizumab Carboplatin	Stroke Cerebral venous thrombosis Myalgias Peripheral neuropathy Hearing loss Transient cortical blindness
Cladribine	Peripheral neuropathy
Cisplatin	Peripheral neuropathy Ototoxicity (high frequency is affected; tinnitus) Encephalopathy
Cytarabine	Cerebellar dysfunction Somnolence Encephalopathy Personality changes Peripheral neuropathy Rhabdomyolysis Myelopathy
Cyclosporin Dacarbazine	PRES Paresthesia
Etoposide	Peripheral neuropathy
5-Fluorouracil	Acute cerebellar syndrome Acute Encephalopathy Seizures
Fludarabine	Visual disturbances
Interleukin-2	Parkinsonism Brachial plexopathy
Isotretinoin	Pseudotumor cerebri
Levamisole	Peripheral neuropathy
Methotrexate	Leukoencephalopathy/chronic encephalopathy Chemical arachnoiditis (if given intrathecally)

(continued)

Nitrourease (Carmustine [BCNU])	Encephalopathy
Paclitaxel (Taxol®)	Peripheral neuropathy
Procarbazine	Peripheral neuropathy Autonomic neuropathy Encephalopathy Ataxia
Suramin	Peripheral neuropathy
Tamoxifen	Decreased visual acuity
Teniposide	Peripheral neuropathy
Thiotepa	Myelopathy
Trimetrexate Glucoronate	Peripheral neuropathy
Vinblastine	Peripheral neuropathy Myalgias Cranial neuropathy Autonomic neuropathy
Vincristine	Peripheral neuropathy Autonomic neuropathy Decreased antidiuretic hormone secretion

VI. Radiation Side Effects

A. Acute reactions: occur during the course of irradiation; include encephalopathy syndrome characterized by headaches, nausea, vomiting, and somnolence. Symptoms due to increased intracranial pressure; reaction is dose related. Rarely, brain herniation.

B. Early delayed reactions: probably secondary to injury to oligodendrocytes; appear a few weeks to 2 to 3 months later; usually transient and disappear without treatment; clinically presents with lethargy and somnolence; pathology: when fulminant, multiple small foci of demyelination with perivascular infiltration by lymphocytes and plasma cells

C. Late delayed reactions: appear from a few months to many years after irradiation; Two major patterns are seen: leukoencephalopathy or a space-occupying gliovascular reaction (*radionecrosis*)

1. Radionecrosis: Severe reaction to radiation affecting white matter; pathologically, coagulative necrosis to foci of demyelination, loss of axons, macrophage, lymphocyte, and plasma cell infiltration; most important change: fibrinoid necrosis and hyalinization of the walls of blood vessels and proliferation of the endothelium. Clinical presentation and MRI findings are similar to tumor progression. Corticosteroids may improve symptoms but lead to steroid dependence.

2. Leukoencephalopathy: patients experience short-term memory deficits, impaired judgement, and visual processing delays, and may progress to dementia. MRI reveals periventricular white-matter changes.

VII. Transplant Neurology

A. Neurological complications of transplantation

TREATMENT	COMPLICATION
Anti-CD3	Aseptic meningitis
Cyclosporine	Anorexia, nausea and vomiting Confusion, psychosis, coma Primary CNS lymphoma Seizures Thrombosis, thrombotic thrombocytopenic purpura (TTP), hemolytic uremic syndrome Tremor
Cytarabine	Cerebellar toxicity (could be reversible) Myelopathy Neuropathy
FK-506	Confusion, psychosis, coma Primary CNS lymphoma Seizures Thrombosis, TTP, hemolytic uremic syndrome
Glucocorticoids	Delirium/Psychosis Opportunistic infections
	Steroid myopathy
Methotrexate Mycophenolate	Intrathecal: aseptic meningitis, myelopathy Intravenous: stroke, epilepsy Progressive multifocal leukoencephalopathy

PHENOMENON	COMPLICATION
Graft versus host disease	Acute transverse myelitis Inflammatory myositis Malignancy Myasthenia gravis

B. CNS infections in transplant recipients

TIME FROM TRANSPLANT	CLASS	INFECTION
Early (0–1 month)	Viral	Herpes Simplex Virus (HSV) encephalitis
	Bacterial Fungal	
Intermediate (1–6 months)	Viral	HSV Cytomegalovirus (CMV) Epstein Barr virus (EBV), varicella zoster virus (VZV) (shingles), adenovirus
	Bacterial	Nocardia Listeria

(continued)

B. CNS infections in transplant recipients (*cont'd*)

TIME FROM TRANSPLANT	CLASS	INFECTION
	Fungal	Mycobacterium tuberculosis Pneumocystis Aspergillus Cryptococcus
	Parasitic	Endemic fungi Strongyloides Toxoplasma Leishmania *Trypanosoma cruzi*
Late (>6 months post-transplantation)	Viral	CMV retinitis/colitis Papillomavirus post-transplantation lymphoproliferative disease
	Fungal	Endemic fungi

KEY WORDS

1p19q deletion	Better response to treatment
Anti-Yo Ab	Cerebellar degeneration; ovarian tumors
Common metastases to brain	Lung, breast, melanoma, renal
Cystic appearance with mural nodule	Hemangioblastoma, pilocytic astrocytoma, ganglioglioma, PXA
Dysplastic cerebellar gangliocytoma	Lhermitte Duclos disease (also Cowden syndrome)
Fried-egg appearance	Oligodendroglioma
Ganglioglioma	Temporal lobe, refractory seizures
Gelastic seizures	Hypothalamic hamartoma
Glioblastoma, gliomatosis, gemistocytic, gliosarcoma	Astrocytic variants with poor prognosis ("G" tumors)
Grade IV	Necrosis + vascular proliferation
Homer-Wright rosettes	Medulloblastoma
Limbic encephalitis (autoimmune)	NMDA-R, LGI1, CRMP-5
Limbic encephalitis (paraneoplastic)	Anti-Ma and anti-Ta antibodies (germ cell tumors)
Most common astrocytic tumor	Glioblastoma

(continued)

KEY WORDS (continued)

Most common CNS tumor	Metastases
Most common nonmetastatic CNS tumor	Meningioma
NF1	Glioma
NF2	Meningioma, schwannoma
Opsoclonus-myoclonus	Neuroblastoma
Psammoma bodies	Cell whorls with calcified center - Meningioma
Ring enhancement	Glioblastoma, lymphoma, toxoplasmosis
Rosenthal fibers	Pilocytic astrocytoma, Also seen with PXA and Alexanders diseases
SEGA	Tuberous sclerosis
Sensory neuronopathy	Anti-Hu Ab
Stiff-person syndrome	GABA-blockage in spine/CNS (GAD-65, amphiphysin, GlyR)
Von Hippel-Lindau disease (VHL)	Chromosome 3 (3 letters)

CHEAT SHEET

Li-Fraumeni cancer susceptibility syndrome	Chromosome 17 p53 tumor suppressor gene
Juvenile pilocytic astrocytoma	Contain Rosenthal fibers
Flexner-Wintersteiner rosettes (true)	Seen in ependymoma, neuroblastoma, retinoblastoma
Oligodendroglioma	Fried-egg appearance
Homer-Wright rosettes	Medulloblastoma
Neurofibromatosis type 1	Multiple schwannomas, plexiform neurofibromas
NF-2	Bilateral acoustic schwannomas
Von Hippel-Lindau syndrome	Hemangioblastoma, retinal angiomatosis, renal cell cancer
Peripheral neuropathy with chemotherapy	Cisplatin, carboplatin, levamisole, Paclitaxel, etc.

(continued)

CHEAT SHEET (continued)

Lambert-Eaton myasthenic syndrome	Blockade of P/Q type voltage-gated calcium channels
Stiff-person syndrome	Associated with either amphiphysin antibodies or GAD 65 antibodies
Subacute cerebellar syndrome	Anti-Yo, GAD-65; may be associated with ovary, breast, uterine carcinoma
Opsoclonus-myoclonus syndrome	Neuroblastoma in young children, anti-Ri antibodies and small-cell lung, breast, gynecologic in adults

Suggested Readings

Dalmau J, Graus F. Paraneoplastic syndromes. *Brain.*2012;135:1650–1653.

Weller M, Wick W. Neuro-oncology 2013: improving outcome in newly diagnosed malignant glioma. *Nat. Rev. Neurol.*2014;10:68–70.

CHAPTER 28

Adult Psychiatry

I. Psychochemistry

A. Neurotransmitters

1. **Dopamine** (DA)

   a. Dopaminergic pathways

PATHWAY	SOURCE (CELL TYPE)	TRACT	DESTINATION
Nigrostriatal	Substantia nigra pars compacta (SNc), midbrain (A8/9)	Medial forebrain bundle	Striatum (D1, D2), amygdala (D1)
Mesolimbic and mesocortical	Ventral tegmentum (A10)	Medial forebrain bundle	Nucleus accumbens (D1, D2, D3), prefrontal cortex, hippocampus, cingulum
Tuberoinfundibular	Hypothalamus (A12)		Portal vessels → pituitary (D2)
Incertohypothalamic	A11/13–15 (hypothalamus)		Hypothalamus

   b. *Synthesis*

   i. Tyrosine—(*tyrosine hydroxylase*) → L-dopa—(dopa decarboxylase) → DA

   ii. Tyrosine hydroxylase is the rate-limiting enzyme

   c. *Catabolism*

   i. DA is broken down by *monoamine oxidase types A and B ($MAO_{A, B}$)* and *catechol-O-methyl-transferase.*

   ii. End products are *homovanillic acid* and *3,4-dihydroxyphenylacetic acid.*

   d. *Receptor* "families" and their distributions

   i. D1 family: characteristics—postsynaptic, excitatory; locations: D1—*striatum, accumbens,* olfactory tubercle, cortex, amygdala; D5—hippocampus, dentate gyrus, thalamus (parafascicular), cortex

   ii. D2 family: characteristics—postsynaptic and presynaptic, inhibitory; locations: D2—striatum, accumbens, olfactory tubercle, lateral septum, SNc, ventral tegmentum, olfactory bulb, zona incerta; D3—olfactory tubercle, accumbens; D4—*cortex* (prefrontal and temporal), dentate gyrus, hippocampus

    d. Receiver "families" and their distributions (cont'd)

        iii. Psychiatric significance: DA's normal functions include movement, perception, motivation, reward, aggression; DA *excess* or *hypersensitivity* is associated with *positive symptoms* of *schizophrenia* (mesolimbic tract), and *tardive dyskinesia (TD)* (nigrostriatal tract); DA *deficiency* or *blockade* is associated with: *extrapyramidal syndromes* ([EPSs] striatum, nucleus accumbens), *hyperprolactinemia* (tuberoinfundibular), *negative symptoms of schizophrenia,* depression.

  2. **Serotonin** (5-hydroxytryptamine [5-HT]): 5-HT is produced in the dorsal and median *raphe nuclei*—periaqueductal gray matter of midbrain and pons, B_{1-9} type cells; raphe neurons project through the *medial forebrain bundle* to hippocampus, hypothalamus, frontal cortex, striatum, and thalamus; receptors are also located on platelets (increase cohesion), sexual organs, and in the gastrointestinal (GI) tract (increase peristalsis).

    a. Synthesis: tryptophan—[*tryptophan hydroxylase*] → 5-hydroxytryptophan—[5-HTPdecarboxylase] → 5-HT

    b. Catabolism: 5-HT—[MAO_A] → 5-hydroxyindoleacetic acid (5-HIAA)

    c. Psychiatric significance

        i. Normal functions of 5-HT include mood and sleep regulation, appetite, and impulse control.

        ii. Stimulation of 5-HT_1 receptors is associated with *antidepressant* activity.

        iii. Stimulation of $5HT_{1D}$ autoreceptors is associated with *migraine* treatment ("triptans").

        iv. Stimulation of 5-HT_2 and 5-HT_3 receptors is associated with *psychosis.*

        v. Blockade of 5-HT_3 receptors is associated with *antiemetics* (ondansetron).

        vi. Decreased levels of 5-hydroxyindoleacetic acid are found in cerebrospinal fluid of violent and suicidal subjects.

        vii. Peripheral 5-HT receptors cause antidepressants side effects (GI distress, sexual dysfunction).

> **NB:** Low levels of CSF 5-HIAA have been reported among patients who have attempted suicide via violent means and in alcoholics with impulsive violent behavior. Norepinephrine and Catechol-O-methyltransferase (COMT) have also been implicated.

  3. **Norepinephrine** (NE): produced by cells in *locus ceruleus;* widely distributed targets (cortex, limbic system, thalamus, hypothalamus, reticular formation, dorsal raphe, cerebellum, brain stem, spinal cord)

    a. Synthesis

        i. Tyrosine—[*tyrosine hydroxylase*] → L-dopa (rate-limiting step)

        ii. L-Dopa—[*dopa decarboxylase*] → DA—[*dopamine β-hydroxylase*] → L-NE

    b. Catabolism is by MAO_A and *catechol-O-methyl-transferase* to 3-methoxy-4-hydroxyphenylglycol

    c. Psychiatric significance

        i. Normal functions include focused attention, stress response, and aggression.

ii. NE reuptake inhibition is associated with treatment of *depression* and *attention deficit hyperactivity disorder.*

iii. *Peripheral* blockade leads to *orthostatic hypotension* (common side effect of psychiatric drugs).

4. **Other neurotransmitters**

a. γ-aminobutyric acid (GABA): GABA is a widely distributed *inhibitory* amino acid neurotransmitter; synthesis: glutamate—[*glutamate decarboxylase*] → GABA; GABA agonists are prescribed for *anxiety, ethanol (ETOH) withdrawal, seizures,* catatonia, and akathisia.

b. Acetylcholine (ACh)

i. *Synthesis:* Choline + acetyl coenzyme A—[*choline acetyltransferase*] → ACh

ii. *Catabolism:* ACh—[*acetylcholinesterase*] → choline + acetate

iii. Psychiatric significance: ACh is heavily involved in cognition and motor function; degeneration of ACh-ergic neurons is associated with cognitive deficits in Alzheimer's and other degenerative dementias; acetylcholinesterase *inhibitors* are prescribed to treat Alzheimer's disease; anticholinergics should be avoided in the elderly and demented.

> **NB:** Alzheimer's disease presents with a decrease of choline acetyltransferase in the basalis nucleus of Meynert.

iv. Central ACh receptor blockade: used to treat EPSs caused by antipsychotics; used to treat parkinsonism; may cause disturbed cognition (particularly in elderly)

v. Peripheral ACh receptor blockade is responsible for side effects of many psychiatric medications; decreased visceral activity: dry mouth, constipation, urinary retention; parasympathetic: blurred vision, tachycardia.

> **NB:** ACh, vital to encoding new memories, is one of the many neurotransmitters deficient in Alzheimer's disease. Medications, including tricyclic antidepressants, antihistamines, and anti-emetics, with strong anticholinergic properties can worsen memory and cause confusion.

c. Glutamate: excitatory amino acid neurotransmitter; **NB:** normal activity associated with memory (*N-methyl-D-aspartate* [NMDA] receptor); antagonism associated with psychosis; **NB:** hyperactivity associated with excitotoxicity

d. Histamine (H): excitatory monoamine neurotransmitter; blockade causes drowsiness, weight gain, cognitive slowing.

B. **Antidepressants: all antidepressants increase monoamine-dependent neurotransmission, most commonly in serotonergic systems; reuptake inhibition at the synapse increases monoamine activity; newer agents are generally more selective and less dangerous in overdose, black-box warning: antidepressants increase the risk of suicidal thinking and behavior in children, adolescents, and young adults (18–24 years of age) with major depressive disorder and other psychiatric disorders.**

B. **Antidepressants** (*cont'd*)

1. **Tricyclic antidepressants** (TCAs): *major indications:* depression, migraine prophylaxis, neuropathic pain, anxiety disorders

   a. Tertiary amines

      i. 5-HT $>$ NE reuptake inhibition

      ii. More antihistaminic and anticholinergic activity than the secondary amines

      iii. Examples: amitriptyline (Elavil®), clomipramine (Anafranil®), imipramine (Tofranil®), doxepin (Sinequan®)

> **NB:** More sedating than other secondary amine classes.

   b. Secondary amines

      i. Secondary amine TCAs are derived from metabolism of tertiary amines.

      ii. Amitriptyline $\rightarrow$ nortriptyline

      iii. Imipramine $\rightarrow$ desipramine

      iv. NE $>>$ 5-HT reuptake inhibition

      v. Examples: nortriptyline (Pamelor®), desipramine (Norpramin®), protriptyline (Vivactil®)

   c. Tetracyclic: these are the only TCAs with some antipsychotic activity; examples: amoxapine (Asendin®), maprotiline (Ludiomil®).

   d. Common *side effects of TCAs*

      i. Potentially lethal in overdose

      ii. Anticholinergic side effects include dry mouth, constipation, blurred vision, urinary retention, delirium, and memory impairment.

      iii. Antiadrenergic (α_1) activity causes orthostatic hypotension.

      iv. Anti-H_1 activity causes sedation and weight gain.

      v. Cardiac toxicity in overdose (*QT prolongation* $\rightarrow$ torsades de pointes)

2. **MAO inhibitors** (MAOIs): examples: phenelzine (Nardil®), tranylcypromine (Parnate®); *work through irreversible inhibition* of $MAO_{A, B}$; resynthesis of the enzymes takes 2 weeks.

   a. Major uses: depression, migraine prophylaxis, borderline personality disorder, anxiety disorders

   b. Side effects: potentially lethal in overdose; *hypertensive crisis:* sudden headache, hypertension, flushing, neck stiffness; associated with ingestion of large amounts of *tyramine-rich food* (aged cheese/meat, cured meats, some alcoholic beverages, sauerkraut); may be caused by MAOI overdose, treat with nifedipine (10 mg orally) or phentolamine; *orthostatic hypotension,* sedation, headache, sexual dysfunction, decreased sleep, fatigue; *serotonin syndrome*

      i. Signs/symptoms: rest tremor, myoclonus, hypertonicity, hyperthermia, hallucinations

      ii. Results from combining serotonergic drugs; combinations including an MAOI are the most dangerous.

      iii. **NB:** *Avoid other serotonergic, adrenergic, or dopaminergic drugs for 2 weeks before or after ingestion of an MAOI.*

3. **Selective serotonin reuptake inhibitors** (SSRIs)

   a. Uses: depressive disorders, anxiety disorders, premenstrual dysphoric disorder

b. Examples:

Fluoxetine (Prozac®)	Paroxetine (Paxil®)
Sertraline (Zoloft®)	Fluvoxamine (Luvox®)
Citalopram (Celexa®)	Escitalopram (Lexapro®)

c. *Distinguishing characteristics:* in most respects, the SSRIs are relatively interchangeable; most differences are pharmacokinetic.

   i. Fluoxetine: **NB:** parent drug has a long half-life ($t_{1/2}$) (5 days) and a long-lived active metabolite (norfluoxetine, $t_{1/2}$ = 10 days); requires 3- to 4-week washout period before initiation of MAOI; cytochrome 2D6 and 3A4 inhibitor.

   ii. Paroxetine: **NB:** *most anticholinergic; very short $t_{1/2}$ can cause severe withdrawal syndrome; cytochrome 2D6 inhibitor; a controlled-release version is now available.*

   iii. Fluvoxamine: initially marketed for obsessive-compulsive disorder; cytochrome 1A2 inhibitor

   iv. Sertraline: can sometimes inhibit warfarin (Coumadin®) metabolism

   v. Citalopram: the most serotonin-specific; U.S. Food and Drug Administration (FDA) issued a black-box warning in 2012: doses greater than 40 mg associated with abnormal heart rhythms—QT interval prolongation

   vi. Escitalopram: the L-isomer of citalopram; has fewer side effects

d. Major side effects of SSRIs

   i. Common, reversible side effects include nausea, diarrhea, sexual dysfunction, headache, and anxiety.

   ii. **NB:** Mania can be induced even in patients without prior history of bipolar disorder.

   iii. Start at low initial dose and titrate slowly to minimize side effects.

   iv. Pregnancy class C (uncertain safety, no adverse effects in studies)

> **NB:** Paroxetine is the most potent SSRI, citalopram is the most selective, and fluoxetine is the longest lasting.

> **NB:** Sertraline is also a potent blocker of the DA transporter.

> **NB:** Serotonin syndrome results from medications that enhance serotonin transmission (via decreased breakdown or increased production). Combinations of MAOIs and SSRIs, TCA, or dextromethorphan should be avoided. Serotonin syndrome can be differentiated from neuroleptic malignant syndrome (NMS) by the presence of shivering and myoclonus.

4. **Serotonin and norepinephrine reuptake inhibitors (SNRIs)**

   a. **NB:** Venlafaxine (Effexor XR®): works through 5-HT reuptake inhibition, but also inhibits NE reuptake at higher doses; side effects: *mild diastolic hypertension* (5–10 mm Hg in 5%–10% of patients); withdrawal syndrome (myalgias, restlessness, poor energy); other side effects similar to the SSRIs

4. **Serotonin and norepinephrine reuptake inhibitors (SNRIs)** (*cont'd*)

   b. Desvenlafaxine (Pristiq®): contains the active metabolite of venlafaxine; similar mechanism of action and side effects

   c. Duloxetine (Cymbalta®): inhibits serotonin and NE reuptake, approved for depression, neuropathic pain, generalized anxiety disorder (GAD), fibromyalgia; side effects similar to other SNRIs; side effects also include elevation of liver enzymes

5. **Other antidepressants**

   a. Bupropion (Wellbutrin®, Zyban®): increases NE activity; also increases DA activity at very high doses; *no sexual dysfunction;* side effects: **NB:** *lowers seizure threshold,* avoid in patients with seizure risk factors, increased seizure risk in patients with eating disorders, increased risk with single doses greater than 300 mg or total daily dose greater than 450 mg; can cause *irritability* and *anxiety;* also used as a smoking cessation aid (Zyban); approved for treatment of attention deficit disorder

   b. Mirtazapine (Remeron®): *enhances 5-HT and NE transmission;* postsynaptic 5-HT$_{1A}$ agonist, presynaptic 5-HT$_2$ and 5-HT$_3$ antagonist, presynaptic α_2 antagonist; *no sexual dysfunction;* anti-H$_1$ side effects *(weight gain, drowsiness)*

   c. Nefazodone (Serzone®): enhances 5-HT and NE neurotransmission: 5-HT reuptake inhibition, presynaptic 5-HT$_2$ antagonism, synaptic NE reuptake inhibition (?); *minimal sexual dysfunction; can cause hepatic dysfunction* and is sedating

   d. Trazodone (Desyrel): mostly serotonergic; 5-HT reuptake inhibition, presynaptic 5-HT$_2$ antagonist, postsynaptic 5-HT agonist at high doses (?); side effects: **NB:** priapism, drowsiness, sexual dysfunction

   e. Vilazodone (Vibryd®): serotonin reuptake inhibitor and 5-HT1A receptor partial agonist; moderate effect on 5-HT4; may have fewer sexual side effects, may help irritable bowel syndrome (IBS); side effects: diarrhea, nausea, vomiting (likely due to 5-HT4), headache (HA)

   f. Vortioxetine (Brintellix®): serotonin reuptake inhibitor, 5-HT1A agonist, 5-HT1B partial agonist, 5-HT3/5-HT1D/5-HT7 antagonist; multimodal action is thought to increase dopamine, norepinephrine, acetylcholine in prefrontal cortex, thought to help with the cognitive deficits associated with depression

   g. **Electroconvulsive therapy** (ECT)

      i. Indications: *medication-resistant depression (80% efficacy), Parkinson's disease (PD),* mania, acute psychosis, neuroleptic malignant syndrome

      ii. Procedure involves delivery of a small current to the brain, under anesthesia, to induce a generalized seizure.

      iii. Mechanism of action unknown: massive monoamine release (?); "resetting" of frontal subcortical systems (?)

      iv. Side effects: *major side effect is temporary anterograde and retrograde amnesia;* other side effects include risks of anesthesia (cardiac arrest, allergic reaction); modern anesthetics and paralytic agents have virtually eliminated risk of broken bones, tongue biting, and broken teeth from the seizure; effect is temporary, usually requires multiple treatments.

C. **Repetitive transcranial magnetic stimulation: application of magnetic field to frontal part of brain, presumably inducing current and neurotransmitter release; may have efficacy in treatment-resistant depression; parameters not fully established**

D. **Antimanic and mood-stabilizing agents**

1. Uses in psychiatry

   a. Treatment of mania; the antipsychotics risperidone and quetiapine can treat acute mania; acute mania and mania prophylaxis:

Lithium (Eskalith®)	Valproate (Depakote®)
Carbamazepine (Tegretol®)	Olanzapine (Zyprexa®)
Lamotrigine (Lamictal®)	

   b. Also used in treatment of *impulse control disorders, agitation, and aggression*

   c. Some can also treat bipolar depression (lithium, lamotrigine).

2. Lithium *(therapeutic levels 0.6–1.2)*

   a. Theories about mechanism of action include effects on second messenger systems, serotonergic neurotransmission, and neuronal ion channels.

   b. Acute side effects: *tremor, ataxia,* acne, weight gain, polyuria, hypokalemia

   c. Chronic side effects: hypothyroidism, psoriasis, weight gain

   d. Reduces the risk of suicide in bipolar disorder and major depression

   e. **NB:** Toxicity: symptoms: *delirium, tremor, ataxia,* diarrhea, seizure, QT prolongation, *renal failure;* risk of toxicity increases with *dehydration, nonsteroidal anti-inflammatory drugs, phenytoin;* dialyze for level greater than 3.0.

3. Antimanic antiepileptics (carbamazepine, valproate, lamotrigine)

4. Antimanic antipsychotics (olanzapine, quetiapine, risperidone)

E. **Review of pharmacology of antipsychotics**

1. **Uses in neurology**

   a. PD-related psychosis: *clozapine* and *quetiapine* have lowest risk of worsening parkinsonism; less D2 blockade; substantial anti-ACh activity, pimavanserin—a 5-HT2A serotonin receptor inverse agonist may be a new option for the treatment of psychosis in PD with little or no extrapyramidal side effects.

   b. Dementia/sundowning: *atypicals preferred;* avoid agents with strong anticholinergic or antihistaminic properties; use low nighttime doses to reduce treatment-emergent side effects; black-box warning: antipsychotics increase the risk of death in patients suffering from dementia.

   c. **NB:** Tic disorders (including Tourette's): high-potency antipsychotic *(pimozide or haloperidol)*

2. Uses in psychiatry

   a. Psychotic disorders (schizophrenia, schizoaffective disorder)

   b. Mood disorders (psychotic depression, mania)

3. **"Typical" antipsychotics** (neuroleptics): work mainly through *D2 blockade*

   a. *Low-potency neuroleptics* (typical daily dose >100 mg)

      i. Significant anti-ACh, anti-NE, and anti-H_1 activity

      ii. Examples: chlorpromazine (Thorazine®), thioridazine (Mellaril®)

      iii. **NB:** The antiemetics prochlorperazine (Compazine®), promethazine (Phenergan®), and metoclopramide (Reglan®) have similar pharmacology and side effects.

   b. *High-potency neuroleptics* (typical daily dose <50 mg)

      i. Higher ratio of anti-DA to anti-ACh—increased risk of EPSs

      ii. Low antiadrenergic and anti-H_1 activity

  b. High-potency neuroleptics (cont'd)

   iii. Examples: haloperidol (Haldol®), thiothixene (Navane®), fluphenazine (Prolixin®)

 4. **"Atypical" antipsychotics**

  a. Defined by 5-HT$_2$ > DA blockade and D4 > D2 blockade; **NB:** much *lower incidence of EPS and TD* than typical agents; increased efficacy for *negative symptoms of schizophrenia and cognition*

   i. Clozapine (Clozaril®): most effective antipsychotic; **NB:** clozapine causes no EPSs; *safely treats PD-related psychosis; approved for treatment of TD; side effects:* **NB:** idiosyncratic *agranulocytosis* (~1% incidence), weekly complete blood count for 6 months, then biweekly complete blood count for duration of treatment, hold or discontinue clozapine if white blood count or neutrophil count declines, **NB:** *lowers seizure threshold* (0.7%–1.0% per 100-mg daily dose), severe anti-ACh and anti-H$_1$ side effects—sialorrhea (excessive salivation)

   ii. Olanzapine (Zyprexa®): *massive weight gain* and moderate sedation because of anti-ACh effects; the only atypical antipsychotic approved for prophylaxis against mania

   iii. Quetiapine (Seroquel®): mostly blocks 5-HT$_2$ receptors; minimal DA blockade at usual doses; **NB:** useful in patients with *PD*; anti-H$_1$ activity causes weight gain and sedation; α_1 blockade causes orthostatic hypotension.

   iv. Risperidone (Risperdal®): the highest D2/5-HT$_2$ blockade ratio of the atypicals; dose-related EPSs at greater than 6 mg/day; *hyperprolactinemia*—caused by tuberoinfundibular DA blockade (DA suppresses prolactin release), decreased libido, gynecomastia, sexual dysfunction; orthostatic hypotension because of α_1 blockade

   v. Ziprasidone (Geodon®): powerful 5-HT$_2$ and DA receptor antagonist; no weight gain; high D2 affinity suggests EPS may prove to be a problem; significant α_1 blockade—may cause hypotension; prolongation of QT interval (clinically insignificant)

   vi. Aripiprazole (Abilify®): new form of antipsychotic—partial agonist; extremely high affinity at D2 and 5-HT$_{2A}$ receptor

   vii. Paliperidone (Invega®): major active metabolite of risperidone; compared to risperidone it has easier dissociation from the D2 receptors; thought less likely to cause EPS; primary renal metabolism, but does not interfere with lithium metabolism

   viii. Asenapine (Saphris®): high-affinity antagonist at 5-HT1A, 5-HT1B, 5-HT2A, 5-HT2B, 5-HT2C, 5-HT5-7, serotonin receptors, as well as D1 to D4 dopaminergic receptors; not recommended in patients with severe hepatic impairment

   ix. Lurasidone(Latuda®): antagonist at D2 and serotonin 5-HT2A and 5-HT7; partial agonist at 5-HT1A; should be administered with food; serum concentration of lurasidone is greatly increased by ketoconazole, rifampin, and diltiazem (CYP3A4 inhibitors).

 5. Quick reference chart: atypical antipsychotic receptor affinities

DRUG	D2	5-HT2	A1	ACH	H1
Clozapine	+	+++	++	++++	++
Risperidone	+++	+++	++++	−	−
Olanzapine	+	+	+	++	+++

(continued)

DRUG	D2	5-HT2	A1	ACH	H1
Quetiapine	+/−	+ +	+ +	+/−	+ + + +
Ziprasidone	+ + + +	+ + + +	+ + + +	+/−	−

+, weak affinity; + +, moderate affinity; + + +, strong affinity; + + + +, very strong affinity.

6. Lasting intramuscular depot formulations

   a. Haloperidol decanoate (3–4 weeks)

   b. Fluphenazine decanoate (2 weeks)

   c. Risperidone (Risperdal Consta®) (2 weeks)

   d. Aripiprazole (Abilify Maintena®) (4 weeks)

7. **NB:** EPS—"3 hours, 3 days, 3 weeks"; likelihood of EPS usually correlates with degree of DA blockade

   a. Acute dystonia (usually occurs within 3 hours): usually occurs with *parenteral high-potency* medications; young men, particularly of African descent, are at higher risk; usually involves midline musculature, oculogyrus, opisthotonus, torticollis, retrocollis; treat with intramuscular/intravenous *diphenhydramine* (Benadryl®) or *benztropine* (Cogentin®).

   b. Akathisia (within 3 days): "inner restlessness"; *most common* EPS; patients fidget, get up and walk around, and are unable to sit quietly; treat with *propranolol* (Inderal®), benzodiazepine, or anticholinergic.

   c. Parkinsonism (approximately 3 weeks): occurs with *high-potency typicals* and *risperidone (usually >6 mg/day)*; features that distinguish EPS from idiopathic PD: EPS parkinsonism is usually symmetric, EPS parkinsonism usually has subacute onset, tremor is typically less prominent than rigidity and bradykinesia; treatment: reduce antipsychotic dose, add anticholinergic, switch to a "more atypical" drug (i.e., lower D2/5-HT$_2$ blockade ratio).

8. **TD:** incidence 3% to 5% per year of treatment with DA-blocking agent; caused by chronic DA blockade, resulting in striatal D2 receptor hypersensitivity; elderly, female patients and those with underlying central nervous system (CNS) disease are at greater risk for developing TD; syndrome consists of choreoathetoid movements that *can occur anywhere in the body*, with the face (buccolingual) being the most commonly affected region; treatment: *decrease dose of antipsychotic*—may cause worsening initially because DA receptors are left unblocked; *switch to atypical antipsychotic;* clozapine does not cause EPS and *is indicated for treatment of TD;* mixed success with benzodiazepines, anticholinergics, gabapentin, and vitamin E.

9. **Neuroleptic malignant syndrome:** incidence less than 1%

   a. Results from *decreased dopaminergic neurotransmission*

      i. Usually results from addition of DA receptor blocker (i.e., antipsychotic)

      ii. Can happen with removal of DA receptor stimulator (i.e., anti-PD medications)

   b. Causes of increased risk of neuroleptic malignant syndrome: affective disorder, concomitant lithium use, sudden decrease of DA agonist or increase of DA antagonist

   c. Symptoms/signs: earliest sign is mental status change (confusion, irritability); physical signs: *rigidity, fever, autonomic instability,* tremor, diaphoresis; labs: ↑ *creatine phosphokinase* (usually >1,000), ↑ white blood count, myoglobinuria

   d. Treatment: *discontinue antipsychotic; supportive care in the intensive care unit, especially cooling and hydration;* bromocriptine (DA agonist), dantrolene (muscle relaxant); ECT in refractory cases; patients usually tolerate rechallenge with antipsychotic

> **NB:** Paroxysmal autonomic instability with dystonia (PAID) is a common symptom cluster similar to NMS and commonly appears following severe traumatic or hypoxic brain injury. Treatment consists of beta-adrenergic blockers, opiod analgesia, DA agonists, and benzodiazepines. DA antagonists can precipitate PAID-like symptoms. Anticholinergics and SSRIs are largely ineffective.

F. **Anxiolytics and hypnotics**

1. *Benzodiazepines*

    a. General properties

        i. All facilitate GABA$_A$ receptor (ligand-gated chloride channel) by binding to its benzodiazepine site.

        ii. Actions include *muscle relaxation, sedation, and amnesia.*

    b. *Indications and uses*

        i. Primary sleep disorders (REM behavior disorder, restless limbs)

        ii. Anxiety disorders (panic disorder, generalized anxiety, phobias, social anxiety disorder)

        iii. Sedation (for agitated patients or medical procedures)

        iv. Muscle spasticity

        v. Alcohol, benzodiazepine, or barbiturate withdrawal

        vi. Epilepsy

    c. Should be used for a brief, well-defined duration

    d. *Tolerance and/or dependence* can develop with all—more likely with rapidly absorbed and short-acting ($t_{1/2}$ <20 hours) compounds.

    e. *Contraindicated in patients with substance use disorders;* can impair memory and cognitive and motor performance

    f. Duration of clinical activity is usually significantly shorter than $t_{1/2}$.

    g. *Quick reference chart: benzodiazepines*

DRUG	BRAND	EQUIVALENT (mg)	ABSORPTION	$t_{1/2}$[a] (hrs)	DOSING (mg/day)	ACTIVE METABOLITES	SPECIAL FEATURES
Midazolam	Versed®	1.25	Intravenous	2	1–5	Yes	Anesthetic, significant amnesia
Triazolam	Halcion®	0.1	Rapid	2	0.25–0.5	No	—
Alprazolam	Xanax®	0.25	Medium	10	0.5–4	Yes	Has anti-depressant activity
Clonazepam	Klonopin®	0.5	Rapid	30	0.5–10	No	Effective against mania
Lorazepam	Ativan®	1	Medium	12	2–8	No[b]	—
Temazepam	Restoril®	5	Medium	10	15–30	No[b]	Typically used for insomnia

(continued)

DRUG	BRAND	EQUIVALENT (mg)	ABSORPTION	$t_{1/2}$[a] (hrs)	DOSING (mg/day)	ACTIVE METABOLITES	SPECIAL FEATURES
Diazepam	Valium®	5	Rapid	100	5–45	Yes	Metabolized to oxazepam
Chlordiaze poxide	Librium®	10	Medium	100	10–100	Yes	Use with caution in hepatic disease
Oxazepam	Serax®	15	Slow	9	20–100	No[b]	—

[a]Benzodiazepines with $t_{1/2}$ <20 hours are considered short acting.
[b]Conjugated metabolites are eliminated in the urine—safer for use in patients with liver disease.

2. Barbiturates: no longer commonly used in psychiatry, but still used as anticonvulsants

   a. Risks: generally similar to those of benzodiazepines; *can cause respiratory depression and severe hypercarbia/hypoxia; can induce hepatic enzymes,* causing rapid elimination of other medications

   b. Modern uses of barbiturates

      i. Amobarbital (Amytal®): used for drug-assisted interviews

      ii. Phenobarbital (Luminal®)

      iii. Seizure prophylaxis

      iv. Medication of choice for barbiturate withdrawal

      v. Methohexital (Brevital®): an ultra-short-acting parenteral barbiturate; the *most popular anesthetic for ECT* and other brief surgical procedures

      vi. Pentobarbital (Nembutal®): used to control status epilepticus

3. Zolpidem (Ambien®) and zaleplon (Sonata®): short-acting *nonbenzodiazepine* compounds that interact with the benzodiazepine binding site; approved for the treatment of insomnia; *cannot be used to treat benzodiazepine withdrawal or muscle spasm;* zolpidem: longer acting

4. Buspirone (BuSpar®): 5-HT$_{1A}$ receptor agonist; requires weeks to obtain therapeutic effect (similar to antidepressants); *no dependence, abuse potential, or withdrawal side effects; not effective for benzodiazepine or barbiturate withdrawal*

G. **Medications for treatment of substance-related disorders**

1. Flumazenil (Mazicon®, Romazicon®): *benzodiazepine receptor antagonist;* used to reverse benzodiazepine toxicity; *may precipitate seizures or severe anxiety* in patients who are epileptic, benzodiazepine-dependent, or have ingested a large quantity of benzodiazepines; $t_{1/2}$ less than 15 minutes; dose in 0.2- to 0.5-mg increments, to max dose of 3 mg/hour

2. Opioid abuse treatments

   a. Naloxone (Narcan®): parenteral opioid antagonist; used to reverse effects of opioid toxicity

   b. Naltrexone (ReVia®): *competitive antagonist* at opioid receptors; used to maintain drug-free state in patients treated for opioid dependence

   c. Methadone (Dolophine®, Methadose®): once-daily opioid agonist; used to replace more illegal, injected, or more addictive opioids; patient remains narcotic-dependent but under a physician's care

   d. Buprenorphine (Buprenex®): partial mu-opioid agonist, alternative to methadone, sublingual and can be prescribed in a clinician's office in the United States; less lethal in overdose than methadone

2. Opioid abuse treatments (*cont'd*)

e. Disulfiram (Antabuse®): used for patients being treated for ETOH dependence; requires high level of motivation and compliance; ETOH—(*ETOH dehydrogenase*) → acetaldehyde—(*aldehyde dehydrogenase*) → acetic acid; disulfiram inhibits aldehyde dehydrogenase, causing accumulation of acetaldehyde; causes multiple unpleasant effects—nausea, headache, diaphoresis, vomiting, tachycardia, vertigo; can cause severe reactions to ETOH in food (desserts, sauces), medicine (cough suppressant), or topical products (aftershave, perfume); can cause death and is contraindicated in patients with pulmonary or cardiac illness; *long $t_{1/2}$ necessitates 2-week washout of disulfiram before ETOH is used again.*

H. β-blockers: effective for social anxiety, medication-induced tremors, and akathisia; used to treat agitation and aggression; propranolol (Inderal®) and metoprolol (Lopressor®) have better CNS penetration because they are more lipophilic; pindolol has been used to augment antidepressants.

I. Psychosurgery: frontal lobotomy, used in the past, is no longer an acceptable therapeutic option; capsulotomy for treatment of obsessive-compulsive disorder (OCD); stereotactic radioablation of small portions of the internal capsule in the region of the caudate; micro-electrode deep-brain stimulation of the same area is being studied.

II. Psychiatric Illnesses:

The *Diagnostic and Statistical Manual of Mental Disorders* (currently in its 5th edition, *DSM-5*) strictly defines psychiatric disorders; for practical purposes, less rigid criteria are often employed with real patients; in general, all diagnoses (except personality disorders) can be made only if there is a change from prior functioning, significant impairment or distress in the patient, and the behavior has no other reasonable cause (medications, medical illness, bereavement, etc.).

A. Mood disorders

1. **Mood states**

a. *Major depressive episode: at least 2 weeks* of symptoms representing a *change from prior functioning;* five or more of the following symptoms (**NB:** *SIGECAPS*):

i. Depressed mood

ii. Alteration in **S**leep patterns (hypersomnia or insomnia)

iii. Diminished **I**nterest or pleasure (anhedonia)

iv. Excessive **G**uilt or feelings of worthlessness

v. Decreased **E**nergy or fatigue nearly every day

vi. Impaired **C**oncentration or unusual indecisiveness

vii. Change in **A**ppetite or weight ($\pm 5\%$)

viii. Unusual **P**sychomotor activity (agitation or retardation)

ix. Thoughts of **S**uicide or death; one of the symptoms must be depressed mood or anhedonia; major depressive episode must not be attributable to depressive symptoms that result from many medications (β blockers), or *medical illnesses* (hypothyroidism, B_{12} deficiency, cancer, lupus, *stroke* [30%], myocardial infarction [30%])

b. *Manic episode: at least 1 week* of symptoms (or need for hospitalization) representing a change from prior functioning; elevated, expansive, or irritable mood; at least three of the following symptoms (**NB:** *DIGFAST*), four if mood is predominantly irritable:

i. **D**istractibility

ii. **I**nsomnia without tiredness

     iii. Grandiose ideas or behavior (exaggerated sense of importance)

     iv. Flight of ideas (constant shifting between connected concepts)

     v. Agitation or increased activity

     vi. Speech excessive and/or pressured (pressure: internal drive to talk)

     vii. Thoughtless or reckless behavior; must cause marked social and/or occupational impairment

   c. **Hypomanic episode**

     i. Requires only *4 days* of manic symptoms

     ii. Symptoms must be observable by others but not severe enough to cause marked impairment.

     iii. *Cannot be severe enough to cause hospitalization and/or psychosis*

   d. **Mixed episode**

     i. Meets criteria for both major depressive and manic episodes almost every day for at least a week

     ii. Symptoms must cause marked impairment.

     iii. Mania, hypomania, or mixed episodes may be induced by *antidepressants, corticosteroids, stimulants,* and *right-sided cerebral damage.*

2. **Mood disorder diagnoses**

   a. Major depressive disorder: one or more major depressive episodes

     i. Epidemiology: 15% lifetime prevalence; twice as common in females

     ii. Risk factors: *genetics* (having a first-degree relative with mood disorder confers risk); other psychiatric illness (personality disorders, anxiety disorders); neurologic illnesses (Parkinson's, 40%–50%; multiple sclerosis, 50%; epilepsy, 40%–50%); pregnancy

     iii. Neuropsychiatric research findings: associated with decreased frontal metabolism on PET scanning; associated with left frontal brain injury; decreased 5-hydroxyindoleacetic acid in cerebrospinal fluid of suicidal patients

     iv. *Suicide risk factors:* genetics (family history of suicide); medical (intoxication, chronic medical illness); gender (successful suicide is 3 times more common in males, suicide attempts are 4 times more common in females); psychiatric: prior suicide attempt, psychosis, substance use disorder; advanced age (peak rates occur in men >45 years old (y/o), and in women >55 y/o, high rate of completion in patients >65 y/o, but remember that suicide is the second-leading cause of death for adolescent males [accidents are the first])

> **NB:** Greater than 50% of epileptics have one or more episodes of significant depression during the course of the disorder, and the suicide rate is greater than that of the general population.

     v. *Treatment:* antidepressants—*avoid tricyclics in the elderly, pregnant, or cardiac compromised; beware of bupropion in patients with seizure disorders;* augmenting agents include lithium and thyroid hormone; *ECT for:* pregnant women; psychotic, medication-resistant, or imminently life-threatening depression; psychotherapy is effective alone but more effective in conjunction with medications; antipsychotics such as aripiprazole are now used as adjunctive treatment for major depressive disorder.

b. **Dysthymic disorder** (*DSM-5*—Persistent Depressive Disorder)

   i. Persistently depressed mood for more days than not and at least two of the following: poor appetite or overeating, insomnia or hypersomnia, low energy, low self-esteem, poor concentration or difficulty making decisions, feelings of hopelessness (new to *DSM-5*, criteria for major depression *may* be continuously present for 2 years)

   ii. Symptoms have been present on most days for *at least 2 years.*

c. **Bereavement** (not a disorder, but should be distinguished from depression): depressive symptoms *within 2 months* of a loved one's death; symptoms *not associated* with normal bereavement

   i. Hallucinations not related to the deceased

   ii. Excessive guilt unrelated to the death

   iii. Morbid preoccupation with one's worthlessness

   iv. Marked functional impairment

   v. Persistent wish for death

   vi. Marked psychomotor retardation

   vii. "Persistent Complex Bereavement Disorder" is now a condition for further study in *DSM-5.*

> **NB:** *Primary melancholia* is characterized by a profound and unremitting autonomous mood change with unnatural sadness, apprehension, or dysphoria, and a pervasive loss of pleasure. At least three of these items must be present for the diagnosis: anorexia, insomnia with early morning awakening, quality of mood distinct from ordinary sadness, diurnal mood swings (worse in the morning), psychomotor retardation or agitation, and feelings of guilt.

d. **Bipolar disorder**

   i. Epidemiology: 2% prevalence; usually presents in 2nd or 3rd decade; approximately 50% of patients have a family history of mood disorder.

   ii. Bipolar I versus bipolar II disorder: any history of a full manic episode → bipolar I; psychosis or hospitalization during elevated mood → bipolar I; mixed episode → bipolar I; hypomanic episodes and major depressive episodes only → bipolar II

   iii. Variants: rapid-cycling—four mood episodes within 1 year; cyclothymic disorder—at least 2 years of alternating between hypomanic and depressive periods that do not meet criteria for mania, hypomania, or a major depressive episode

   iv. Treatment: treat manic symptoms with antimanic agent (see Section I.D); lithium and valproic acid are first-line agents; broad efficacy in different types of bipolar illness; valproate is relatively safe; clonazepam may be used as an adjunctive agent; antidepressants during manic or mixed phases can cause rapid cycling; addition of an antipsychotic may be necessary to control psychotic symptoms; antipsychotics such as quetiapine and aripiprazole are now used for bipolar disorder.

> **NB:** Catatonia is a marked psychomotor disturbance that may be seen in over 10% of inpatients in the psychiatric ward. It is more prevalent in mood disorders, especially bipolar disorder, compared to schizophrenia. It may have a "retarded stuporous" form or an "excited delirious" form and is characterized by cataplexy, waxy flexibility, echophenomena, and negativism. Catatonia is 3 or more of 12 psychomotor features: stupor, catalepsy, waxy flexibility, mutism, negativism, posturing, mannerism, stereotypy, agitation, grimacing, echolalia, echopraxia. Treatments include benzodiazepines, barbiturates, and ECT. DA antagonists and baclofen can worsen catatonia.

B. **Psychotic disorders**

1. **Psychotic symptoms**

   a. Delusions: false, fixed, idiosyncratic beliefs (bizarre delusions are totally implausible)

   b. Thought disorganization: illogical progression of thoughts, association of unrelated ideas

   c. Disorganized behavior: behavior incongruous with surrounding stimuli and events

   d. Catatonia: motor immobility, motiveless hyperactivity or resistance to movement, or posturing

   e. Hallucinations (perception of nonexistent stimuli in any sensory modality)

   f. Illusions (misinterpretation of real stimuli)

   g. Negative symptoms: most common in schizophrenia; diminished emotional expression, avolition, alogia, anhedonia, and asociality

2. **Psychosis due to physical illness**

   a. Neurologic: Wilson's, Huntington's, Parkinson's, encephalitis, epilepsy

> **NB:** Forced normalization is a psychotic phenomenon occurring after achievement of good clinical seizure control or resolution of epileptiform discharges.

   b. General medical: hepatic encephalopathy, steroid use, AIDS, lupus, B_{12} deficiency, tertiary syphilis, porphyria

3. **Schizophrenia**

   a. Epidemiology: approximately 1% (0.3%–0.7%) of the population

   b. Genetics: approximately 50% concordance in twin studies; increased risk of schizophrenia in first-degree relatives of schizophrenics; increased risk of other psychotic disorders (schizotypal, schizoaffective, schizophreniform) in relatives of schizophrenics

   c. **Neuropsychiatric research findings**

      i. Anatomic: *increased size of lateral and third ventricles; decreased size of temporal lobes,* caudate nucleus increases in size with treatment

      ii. Functional: altered metabolism in prefrontal cortex and striatum; saccadic breakdown of ocular tracking; poor working memory

c. **Neuropsychiatric research findings** (*cont'd*)

    iii. Neurochemical: suggestions of *dopaminergic* hyperactivity in striatum come from hallucinations in parkinsonism and the efficacy of DA antagonists; studies of hallucinogens and antipsychotics suggest a role for *serotonin;* effects of phencyclidine (PCP; NMDA glutamate antagonist) and glutamate receptor agonists suggest a role for *glutamate* in pathogenesis of schizophrenia.

d. Diagnosis

    i. *At least 1 month of two of the following symptoms:* delusions, hallucinations, disorganized speech, disorganized behavior or catatonia, negative symptoms

    ii. Decline in function in one or more areas: work, social relationships, or self-care

e. Differential diagnosis

    i. *Brief psychotic disorder: 1 month or less* of one psychotic symptom

    ii. *Schizophreniform disorder: 1 to 6 months* of schizophrenia

    iii. *Schizoaffective disorder:* schizophrenia with criteria simultaneously met for major depressive and/or manic episode

    iv. *Delusional disorder:* at least 1 month of *nonbizarre* delusions, without other symptoms of schizophrenia

    v. *Shared psychotic disorder (folie à deux):* a psychotic individual draws another into believing his or her delusions.

    vi. *Major depression or bipolar disorder with psychotic or catatonic features*

f. Course of illness

    i. Onset: late teens to mid-30s, peak in males early to mid-20s; bimodal with peaks in females in late 20s and early 50s

    ii. Social function usually is better preserved in women.

    iii. *Progressive decline in social, cognitive, and occupational function*

    iv. Prevention of exacerbations may slow deterioration.

    v. *Approximately 5% to 6% die of suicide; 20% attempt suicide.*

    vi. *The most common cause of exacerbations is treatment noncompliance.*

g. Treatment

    i. Antipsychotic medication: *atypical agents are first-line treatment because of their reduced risk of EPSs and TDs;* patient must be informed about risk of TDs; intramuscular depot agents increase compliance.

    ii. Augmenting agents include antimanic agents and benzodiazepines.

    iii. Social support (housing, employment, group therapy)

C. **Anxiety disorders: almost all can be treated with benzodiazepines and/or antidepressants.**

1. Evidence for neurotransmitter involvement

    a. NE

        i. Ablation of locus ceruleus in primates abolishes fear.

        ii. β-Agonists and α_2 antagonists can induce panic in humans.

    b. Serotonin (5-HT)

        i. Serotonergic agents (SSRIs, tricyclics) are effective for treating anxiety.

        ii. Rapid titration of SSRI can cause acute anxiety.

    c. GABA

        i. GABA agonists can immediately relieve anxiety.

      ii. Flumazenil (GABA antagonist) can rapidly induce panic attacks.

     iii. Withdrawal from barbiturates or benzodiazepines causes anxiety.

2. Anxiety caused by medical illness or medications

    a. Neurologic: Parkinson's, multiple sclerosis, neoplasm, stroke, migraine

    b. General medical: pheochromocytoma, allergic reactions, syphilis, carcinoid

    c. Medications: steroids, stimulants (xanthines), thyroid hormone

3. Descriptions of the anxiety disorder diagnoses

    a. **Panic disorder:** recurrent unexpected panic attacks

      i. *Panic attack:* abrupt onset and peak (within 10 minutes) of four of the following: cardiac symptoms, sweating, tremor, dyspnea, choking, chest discomfort, GI distress, dizziness, derealization/depersonalization, fear of losing control, fear of dying, paresthesias, chills, or hot flushes

      ii. Can occur with or without *agoraphobia* (fear and avoidance of being in situations from which escape might be difficult or embarrassing)

     iii. May be an overreaction to internal fight-or-flight cues; breathing CO_2 can induce panic attacks in susceptible individuals; lactate infusion may cause panic attacks.

     iv. Treatment: *antidepressants are the drugs of choice—start at low dose and titrate slowly, because they can induce panic attacks,* they take a few weeks to establish maximum effect; *benzodiazepines* work most rapidly—they are often started concurrently with an antidepressant and tapered after a few weeks; psychotherapy (cognitive behavioral therapy, relaxation, exposure/desensitization).

    b. **Phobias:** irrational fear of a subject or situation

      i. *Specific phobia (social anxiety disorder):* a particular object or situation causes immediate and disabling anxiety. The anxiety or the patient's avoidance of the situation interferes significantly with his or her activities or daily functioning.

      ii. *Social phobia:* similar to specific phobia but cued by situations in which the patient feels he or she will be scrutinized or embarrassed.

     iii. Prevalence for specific phobia: 7% to 9%; social phobia: 7%

     iv. Treatment: medications: antidepressants, benzodiazepines, → blockers; therapy: hypnosis, exposure/response-prevention, cognitive behavioral

    c. **Obsessive-compulsive disorder (OCD)**

      i. *Obsession:* persistent and recurrent ideas, urges, or images that are often unwanted and intrusive and produce anxiety or distress even though the patient attempts to ignore or suppress them (e.g., fear of contamination, irrational self-doubt, need for symmetry)

      ii. *Compulsion:* conscious, stereotyped behavior that the patient feels driven to carry out to reduce or "undo" the distress caused by obsessions (e.g., washing hands, counting ceiling tiles)

     iii. Prevalence: 1.2%

     iv. Treatment: serotonin reuptake inhibitors (clomipramine, SSRIs) are the first-line treatment; benzodiazepines can be used as augmentation; DA blockade (risperidone, haloperidol); cognitive behavioral therapy may be as effective as medications.

    d. **Posttraumatic stress disorder:** diagnostic features

      i. *Exposure* to an event involving a threat of serious injury to self or others; during the event, the person felt terrified, horrified, or helpless. Exposure can be direct or through witnessing or learning about the traumatic event from others or through exposure to details of the traumatic event.

    d. **Posttraumatic stress disorder:** diagnostic features (*cont'd*)

        ii. *Re-experiencing* of the event through nightmares, flashbacks, dissociation, event-related hallucinations, or excessive reactivity when exposed to reminders

       iii. *Avoidance* of stimuli associated with the event: patients may avoid any thoughts, activities, conversations, places, or people that recall the event; they may fail to recollect an important aspect of the trauma.

       iv. *General emotional numbing,* as exemplified by restricted affect, detachment from others, decreased participation in significant activities, and no expectations/hopes about the future

       v. *Increased arousal,* exhibited as exaggerated startle, insomnia, irritability, poor concentration, and hypervigilance

      vi. Treatment: there is no clearly established or overwhelmingly effective treatment; antidepressants: paroxetine, sertraline, venlafaxine, imipramine, amitriptyline; symptom-directed treatments: anxiety may be treated with benzodiazepines; insomnia can be addressed with sedatives and hypnotics, sedating antidepressants (e.g., trazodone, mirtazapine); flashbacks and hallucinations sometimes respond to antipsychotics; hyperarousal can be muted with clonidine (Catapres®), → blockers; aggression/agitation: antipsychotics, antimanic agents, antidepressants.

    e. **Generalized anxiety disorder:** diagnosis

       i. Persistent and excessive anxiety on most days, for at least 6 months

       ii. Lack of control over the anxiety

       iii. At least three of the following: restlessness, easy fatigability, poor concentration, irritability, muscle tension, insomnia

       iv. Treatment: antidepressants, buspirone, benzodiazepines (use on a limited basis)

  D. **Substance-related disorders: the board examination tends to focus on symptoms of withdrawal and intoxication and their treatment; however, you should also be familiar with persistent neurologic deficits that can be caused by substances of abuse and associated conditions (such as nutritional deficiency states).**

    1. **ETOH (alcohol use disorder in *DSM-5*)**

      a. Epidemiology

        i. Alcoholics: 10% of Americans who drink (they consume 50% of all alcohol)

        ii. Men 3 times more likely to be affected with ETOH-related disorder

       iii. ETOH is involved in 30% of suicides, 50% of homicides, 41% of highway crashes, and 86% of highway deaths.

       iv. ETOH accounts for 25% of hospitalizations in the United States (third, behind heart disease and cancer).

      b. Pharmacology

        i. Unknown neuronal effects; some believe that ETOH causes *changes in cell membranes,* perhaps acutely increasing their fluidity, but chronically causing rigidity; *potentiation of GABA neurotransmission* is suspected, because of the similar effects of ETOH, benzodiazepines, and barbiturates. *GABA agonists are the only reliable treatment for ETOH withdrawal.*

        ii. Metabolism

          (A) ETOH—[*ETOH dehydrogenase*] → acetaldehyde—[*aldehyde dehydrogenase*] → acetic acid

(B) Average metabolism is 15 mg/dL/hour (faster in men and in chronic drinkers)

(C) 90% metabolized by the liver; 10% excreted unchanged in breath and urine

(D) The lower amount of serum ETOH dehydrogenase in women and some Asian populations causes easier intoxication.

(E) Aldehyde dehydrogenase deficiency (Asian populations) may cause quicker toxicity.

(F) Chronic alcohol users upregulate ETOH-metabolizing enzymes.

c. **Intoxication**

i. *Legal limit for driving is 0.08% in most states.*

ii. General symptoms (blood alcohol concentration >0.05%): disinhibition, inappropriate sexual behavior, aggression, mood lability, impaired judgment, and one or more of the following: dysarthria, incoordination, unsteady gait, nystagmus, impaired attention or memory, stupor or coma

iii. "Blackouts" (conscious amnestic periods)

iv. Severe symptoms: hypotension, hypothermia, loss of gag reflex

v. Treatment

(A) Supportive: *airway protection, fluid resuscitation, electrolyte replacement, nutrition,* warming

(B) Protective: *thiamine* (to prevent Wernicke's encephalopathy), antipsychotics for agitation/aggression

(C) Evaluate for presence of other substances.

d. **ETOH withdrawal** (can last for 14 days)

i. Typical progression

(A) Tremor (4–8 hours after last drink) is the earliest, most common symptom.

(B) Autonomic arousal (6–8 hours): anxiety, agitation; tachycardia, mild hypertension; facial flushing, diaphoresis, mydriasis; *may be treated with clonidine or β blockers*

(C) Agitation, perceptual disturbances (8–12 hours)

(D) Seizures (12–36 hours): ETOH withdrawal seizures are generalized. *A partial seizure should raise suspicion for an underlying CNS lesion or seizure disorder;* treat with parenteral benzodiazepines. Other antiepileptics are unnecessary and sometimes ineffective; *failure of benzodiazepines should initiate a search for other causes for the seizures.*

ii. **Treatment of uncomplicated ETOH withdrawal**

(A) Benzodiazepines: lorazepam (Ativan®), 2 to 4 mg q2 to 4h; chlordiazepoxide (Librium®), 25 to 50 mg q2 to 4h; diazepam (Valium®), 15 to 30 mg tid; benzodiazepine oxidation is decreased in hepatic failure; use lorazepam, temazepam, or oxazepam, which are minimally affected by liver disease.

(B) Antipsychotics: for severe agitation or hallucinations if benzodiazepines are ineffective; haloperidol, 1 to 2 mg q4h

iii. **Delirium tremens** (*72 hours to 1 week*)

(A) Occurs in 5% of hospitalized alcoholics

(B) *Mortality: 20%;* death usually caused by intercurrent illness: cardiovascular collapse, pneumonia, renal or hepatic insufficiency

iii. **Delirium tremens** (*cont'd*)

    (C) Can appear without prior signs of withdrawal

    (D) Rarely occurs in otherwise healthy individuals

    (E) Hallmark symptoms: fluctuating arousal, from excitability to lethargy; autonomic instability; severe perceptual disturbances, paranoia, anxiety; dehydration, electrolyte imbalances

    (F) Treatment: aggressive pharmacologic treatment for withdrawal; reduced stimulation (private room, lights low, reassurance); supportive care (hydration, correction of electrolyte and autonomic abnormalities)

e. **Other ETOH-related syndromes**

  i. **Thiamine (B$_1$) deficiency syndromes**

    (A) *Wernicke's encephalopathy:* develops over hours to days; pathology: petechial hemorrhages of periventricular structures; extrinsic oculomotor nuclei (III, VI); vestibular nuclei, cerebellar vermis; *clinical triad:* confusion, ophthalmoparesis (usually cranial nerve VI palsy), and gait disturbance (wide-based, lurching); treatment: *large doses (300–500 mg intravenously/intramuscularly qd) of thiamine for 3 days; glucose should not be given without thiamine.*

> **NB:** There may also be damage to the mamillary nucleus.

    (B) *Korsakoff's amnesia:* the chronic stage of Wernicke-Korsakoff syndrome; pathology: lesions of Wernicke's, damage to inferomedial temporal lobes, thalamus, mamillary bodies; clinical features: anterograde and retrograde amnesia; disorientation, *other cognitive functions relatively preserved, confabulation* sometimes prominent, sometimes absent; treatment: *abstinence* from alcohol for life, *supplemental thiamine,* long-term nutritional support; improvement possible, but patients do not usually return to baseline

    (C) *Beriberi:* develops over weeks to months; length-dependent *axonal* polyneuropathy (wallerian degeneration): frequent clinical features: paresthesias and/or pain of lower extremities, distal muscle weakness, decreased distal reflexes; other clinical features: cardiac dysfunction (tachycardia, palpitations, dyspnea), wet beriberi: pedal edema due to cardiac failure, blindness (optic neuropathy), hoarseness (laryngeal nerve dysfunction)

  ii. **Niacin (B$_3$) deficiency—pellagra**

    (A) Mnemonic: five Ds—dermatitis, diarrhea, delirium, dementia, death

    (B) Psychiatric: irritability, insomnia, depression, delirium

    (C) Medical/neurologic: dermatitis, peripheral neuropathy, diarrhea

  iii. **Fetal alcohol syndrome (FAS)**

    (A) Caused by fetal exposure to ETOH: usually occurs when mother drinks more than 80 g ETOH/day; milder forms are possible in social- or binge-drinking mothers.

    (B) NB: *FAS is the leading known cause of mental retardation in United States.*

    (C) Second most common cause of agenesis of corpus callosum

    (D) Clinical features: growth retardation (height and weight <10th percentile); craniofacial anomalies: short palpebral fissures, smooth and/or long philtrum, thin upper lip; any of a number of cerebral abnormalities: developmental delay, hyperactivity, seizures

(E) Prognosis: facial features become less prominent over time; small size and developmental delay persist

iv. **Cerebellar degeneration**

(A) ETOH is the most common cause of cerebellar degeneration.

(B) Progresses subacutely, over weeks to months

(C) Pathology: atrophy of cerebellum, most prominent in vermis; cell loss, particularly among Purkinje cells

(D) Clinical features: marked truncal ataxia; other signs of cerebellar dysfunction are usually absent; if limb ataxia is present, legs are worse than arms.

(E) Treatment: *abstinence* from ETOH and adequate nutrition

v. **Marchiafava-Bignami disease**

(A) *Demyelination of the middle portion of corpus callosum*

(B) Variable presentations: bilateral frontal lobe dysfunction; sexual disinhibition

vi. **Alcohol-induced persistent dementia:** it is unclear whether the dementia results specifically from exposure of the brain to ETOH or from the accumulation of known effects of ETOH on all organ systems, combined with chronic nutritional deficiencies, CNS trauma (e.g., from falls, fights, or automobile accidents), and other maladies that affect alcoholics; cause notwithstanding, patients with chronic ETOH use often develop early and severe dementia.

vii. **Neuropathy:** clinically indistinguishable from neuropathy of beriberi

> **NB:** Chronic alcoholic hallucinosis consists of auditory hallucinations that may persist during sobriety.

2. **Amphetamine and related stimulants**

   a. Types

      i. "Classic" stimulants: dextroamphetamine (Dexedrine®), methamphetamine (Desoxyn®), methylphenidate (Ritalin®)

      ii. "Designer" stimulants: *3,4-methylenedioxy methamphetamine (Ecstasy),* N-ethyl3, 4-methylenedioxyamphetamine (MDEA), 5-methyoxy-3,4-methylenedioxyamphetimine (MMDA), 2,5-dimethoxy-4-methylamphetamine (DOM)

   b. Epidemiology

      i. Experimental use in 2% of general population; stimulant use disorder in 0.2%

      ii. Young adults particularly affected (9% of 18–25 y/o report use)

   c. Pharmacology

      i. **NB:** *Classic drugs increase presynaptic release of catecholamines (DA > NE).*

      ii. Designer drugs cause catecholamine release, but additional 5-HT release probably makes them more hallucinogenic.

   d. Intoxication

      i. Behavioral symptoms: euphoria or affective blunting, hypervigilance, anxiety/tension/anger, stereotypies, poor judgment, *psychotic paranoia*

      ii. Physiologic symptoms (*autonomic arousal*): tachycardia/bradycardia, mydriasis, altered blood pressure, weight loss, diaphoresis, chills, dyskinesia, dystonia

    d. Intoxication (*cont'd*)

        iii. Severe symptoms: seizures, respiratory depression, cardiac dysrhythmias, myocardial infarction

        iv. Symptoms typically resolve within 48 hours.

    e. Withdrawal

        i. Progresses to peak in 72 hours, resolves in approximately 1 week

        ii. Depression, suicidality, anxiety, tremulousness, lethargy, fatigue, nightmares, gastrointestinal (GI) cramping, severe hunger

        iii. The best-documented cases of substance-induced *cerebral vasculitis* have occurred in amphetamine users.

3. **Caffeine**

    a. Epidemiology

        i. An average American adult consumes 200 mg caffeine per day.

        ii. 20% to 30% of adults: consume more than 500 mg/day

    b. Pharmacology: belongs to the methylxanthine family; acts as an antagonist at inhibitory G-coupled adenosine receptor, thus increasing intraneuronal cyclic adenosine monophosphate formation; probably hyperactivates DA and NE neurons

    c. Intoxication: restlessness, nervousness, insomnia, facial flushing, diuresis, GI disturbance, muscle twitching, tachycardia, agitation

    d. Withdrawal: headache, fatigue, depression, impaired motor performance, caffeine craving

4. **Marijuana (cannabis)**

    a. Epidemiology

        i. Probably the world's most-used illicit substance

        ii. Used in the past month by 4.7% of the population greater than 11 y/o

        iii. Used by 2.5% of the population more than 50 days per year

    b. Pharmacology

        i. Tetrahydrocannabinol binds to inhibitory G-protein–linked *cannabinoid receptors (hippocampus, basal ganglia, cerebellum).*

        ii. Affects monoamine and GABA neurons

    c. Intoxication

        i. Variable effects

        ii. Behavioral: ataxia, *euphoria, silliness,* temporal distortion, *poor judgment,* perceptual distortions

        iii. Physiologic: *conjunctival injection, hunger, dry mouth,* tachycardia

        iv. Euphoria from acute dose lasts up to 4 hours; psychomotor symptoms may last for 12 hours.

    d. No well-recognized withdrawal syndrome, although chronic users can have psychologic dependence

    e. Other marijuana-related syndromes

        i. May cause a depression-like state with chronic use (*apathy,* decreased energy, sleep disturbance, poor attention/concentration, weight gain)

        ii. Can cause psychosis or anxiety

        iii. Causes acute and chronic pulmonary effects similar to tobacco smoking

5. **Cocaine**

    a. Epidemiology

        i. Used by approximately 0.7% of population greater than 11 y/o

      ii. Frequent use by 0.3% (thus, almost one-half of all users are addicted)

     iii. Highest use in 18 to 25-y/o age group (1.3% reported use)

  b. Pharmacology

       i. Can be injected, smoked ("freebasing" or smoking "crack rocks"), inhaled (by "snorting" or "tooting" the fine powder), ingested (rarely)

      ii. **NB:** *Blocks presynaptic DA reuptake,* causing hyperactivation of mesolimbic dopaminergic system

  c. Intoxication

       i. Behavioral: euphoria, *hypervigilance, tension/anger,* poor judgment, hallucinations and paranoia, impulsivity, hypersexuality

      ii. Physiologic: *tachycardia, mydriasis, hypertension, weight loss, psychomotor agitation*

     iii. Severe: seizures, delirium, movement disorders, coma

     iv. Treatment: antipsychotics for paranoia, agitation, and hallucinations

  d. Withdrawal: depression and suicidality, fatigue, nightmares, altered sleep, increased appetite, psychomotor changes

  e. Other cocaine-related syndromes

       i. Cocaine is the most important cause of drug-related cerebrovascular accident; most often causes ischemic lesions; infarction can occur hours to days after use; spinal ischemia can be a complication of cocaine use.

      ii. *Seizures* account for approximately 5% of cocaine-related emergency department visits.

     iii. Users are at risk for *myocardial infarction,* dysrhythmias, and cardiomyopathy.

     iv. May cause cerebral vasculitis

6. **Hallucinogens**

  a. Synthetic: *lysergic acid diethylamide (LSD)*

  b. Natural: *mescaline* (peyote cactus), *psilocybin* (mushrooms)

  c. Epidemiology: most commonly used by young adults (~1% report recent use)

  d. *Pharmacology*

       i. Data based on findings from LSD in animals

      ii. **NB:** LSD is a postsynaptic *5-HT receptor agonist.*

     iii. Acute effects last 8 to 12 hours.

  e. No recognized dependence or withdrawal syndrome; tolerance develops rapidly with continual use

  f. Intoxication

       i. Behavioral: anxiety/depression, paranoia, poor judgment, fear of losing one's mind

      ii. Perceptual: derealization, intensification of sensory experiences, hallucinations, illusions, synesthesia

     iii. Physiologic: diaphoresis, tachycardia, mydriasis, tremor, ataxia

     iv. Treatment: gentle reassurance ("talking down"), antipsychotics

7. **PCP**

  a. Pharmacology

       i. May be smoked (usually with marijuana) or injected

      ii. Effects peak in 30 minutes, can last for weeks

     iii. **NB:** PCP acts as *antagonist at NMDA glutamate receptor.*

     iv. Also activates dopaminergic neurons in ventral tegmentum *b.* Intoxication

        i. Behavioral: *assaultiveness, belligerence, paranoia,* impulsivity, poor judgment, hypersexuality, inappropriate laughter, amnesia

        ii. *Physiologic:* **NB:** *vertical or horizontal nystagmus, hypertension, tachycardia, decreased pain response,* ataxia, dysarthria, seizures, hyperacusis, muscle rigidity, excess salivation

        iii. Patients can be extremely dangerous and often exhibit seemingly superhuman strength.

        iv. Treatment

            (A) Supportive: observe for rhabdomyolysis (from rigidity and hyperactivity), hydrate, decrease stimulation, attempt "talking down," protect airway.

            (B) Pharmacologic

                (1) Benzodiazepines: preferred for muscle spasms and seizures

                (2) DA blockade (antipsychotic): may be necessary to treat aggression

8. **Inhalants:** volatile substances (glue, solvents, aerosol propellants, thinners, fuel) and nitrous oxide

    a. Epidemiology

        i. More common in whites, the poor, and adolescents; prevalence 0.02% up to 0.4% in ages 12 to 17 years

        ii. Account for 1% of all substance-related deaths (respiratory depression, cardiac dysrhythmias, aspiration)

    b. Pharmacology

        i. May be sniffed or "huffed" (inhaled orally) from a tube, soaked rag, or plastic bag

        ii. Effects peak in minutes, may last for hours with repeated inhalations.

        iii. Mechanism of action unknown: may enhance GABA activity or alter cell membranes

    c. Intoxication

        i. Behavioral: belligerence, assaultiveness, apathy, poor judgment, euphoria, psychosis, sensory distortions

        ii. Physiologic: dizziness, nystagmus, dysarthria, tremor, lethargy, ataxia, coma

    d. Other inhalant-related syndromes

        i. **NB:** *Neurologic*

            (A) **NB:** Subacute combined degeneration (nitrous oxide)

            (B) Lead intoxication (gasoline)

            (C) **NB:** Peripheral neuropathy (n-hexane)

            (D) Dementia, epilepsy, brain atrophy

        ii. General medical: renal failure, hepatic failure, fetal effects

9. **Nicotine**

    a. Epidemiology

        i. Smokers: 25% of Americans

        ii. 1 billion smokers worldwide

        iii. Accounts for 60% of health care costs in the United States

        iv. Associated with 400,000 U.S. deaths per year

(A) 25% of all deaths

(B) 30% of cancer deaths (most lethal carcinogen)

v. Demographics

(A) Rate of smoking in women now almost equals rate in men.

(B) No race difference

(C) Inverse correlation with education (17% of college grads versus 37% of individuals who did not finish high school)

(D) 50% in psychiatric patients (70% and 90% in bipolar I and schizophrenia, respectively)

b. **Pharmacology**

i. Acts as an *agonist at nicotinic ACh* receptors

ii. Increases concentration of circulating catecholamines

iii. Increases mesolimbic dopaminergic activity

iv. Most commonly used form is tobacco, which can be smoked or chewed

c. Intoxication (no specific criteria defined by *DSM-5*)

i. Behavioral: improved concentration and attention, decreased reaction time, elevation of mood

ii. Physiologic: increased heart rate, increased cerebral blood flow, relaxation of skeletal muscle

iii. Toxicity: sialorrhea, diaphoresis, increased peristalsis, tachycardia, confusion

d. Withdrawal

i. Occurs within 24 hours of cessation

ii. Depressed mood, insomnia, irritability, restlessness, poor concentration, decreased heart rate, hunger, or weight gain

e. Other nicotine-related syndromes

i. Direct

(A) Lung cancer (8 times risk; 106,000 deaths per year)

(B) Emphysema, chronic bronchitis (51,000 deaths per year)

(C) Oropharyngeal cancer (from chewing tobacco)

ii. Indirect

(A) *Increases risk of ischemic stroke 2 to 3 times*

(B) 35% of myocardial infarctions partially attributed to smoking

(C) Increases risk of bladder, esophageal, pancreatic, stomach, kidney, and liver cancer

f. Treatment of dependence

i. Nicotine replacement, with gum or patch

ii. Encouragement from nonsmoking physician is correlated with abstinence.

iii. Decrease nicotine withdrawal symptoms.

(A) Bupropion (Zyban®) approved by FDA

(B) Clonidine, fluoxetine, and buspirone may be helpful.

10. **Opioids**

a. Epidemiology

i. Heroin is the most commonly abused opioid (1.3% of population have used), opioid use disorders occur in 0.37% of adults and affect men more than women.

ii. Of opioid abusers, 90% have another psychiatric diagnosis.

a. Epidemiology (*cont'd*)

    iii. Tolerance and dependence can develop rapidly, even in individuals who are using prescription opioids appropriately.

    iv. Opioid use disorders are 3 times more common in males.

b. Pharmacology

    i. Opioids: available in injectable, smokeable, transdermal, and ingestible forms

    ii. Opioid receptors

        (A) μ Receptor: analgesia, respiratory depression, constipation, dependence

        (B) κ Receptor: analgesia, diuresis, sedation

        (C) δ Receptor: analgesia (?)

        (D) Also inhibit locus ceruleus (noradrenergic) activity

    iii. Addiction probably mediated through enhanced mesolimbic dopaminergic transmission

    iv. *Endogenous opioids* (endorphins and enkephalins): related to euphoria, pain suppression, and neural transmission; released on injury

c. *Intoxication*

    i. Behavioral: euphoria followed by apathy, poor judgment, psychomotor changes (usually retardation)

    ii. Physiologic: *miosis, constipation,* dysarthria, drowsiness, impaired cognition

d. *Withdrawal*

    i. *Physiologic withdrawal: an expected phenomenon, regardless of the reason (recreational or therapeutic) for opioid use*

    ii. Withdrawal may develop within minutes of cessation, usually peaks in 2 days; with meperidine (Demerol®), withdrawal symptoms can peak in 12 hours.

    iii. Symptoms: dysphoria, *nausea/vomiting,* diarrhea, *lacrimation/rhinorrhea, yawning, mydriasis,* piloerection ("cold turkey"), diaphoresis, *myalgia,* headache, autonomic instability, *severe opioid craving*

    iv. Opioid withdrawal, although intensely uncomfortable, is *not life threatening.*

e. **NB:** *Toxicity*

    i. *Symptoms: pinpoint pupils, respiratory depression, coma, vascular shock*

    ii. *Treatment*

        (A) Supportive care: airway protection, telemetry, cardiovascular support

        (B) *Opioid antagonist—naloxone (Narcan®), 0.4 mg intravenously*

            (1) Doses may be repeated to total dose of 2 mg in 45 minutes.

            (2) Can induce instant and severe withdrawal syndrome

            (3) *Short $t_{1/2}$—patient on long-acting opioid may suddenly relapse into coma.*

f. Other opioid-related syndromes

    i. **NB:** Meperidine can induce seizures.

    ii. *Needle-related complications*

        (A) *Most common and most dangerous complication of opioid use*

        (B) *Transmission of HIV and hepatitis*

        (C) *Infective endocarditis* (20% progress to have stroke)

(D) Abscesses at injection points

(E) Injection and embolism of crushed pills

iii. May cause CNS vasculitis

iv. Anoxia and ischemia from respiratory/cardiovascular collapse

v. The best-documented cases of substance-induced *myelopathy* have occurred in heroin users; resembles anterior spinal artery syndrome.

vi. *1-Methyl-4-phenyl-1,2,3,6-tetrahydropyridine (MPTP)*

(A) Synthetic opioid manufactured in the 1970s

(B) Converted in vivo to MPP+, a toxin taken up by dopaminergic neurons

(C) *Induces parkinsonism*

g. Treatment of dependence

i. Gradual decrease of opioid dosage

(A) Clonidine to control withdrawal symptoms

(B) Usually unsuccessful if not monitored closely

ii. Replacement opioid

(A) Methadone most frequently used

(1) Eliminates needle-related complications

(2) Easier to detoxify than heroin or morphine

(3) Produces minimal euphoria or drowsiness but prevents withdrawal

(4) Problems

(a) Patient remains narcotic dependent.

(b) In some programs, the patient must obtain the daily dose at the clinic.

(B) Buprenorphine (Subutex®): FDA approved in 2002 for opioid addiction treatment; sublingual tablet, opioid partial agonist

(C) Levo-α-acetylmethadol is longer-acting than methadone and can be taken every other day.

iii. Opioid antagonist

(A) Attempt to decrease opiate use by blocking pleasant effects

(B) Naltrexone (ReVia®) has $t_{1/2}$ of 72 hours.

(C) Requires strong motivation and compliance from patient

Quick Reference Chart: Substances of Abuse

SUBSTANCE	RECEPTOR OR NEUROTRANSMITTER	URINE DETECTION	NEUROLOGIC ACUTE	TOXICITY CHRONIC
Alcohol	Cell membrane, GABA receptor	N/A	Wernicke	Korsakoff, beriberi, cerebellar atrophy, dementia, neuropathy
Amphetamine	Catecholamine release	48 hrs	Seizures	Vasculitis
Caffeine	Adenosine antagonist	N/A	None	None

(continued)

SUBSTANCE	RECEPTOR OR NEUROTRANSMITTER	URINE DETECTION	NEUROLOGIC ACUTE	TOXICITY CHRONIC
Marijuana	Cannabinoid receptor, GABA, catecholamines	4–5 days	None	None
Cocaine	Inhibits DA reuptake	48 hrs	Cerebrovascular accident, spinal ischemia	Vasculitis
Hallucinogens	5-HT receptor agonist	N/A	None	None
PCP	NMDA antagonist	14 days	Rhabdomyolysis	None
Inhalants	Cell membrane, GABA receptor (?)	N/A	None (?)	Neuropathy, subacute combined degeneration, lead poisoning, dementia, epilepsy
Nicotine	Nicotinic ACh agonist	N/A	None	Cerebrovascular accident
Opioids	Opioid receptors	2–5 days[a]	Coma	Human immunodeficiency virus, myelopathy, embolic stroke
Benzodiazepines[b]	GABA inducer	5–7 days[a]	None	Psychomotor slowing
Barbiturates[b]	GABA inducer	1–7 days[a]	None	None

N/A, not applicable.
[a]Depends on $t_{1/2}$ of specific compound.
[b]For more information on benzodiazepines and barbiturates, refer to Section I.F.

E. **Somatoform disorders:** these illnesses present with physical complaints for which there is no adequate physiologic or anatomic explanation; they are presumed to allow patients to express their psychological discomfort in a culturally acceptable fashion (i.e., physical illness); they may be present in up to 15% of patients in primary care settings; in somatoform disorders, the symptoms are not feigned or consciously produced; the patients are subconsciously seeking primary gain, the resolution of internal conflict. In *DSM-5* these have been renamed Somatic Symptom and Related Disorders and rely less on medically unexplained symptoms and are now defined by distressing somatic symptoms, with abnormal thoughts and emotional and behavioral responses to the experienced symptoms. This new definition is thought to better describe the scenario when somatic symptom disorders accompany diagnosed medical or neurological disorders (i.e., functional overlay).

1. **Somatization disorder** (preoccupation with *multiple, diffuse symptoms*) (now somatoform symptom disorder)

   a. Demographics: young; female (20:1)

   b. Description: 2 years of more than five physical symptoms that are not fully explained by any detectable abnormality; the review of systems (particularly GI, genitourinary, cardiovascular, neurologic) is extremely positive; the patient is unable to accept medical reassurances of good health for more than a few weeks.

    c. **NB:** *Treatment:* regular appointments, regardless of symptoms, will reduce the patient's need for "crisis" appointments.

  2. **Hypochondriacal disorder** (preoccupation with having *a particular defined disease*) (new to *DSM-5*: approximately 75% now diagnosed as somatic symptom disorder and 25% as illness anxiety disorder)

    a. Demographics: middle-aged or elderly; history of physical illness; no gender specificity

    b. Description: at least 5 months of persistent preoccupation about having no more than two serious medical illnesses; worry about the illness impairs function or causes distress and *cannot be alleviated by medical reassurance.*

    c. Treatment: avoid tests and treatment for nonobjective signs; regular appointments to reassure the patient he or she is not being abandoned.

  3. **Body dysmorphic disorder** (preoccupation with an *imagined flaw*)

    a. Demographics: usually begins in 2nd or 3rd decade of life

    b. Most frequent body parts are hair, nose, skin, and eyes

    c. Treatment: antidepressants, stress management techniques

  4. **Conversion disorder** (presentation with a *pseudoneurologic symptom*)

    a. Demographics: more prevalent in rural, poorly educated, and low socioeconomic classes; female predominant; psychologically immature

    b. Description: patient presents with sudden onset of blindness, paralysis, numbness, or other condition that does not follow a known physiologic pattern; the onset is often preceded by a psychologically conflicting event or situation; patients sometimes seem strangely unconcerned *(la belle indifférence)*

    c. Treatment: reassurance, symptom-directed therapy (e.g., physical therapy for paralysis), psychotherapy; *do not tell patients their symptoms are imaginary;* prognosis is excellent with prompt therapy.

F. **Factitious disorder**

  1. Symptoms are consciously feigned, but for primary gain (assuming the sick role).

  2. May also be *by proxy* (Munchausen syndrome), in which the mentally ill person causes signs and symptoms in another (usually mother inflicts illness on child).

G. **Malingering:** symptoms are consciously feigned for a conscious *secondary gain*, such as financial gain, avoiding work, or escaping legal consequences.

Quick Reference Chart: Patients With Pseudosymptoms

	CONVERSION	FACTITIOUS	MALINGERING
Feigned symptoms	–	+	+
Conscious gain	–	–	+

+, present; –, absent.

H. **Dissociative disorders**

  1. **Dissociative fugue:** patient goes on an unexpected journey away from familiar surroundings; behavior is organized, and self-care is maintained; patient often experiences amnesia for his or her prior identity during the trip, and amnesia about the journey once he or she returns home.

  2. **Dissociative identity disorder:** *"multiple personality disorder,"* the presence of multiple personality states that recurrently take control of the patient's behavior; each personality has its own distinct preferences and memories that may be inaccessible to the other personalities.

I. **Eating disorders**

   1. *Anorexia nervosa*

      a. Diagnosis

         i. Persistent intake restriction; refusal to maintain body weight greater than *85% of expected*

         ii. Irrational fear of gaining weight

         iii. Self-image influenced by *distorted perception* of weight and/or shape

         iv. *Amenorrhea is common.*

      b. Treatment

         i. Medical: restore nutritional status, rehydrate, correct electrolyte imbalances.

         ii. Psychiatric: psychotherapy, behavioral management; *no reliable medication*

   2. *Bulimia nervosa*

      a. Diagnosis

         i. Recurrent episodes of eating a larger-than-normal amount during a discrete period, with a feeling of distress and lack of control over the binges

         ii. Compensation for bingeing (vomiting, excessive exercise, laxative abuse, fasting)

         iii. Self-esteem unduly influenced by weight and shape (patients are often normal or slightly overweight)

      b. Treatment

         i. Medical: sequelae of vomiting (dental decay, esophageal erosions, gastritis, hypokalemia, metabolic alkalosis) and laxative overuse (hemorrhoids, fissures) should be evaluated and repaired.

         ii. Psychiatric: psychotherapy, antidepressant medications (not bupropion)

J. **Personality disorders: these disorders describe an individual's pattern of responding to people and events in his or her environment; usually formed early in life and tend to be predictable and durable; patients with personality disorders do not recognize the maladaptive nature of their behaviors; treatment consists mainly of psychotherapy; medications are used to treat symptoms or comorbidities.**

   1. **Cluster A: odd, suspicious**

      a. Paranoid: suspects deception in others; doubts loyalty of friends and partner; believes others intend malice; persistently bears grudges; perceives nonexistent attacks on character/reputation; reads threats or injuries into benign statements

      b. Schizoid: no desire for close interpersonal relationships; chooses solitary activities; little interest in sex; little pleasure; few nonfamilial friends; indifferent to others' opinions; emotionally cold

      c. Schizotypal: ideas of reference; magical thinking or odd beliefs; perceptual distortions; odd thinking and speech; paranoia; inappropriate affect; unusual behavior; few close friends; social anxiety

   2. **Cluster B: dramatic, impulsive**

      a. Histrionic: strives to be center of attention; sexually provocative behavior; shifting, shallow emotions; uses physical appearance to draw attention; impressionistic speech; theatrical; suggestible; overvalues relationships

      b. Narcissistic: inflated self-importance; fantasizes about unlimited success, power, or ideal love; believes he or she is special and should only associate with other special people; requires admiration; entitled; treats others as objects to satisfy his or her needs; lacks empathy; envious or suspects others of envying him or her; arrogant attitude

c. *Antisocial:* repeated unlawful acts; deceitfulness; impulsivity; aggressiveness; irresponsibility; disregard for safety of self or others; lack of remorse; *history of conduct disorder as a child*

d. *Borderline:* frantic avoidance of perceived abandonment; unstable and intense relationships; unstable self-image; impulsivity; recurrent suicidal behavior or self-mutilation; affective instability; chronic feelings of emptiness; difficulty controlling anger; stress-related paranoia or dissociation

> **NB:** Instability of mood is the most consistent finding in borderline personality disorder.

3. **Cluster C:** anxious

a. *Avoidant:* avoids activities involving interpersonal contact; unwilling to form friendship unless assured of being liked; fears shame/ridicule in intimate relationships; preoccupied with fears of criticism/rejection; feels inadequate in new situations; poor self-image; does not take risks that may cause embarrassment

b. *Dependent:* requires reassurance/advice to make decisions; needs others to be responsible for his or her life; unable to express disagreement; unable to initiate projects; does anything for approval of others; uncomfortable when alone; must be involved in relationship; preoccupied with fears of having to take care of him- or herself

c. *Obsessive compulsive: not related to obsessive-compulsive disorder;* preoccupation with rules, details, order instead of the main point; perfectionism interferes with progress; excessively devoted to work; inflexible about morality, ethics, or values; unable to discard worthless objects; reluctant to delegate; miserly; rigid and stubborn

III. Medical Ethics in Psychiatry: For the most part, laws governing ethical conduct are state specific; we have included some general principles that guide appropriate behavior vis-à-vis psychiatric patients.

A. **Informed consent**

1. Issues of informed consent are usually taken more seriously in psychiatry than in other fields, because patients with mental illnesses are vulnerable to exploitation.

2. Definitions

a. Capacity: the ability to make informed decisions

i. Mental illness is only one factor that can affect a patient's capacity.

ii. Any physician can submit an opinion about whether a patient has capacity; a psychiatrist is usually asked to decide whether mental illness limits the patient's capacity.

iii. Patients may have capacity for directing some aspects of care and lack capacity for others.

b. Competence: a *judicial determination* about whether a patient is authorized to make decisions; if the patient is judged incompetent, a guardian is assigned to make decisions *in the patient's best interest.*

3. Consent for hospitalization

a. In most states, a person being admitted to a psychiatric ward must give written consent to his or her admission, general medical treatment, and, *specifically,* for psychiatric treatment.

b. When a patient requires hospitalization but is unable to give informed consent, a legal mechanism allows for involuntary admission to the hospital. In general, this requires evidence that the patient has a mental illness *and* presents an *imminent* risk of harm to him- or herself or others.

    c. *A patient's acceptance of hospitalization or treatment does not qualify as informed consent for hospitalization or treatment.*

        i. The patient must understand the reason for his or her hospitalization and treatment.

        ii. The patient must understand the likely outcome of accepting or refusing treatment.

    4. The presence of a severe mental illness does not automatically indicate that a patient lacks capacity to make decisions concerning his or her psychiatric or medical care.

B. Privacy

1. As with all medical records, privacy should be preserved at all costs.

2. Health Insurance Privacy and Portability Act (HIPPA) guidelines *do* allow exchange of information to improve patient care, for operational purposes, and for third-party payment.

3. The requirement to inform a potential victim of a psychiatric patient's intent to harm him or her, or "duty to warn," was established in California in the *Tarasoff* case; that ruling, however, did not establish the same requirement in other states.

C. Restraints

1. The use of "chemical restraints" is no longer considered appropriate.

    a. Treatment of agitated or aggressive behavior should be directed at the root cause, when possible.

    b. The first priority of emergency pharmacotherapy should be to reduce the risk of harm to the patient, and those around him or her—*not* to sedate or mute the patient.

    c. The patient should be given the option of accepting the medication, *if conditions permit a safe conversation.*

    d. Address escalation early, not before it becomes unsafe.

        i. Try redirection, "talking down"; offer the patient an empty room to calm down.

        ii. Offer medication to help calm the patient. Listen to the patient's suggestions about what he or she thinks may help.

        iii. Separate the patient from others and de-stimulate (move to quite calm area).

2. Physical restraints

    a. Should be used as a last resort, only if less restrictive interventions are determined to be ineffective

    b. Re-evaluate the need for restraints frequently.

    c. If improperly applied (too loose or too tight), restraints can be very dangerous for the patient.

    d. Physical restraints should always be used in combination with behavioral and pharmacologic approaches.

D. Absolutely unethical behavior

1. A romantic relationship with a patient

2. Lying to a patient

3. Altering the medical record

4. Exploitation of patients (e.g., getting free goods or services, requesting gifts)

CHEAT SHEET

Dopamine pathways	Nigrostriatal, mesolimbic and mesocortical, tuberoinfundibular, incertohypothalamic
Serotonin	Produced in dorsal and median raphe nuclei and project to hippocampus, hypothalamus, frontal cortex, striatum, thalamus
Acetylcholine	Involved in cognition, motor function, memory
SIGECAPS	Mnemonic for major depressive episode
DIGFAST	Mnemonic for manic episode

Suggested Readings

American Psychiatric Association. *Diagnostic and statistical manual of mental disorders* (5th ed.). Arlington, VA: American Psychiatric Publishing;2013.

Lieberman JA, Stroup TS, McEvoy JP, et al. Effectiveness of antipsychotic drugs in patients with chronic schizophrenia. *N. Engl. J. Med.*2005;353:1209–1223.

Nierenberg AA, Ostacher MJ, Calabrese JR, et al. Treatment-resistant bipolar depression: a STEP-BD equipoise randomized effectiveness trial of antidepressant augmentation with lamotrigine, inositol, or risperidone. *Am. J. Psych.*2006;163(2):210–216.

Rush AJ, Trivedi MH, Wisniewski SR, et al. Bupropion-SR, sertraline, or venlafaxine-XR after failure of SSRIs for depression. *N. Engl. J. Med.*2006;354(12):1231–1242.

CHAPTER 29

Child Psychiatry

Child Pharmacology

I. General Concepts

A. **Pharmacokinetics: different in children**

1. Drug distribution

   a. Less fatty tissue (less drug storage in fat)

   b. Protein binding may be unpredictable.

   c. Weight changes more rapidly, and changes are a greater percentage of total weight.

2. Elimination is generally faster than in adults.

   a. Higher glomerular filtration rate

   b. Larger hepatic capacity

B. **Pharmacodynamics**

1. Central nervous system (CNS) is still developing; effects of medications may change with CNS maturation.

2. Surprising or paradoxic side effects may occur.

3. Therapeutic drug levels may not apply.

C. **Diagnosis: may be more difficult in children (e.g., attention deficit hyperactivity disorder [ADHD] or bipolar? schizophrenia or autism?)**

1. Sometimes the diagnosis is established only after a response to pharmacotherapy.

2. Symptom-directed treatment is common.

3. Many childhood disorders have no specific treatment (autism, retardation, etc.).

D. **Most psychotropics: not approved by the U.S. Food and Drug Administration (FDA) for use in children**

E. **Electroconvulsive therapy and psychosurgery: generally not indicated**

F. **Children are minors: the child's parents or guardians are the ultimate decision makers; treatment of any kind requires their informed consent.**

II. Psychotropics Used Mostly in Children

A. **Medications for ADHD**

1. *Amphetamines*

   a. Effects

      i. Increased release of catecholamines (norepinephrine [NE] and dopamine [DA])

      (A) Increased attention and concentration

      (B) Increased motivation

      a. Effects (*cont'd*)

        ii. Reduced hyperactivity, aggression

        iii. Similar behavioral responses occur in children without ADHD (i.e., improvement with amphetamine is not diagnostic of ADHD).

      b. Specific drugs

        i. Methylphenidate (Ritalin®, Metadate®, Concerta®): the most frequently used

        ii. Dextroamphetamine (Dexedrine®)

        iii. Mixed amphetamine salt (Adderall®)

      c. Adverse effects

        i. Can worsen tics (which are often comorbid)

        ii. Insomnia, anorexia, nervousness

        iii. Potentially habit forming

        iv. If stimulants suppress growth, the effect is minimal, and growth catches up eventually.

        v. Toxicity: hallucinations and seizures

  2. Pemoline (Cylert®)

      a. Nonamphetamine stimulant

      b. Longer-acting than most amphetamines

      c. Withdrawn from U.S. markets in 2005 due to liver toxicity

  3. Antidepressants: *black-box warning: antidepressants increase the risk of suicidal thinking and behavior in children, adolescents, and young adults (18–24 years of age) with major depressive disorder and other psychiatric disorders.*

      a. Tricyclics

        i. Likely work through NE reuptake inhibition

        ii. Therapeutic effects may be evident within days (unlike in depression).

        iii. *Desipramine: effective but associated with sudden cardiac death*

      b. Bupropion (Wellbutrin®)

        i. Increased NE and DA transmission

        ii. *Decreases seizure threshold*

  4. Atomoxetine (Strattera®)

      a. Nonstimulant; selective NE reuptake inhibitor

      b. May cause drowsiness

  5. Presynaptic α_2-noradrenergic agonists (not FDA approved)

      a. Clonidine (Catapres®), also available as a patch

      b. Guanfacine (Tenex®) may be more frontal lobe specific than clonidine

      c. Can cause hypotension, dysrhythmias, sedation

      d. Rebound hypertension can occur if discontinued suddenly

B. NB: Medications for Tourette's disorder

  1. Antipsychotics are the most effective treatments—probably work through DA blockade

      a. **NB:** Pimozide (Orap®): not frequently used but is a test answer

      b. **NB:** Haloperidol (Haldol®)

      c. Risperidone (Risperdal®)

   d. Risks

       i. *Extrapyramidal side effects, tardive dyskinesia*

      ii. *QT prolongation*—monitor with serial electrocardiographies.

   2. Clonidine (less effective, but no risk of tardive dyskinesia)

C. **Medications for enuresis**

   1. Tricyclics

      a. Effective in 60% of patients

      b. Low doses, given approximately 1 hour before bedtime

      c. Clomipramine (Anafranil®): most commonly used

   2. Desmopressin

      a. Analogue of antidiuretic hormone

      b. Effective in approximately 50% of cases

      c. Dosed intranasally

      d. Can cause water retention

D. **Medications for self-injury (in developmental disorders)**

   1. Antimanic agents, such as *lithium and anticonvulsants*

   2. Antipsychotics—risperidone and aripiprazole in autism spectrum disorders

   3. Nonspecific sedatives, such as benzodiazepines and antihistamines

   4. β-Blockers sometimes have a calming effect.

   5. Opioid antagonists naloxone (Narcan®) and naltrexone (Revia®)

Childhood Psychiatric Illnesses

Childhood psychiatric illnesses differ from adult illnesses in two ways. First, children may present with unusual symptoms of adult illnesses. Second, as in neurology, children have their own unique diagnoses that rarely present in adulthood. This chapter is not intended to be a comprehensive review of these illnesses but to present those that are likely to come to the attention of a neurologist (in real life or on an examination).

III. Mental Retardation (Now Called Intellectual Disability; Renamed by Federal Statue 111-256, Rosa's Law)

A. *Categorization*

   1. Mild

      a. Intelligence quotient (IQ): 50 to 70

      b. 6th-grade educable

      c. May be able to hold simple job

   2. Moderate

      a. IQ: 35 to 50

      b. 2nd-grade educable

      c. May be able to function in sheltered workplace

A. *Categorization* (*cont'd*)

   3. Severe

     a. IQ: 20 to 35

     b. May be able to talk or otherwise communicate

     c. Unlikely to benefit from vocational training

     d. May be able to protect self and perform simple hygiene

   4. Profound

     a. IQ: less than 20

     b. May develop rudimentary speech in adulthood

     c. Will require nursing care

B. **Causes**

   1. **NB:** Down syndrome

     a. *Trisomy 21:* most common cause

     b. Incidence: 1/700 live births (1 in 100 if mother >32 years old [y/o])

     c. Signs

        i. Physical examination: hypotonia, oblique palpebral fissures, extra neck skin, protruding tongue, single palmar crease (simian crease)

        ii. Mental development seems normal until 6 months; IQ decreases after age 1 year.

        iii. As children, they are usually quite pleasant and placid.

        iv. Various behavioral problems can develop in adolescence.

     d. Prognosis/complications

        i. Frequent childhood infections (depressed immune system)

        ii. Outcome can range from holding jobs to lifelong institutionalization (10%).

        iii. **NB:** *Early-age Alzheimer's symptoms and neuropathology (age 30–40 years)*

        iv. *Atlantoaxial instability may cause myelopathy.*

   2. **NB:** Fragile X syndrome

     a. Caused by *trinucleotide repeat* at chromosomal locus Xq27.3

     b. Incidence: 1/1,000 males, 1/2,000 females

     c. Diagnosis

        i. Long head, large ears, hyperflexible joints, *macroorchidism,* short stature

        ii. Mild to severe intellectual disability

        iii. These patients are often gregarious and pleasant.

        iv. Females are usually less severely affected.

        v. High frequency of ADHD and pervasive developmental disorders

> **NB:** Fragile X is the most common cause of inherited intellectual disability. Nearly all affected boys manifest attention deficit disorder (ADD) and have learning disabilities. The most common neurocognitive symptoms are abstract reasoning, complex problem solving, and expressive language; 33% meet criteria for autism. Female carriers can have a milder form of the disease.

3. **Prader-Willi syndrome**

   a. **NB:** *Paternal* chromosome 15q12 deletion

   b. Prevalence: 1/10,000

   c. Signs

      i. **NB:** *Compulsive eating (obesity)*

      ii. Can be oppositional, aggressive, and behaviorally labile

      iii. Hypogonadism

4. **Angelman's syndrome**

   a. **NB:** *Maternal* chromosome 15q12 deletion

   b. Diagnosis

      i. Developmental delay at 6 to 12 months

      ii. *Microcephaly* and seizures at early age

      iii. Speech impaired but often able to understand and communicate otherwise

      iv. **NB:** *Happy puppet*

         (A) Posture impairment and jerky gait

         (B) Flapping movements of hands

         (C) Excitable and tend to smile and laugh frequently

5. **Lesch-Nyhan syndrome**

   a. **NB:** *X-linked recessive (essentially affects only males)*

      i. Deficiency of hypoxanthine-guanine phosphoribosyl transferase

      ii. Causes accumulation of uric acid

   b. Incidence: 1/380,000

   c. Diagnostic features

      i. Patients typically present around 6 months old, with motor delay.

      ii. *Medical:* uric acid tophi, nephrolithiasis, gout

      iii. *Neurologic:* microcephaly, seizures, movement disorders, pyramidal signs

      iv. *Psychiatric:* **NB:** *severe self-mutilation (biting lips, tongue, fingers),* mental retardation

   d. Treatment

      i. Decrease uric acid

      ii. Allopurinol is used but fails to prevent progression.

   e. Most patients die before 40 y/o.

IV. Specific Learning Disorders

A. Diagnosed when one specific area of cognitive achievement is significantly below what would be expected for the child's age, schooling, and performance in other areas

B. Types

1. Reading disorder

   a. 4% of children

   b. Impaired word recognition and comprehension

   c. If associated with right/left confusion, called *dyslexia*

2. Mathematics

   a. 5% of children

   b. May present as simply as inability to count, or as complexly as failing geometry

3. Written expression

    a. 3% to 10% of children

    b. Possible genetic influence

4. Other types: spelling, mixed

V. Pervasive Developmental Disorders (in *Diagnostic and Statistical Manual of Mental Disorders*, 5th Edition [*DSM-5*], Now Called Autism Spectrum Disorders)

A. Characterized by severe, persistent impairment in developmental areas, particularly socialization

B. Cognitive skill: usually better than functional impairment would predict

C. Autistic disorder

1. Abnormal or failed development, before age 3 years, of language and communication, social attachment and interaction, or symbolic play

2. Incidence: 5/10,000 (males affected 3 times more often than females)

3. Diagnosis: symptoms of dysfunction in three main areas

    a. Reciprocal social interaction: poor eye contact; impaired use of body language; failure to develop peer relationships; lack of interest in sharing enjoyment; deviant responses to social cues

    b. Communication: lack of language output, inability to maintain conversation; stereotyped or idiosyncratic use of language; lack of imitative play

    c. Repetitive or restricted patterns of behavior: intense preoccupation with an unusual topic; compulsive adherence to rules or rituals; stereotyped motor mannerisms; preoccupations with object parts or nonfunctional elements of objects (color, texture, etc.)

4. Other symptoms

    a. Seizures: 10% to 30%

    b. Intellectual disability: 60%

    c. Treatment

        i. Behavioral therapy

        ii. Symptomatic

            (A) Antidepressants for compulsions, affective lability

            (B) D2-blocking agents for tics

            (C) Antimanics and antipsychotics for agitation and aggression

        iii. Self-mutilation: data have shown efficacy of *risperidone.*

D. Asperger's syndrome: autism without language or intellectual disturbance

1. Incidence unclear because diagnostic criteria have changed frequently

2. Comparison to autism

    a. Similar criteria for abnormal social interaction and repetitive patterns of behavior

    b. **NB:** *No significant language delay*

    c. Child maintains normal curiosity about environment and has normal nonsocial adaptive behavior.

E. **Rett's disorder**

1. **NB:** *X-linked dominant*

2. **NB:** *Affects only females* (males die in utero or at birth)

3. Incidence: 1/20,000

4. Diagnosis

    a. **NB:** *Normal development until 5 months old*

    b. **NB:** *Deceleration of head growth between 5 and 48 months*

    c. **NB:** Characteristic wringing of hands (actually apraxic movements)

    d. Loss of social engagement

    e. Ataxia of trunk and gait

    f. Gait disturbance, scoliosis, seizures

VI. Attention Deficit and Disruptive Disorders

A. **ADHD**

1. Approximately 5% in American school-aged children

2. Can persist into adulthood (15% of cases)

3. Males affected 2 to 1; females tend to have inattentive type.

4. Causes

    a. Some evidence for genetic cause (increased risk in twins and siblings)

    b. Hypofunction of NE?

    c. Hypofunction of DA?

    d. Impaired frontal lobe function?

> **NB:** DA pathways have been recently implicated in the pathogenesis of ADHD, including the association between ADHD and polymorphisms in DRD4, DRD5, and SLC6A4, which encode D4 and D5 receptors and the DA transporter.

5. Diagnosis

    a. *Inattention:* poor attention to detail; unable to sustain concentration; seems not to listen when spoken to; fails to follow through on instructions; poor organization; dislikes tasks that require attention; loses things; forgetful; easily distracted by extraneous stimuli/information

    b. *Hyperactivity/impulsivity:* fidgety; difficulty remaining seated; excessive running/climbing; difficulty playing quietly; talks excessively; on the go; has trouble waiting turn; intrusive

    c. Some evidence of symptoms before age 7 years

    d. Impairment in social, academic, or occupational function

    e. May be predominantly inattentive, predominantly hyperactive, or combined type

6. Treatment

    a. Pharmacotherapy, (see Section II.A)

        i. Many clinicians give drug holidays on weekends and in the summer.

        ii. Beware of rebound hyperactivity when medication is discontinued.

6. Treatment (*cont'd*)

   b. Therapy

      i. Family therapy

         (A) Instruct parents not to be overly permissive or punitive.

         (B) Help parents develop useful behavioral interventions.

      ii. Individual and group therapy

         (A) Help build self-esteem

         (B) Help refine interpersonal skills

   c. Associated illnesses

      i. Comorbidities: conduct disorder, depression, tics

      ii. Differential diagnosis: learning disorder, pervasive developmental disorder, bipolar disorder

B. Oppositional defiant disorder

1. Diagnosis

   a. *Negative and hostile behavior*: loses temper; argues with adults; deliberately annoys people; defies adults' requests or rules; angry, resentful, and vindictive; irritable; blames others for his/her behavior

   b. Behaviors occur more frequently than would be expected for age and developmental level

   c. Behaviors last for at least 6 months

2. Differential diagnosis: depression, conduct disorder, bipolar disorder, ADHD

3. Treatment

   a. Family and behavioral therapy

   b. Symptom-directed pharmacotherapy, if necessary

C. Conduct disorder

1. Diagnosis

   a. *Aggression*: bullies or threatens others; starts fights; has used a weapon; physically cruel to people or animals; has stolen while confronting the victim

   b. *Property destruction*: deliberate fire setting or other property destruction

   c. *Deceitfulness/theft*: has broken into a building or car; frequently lies; has stolen without confrontation

   d. *Rules violations*: stays out past curfew (before 13 y/o); has run away overnight at least twice; often truant (before 13 y/o)

   e. Must be less than 18 y/o

2. 50%: progress to antisocial personality disorder

3. Treatment

   a. Poor prognosis

   b. Treat comorbidities (depression, ADHD, learning disorder)

   c. Individual therapy to improve problem-solving skills

   d. Family therapy

   e. Psychopharmacology directed at aggression (antimanics, antipsychotics, clonidine, antidepressants)

VII. Tic Disorders

    A. **NB: Tourette's disorder**

        1. Prevalence: 4/10,000

        2. Males are affected 3 times more often than females.

        3. Causes

            a. Genetic: higher coincidence in twins; autosomal dominant in some families

            b. Likely some degree of *DA hyperactivity* present

            c. May be *exacerbated by stimulants and cocaine* (both increase synaptic DA)

            d. Can be a tardive side effect of antipsychotic treatment

        4. **NB: Diagnosis**

            a. A *vocal tic* and *multiple motor tics* (not necessarily concurrent)

            b. Tics occur several times each day for at least 1 year, with no tic-free period longer than 3 months.

            c. Onset before age 18 years

            d. Differential: other movement disorders, Sydenham's chorea, Wilson's disease, obsessive-compulsive disorder, myoclonic disorders

        5. Comorbidities: depression, obsessive-compulsive disorder (OCD), ADHD, impulsivity/rage attacks

        6. **NB: Treatment**

            a. Low-dose, high-potency antipsychotics, or clonidine

            b. Psychotherapy generally ineffective

            c. Treatment of comorbidities can sometimes improve the tic.

    B. **Motor or vocal tic disorder**

        1. Prevalence: 1/1,000

        2. Single or multiple vocal or motor tics

        3. *Treatment*

            a. As with Tourette's disorder

            b. Psychotherapy sometimes effective

VIII. Miscellaneous Childhood Disorders

    A. **Separation anxiety**

        1. Epidemiology

            a. Most common anxiety disorder in children

            b. Prevalence: 3% to 4% of all school-age children; 1% of adolescents

            c. No gender difference

        2. Diagnosis

            a. Excessive worry about becoming separated from loved ones; distress when separated; fear/refusal to go to school or elsewhere; separation nightmares; fear of being alone

            b. Occurs for a minimum of 4 weeks

            c. Onset before age 18 years

B. **Selective mutism**

1. Psychologically driven refusal or inability to speak in *some* situations
2. Of affected children, 90% have some degree of social anxiety
3. Treatment: family and behavioral therapy, fluoxetine (?)

IX. Differences From Adult Diagnostic Criteria

A. **Depression**

1. *Irritability* may replace depressed mood.
2. *Failure to achieve appropriate weight gain* may replace loss of appetite or weight.
3. Children often exhibit physical complaints.
4. Children less frequently have trouble with sleep or appetite.
5. Withdrawal from social and family activities may be more prominent.

B. **Dysthymia and cyclothymia**

1. Irritability can replace depressed mood.
2. Symptoms present for 1 year (instead of 2).

C. **Schizophrenia**

1. Very rare in children less than 5 y/o
2. Must be distinguished from pervasive developmental disorder or fantasy play

D. **Bipolar disorder**

1. Rare before adolescence
2. Manic episodes may be less discrete than in adults.

CHEAT SHEET

Intellectual disability	Renamed by Rosa's Law
Down syndrome	Usually trisomy 21, early-onset Alzheimer's
Fragile X syndrome	Trinucleotide repeat at Xq27.3; long head, large ears, macroorchidism, ADD
Angelman's syndrome	Maternal 15q12 deletion, "happy puppet"
Lesch-Nyhan syndrome	X-linked recessive, deficiency hypoxanthine-guanine phosphoribosyl transferase, severe self-mutilation
Asperger's syndrome	Autism without language or intellectual disturbance
Rett's syndrome	X-linked dominant, females, normal development until 5 months then decelerating head growth, characteristic wringing of hands

Suggested Readings

Almandii NB, Wong IC. Review on the current use of antipsychotic drugs in children and adolescents. *Arch. Dis. Child. Educ. Pract. Ed.*2011;96(5):192–196.

Constantino JN, Charman T. Diagnosis of autism spectrum disorder: reconciling the syndrome, its diverse origins, and variation in expression. *Lancet Neurol.*2015;Oct.20;Epub ahead of print.

Hopkins K, Crosland P, Elliot N, Bewley S. Diagnosis and management of depression in children and young people: summary of updated NICE guidance. *BMJ.*2015;350:h824.

Stroeh O, Trivedi HK. Appropriate and judicious use of psychotropic medications in youth. *Child Adoles. Psych. Clin. N. Am.*2012;21(4):703–711. Up to one third of patients with the symptoms lasting less than 24 hours are found to have a infarction.

CHAPTER 30

Neurobehavior and Neuropsychology

I. **Functional-Anatomic Correlations:** Review Chapter 4 to identify vessels supplying these important regions of the brain.

A. **Frontal lobes**

    1. Luria description of functions

        a. Identification of problems or objectives

        b. Formulation of strategies and selection of an appropriate plan

        c. Execution of the plan

        d. Evaluation of outcomes

    2. Specific behavioral signs and symptoms of frontal damage

        a. Lateralized signs/symptoms

            i. Either frontal lobe: release of primitive reflexes (grasp, root, palmomental, suck, glabellar, snout); witzelsucht (inappropriate jocularity); depression

            ii. *Dominant frontal lobe: left-hand apraxia* (inability to perform learned patterned movements); poor verbal fluency, including *Broca's aphasia*

            iii. *Nondominant frontal lobe:* decreased attention; loss of prosody (emotional content of speech); nonspecific behavioral symptoms; mania

            iv. **NB:** Bilateral damage: abulia, mutism; poor attention; rigid thinking; gait and sphincter disturbances

        b. By specific region

            i. *Orbitofrontal*—the region of social and interpersonal function: disinhibition, lability, euphoria, lack of remorse or social propriety/comportment

> **NB:** *Witzelsucht (inappropriate jocularity) is seen in patients with orbitofrontal cortex lesions.*

            ii. *Dorsolateral*—executive function: poor planning, decreased motivation and flexibility, unable to resist reaction to environmental stimuli

            iii. *Medial:* apathy, akinetic mutism

> **NB:** Pseudobulbar affect: exaggerated emotional response incongruent to mood. Treat with dextromethorphan/quinidine sulfate.

B. **Parietal lobes: carry out diverse functions that help us to interpret the environment and our place within it; perform higher-order and multimodal processing of incoming sensory information**

1. Damage to either side
   a. Sensory extinction of the contralateral side of the body
   b. **NB:** *Hemineglect* of the opposite side of space
      i. May include neglect of body parts (amorphosynthesis)
      ii. Hemineglect is sometimes accompanied by anosognosia (unawareness of deficits). **NB:** More common with right-sided parietal lesions. Left-sided lesions may produce transient right-sided neglect, but resolve within a few days.

2. **Dominant parietal lobe damage**
   a. Alexia (impaired ability to read)
   b. *Bilateral astereognosis*
   c. *Bilateral ideomotor apraxia*
   d. **NB:** Gerstmann syndrome: tetrad—dysgraphia, dyscalculia, right–left disorientation, finger agnosia; the individual signs of the syndrome are not localizing.
   e. **NB:** Alexia without agraphia: intact writing with impaired reading due to damage to dominant occipital, parietal, and forceps major of corpus callosum

3. **Nondominant parietal lobe damage**
   a. Constructional apraxia (impaired ability to draw or copy figures)
   b. Difficulty with visuospatial memory
   c. Confusion (especially with acute damage, such as cerebrovascular accident)
   d. Apraxia of eyelid opening—difficulty opening eyes despite normal consciousness and strength

> **NB:** *Reduplicative paramnesia* (reduplication of place) has been associated with combined lesions in the right parietal and bifrontal areas.

> **NB:** *Anosodiaphoria* (indifference to the condition despite recognition of the deficit) is seen with right-hemisphere lesions.

4. **Bilateral parietal damage**
   a. **NB:** Balint's syndrome
      i. Caused by damage to posterior superior watershed areas (Brodmann's areas 19 and 7)
      ii. *Simultanagnosia*—inability to relate objects presented together, or appreciate the sum for the parts (e.g., looking at an American flag, a patient might say, "I see a white star," then, "I see a stripe")
      iii. *Oculomotor apraxia*—inability to direct oculomotor function; paralysis of optic fixation—inability to purposefully direct one's eyes to a target in a logical fashion
      iv. *Optic ataxia*—misreaching in response to visual stimuli, inability to visually direct to a target (patients experience dysmetria with overshooting and undershooting target until they receive proprioceptive or auditory cues, then are able to do task)
   b. Spatial disorientation

C. **Temporal lobes:** the major functions associated with the temporal lobes are memory, language, and auditory processing.

1. **Hemispheric dominance**

   a. "Dominant" is defined by the hemisphere responsible for language.

   b. *Left-hemisphere dominance* in 96% of right-handers, 70% of left-handers

   c. *Right-hemisphere dominance* in 4% of right-handers, 15% of left-handers

   d. *Bilateral dominance* in 0% of right-handers, 15% of left-handers

2. **Damage to either temporal lobe**

   a. Hallucinations (any sensory modality)

   b. Delirium

   c. Distortions in time perception

3. **Damage to dominant temporal lobe**

   a. Aphasias

   b. Verbal amnesia

> **NB:** Aphasias.

TYPE	SPEECH	COMPREHENSION	REPETITION	PARAPHASIA	LOCALIZATION
Wernicke's (sensory)	Fluent	−	−	+	Superior temp gyrus (area 22)
NB: Transcortical sensory	Fluent	−	+	+	Watershed zone between MCA and PCA (areas 40, 41, 42)
Broca's (motor)	Nonfluent	+	−	−	Inferior Frontal Gyrus (area 44)
Transcortical motor	Nonfluent	+	+	−	Anterior watershed (above areas 44 and 45); **NB:** Supplementary motor area
Global	Nonfluent	−	−	+	Perisylvian/large area of dominant hemisphere
Transcortical mixed	Nonfluent	−	+	−	Both watershed zones; spares arcuate fasciculus
Anomic	Fluent	+	+	−	Angular gyrus (area 39)
Conduction	Fluent	+	−	+	Arcuate fasciculus

+, normal; −, abnormal.

> **NB:** Naming is poor in all of these syndromes; note that the transcortical (also called *extrasylvian*) aphasias have spare repetition.

> **NB:** In advancing Alzheimer's disease, speech remains intact as language deteriorates. The result is an aphasia in which the patient is fluent but makes paraphasic errors, with poor comprehension but preserved repetition, similar to transcortical sensory aphasia.

4. **Damage to nondominant temporal lobe**
   a. Impaired performance with visual testing
   b. Impaired visual memory
   c. Impaired recognition of harmony and melody/prosody of language

> **NB:** Topographic disorientation (impaired orientation and navigation in the environment) occurs with a lesion in the right posterior parahippocampal region or the infracalcarine cortex, but a milder form may be seen with a lesion in the right parietal area.

5. **Bilateral temporal damage**
   a. Korsakoff's dementia
   b. **NB:** *Klüver-Bucy syndrome*
      i. Usually with anterior temporal damage
      ii. Hyperorality, hypersexuality, apathy, hypermetamorphosis (overly sensitive or acutely aware of minute stimuli in the environment, resulting in preoccupation with these stimuli), and visual agnosia.
      iii. Aggression is not a component of the syndrome!
   c. Inability to ignore visual stimuli

D. **Occipital lobes: receive visual input and perform visual processing; information encoded with the identity of objects is routed ventrally ("what" stream) toward temporal lobes; data about the location and movement of environmental objects ("where" stream) are routed dorsally, to the parietal lobes.**

1. Damage to either occipital lobe can cause simple visual hallucinations.

2. **Damage to dominant occipital lobe**
   a. Visual object agnosia (inability to identify objects by sight)
      i. **NB:** Interhemispheric fibers (from/to splenium) may be involved; disconnects primary visual cortex from language areas; signs: often associated with *color anomia, alexia without agraphia* (pure word blindness)
      (A) Patient *unable to read words*
      (B) Patient *able to write, speak, and spell*
      (C) Patient may be able to read individual letters and numbers

3. **Damage to nondominant occipital lobe**
   a. May cause contralateral visual neglect
   b. Visuospatial disorientation
   c. Visual illusions and hallucinations

4. **Bilateral occipital damage**
   a. **NB:** *Cortical blindness:* patient is unable to see; no response to visual threat; pupils remain reactive; **Anton's syndrome**—anosognosia for cortical blindness.
   b. Achromatopsia (loss of color perception)
   c. **NB:** Balint's syndrome (see Section I.B.4.*a*)

  d. **NB:** *Prosopagnosia* (inability to recognize faces)

   i. Can occur in the absence of other visual deficits

   ii. Commonly associated with achromatopsia

   iii. **NB:** Requires ventral occipitotemporal lesion ("what" pathway)

E. Disconnection syndromes

 1. *Callosal disconnection*

  a. **NB:** *Left posterior cerebral artery territory and splenium*

   i. Right homonymous hemianopsia—all visual information enters right hemisphere.

   ii. Damaged posterior corpus callosum prevents right occipital lobe from communicating with language centers on the left; alexia (inability to read), color anomia (inability to name colors); the ability to copy words is spared—motor information crosses in anterior corpus callosum.

  b. Anterior corpus callosum: disconnects right-hemisphere motor and sensory integration centers from left-hemisphere language areas: signs: apraxia of left hand, agnosia of fingers of left hand

> **NB:** Callosal apraxia results from a lesion in the genu of the corpus callosum, resulting in limb kinetic apraxia. Tactile and auditory input cross the corpus callosum posteriorly and are therefore unaffected by a genu lesion!

  c. Complete callosotomy

   i. Alien hand (nondominant hand performs apparently independent acts)

   ii. Disconnection of dominant-sided sensory input (going to the nondominant side of the brain) from the patient's ability to describe or name the phenomena

 2. **NB:** *Arcuate fasciculus*—conduction aphasia

 3. *Subcortical fibers in dominant temporal lobe*

  a. Damages Wernicke's area and interhemispheric fibers

  b. No access of auditory input to language area

  c. Causes *pure word deafness*—sounds are appreciated, but not speech

II. Medical Diseases Causing Psychiatric Symptoms

A. Cerebrovascular disease

 1. Most common sequela is *depression.*

  a. Of stroke victims, 30% to 40% have depression.

  b. Previously associated with *left frontal* infarction in particular.

 2. Poststroke *mania associated with right-sided lesions*

B. Epilepsy

 1. 30% to 50% have psychiatric illness

 2. Increased risk of suicide

 3. Auras—hallucinations and affective changes

 4. Ictal—rarely, complex partial seizures cause violent behavior.

 5. Postictal—psychosis, confusion

B. **Epilepsy** (*cont'd*)

   6. Interictal

     a. Personality disturbances

       i. Hyper-religiosity

       ii. Viscous ("complex partial personality"); circumstantial, pedantic, ponderous speech; hypergraphia

       iii. Sexual behavior: hyposexuality most common; fetishism, transvestism, deviant interests

     b. Psychosis

       i. Usually develops after years of epilepsy

       ii. Often preceded by other personality changes

   7. Medications: all compounds that suppress cerebral activity can cause changes in energy, sleep, appetite, and concentration.

     a. **NB:** Topiramate

       i. Psychosis

       ii. Cognitive slowing

       iii. Anomia

     b. Benzodiazepines and barbiturates

       i. Cognitive impairment

       ii. Depression

     c. Keppra

       i. Irritability

       ii. Depression

     d. Anticholinergics

       i. Memory loss

       ii. Hallucinations

C. **Multiple sclerosis**

   1. Depression

     a. 25% to 50% of patients

     b. Carries a higher risk of suicide

   2. Witzelsucht

     a. Frontal subcortical dementia

     b. Subsyndromal mania

   3. Personality change—irritability or apathy

D. **Movement disorders**

   1. **NB:** *Parkinson's disease*

     a. Depression: may be difficult to distinguish from masked facies and generalized bradykinesias that are part of the motor manifestations of Parkinson's disease

       i. Present in 30% to 45% of patients

       ii. It may be presenting symptom, and it may not be correlated with motor severity.

     b. Dementia in 30%

     c. Psychosis

       i. Associated with dopamimetics, but can occur without

ii. Approach

(A) Rule out concurrent medical illness causing delirium.

(B) Decrease anti-Parkinson's medications, if possible.

(C) **NB:** Treat with *low-dose atypical antipsychotics (quetiapine or clozapine).*

2. **NB:** *Huntington's disease*

a. Can be accompanied by severe depression and suicidality

b. Dementia, psychosis, or irritability may precede motor dysfunction.

3. **NB:** Wilson's disease

a. Irritability and excessive emotionality may be first symptoms.

b. Delirium and dementia may present late or early.

4. Essential tremor

a. Associated with anxiety

b. Because of beneficial effects of ethanol, abuse may result.

E. **NB: Acute intermittent porphyria**

1. Affects females more than males; between ages 20 and 50 years

2. **NB:** *Recurrent triad:* abdominal pain, motor polyneuropathy, psychosis

3. Seizures in 15%

4. **NB:** Barbiturates and antiepileptics can exacerbate or precipitate attacks.

5. Treatment

a. Glucose and hematin infusions (to inhibit aminolevulinic acid [ALA] synthetase)

b. Gabapentin for seizures

F. **NB: B$_{12}$ deficiency (subacute combined degeneration)**

1. Usually results from poor absorption

a. Failure to secrete required intrinsic factor, or

b. Dysfunction of terminal ileum (absorption site)

2. Psychiatric: depression, dementia, delirium, psychosis

3. Neurologic abnormalities (present in 80%)

a. Length-dependent demyelinating polyneuropathy

b. Myelopathy (demyelination of posterior columns and lateral corticospinal tracts)

4. Hematologic abnormalities

a. Megaloblastic ("pernicious") anemia

b. Hypersegmented neutrophils

c. *May follow neuropsychiatric symptoms*

G. HIV

1. Depression very common

2. Dementia

3. Neuropsychiatric disturbances from secondary infections—neuropsychological assessment

4. HAND: HIV-associated neurocognitive disorder: associated with widespread white-matter involvement

H. **Thyroid disorders**

1. Hyperthyroidism

    a. Anxiety

    b. Apathy in elderly

2. Hypothyroidism

    a. Depression

    b. Cognitive decline

III. Intelligence

A. **Wechsler Adult Intelligence Scale and Wechsler Intelligence Scale for Children**

1. **NB:** Most common test used in clinical practice

2. Six verbal subtests: Information, Comprehension, Arithmetic, Similarities, Digit Span, Vocabulary

3. Four performance subtests: Block Design, Picture Arrangement, Object Assembly, Digit Symbol

4. Scores

    a. Mean = 100

    b. Standard deviation = 10

    c. Average range: 90 to 110

    d. Intelligence quotient less than 70 defines mental retardation (2.2% of population)

5. Advantages

    a. Extremely high reliability

    b. High validity for detecting mental retardation and predicting school performance

    c. Can be used to localize cerebral dysfunction

    d. Can compare function in different domains

6. Disadvantages

    a. Performance subtest is age-sensitive

    b. Some false lateralization with subcortical or parietal lesions

B. **Stanford-Binet Test**

1. Once the gold standard for children, but now less popular than Wechsler Intelligence Scale for Children

2. Mostly used in psychiatry and education

IV. Frontal Lobes

A. **Executive functioning and reasoning**

1. **NB:** Wisconsin Card Sorting Test

    a. Subject sorts cards with objects of different shape, color, form, and number

        i. Initially, the patient does not know the rule.

        ii. The examiner tells the patient whether the sorting is correct.

        iii. Scored by the number of trials required to obtain 10 consecutive correct responses

        iv. Once goal is achieved, the examiner changes the rule again.

    b. Tests *cognitive flexibility* (ability to avoid perseveration) and *abstract thought*

        i. Sensitive to *frontal lobe* dysfunction

        ii. Also abnormal in patients with schizophrenia and caudate lesions

  2. Tower of Hanoi, Tower of London

    a. Subject moves blocks from starting arrangement to goal arrangement.

    b. Scored by number of moves required (the fewer moves, the better)

    c. Excellent test of planning abilities/executive function

  3. **Bedside maneuvers**

    a. Ability to perform nonutile motor sequences (Luria tests): with minimal or no practice, the intact brain can learn simple motor sequences simply by mimicry; the more complex or variable the rhythm or sequence, the more sensitive the test is for frontal lobe dysfunction.

        i. Two-step hand sequence (reciprocally alternating fists and prone hands)

        ii. Three-step hand sequence ("fist-edge-palm")

        iii. Rhythm tapping

        iv. Alternating pattern (drawing alternating peaks and blocks)

    b. Suppression of motor impulses: the intact frontal lobes should be able to suppress the instinctive tendency to direct activity toward novel stimuli.

        i. Crossed response inhibition ("raise the hand that I don't touch")

        ii. Antisaccades ("look away from the finger that moves")

        iii. "Go/no-go" evaluates for errors of commission (e.g., tapping when asked not to)

    c. Creativity: the normal frontal lobes are able to categorize and retrieve items in memory that have concrete or abstract relationships to one another.

        i. "Thurstone" Controlled Oral Word Association Test ("all the words that start with the letter __")

        ii. Category fluency ("name all the [farm animals, cities] you can in 1 minute")

    d. Suppression of primitive reflexes: glabellar (Myerson's), snout, rooting, suck, Babinski, grasp (palmar and plantar), and palmomental reflexes are present in early life but sequentially extinguish as the frontal lobes myelinate and organize their function.

B. Attention

  1. Three types of attention

    a. Focused attention—seeking and finding an objective

    b. Sustained attention or vigilance—extended monitoring of an objective

    c. Divided attention—ability to perform two tasks simultaneously

  2. Tests

    a. **Trail making** (connect the dots)

        i. *Trails A*—connect dots in simple numerical order (focused attention)

        ii. *Trails B*—connect dots with alternating sequence of numerical and alphabetical order (i.e., 1-A-2-B-3-C. . . .) (divided attention)

        iii. Scored based on time to perform each test and difference in performance between A and B

    b. **Stroop test**

        i. Reading of words on cards with increasingly difficult-to-ignore distractors

    b. **Stroop test** (*cont'd*)

        ii. Most difficult is reporting the color in which a word representing a different color is printed (e.g., for the word "black" printed in green, the correct response is "green")

    c. NB: **Digit span: good bedside exam of attention**

        i. **Count backwards from 100 by 7, or 30 by 3**

V. Memory

A. **Temporal categorization**

    1. Working memory: a temporary storehouse for recently acquired (within the past minute) information; managed by the frontal lobes; usually able to store about seven or eight "chunks" of information

        a. Digit span and reverse digit span

        b. Memory for designs

        c. "N-back" test

    2. **Recent memory:** the collection of events over the past few minutes to hours

        a. Verbal memory: word lists (Hopkins Verbal Learning Test, Rey Auditory Verbal Learning Test)

        b. Visual memory: diagrams (Rey-Osterrieth Complex Figure)

    3. **Recent past memory:** extends over the past few months; asking about recent events in the patient's life or in the news is a useful test.

    4. **Remote memory:** concerns events in the distant past

        a. Although preserved (relative to more recent memories) in dementias and amnesias, usually not intact

B. **Categorization by type of data**

    1. Episodic memory: the recall of specific events (e.g., what you ate for breakfast today)

    2. Semantic memory: the storage of knowledge and facts (e.g., semantic memory is the storage of knowledge and facts)

    3. Procedural or implicit memory: preservation of learned automatic skills (e.g., riding a bicycle)

    4. *Semantic and implicit memories do not deteriorate with normal aging;* episodic memory may decline slightly because of age-related inefficiency of frontal processing.

VI. Perceptual and Motor Performance

A. **Bender Visual Motor Gestalt**

    1. Originally developed to test cognitive maturity of children

    2. Normal 12-year-old children can complete the test well.

    3. Consists of nine simple diagrams, which are directly copied by the patient

    4. Used to screen for cerebral dysfunction (*sensitive, but nonspecific*)

B. **Benton Facial Recognition Test**

    1. The patient is shown a head-on photograph of an unfamiliar face.

    2. The patient is shown the same face photographed in different ways (changed lighting or angle) and scored on the number of previously presented faces he or she recognizes

    3. Specific for *posterior right-hemisphere* lesions

C. **Hooper Visual Organization Test: subject names fragmented objects**

VII. Language Function

A. Lengthy, comprehensive tests

1. Boston Diagnostic Aphasia Examination
2. Western Aphasia Battery
3. Porch Index of Communicative Ability

B. Brief, but fairly complete: Reitan Aphasia Screening Test

C. Specific tests

1. Token Test: verbal comprehension
2. Boston Naming Test: naming pictured objects
3. Peabody Picture Vocabulary Test: auditory comprehension

VIII. Comprehensive Tests of Brain Function

A. Halstead-Reitan Battery

1. Domains tested
   a. Tactile perception (stereognosis, manual dexterity, finger localization, graphesthesia, simultaneous tactile stimulation)
   b. Auditory perception (rhythm discrimination, speech-sounds test)
   c. Abstraction (categorization test)
   d. Aphasia screening (naming, speech sounds, body part identification)
   e. Attention (trail-making test, flickering light)
   f. Visual perception (flickering light)
   g. Dexterity and motor speed (finger oscillation)
2. Long, intense test procedure
3. Reliably identifies subjects with brain damage

B. Luria-Nebraska Neuropsychological Battery

1. Tests broad range of cerebral function
2. Can localize dysfunction and identify particular disorders (i.e., sensitive and specific)
3. Can define hemispheric dominance

CHEAT SHEET

A. Main divisions

1. Left—language/praxis
2. Right—prosody, spatial representation, attention
3. Anterior of Sylvian fissure—action
4. Posterior of Sylvian fissure—perception
5. Dorsal—where
6. Ventral—what

(continued)

B. Language anatomy

1. Broca's area: inferior frontal (nonfluent, nonrepetitive, with intact comprehension)
2. Wernicke's area: superior temporal (fluent, nonrepetitive, with loss of comprehension)
3. Conduction: arcuate fasciculus (fluent, comprehension intact, with loss of repetition)

C. Frontal lobe: executive function

1. *Witzelsucht (inappropriate jocularity) is seen in patients with orbitofrontal cortex lesions.*
2. Pseudobulbar affect: exaggerated emotional response incongruent to mood; treat with dextromethorphan/quinidine sulfate

D. Parietal lobe: higher-order sensory processing

1. Gerstmann syndrome: tetrad—dysgraphia, dyscalculia, right-left disorientation, finger agnosia
2. Alexia without agraphia: intact writing with impaired reading due to damage to dominant occipital, parietal, and forceps major of corpus callosum
   i. Left PCA stroke
3. Balint's syndrome: Simultanagnosia, oculomotor apraxia, and optic ataxia

E. Temporal lobe: memory, language, and auditory processing

1. Klüver-Bucy syndrome: hyperorality, hypersexuality, apathy, hypermetamorphosis, and visual agnosia

F. Occipital lobe: visual processing

1. Anton syndrome: anosognosia for cortical blindness

G. Neuropsychological testing

1. Intelligence: Wechsler Intelligence Scale
2. Executive Functioning: Wisconsin Card Sorting, Tower of Hanoi
3. Attention: Stroop Color Naming, trail making, digit span
4. Memory: digit span, Rey-Osterrieth Complex Figure
5. Language: Boston Diagnostic Aphasia Exam

Suggested Readings

Behavioral neurology and neuropsychiatry [Entire issue]. *Continuum*.2015;21(3).

Darby D, Walsh K. *Walsh's Neuropsychology*, 5th ed. New York, NY: Elsevier;2005.

Lezak M. *Neuropsychological Assessment*, 4th ed. New York, NY: Oxford University Press;2004.

Snyder P, Nussbaum P, Robins D. *Clinical Neuropsychology: A Pocket Handbook for Assessment*, 2nd ed. Washington DC: American Psychological Association Press;2006.

50 Practice Questions With Answers

Practice Questions and Answers

Questions

1. Activation of a postsynaptic acetyl choline receptors results in which of the following?

   a. An efflux of Na^+ into the cell and an efflux of K^+, depolarizing the postsynaptic neuron

   b. An influx of Na^+ into the cell and an efflux of K^+, depolarizing the postsynaptic neuron

   c. An influx of Na^+ into the cell and an influx of K^+, depolarizing the postsynaptic neuron

   d. An influx of Na^+ into the cell and an efflux of K^+, repolarizing the postsynaptic neuron

   e. An efflux of Na^+ into the cell and an influx of K^+, repolarizing the postsynaptic neuron

2. Atropine and scopolamine

   a. block ACh actions only at muscarinic receptors.

   b. inhibit the release of AChr.

   c. prevent Ach receptor channel opening.

   d. prevent Ach receptor channel opening at motor end plate.

   e. block presymptomatic vesicle mobility.

3. Of the four main dopaminergic tracts, the

   a. nigrostriatal tract accounts for only a small part of the brain's dopamine.

   b. tuberoinfundibular tract controls release of prolactin via D3 receptors.

   c. tuberoinfundibular tract controls release of prolactin via D2 receptors.

   d. mesolimbic tract controls release of prolactin via D3 receptors.

   e. mesocortical tract controls release of prolactin via D2 receptors.

4. Raphe nuclei

   a. project rostrally, mainly in the medulla and spinal cord.

   b. project caudally to the limbic structures and the cerebral cortex.

   c. project caudally, mainly to the medulla and spinal cord.

   d. stimulation produces effects similar to those of glutamate.

   e. lie dorsally in the diencephalon.

5. Which of the following is true regarding Prader-Willi syndrome and Angelman's syndrome?

   a. Prader-Willi syndrome is paternally inherited with maternal imprinting; Angelman's syndrome is paternally inherited with maternal imprinting.

   b. Prader-Willi syndrome is maternally inherited with maternal imprinting; Angelman's syndrome is paternally inherited with paternal imprinting.

   c. Prader-Willi syndrome is maternally inherited with paternal imprinting: Angelman's syndrome is paternally inherited with maternal imprinting.

   d. Prader-Willi syndrome is paternally inherited with maternal imprinting; Angelman's syndrome is maternally inherited with paternal imprinting.

   e. In both Prader-Willi syndrome and Angelman's syndrome, genes inherited from the father are silenced via methylation.

6. Trinucleotide repeats are seen in which of the following genetic conditions?

   a. Alzheimer's disease; fragile X; Huntington's disease

   b. Friedreich's ataxia; AR torsion dystonia; myotonic dystrophy

   c. FTD; Segawa syndrome; fragile X

   d. Myotonic dystrophy; adult-onset focal dystonia; Alzheimer's disease

   e. Fragile X; myotonic dystrophy; Friedreich's ataxia

7. Which of the following clinical syndromes is matched with the appropriate region of protein/ gene abnormality?

   a. Kallmann's anosmia-hypogonadism: ATP-binding cassette transporter 7(ABCB7)

   b. Rett syndrome: cyclin-dependent kinase-like 5 (CDKL5)

   c. LIS1: reelin (RELN)

   d. LISX1: alpha-1-tubulin (TUBA1A)

   e. Holoprosencephaly: sonic hedgehog (SHH)

8. Which of the following statements related to disorders of primary neurulation is (are) correct?

   a. Spina bifida results from failure of the anterior neuropore to form.

   b. Spina bifida aperta is associated with a neurological deficit in 90% of those affected.

   c. Meningocele is a herniation of a cerebrospinal-fluid-filled sac with neural elements.

   d. Meningocele is a herniation of a cerebrospinal-fluid-filled sac without neural elements.

   e. B and D

   f. A, B, and C

9. Dandy-Walker syndrome is characterized by which of the following?

   a. Failure of foramen Magendie development; enlarged cerebellar vermis; agenesis of the corpus callosum

   b. Depression of the inion; cardiac abnormalities; increased migrational disorders

   c. Failure of foramen of Magendie development; cystic dilation of 4th ventricle; cerebellar vermis agenesis with enlarged posterior fossa

   d. Holoprosencephaly; elevation of the inion; agenesis of corpus callosum

   e. Absent septum pellucidum; hypoplastic optic nerves: schizencephaly

10. The shaded area represents which brain area?

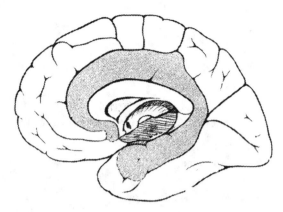

    a. Somatosensory association cortex

    b. Parahippocampal gyrus

    c. Hippocampal gyrus

    d. Prefrontal cortex

    e. Limbic system

11. Which of the following thalamic nuclei is matched with the appropriate inputs and projections?

    a. Anterior: mammillary nucleus of the hypothalamus; cingulate gyrus

    b. Anterior: globus pallidus; striatum

    c. Pulvinar: association areas; striatum

    d. Ventroposterolateral: trigeminothalamic tracts; sensory cortex

    e. Lateral geniculate body: auditory input; primary auditory cortex

12. Which of the following superior-division middle cerebral artery branches is matched to the correct clinical syndrome?

    a. Ascending frontal branch: brachial monoplegia

    b. Ascending parietal: conduction aphasia

    c. Cortical-subcortical: brachial monoplegia

    d. Rolandic: primarily cortical sensory deficit

    e. Ascending parietal: agrammatic speech with normal comprehension

13. Which aphasia type is matched with the correct characteristics of comprehension, fluency, repetition, and naming?

    a. Transcortical sensory: spared comprehension, normal fluency, normal repetition, impaired naming

    b. Global aphasia: impaired comprehension, impaired fluency, spared repetition, impaired naming

    c. Broca: impaired comprehension, impaired fluency, impaired repetition, impaired naming

    d. Transcortical motor: spared comprehension, impaired fluency, normal repetition, impaired naming

    e. Conduction: spared comprehension, impaired fluency, normal repetition, impaired naming

14. Balint's syndrome of oculomotor apraxia, optic ataxia, and asimultagnosia can be due to

    a. bilateral mesial frontal infarction.

    b. mesial hippocampal infarction.

    c. lateral temporal infarction.

    d. infarction of Striae of Gennari.

    e. bilateral occipito-parietal infarctions.

15. Contralateral paralysis of the arm and leg, contralateral impaired tactile and proprioceptive sense, and ipsilateral tongue paralysis are seen in which of the following syndromes?

    a. Posterior medullary region

    b. Avellis syndrome

    c. Wallenberg syndrome

    d. Jackson syndrome

    e. Medial medullary syndrome

16. IV thrombolysis with tissue plasminogen activator is approved by the FDA for which of the following?

    a. Ischemic stroke presenting within 4.5 hours

    b. Ischemic stroke presenting within 3 hours

    c. Hemorrhagic stroke presenting within 3 hours

    d. TIA presenting within 3 hours

    e. Lacunar stroke presenting within 3 hours

17. Concussion is defined as

    a. bruising of the brain without interruption of its architecture.

    b. contre-coup injury.

    c. violent shaking or jarring of the brain with transient functional impairment.

    d. head injury with definite loss of consciousness.

    e. focal injury at the site of impact.

18. Which of the following statements is correct regarding minor head injury?

    a. CT imaging is mandatory with minor head injury.

    b. All minor head injuries should be evaluated by a neurologist.

    c. There is a 1-in-1,000 chance of intracranial hemorrhage if no fracture and mentally clear.

    d. There is a 1-in-500 chance of intracranial hemorrhage if no fracture and mentally clear.

    e. There is a 1-in-100 chance of intracranial hemorrhage if no fracture and mentally clear.

19. Chronic subdural hematomas

    a. occur after a lucid period.

    b. generally occur weeks after a well-defined head injury.

    c. can cause aphasia as a common presentation.

    d. require immediate burr-hole evacuation.

    e. may be accompanied by giddiness, slowness of thinking, confusion, or apathy.

20. Which of the following is correct regarding treatment of refractory hypertension in the neurological ICU?

    a. Blood pressure should be reduced if SBP $>$185, regardless of baseline blood pressure.

    b. Nitroprusside is an acceptable treatment for hypertension in this setting.

    c. Nicardipine, hydralazine, or labetalol is recommended for the NICU setting.

    d. Aim is to keep MAP $<$90.

    e. Aim is to keep MAP $<$110.

21. Which of the following is true regarding intracranial hematoma expansion?

    a. It does not occur after first presentation except in rare circumstances.

    b. It is less likely in poorly controlled diabetics

    c. Patients may show the "spot sign."

    d. Patients may show the "dot sign."

    e. Antiplatelets increase the risk for ICH expansion.

22. Mild cognitive impairment (MCI) differs from dementia in that

    a. language disorders are uncommon in MCI.

    b. activities of daily living are generally spared.

    c. patient retains insight into problems with memory.

    d. MRI imaging differs between MCI and dementia.

    e. α beta 42 CSF levels are normal in MCI.

23. Alzheimer's disease is

    a. more likely with higher education.

    b. more likely with moderate drinking.

    c. more likely with apolipoprotein E2 allele.

    d. less common with Down syndrome.

    e. more common with midlife obesity.

24. Which of the following is true regarding Lewy body disease (LBD) pathology?

    a. It consists of amyloid deposition in the striata nigra.

    b. Patient has antibodies against ubiquitin or alpha-synuclein.

    c. It never occurs with Alzheimer's pathology.

    d. Patient has Lewy bodies (intracellular eosinophilic core with peripheral halo).

    e. Defects in NMDA have been described in LBD.

25. Frontotemporal dementia can present with which of the following?

    a. Semantic dementia; apathy; nonfluent aphasia

    b. ALS and behavioral disorders; cortical blindness; ataxia

    c. Nonfluent aphasia; memory disorder; myoclonic seizures

    d. Diffuse myoclonus; logopenic aphasia; simultanagnosia

    e. Depression; apraxia for limb kinetic activities; abulia

26. Migraine without aura includes

    a. headache attacks lasting 1 to 3 hours.

    b. improvement with exercise.

    c. bilateral temporal distribution.

    d. pulsatile quality.

    e. mild pain intensity.

27. A 54-year-old male patient comes to your practice. He has recurrent unilateral supraorbital attacks of pain lasting 2 minutes. These occur from 5 to 25 times a day. During the pain, he notices he has increased tearing. He has had these attacks for the past year and has had a workup for mass lesions, which was negative. You diagnose which of the following?

    a. Temporal arteritis

    b. Paroxysmal hemicranias

    c. Migraine with autonomic features

    d. Secondary headache due to undiagnosed orbital pseudotumor

    e. SUNCT

28. Which of the following is the most appropriate match between muscle fiber type and characteristics?

    a. Type 1: tonic; dark color; small fiber diameter; slow twitch speed; low fatigability

    b. Type 1: phasic; dark color; small fiber diameter; fast twitch speed; low fatigability

   c. Type 2a: phasic; pale color; largest fiber diameter; fast twitch speed; low fatigability

   d. Type 2b: Tonic; dark color; small fiber diameter; slow twitch speed; low fatigability

   e. Type 2b; Phasic; pale color; largest fiber diameter; slow twitch speed; high fatigability

29. In differentiating a peroneal nerve lesion from an L5 root lesion, which of the following signs is most useful?

   a. Knee flexion weakness

   b. Knee extension weakness

   c. Foot everter weakness

   d. Intrinsic foot muscle weakness

   e. Foot inverter weakness

30. Meralgia paresthetica

   a. is a psychiatric dissociation disorder.

   b. was described by Karl Jung.

   c. is due to entrapment of the lateral femoral cutaneous nerve.

   d. can be reliably diagnosed by electrophysiology.

   e. is usually treated surgically.

31. A 15-year-old boy comes into your clinic with his mother. He had an early morning generalized tonic-clonic seizure 2 weeks ago and is now on phenytoin 100 mg three times a day. His mother notes that in the mornings, he may have episodes of staring for a few seconds, and tends to jerk his arms for an hour after awakening. There is no developmental or family history of significance. His EEG shows 4- to 5-Hz generalized spike and wave. The mother notes that the jerks and staring spells are more prominent since beginning the medicine. Your next move is to

   a. raise the phenytoin to 200 mg twice a day

   b. switch to carbamazepine.

   c. switch to lacosamide.

   d. switch to valproic acid.

   e. switch to topiramate.

32. A 1-year-old child is brought to your clinic by his parents. At age 4 months he began to have episodes of suddenly flexing his body and arms. Development has slowed, and he has episodes hundreds of times a day. His EEG shows hypsarrhythmia. Imaging has not yet been done. Your diagnosis is which of the following?

   a. Aicardi's syndrome

   b. Lennox-Gastaut syndrome

   c. MERRF

   d. Sialidosis type 1

   e. West's syndrome

33. A 23-year-old female known to have complex partial seizures treated with carbamazepine is brought to the emergency room after having had three seizures in the past half hour. She remains unconscious, breathing shallowly. After ABCs, insertion of an IV, and institution of monitoring, you decide to treat her by

   a. giving diazepam 10 mg IV.

   b. giving pentobarbital due to refractory status.

   c. giving midazolam due to refractory status.

    d. loading IV carbamazepine.

    e. giving lorazepam 0.1-mg/kg bolus.

34-38.   Match each movement disorder with the appropriate MRI finding.

34.	PKAN	a. "Hot cross bun" sign
35.	PSP	b. "Eye of the tiger" sign
36.	MSA	c. Hummingbird sign
37.	CBD	d. Asymmetric MRI atrophy
38.	Variant CJD	e. Pulvinar sign

39. You have a 34-year-old patient with relapsing-remitting MS who has had three relapses treated with high-dose IV solumedrol in the past year. Her MRI continues to show new lesion activity with gadolinium-positive lesions despite treatment with a low-dose interferon. Your next treatment strategy might include the following, but will be tempered by the risk of the linked complication:

    a. Natalizumab; treatment-related acute leukemia

    b. Fingolimod; autoimmune hepatitis

    c. Alemtuzumab; idiopathic thrombocytopenic purpura

    d. Cyclophosphamide; Grave's disease

    e. Mitoxantrone: progressive multifocal leukoencephalopathy

40. You have a 12-year-old patient who, after an initial viral illness, develops confusion, fever and tachycardia, nystagmus, brisk reflexes, pale optic discs, and upgoing toes. The MRI shows diffuse white-matter lesions that also affect the basal ganglia and spinal cord. CSF shows 34 white cells 90% lymphs, protein slightly elevated, and normal CSF glucose with no oligoclonal bands. You make which diagnosis?

    a. Acute necrotizing hemorrhagic encephalomyelitis

    b. Schilder's disease

    c. Neuromyelitis optica spectrum disorder

    d. Acute disseminated encephalomyelitis

    e. Bal\u00f3's concentric sclerosis

41. West Nile virus infection

    a. usually causes a Guillain-Barre-like illness.

    b. causes symptoms in most affected individuals.

    c. occurs primarily in young, healthy teenagers.

    d. shows characteristic lesions on MRI.

    e. rarely causes a syndrome of acute flaccid paralysis.

42. A 16-year-old male develops behavioral and personality changes followed 1 month later by myoclonus, ataxia, and difficulty with language. After 3 months the patient develops visual loss and quadriparesis, and gradually slips into a coma. Late in his course the EEG shows burst suppression. This condition

    a. is a delayed response to herpes zoster infection.

    b. is due to a slow virus infection.

c. can be effectively treated by rituximab.

d. is due to a rubella.

e. is due to defective viral maturation in the brain.

43–46.   Match each neurotoxin to the appropriate clinical finding.

43. Arsenic poisoning   a. Alopecia

44. Thallium poisoning   b. Mees' lines

45. Lead poisoning   c. Bradykinesia

46. Manganese poisoning   d. Burtonian line

47. Triphasic waves

   a. are pathognomonic of hepatic encephalopathy.

   b. are pathognomonic for CJD.

   c. are a late finding of status epilepticus.

   d. are seen in a variety of encephalopathies.

   e. respond to benzodiazepine treatment.

48. Which of the following is true regarding the hypogastric nerve?

   a. It provides striated muscle relaxation via beta-adrenergic receptors.

   b. The postganglionic efferent nerves exit at T10-L2.

   c. The nerves travel via the hypogastric nerve to the superior pelvic plexus.

   d. It provides smooth muscle relaxation via alpha-adrenergic receptors.

   e. It provides smooth muscle relaxation via beta-adrenergic receptors.

49. Downbeat nystagmus is a sign of which of the following?

   a. A lesion of the parasellar region

   b. A lesion of the dorsal midbrain

   c. Lesion of Mollaret's triangle

   d. A massive pontine lesion

   e. A lesion of the cervicomedullary junction

50. Ménière's syndrome

   a. causes persistent hearing loss from onset.

   b. causes positional vertigo.

   c. is due to reduction of endolymph pressure.

   d. causes episodic vertigo.

   e. causes vertigo with compression of the tragus.

And 10 More Bonus Questions

1. Which of the following is true regarding SIADH?

   a. Laboratory findings show hyponatremia with inappropriate urine osmolality.

   b. Laboratory findings show hypernatremia with inappropriate urine osmolality.

   c. Laboratory findings show euvolemia with inappropriate urine osmolality.

    d. It is improved by increased free water.

    e. It is often seen after severe head injury.

2. Which of the following is true regarding oligodendrogliomas?

    a. They account for 25% of intracranial gliomas.

    b. They usually affect the brainstem.

    c. Deletion of 1p19q causes a better treatment response.

    d. They rarely calcify.

    e. They cause a scrambled-egg appearance on pathology.

3–6.   Match each syndrome with the most common antibody syndrome.

3. Progressive encephalomyelitis   a. GAD-65

4. Sensory neuropathy   b. anti-Hu

5. Stiff-person syndrome   c. VGCC

6. Lambert-Eaton syndrome   d. GlyR

7. Features related to clozapine include which of the following?

    a. Lack of EPS; agranulocytosis; elevated seizure threshold

    b. More dopamine than 5-HT blockade

    c. Approved for treatment of TD: most effective antipsychotic

    d. Mild anticholinergic effects; lowers seizure threshold

    e. Agranulocytosis: primarily D3 blockade

8. Fragile X syndrome is caused by a

    a. binucleotide repeat at chromosomal locus Xq27.3.

    b. trinucleotide repeat at chromosomal locus Xq27.3.

    c. trinucleotide repeat at chromosomal locus Xq26.3.

    d. tetranucleotide repeat at chromosomal locus Xq26.3.

    e. trinucleotide repeat at chromosomal locus Xq25.3.

9. Anton's syndrome causes

    a. right homonymous hemianopsia.

    b. apraxia of the left hand.

    c. retention of reactive pupils.

    d. prosopagnosia.

    e. visuospatial disorientation.

10. Klüver-Bucy syndrome

    a. is usually seen with posterior temporal damage.

    b. may be seen with unilateral temporal damage.

    c. is associated with hyposexuality.

    d. is associated with hyperorality.

    e. results in inattention to stimuli in the environment.

Answers

1. *b. An influx of Na$^+$ into the cell and an efflux of K$^+$, depolarizing the postsynaptic neuron*

   The voltage-gated calcium channel is open as the action potential (AP) reaches the terminal bouton of the presynaptic neuron, producing an influx of calcium ions that allows exocytosis of presynaptic vesicles containing ACh into the synaptic cleft. The activation of postsynaptic ACh receptors results in an influx of Na$^+$ into the cell and an efflux of K$^+$, which depolarizes the postsynaptic neuron, propagating a new AP.

2. *a. Block ACh actions only at muscarinic receptors.*

   Atropine and scopolamine block ACh actions only at muscarinic receptors. Botulinum toxin inhibits the release of ACh. Beta bungarotoxin prevents ACh receptor channel opening. D-Tubocurarine prevents ACh receptor channel opening at motor endplates. Botulinum toxin blocks presymptomatic vesicle mobility.

3. *c. tuberoinfundibular tract controls release of prolactin via D2 receptors.*

   The nigrostriatal tract accounts for most of the brain's dopamine. The tuberoinfundibular tract controls release of prolactin via D2 receptors.

4. *c. project caudally, mainly to the medulla and spinal cord.*

   The raphe nuclei also project rostrally to the limbic structures and cerebral cortex. Stimulation of the raphe nuclei produces effects similar to those of lysergic acid diethylamide (LSD). Raphe nuclei are located in the brainstem.

5. *d. Prader-Willi syndrome is paternally inherited with maternal imprinting; Angelman's syndrome is maternally inherited with paternal imprinting.*

   DNA and histone methylation allow transcriptional silencing of individual genes, as well as regions of chromosomes. Genomic imprinting is the regulation of gene expression depending on the parental origin of the gene. In paternal imprinting, genes inherited from the father are silenced through methylation, and only those from the mother are expressed. Maternal imprinting is the opposite.

6. *e. Fragile X; myotonic dystrophy; Friedreich's ataxia*

   CAG repeat diseases are the most common trinucleotide repeat syndromes in neurology. Examples include Huntington's, spinocerebellar ataxia type 1 and other SCAs, spinobulbar muscular atrophy, and dentatorubropallidoluysian syndrome. Fragile X is a CGG repeat ("Child with Giant Gonads"). Myotonic dystrophy is due to a CTG repeat ("Continues To Grasp"). Friedreich's ataxia is due to a GAA repeat ("German [name] AtaxiA").

7. *e. Holoprosencephaly: sonic hedgehog (SHH)*

   Kallmann's syndrome (anosmia, hypogonadism) is an X-linked recessive disorder related to abnormalities in the enzyme anosmin related to the gene KAL1. Rett syndrome is an X-linked dominant condition related to abnormalities in methyl-CpG-binding protein 2 (gene MECP2). LIS1 (Miller-Dieker syndrome) is autosomal recessive and related to abnormalities in the enzyme LIS1 (gene PAFAH1B1). LISX1 is an X-linked dominant condition related to abnormalities of doublcortin (gene DBX).

8. *e. B and D*

   Spina bifida aperta is associated with a neurological deficit in 90% of cases. **Meningocele** is a herniation of a cerebrospinal-fluid-filled sac without neural elements. Spina bifida results from failure of the posterior neuropore to form. **Myelomeningocele**: herniated neural elements covered by meningeal sac; 80% are lumbar; 90% have hydrocephalus if lumbar is involved; symptoms include motor, sensory, and sphincter dysfunction. **Myeloschisis**: neural elements at surface completely uncovered; associated with malformed skull base; most babies are stillborn. **Myelocystocele**: herniation of meninges and cord with dilated central canal.

9. c. *Failure of foramen of Magendie development; cystic dilation of 4th ventricle; cerebellar vermis agenesis with enlarged posterior fossa*

   Dandy-Walker malformation is association with failure of foramen of Magendie development; cystic dilation of 4th ventricle; cerebellar vermis agenesis with enlarged posterior fossa; elevation of the inion; agenesis of the corpus callosum; 70% with migrational disorders; associated with cardiac abnormalities and urinary tract infections; frequency: 1:25,000; may result from riboflavin inhibitors, posterior fossa trauma, or viral infection. **Septo-optic dysplasia** is associated with absent or hypoplastic septum pellucidum, hypoplastic optic nerves, schizencephaly in approximately 50% but normal-sized ventricles, pituitary axis dysfunction (50% with diabetes insipidus).

10. e. *Limbic system*

    The limbic system incorporates several structures involved in emotion, memory, olfaction, and other evolutionarily ancient functions. The limbic pathways include the circuit of Papez: subiculum–fornix–mamillary body–mamillothalamic tract–anterior nucleus of thalamus–anterior limb of internal capsule–cingulate gyrus–cingulum–entorhinal cortex–perforant pathway–subiculum and hippocampus; olfactory projections; hippocampal formation projections and amygdalar connections.

11. a. *Anterior: mammillary nucleus of the hypothalamus; cingulate gyrus*

    The anterior thalamic nuclei have inputs from mammillary nuclei of the hypothalamus and projections to the cingulate gyrus. The pulvinar connects reciprocally with large association areas of the parietal, temporal, and occipital lobes. The ventroposterolateral nuclei have inputs from the spinothalamic tracts and medial lemnisci, and project to the sensory cortex. The ventroposteromedial nuclei receive input from trigeminothalamic tracts and nucleus solitarius and project to the sensory cortex. The lateral geniculate body has inputs from the retina via the optic tract, and projects to the visual cortex. The medial geniculate body receives auditory input via the brachium of the inferior colliculus and projects to the primary auditory cortex.

12. c. *Cortical-subcortical: brachial monoplegia*

    The **cortical-subcortical branches** of the superior division of the MCA cause a brachial monoplegia. **Ascending frontal branches** cause initial mutism and mild comprehension defect, then slightly dysfluent, agrammatic speech with normal comprehension. **Rolandic branches** are associated with sensorimotor paresis with severe dysarthria but little aphasia. **Ascending parietal**: no sensorimotor defect, only a conduction aphasia.

13. d. *Transcortical motor: spared comprehension, impaired fluency, normal repetition, impaired naming*

Type	Comprehension	Fluency	Repetition	Naming
Broca	Normal	Impaired	Impaired	Impaired
Wernicke	Impaired	Normal	Impaired	Impaired
Conduction	Normal	Normal	Impaired	Normal/impaired
Transcortical motor	Normal	Impaired	Normal	Impaired
Transcortical sensory	Impaired	Normal	Normal	Impaired
Mixed transcortical	Impaired	Impaired	Normal	Impaired
Global	Impaired	Impaired	Impaired	Impaired

14. e. *bilateral occipito-parietal infarctions.*

    Balint's syndrome is usually caused by watershed infarctions between the posterior and middle cerebral artery territories caused by hypoperfusion. It causes oculomotor apraxia (inability to direct eyes to object of interest), optic ataxia (failure to grasp objects under visual guidance), and simultanagnosia (inability to perceive more than a single object at a time in a scene that contains more than one object).

15. e. *Medial medullary syndrome*

Lateral medullary syndrome/Wallenberg syndrome: vestibular nuclei (nystagmus, oscillopsia, vertigo, nausea, vomiting); spinothalamic tract (contralateral impairment of pain and thermal sense over one-half the body); descending sympathetic tract (ipsilateral Horner's—ptosis, miosis, anhidrosis); cranial nerves (CNs) IX and X (hoarseness, dysphagia, ipsilateral paralysis of palate and vocal cord, diminished gag); otolithic nucleus (vertical diplopia and illusion of tilting of vision); olivocerebellar and/or spinocerebellar fibers/restiform body (ipsilateral ataxia of limbs, falling to ipsilateral side); nucleus and tractus solitarius (loss of taste); descending tract and nucleus of V (pain, burning, impaired sensation on ipsilateral one-half of face; rarely nucleus cuneatus and gracilis (ipsilateral numbness of limbs); most likely due to occlusion of vertebral artery (eight-tenths) or posterior-inferior cerebellar artery. **Opalski syndrome**: considered a variant of lateral medullary syndrome with ipsilateral hemiplegia, likely due to caudal extension of the infarct due to involvement of perforator branches arising from the distal vertebral artery. **Medial medullary syndrome**: involves medullary pyramid (contralateral paralysis of arm and leg); medial lemniscus (contralateral impaired tactile and proprioceptive sense over one-half the body); CN XII (ipsilateral paralysis and, later, hemiatrophy of the tongue). **Hemimedullary infarction (Babinski–Nageotte syndrome)**: occlusion of the ipsilateral vertebral artery proximal to the posterior-inferior cerebellar artery and its anterior spinal artery causes medial medullary syndrome and lateral medullary syndrome simultaneously. **Posterior medullary region**: ipsilateral cerebellar ataxia and, rarely, hiccups. **Avellis syndrome**: tegmentum of medulla: CN X, spinothalamic tract (paralysis of soft palate and vocal cord and contralateral hemianesthesia). **Jackson syndrome**: tegmentum of medulla: CN X, XII, corticospinal tract (Avellis syndrome plus ipsilateral tongue paralysis).

16. b. *Ischemic stroke presenting within 3 hours*

The NINDS Tissue Plasminogen Activator (tPA) trial established the efficacy of intravenous (IV) tPA for patients presenting within 3 hours from symptom onset. Compared to placebo, patients treated with tPA had a 16% absolute increase in favorable outcomes at 3 months. IV tPA is approved by the FDA for ischemic stroke presenting within 3 hours from last known normal. No consent is required for this time window. For patients presenting after 3 hours but before 4.5 hrs, ECASS III was the first study to show a statistical benefit for IV tPA use, with a slightly higher intracranial hemorrhage rate. The American Heart Association and American Stroke Association recommend the use of IV tPA for patients presenting between 3 and 4.5 hours from last known normal; however, this is not FDA approved.

17. c. *violent shaking or jarring of the brain with resulting transient functional impairment.*

Loss of consciousness is not required for the diagnosis of concussion. **Contusion** is bruising of the brain without interruption of its architecture. A **coup injury** usually occurs when the head is immobilized, and damage is focused at the site of impact. A **contre-coup injury** is injury opposite to the site of impact due to the head not being immobilized (brain thrown into opposite region of the skull).

18. c. *There is a 1-in-1,000 chance of intracranial hemorrhage if no fracture and mentally clear.*

CT imaging is not mandatory with minor head injury. Neurologists are not needed in the evaluation of all minor head injuries.

19. e. *May be accompanied by giddiness, slowness of thinking, confusion, or apathy*

Chronic subdural hematomas are generally due to traumatic injury that was trivial or forgotten. A period of weeks passes before onset of headaches, giddiness, slowness of thinking, confusion, apathy, drowsiness, or seizures. CSF may be clear, bloody, acellular, to xanthochromic (generally not recommended due to mass effect; diagnosis usually by CT or MRI). A subdural hygroma (collection of blood and CSF in subdural space) may form in the potential space created by the SDH.

20. *c. Nicardipine, hydralazine, and labetalol are recommended for the NICU setting.*

Blood pressure reduction should take into account prehospitalization baseline blood pressures. Nitroprusside may cause venodilation, which may lead to increased intracranial pressure. Aim is to keep MAP (mean arterial pressure) less than 130.

21. *c. Patients may show the "spot sign."*

CT may show a hyperdense spot within a hematoma, suggesting active bleeding. CTA may assist in locating a bleeding source. Nearly half of all ICHs expand in size from presentation within first few hours. Most stabilize in 24 hours. Most ICH patients should be monitored in an appropriate ICU. Antiplatelets have not been shown to increase risk for ICH expansion.

22. *b. activities of daily living are generally spared.*

Patients with MCI can have language disorders, although usually they present with memory impairment. Patients may not retain insight into memory problems, although issues with insight tend to be less than with dementia. MRI imaging does not discriminate between MCI and dementia. α-beta 42 CSF levels may be reduced in MCI prior to onset of dementia. They may predict Alzheimer's pathology but do not indicate present severity of cognitive deficit.

23. *e. more common with midlife obesity.*

Alzheimer's disease is the most common degenerative disease of the brain. The incidence increases sharply with age after 65. Age is the most important risk factor. Other risk factors include Down syndrome (patient 30–45 y/o shows similar pathologic changes), midlife obesity, diabetes mellitus, current tobacco use, head injury, apolipoprotein E 4 genotype; reported protective factors: education, Mediterranean-type diet, low or moderate alcohol intake, physical activity, inheritance of apolipoprotein E2 allele. Dominant AD can occur with multiple genetic mutations (presenilin 1 [PS1] most common, presenilin 2 [PS2], amyloid precursor protein [APP], C9 open reading frame 72, Trem2, etc.).

24. *b. Patient has antibodies against ubiquitin or alpha-synuclein.*

LBD shows Lewy bodies in brainstem nuclei, subcortical regions, and cerebral cortices. In the brainstem, pigmented neurons often present with the classic morphology of intracellular LBs, comprising an eosinophilic core with a peripheral halo; immunohistochemistry using antibodies against ubiquitin or α-synuclein has been shown to be more sensitive and specific in the detection of cortical LB; the clinical overlap of AD, DLB, and PD with dementia similarly extends to their pathology—most cases of DLB have varying degrees of AD pathology, including deposits of β-amyloid protein and neurofibrillary tangles. Neurochemistry: substantial loss of cholinergic neurons in the nucleus basalis of Meynert, suggesting a cholinergic mechanism of cognitive impairment in DLB, similar to that of AD; deficits in γ-aminobutyric acid (GABA), dopamine, and serotonin neurotransmission have also been described in DLB; neocortical choline acetyltransferase, a synthetic enzyme for acetylcholine, is decreased significantly, similar to that seen in AD or PD with dementia; reduced dopamine and its metabolites have been shown in DLB brains, possibly accounting for its parkinsonian features.

25. *a. Semantic dementia; apathy; nonfluent aphasia*

Frontotemporal dementia can have various presentations. Most commonly presents with behavioral variant, either disinhibition or apathy, often with personality change, loss of judgment, altered appetites (often bizarre appetites), difficulty with decision making, and sometimes sexual disinhibition. Other variants include semantic dementia, with problems with fluent empty speech, naming impairment, and difficulty with identifying objects. Occasionally patients have a progressive nonfluent aphasia. Some patients can have ALS and FTD in combination.

26. *d. pulsatile quality,*

    Migraine without aura:

    At least five attacks fulfilling criteria

        Headache attacks lasting 4 to 72 hours

        Headache has at least two of the following characteristics:

            Unilateral location

            Pulsating quality

            Moderate or severe pain intensity

    Aggravation by or causing avoidance of routine physical activity

        During headache at least one of the following:

            Nausea and/or vomiting

        Photophobia and phonophobia

        Not attributed to another disorder

27. *e. SUNCT*

SUNCT (short-lasting unilateral neuralgiform headache with conjunctival injection and tearing) is a rare headache syndrome, most common men over 50, involving bursts of moderate to severe burning, piercing, throbbing pain around eye or temple one side. Peaks in seconds lasts from 5 seconds to 4 minutes. Associated with conjunctival injection, nasal congestion, runny nose, sweaty forehead, swelling of the eyelid, and pressure in the eye. May occur up to 5 to 6 times per hour. Corticosteroids, gabapentin, lamotrigine, and carbamazepine may be helpful. Glycerol injections have been used in severe cases. Temporal arteritis causes persistent headache without autonomic features. **Paroxysmal hemicrania** is a rare adult-onset headache syndrome. Pain is severe throbbing or boring pain on one side of face. Associated with red and tearing eyes, drooping eyelid. Episodes occur 5 to 30 times per day and last 2 to 30 minutes. NSAIDs, particularly indomethacin, provide relief, but dosing may need to be high. Migraines last longer than this headache syndrome. Orbital pseudotumor has been ruled out.

28. *a. Type 1: tonic; dark color; small fiber diameter; slow twitch speed; low fatigability*

Types of muscle fibers

	Type 1	Type 2a	Type 2b
Axon innervating	Smaller	Larger	Larger
Type	Tonic	Phasic	Phasic
Color	Dark	Dark	Pale
Fiber diameter	Small	Larger	Largest
Twitch speed	Slow	Fast	Fast
Fatigability	Low	Low	High

29. *e. Foot inverter weakness*

Everters and dorsiflexors of the foot are innervated by peroneal nerve muscles. Foot inverters are innervated by the tibial nerve. Both are partially supplied by L5. Thus in a peroneal nerve palsy, foot inverters will be spared, but will be weak in L5 root disorder.

30. *c. is due to entrapment of the lateral femoral cutaneous nerve.*

Meralgia paresthetica is an entrapment of the lateral femoral cutaneous nerve, usually as it enters the pelvis between the inguinal ligament and its attachment to the anterior superior iliac spine. It was described by Sigmund Freud in the 1800s. It cannot be reliably diagnosed by electrophysiology in many cases. It is usually treated conservatively with looser garments and belts, weight reduction, reposition of seats, and possibly medications to reduce burning paresthesias.

31. *d. switch to valproic acid.*

This case is characteristic of juvenile myoclonic epilepsy. This subtype of myoclonic epilepsy usually begins at age 12 to 16 with myoclonic events and tonic-clonic seizures with occasional atypical absence. Genetic localization is chromosome 6p. May be increased by photic stimulation and sleep deprivation. The treatment of choice is valproic acid, and patients may not respond to other, older antiepileptics.

32. *e. West's syndrome*

This patient has typical age of onset and clinical manifestations of West's syndrome. This begins between age 3 months and 3 years, with tonic spasms (brief, rapid tonic contractures of trunk and limbs lasting few seconds), which may be flexor, extensor, or mixed. These may occur up to hundreds of times a day. Patients experience mental retardation. EEG shows hypsarrhythmia, a characteristic pattern with chaotic high- to extremely-high-voltage delta and theta with superimposed multiple spike and wave. Treatment consists of ACTH or vigabatrin. **Aicardi's syndrome** is an X-linked disorder with onset at birth presenting with infantile spasms, hemiconvulsions, agenesis of the corpus callosum, coloboma, and vertebral anomalies. **MERRF** (mitochondrial epilepsy with ragged red fibers) is a mitochondrial disorder with onset at age 3 to 65 that presents with myoclonic epilepsy, cerebellar dysfunction, and other features suggestive of a mitochondrial disorder. **Sialidosis I** is an autosomal recessive disorder due to decreased alpha-neuraminidase. Onset is in adolescence, with severe myoclonus, visual impairment, and cherry-red spots in the fundi. **Lennox-Gastaut** is a disorder with an onset of age 1 to 10 years presenting with multiple seizure types, with slow spike and wave pattern.

33. *e. giving lorazepam 0.1-mg/kg bolus.*

After evaluating and treating ABCs, the next step in the treatment of status epilepticus is giving lorazepam 4 to 10 mg IV (0.1-mg/kg bolus), as this is the most rapid and effective treatment for status epilepticus. Fosphenytoin may be given after this. Carbamazepine is not available IV. Pentobarbital and midazolam have been used for refractory status, but this patient does not meet this criterion. Diazepam redistributes to fatty tissues within minutes, so is not an optimal therapy for initial status treatment.

34. *b*

35. *c*

36. *a*

37. *d*

38. *e*

34–38.   **Pantothenate kinase-associated neurodegeneration** (PKAN) was formerly known as Hallervorden-Spatz syndrome; it is one of the rare neurodegeneration disorders with brain iron accumulation. Imaging shows decreased T2-weighted signal in the globus pallidus and substantia nigra, sometimes accompanied by hyperintense area within the hypodense zone ("eye of the tiger"). **Progressive supranuclear palsy** (PSP) is a progressive neurodegenerative disorder primarily affecting the midbrain and causing toppling gait, dysarthria, vertical gaze disorder, and other findings. MRI may show thinning of the midbrain, causing a "hummingbird sign" on sagittal imaging. **Multiple-system atrophy** (MSA) is a degenerative disorder affecting multiple systems. It may show a sign of crisscross linear atrophy on MRI of the pons, the so-called "hot cross bun" sign. **Corticobasal degeneration** (CBD) is a group of disorders that manifest with focal cortical symptoms such as apraxia and visuospatial deficits, dystonic limb with stimulus sensitive myoclonus, and cortical sensory findings. Focal brain atrophy in parietal regions on MRI may accompany this. **Creutzfeldt-Jakob disorder** (CJD) is a rapidly progressive prion disorder. On imaging, variant CJD may show the "pulvinar sign" with altered signal in the dorsal thalamus.

39. *c. Alemtuzumab; idiopathic thrombocytopenic purpura*

Natalizumab, a monoclonal that blocks lymphocyte entry into the CNS, increases the risk of progressive multifocal leukoencephalopathy, particularly when patients are positive for

John Cunningham virus antibody (JCVAB +). **Fingolimod** binds to the SIP receptor of the lymphocyte, internalizing the receptor and interfering with the exit of lymphocytes from the lymph nodes. Risks include first-dose bradycardia, disseminated zoster infections, and macular edema. **Alemtuzumab** is a monoclonal antibody that depletes B and T cells for months after initial treatment. It can cause Grave's disease or ITP due to return of certain B-cell lines predisposing to immune disorders. **Cyclophosphamide** is a chemotherapy that can cause immunosuppression and hair loss. **Mitoxantrone** is a chemotherapy that can cause treatment-related acute leukemia and cardiomyopathy.

40. *d. Acute disseminated encephalomyelitis*

ADEM is an autoimmune demyelinating disorder usually seen in children after a viral illness or a vaccination. It is acute, usually with encephalopathy and systemic symptoms, with diffuse white-matter lesions in the spinal cord and brain that can include basal ganglia and brainstem. **Schilder's disease** is a poorly characterized demyelinating disorder of children; it had a progressive course leading to death with elevated CSF myelin basic protein. **Neuromyelitis optica spectrum disorders** are caused by antibodies directed at aquaporin-4 located at astrocytic foot processes. Course is relapsing primarily with optic neuritis or myelitis, but occasionally with atypical brain events such as refractory vomiting due to lesions near the fourth ventricle. **Acute necrotizing hemorrhagic encephalomyelitis** is a rare fulminant form of demyelination with hemorrhagic brain lesions. **Balo's concentric sclerosis** is a type of demyelination with pathologically alternative bands of demyelination and preserved myelin.

41. *e. rarely causes a syndrome of acute flaccid paralysis.*

West Nile virus infection is usually asymptomatic; less than 1% develop neurological symptoms. Elderly and immunocompromised patients are at most risk for neurological complications. Imaging is nonspecific but may show changes on MRI in the basal ganglia, thalami, brainstem, and cerebellum. T2 signal change may be seen in the spinal cord. It can cause a polio-like acute lower motor neuron syndrome with flaccid paralysis. It can also present with meningitis, encephalitis, or myelitis.

42. *e. is due to defective viral maturation in the brain.*

This syndrome is known as subacute sclerosing panencephalitis (SSPE). There is no treatment, and prognosis is progression to death over 1 to 3 years. EEG shows high-amplitude spike or slow-wave bursts correlating with myoclonus progressing to burst-suppression pattern. Slow viral infections cause conditions such as CJD, fatal familial insomnia, and Gerstmann-Straussler-Scheinker syndrome. Congenital rubella syndrome can cause mental retardation, cataracts, sensorineural hearing loss, and congenital heart disease.

43. *b. Mees' lines*

44. *a. Alopecia*

45. *d. Burtonian line*

46. *c. Bradykinesia*

43–46.   Arsenic causes acute GI symptoms, an axonal sensory neuropathy beginning 5 to 10 days after ingestion, nail changes called Mees' lines, and hyperkeratosis and sloughing of skin from the palms and soles. Thallium poisoning has a hallmark of alopecia and may cause cranial nerve and autonomic neuropathy. Lead poisoning may cause Burtonian lines or lead lines in the gums, and causes a chronic axonal motor neuropathy, abdominal pain, and anemia. Manganese poisoning may cause an extrapyramidal syndrome.

47. *d. are seen in a variety of encephalopathies.*

Triphasic waves on EEG are seen in hepatic encephalopathy but may be seen in other acute encephalopathies and are evidence of diffuse brain dysfunction. CJD may cause periodic sharp waves that can sometimes be mistaken for triphasic waves. A burst-suppression pattern may be seen as a late finding in status epilepticus. Triphasic waves do not suppress with benzodiazepines, but epileptiform sharp waves may at times suppress with this treatment.

48. *e. It provides smooth muscle relaxation via beta-adrenergic receptors.*

The hypogastric nerve provides smooth muscle relaxation via beta-adrenergic receptors. The preganglionic efferent nerves exit T10-L2. Ganglia are paraganglia (next to vertebrae), pre-ganglia (between vertebrae and end organ) or peripheral ganglia (in end organ).

Nerves travel within hypogastric nerve to the inferior pelvic plexus, where they modulate urethral smooth muscle contraction and inhibit parasympathetic activity.

Release of norepinephrine stimulates beta-3 adrenergic receptors in the bladder, causing relaxation (storage). Release of norepinephrine stimulates alpha-1 adrenergic receptors in the involuntary sphincter, causing sphincter contraction (storage).

49. *e. A lesion of cervicomedullary junction*

Downbeat nystagmus is characteristic of a cervicomedullary lesions and is often seen in a Chiari malformation. A lesion of the dorsal midbrain can cause Parinaud's syndrome with limited of vertical gaze and convergence retraction nystagmus. A lesion of Mollaret's triangle may cause palatal nystagmus (Mollaret range red nucleus, inferior olive, dentate nucleus). A massive pontine lesion can cause ocular bobbing. A lesion of the parasellar region may cause seesaw nystagmus.

50. *d. causes episodic vertigo.*

Ménière's syndrome is caused by distension of the endolymphatic system (endolymphatic hydrops). Symptoms include fluctuating hearing loss at low frequencies, tinnitus, episodic vertigo, and a sensation of pressure in the affected ear.

Bonus Answers

1. *b. Laboratory findings show hypernatremia with inappropriate urine osmolality.*

Syndrome of inappropriate antidiuretic hormone secretion: usually a diagnosis of exclusion; hyponatremia with plasma osmolality less than 275 mOsm/kg H_2O and inappropriate urine osmolality (>100 mOsm/kg H_2O); with normal renal function; with euvolemia; without adrenal insufficiency, hypothyroidism, or diuretics. It is caused by CNS infections, tumors, and trauma; pulmonary and mediastinal infection and tumors; and drugs—phenothiazines, tricyclic antidepressants, desmopressin, oxytocin, salicylates, nonsteroidal anti-inflammatory drugs. Diagnosis in difficult cases can be aided by water loading test (oral water load of 20 mL per kg body weight in 15–20 minutes, inability to excrete 80%–90% of the oral load in 4–5 hours, and inability to suppress the urine osmolality to <100 mOsm/kg H_2O). Treatment: 3% NaCl in acute severe symptomatic hyponatremia; restriction of free water intake if chronic, with option of vasopressin 2 receptor antagonist if not responding.

2. *c. Deletion of 1p19q causes a better treatment response.*

Oligodendrogliomas account for 5% of intracranial gliomas. They usually occur in the cerebral hemispheres and are most frequent between 30 and 50 years of age. The pathology shows a typical fried-egg appearance, delicate vessels, and calcification. Deletion of 1p19q provides a better treatment response.

3. *d. GlyR*

4. *b. anti-Hu*

5. *a. GAD-65*

6. *c. VGCC*

3–6. A progressive encephalomyelitis can be seen in Hodgkin's lymphoma associated with GlyR antibody. A sensory neuropathy can be seen with anti-Hu (ANNA 1) antibodies. Stiff-person syndrome is commonly associated with GAD-65 antibodies. Lambert-Eaton syndrome commonly is associated with voltage-gated calcium channel antibodies.

7. *c. Approved for treatment of TD: most effective antipsychotic*

    Clozapine (Clozaril®) is the most effective antipsychotic; NB: clozapine causes no EPS; safely treats PD-related psychosis; approved for treatment of TD; side effects: NB: idiosyncratic agranulocytosis (~1% incidence), weekly complete blood count for 6 months, then biweekly complete blood count for duration of treatment, hold or discontinue clozapine if white blood count or neutrophil count declines; NB: lowers seizure threshold (0.7%–1.0% per 100-mg daily dose), severe anti-ACh and anti-H1 side effects—sialorrhea (excessive salivation).

8. *b. trinucleotide repeat at chromosomal locus Xq27.3.*

    Fragile X syndrome is caused by trinucleotide repeat at chromosomal locus Xq27.3. Incidence: 1/1,000 males, 1/2,000 females. Diagnostic features include long head, large ears, hyperflexible joints, macroorchidism, short stature, and mild to severe intellectual disability; patients are often gregarious and pleasant; females are usually less severely affected. There is a high frequency of comorbidity with ADHD and pervasive developmental disorders. Fragile X is the most common cause of inherited intellectual disability. Nearly all affected boys manifest attention deficit disorder (ADD) and have learning disabilities. The most common neurocognitive symptoms are problems with abstract reasoning, complex problem solving, and expressive language; 33% meet criteria for autism.

9. *c. retention of reactive pupils.*

    Anton's syndrome is due to bilateral occipital lobe lesions. It causes inability to see with absent response to visual threat. Patients are often unaware of having a deficit and may confabulate reasons for inability to identify objects. Pupillary reactions are spared, as this pathway bypasses the neocortex (Edinger-Westphal nucleus of the midbrain). Apraxia of the left hand may occur with anterior corpus callosum lesions. Right homonymous hemianopsia occurs with left retrochiasmal lesions. Prosopagnosia may occur with ventral occipitotemporal lesions. Visuospatial disorientation often occurs with parietal lesions.

10. *d. is associated with hyperorality.*

    Klüver-Bucy syndrome can be seen with bilateral temporal lobe damage, usually in the anterior temporal regions. Hyperorality, hypersexuality, apathy, hypermetamorphosis (overly sensitive to minute stimuli in the environment with preoccupation with these stimuli), and visual agnosia are common. Patients are unable to ignore visual stimuli.

Index

Note: Page numbers followed by "*f*" indicate figures and "*t*" indicate tables

acetylcholine (ACh), 2–5, 563
acromegaly, 537
acrylamide, 380
action potential (AP) generation, 401
active sleep, 421
acute disseminated encephalomyelitis, 335
acute dystonia, 569
acute intermittent porphyria, causing
    psychiatric symptoms, 613
acute intracerebral hemorrhage,
    150–154
acute ischemic stroke, 147–149
acute necrotizing hemorrhagic
    encephalomyelitis, 335–336
acute stroke therapy, 125–127
AD ataxias, 36*t*
Adie's pupil, 104
adult psychiatry
    medical ethics in, 591–592
    psychiatric illnesses, 572–591
    psychochemistry, 561–572
advanced sleep phase disorder, 393
afferent fibers, 95
akathisia, 569
alemtuzumab, 334
alexander disease, 476*t*
alleles, 23
Alpers Huttenlocher disease, 477*t*
α-fetoprotein, 55
α-fluoromethylhistidine, 16
α-latrotoxin, 4*t*
alphaviruses, 346
alport's syndrome, 530*t*
ALS. *See* Amyotrophic lateral sclerosis
    (ALS)
Alzheimer's disease, 171–172, 610
    ACh deficiency and, 563
    treatment, 173*t*
amantadine, 304
American Academy of Neurology
    (AAN) guidelines, 278*t*
american trypanosomiasis, 371
aminoacidopathies
    Hartnup disease, 473*t*
    phenylketonuria, 472*t*

amino acids, 1
    disorders of, 472–473*t*
1-amino-1,3-cyclopentone dicarboxylic
    acid (ACPD), 12
aminoglycosides, 529
amino-oxalyl aminobutyric acid, 383
amino-β-oxalyl aminopropionic acid, 383
4-aminopyridine, 20
amiodarone, 206
AMPA (α-amino-3-hydroxyl-5-methyl-
    4-isoxazolepropionate), 12
amphetamines, 9
    adverse effects, 596
    effects, 595–596
    related disorder, 581–582
    specific drugs, 596
amphiphysin, 559*t*
amplifiers, 418
amplitude, 402
amplitude of sensory nerve AP (SNAP),
    402
amygdala, 109
amyloid, 172
amyotrophic lateral sclerosis (ALS),
    224–225
anaplastic astrocytoma, 541*t*, 542*t*
anaplastic ependymomas, 543*t*
anaplastic oligodendroglioma, 544*t*
anatomic reorganization, 531
anencephaly, 56
Angelman's syndrome, 599
angiokeratoma corporis diffusum, 468*t*
angioplasty, 157
animal toxins
    ciguatoxin toxin, 381–382
    latrodectism, 382
    saxitoxin, 382
    snake venoms, 381
ANNA-1 (antineuronal nuclear Ab
    type 1), 204–205
ANNA-2 (antineuronal nuclear Ab
    type 2), 205
anorexia nervosa, 590
anosodiaphoria, 608
anterior cerebral artery (ACA), 120

anterior chiasm lesion. *See* Willebrand's
    knee
anterior choroidal artery, 120–121
anterior compartment syndrome, 87
anterior horn cell/muscle disorders,
    479–482
anterior interosseous nerve syndrome, 81
anterior ischemic optic neuropathy
    (AION), 515–516
anterior median fissure, 68
anterior pituitary hormones, disorders
    of, 536*t*
    acromegaly, 537
    Cushing's disease, 537–538
    hyperprolactinemia, 537, 537*t*
    hypopituitarism, 538–539
    thyrotropinomas, 538
anterior tarsal tunnel syndrome, 87
anterior visual pathways, function of, 443
anterolateral sulcus, 68
antibiotics
    for bacterial meningitis, 339*t*
    for botulism, 358–359, 384–385
anticholinergic agents, 304
anticholinesterases, 5
anticoagulants, 118
    reversal, 152–153
anticoagulation, 148
anticonvulsants, drug-drug interactions
    of, 279–280*t*
antidepressants, 563, 566, 596
    MAOIs, 564
    SNRIS, 565–566
    SSRIs, 564–565
    TCAs, 564
antidiuretic hormone secretion, syndrome
    of inappropriate, 539–540
antiepileptic drugs (AEDs), 149, 152
    adjunctive use of, 278*t*
    adverse events of, 279*t*
    CBZ, 268–269*t*
    ethosuximide, 271*t*
    gabapentin, 273*t*
    lamotrigine, 272–273*t*
    levetiracetam, 274*t*

antiepileptic drugs (AEDs) (*cont.*)
    oxcarbazepine, 272*t*
    phenobarbital, 270*t*
    PHT, 265–266*t*
    primidone, 271*t*
    sodium valproate (valproic acid [VA]),
        267–268*t*
    for status epilepticus, 285*t*
    topiramate, 274–275*t*
    zonisamide, 273–274*t*
anti-Hu Ab syndrome, 204
antimanic agents, 567
anti-Nova Ab syndrome, 205
antiphospholipid antibodies syndrome,
    134
antipsychotics, 175, 567–568, 596–597
    atypical, 568, 568–569*t*
    EPS, 569
    for EtOH withdrawal, 579
    for lasting intramuscular depot
        formulations, 569
    for neuroleptic malignant
        syndrome, 569
    TD, 569
anti-Purkinje cytoplasmic Ab type 1
    (PCAb1), 205
antiretroviral therapy, 350
anti-Ri antibodies, 546*t*, 560*t*
anti-Ri syndrome, 205
antithrombin III activator, 152–153
antiviral treatment, 341*t*
anti-YoAb syndrome, 205
antoni type A, 547*t*
antoni type B, 547*t*
Anton's syndrome, 610
anxiety disorders, 577–578
anxiolytics, 570–571
aphasia, 532
apnea/hypopnea index (AHI), 394
apomorphine, 305
appetite, 535
approach to the patient with head injury,
    139–143
aprosencephaly, 57
aqueductal stenosis, 59
AR ataxias with known gene loci, 36*t*
arginine vasopressin, 539–540
Argyll-Robertson pupil, 103
Argyll-Robertson syndrome, 520
aripiprazole, 568
Arnold-Chiari malformation, 57
arousal system, 391
arsenic, 487
    neuropathy, 207
    neurotoxicity of, 375
arterial supplies, 62*f*
arteriovenous malformations, 157–158
arthropod-borne infections, 346–348
artifacts
    antidromic versus orthodromic, 403
    nonphysiologic, 403, 419–420

    physiologic, 403, 419
    stimulus, 403
    theories, 531
asenapine, 568
asomatognosia, 66
aspartate, 2, 15
Asperger's syndrome, 600
aspergillosis, 365–366
astrocytes, 52
astrocytic tumors, 542–543*t*
astrocytomas, 542–543*t*
asymmetric polyradiculoneuropathy, 197
ataxia, 320–323, 533
    telangiectasia, 484
atelencephaly, 57
atomoxetine, 596
atropine/scopolamine, 4*t*
attention deficit hyperactivity disorder
    (ADHD), 487, 595–596, 601–602
attention, types of, 615
auditory dysfunction, examination, 527
auditory evoked potentials (AEPs)
    early, 429–430
    late, 435
    middle latency, 435
auditory system, 99–101, 100*f*
aural impairment, 532
autism, 487, 600
autistic disorder, 600
autoimmune encephalitis, 160
autonomic dysreflexia, 75
autonomic nervous system, 494
autonomic neuropathy, 198
autosomal dominant (AD)
    ataxias, 36*t*, 322–323*t*
    inheritance pattern, 27, 466
autosomal recessive (AR) inheritance,
    27, 466
axillary nerve, 78
axonal transport, 51
axonotmesis, 186
azathioprine, 220

bacterial meningitis, 160, 337–339
bacterial toxins, 383–385
BAERs. *See* brainstem auditory-evoked
    responses (BAERs)
bag₂, 88
Balint's syndrome, 522, 608
baltic myoclonus. *See* Unverricht-
    Lundborg disease
barbiturates, 13, 571
    coma, 522
Barrington nucleus, 493
basal ganglia, 89–92, 105–109
basilar artery, 122–123
B cell, 549*t*
Becker's muscular dystrophy, 228, 480
bedside maneuvers, 615
behavioral modification, 532
behavioral substitution, 531

behavioral variant FTD (bvFTD), 175
Behçet's disease, 523
bender visual motor gestalt test, 616
benign paroxysmal positional vertigo
    (BPPV), 528
benign paroxysmal vertigo, 180
benign rolandic epilepsy, 263
benton facial recognition test, 616
benzodiazepines, 13, 570–571
    for EtOH withdrawal, 579
    treatment, 423*f*
bereavement, 574
Beriberi, 580
β-blockers, 572
β-bungarotoxin, 4*t*
β-galactosidase deficiency. *See* GM1
    gangliosidosis
β-noradrenergic receptors, 6
β-N-oxalyl amino-L-alanine, 383
biotinidase deficiency disease, 258
bipolar disorder, 574, 604
bladder, neurologic lesion and effect
    on, 494
blastomycosis, 367
blepharospasm, 502, 505
blindness, cortical, 610
blood aging determination, 154*t*
blood–brain barrier, 52
blood-cerebrospinal fluid barrier, 52
blood pressure
    augmentation/reduction, 149
    control, aggressive, 153
B-lymphocytes, 327
body dysmorphic disorder, 589
boston naming test, 617
botulinum toxin, 4*t*
botulism, 223, 487, 358–359, 384–385
brachial plexopathy, 195–196, 439
brachial plexus
    lesions of, 78
    muscles innervated by, 79–80*t*
    structure of, 76*f*
    trunks of, 76
brain abscess, 357–358
    toxoplasmosis. *See* toxoplasmosis
        abscess
brain arteries, inflammatory disease of,
    129–130
brain death, 164–165
brain function, 617
brain herniation, 161–162
brain injury, mechanisms of, 139
brainstem, 93–105
    auditory, 527
brainstem auditory-evoked responses
    (BAERs), 429–435
    audiometry, 434–435
    classification of, 429*t*
    clinical applications, 432–435
    general interpretation of, 433
    in infants and children, 434

intraoperative monitoring, 434
physiology, 430–431
recording and stimulus parameters,
431–432
waves, 430*t*, 430*f*
brain tumors, genetic syndromes
associated with, 41–42*t*
branched-chain amino, 472*t*
Brown-Sequard syndrome, 75
brucellosis, 359–360
bulimia nervosa, 590
bunyaviruses, 347–348
buprenorphine, 571, 587
bupropion, 566, 596
burning feet syndrome, 201
burst suppression, 427, 427*f*
buspirone, 571

CADASIL, 132
caffeine, 12, 13
related disorder, 582
withdrawal, 180
calcium channel disorders, 20
calibration, 418
California encephalitis virus, 347–348
callosal disconnection, 611
calmodulin, 18
caloric testing, 526
candidiasis, 366
cannabis, related disorder, 582
capillary telangiectasia, 158
capsaicin, 17
carbamoyl phosphate synthetase
deficiency, 474*t*
carbon monoxide poisoning, 379
carcinomatous/paraneoplastic
neuropathy, 204–206, 205*t*
carnitine deficiency, 241
carnitinepalmitoyltransferase
deficiency, 241
carpal tunnel syndrome (CTS), 192–193
symptoms of, 81
cataplexy, medications for, 398
catatonia, 575
catecholamines, 5–9
Catechol-O-methyltransferase
inhibitors, 305
catheter angiogram, 156
cauda equina syndrome, 76, 197*t*
Caudal-Edinger-Westphal nucleus, 105
caudal regression syndrome, 57
caudate, 89
cavernous malformations, 158
cavernous sinus syndromes, 98, 508–509
CBZ (Tegretol®/Tegretol XR®/
Carbatrol®), 268–269*t*
central apnea, 394
central cord syndrome, 72
central core disease, 235, 481
central dogma of genetics, 23–28
central hearing disorders, 528

central lesion, 72
central nervous system (CNS), 493
tumors, oncogenes and chromosomal
aberrations in, 31–32, 541
central neurocytoma, 545*t*
central scotoma, 523
centronuclear myopathy, 234
ceramidase deficiency. *See*
lipogranulomatosis
cerebellar cortex, 91
corpus callosum, 67
frontal lobe, 65
functional areas, 64*f*, 65*f*
layers of neocortex, 64
occipital lobe, 67
parietal lobe, 65–67
temporal lobe, 67
cerebellar degeneration, 581
cerebellar peduncles, 91
cerebellum, 89–92, 551*t*
cerebral amebiasis, 370
cerebral arterial vasospasm
management, 156
cerebral autosomal dominant
arteriopathy with subcortical
infarcts and
leukoencephalopathy
(CADASIL), 132
cerebral autosomal recessive arteriopathy
with subcortical infarcts and
leukoencephalopathy
(CARASIL), 132
cerebral blood flow (CBF), 116*t*
cerebral contusion, 142
cerebral death, 424
cerebral palsy, 465, 465*t*
cerebral vasculature, diseases involving,
131–132
cerebral veins, thrombosis of, 133–134
cerebrovascular accident, 533*t*
cerebrovascular disease
causing psychiatric symptoms, 611
genetic syndromes in, 132–133
cervical artery dissection, 131
cervical radiculopathies, 194*t*
Chagas disease, 371
channelopathies, neurologic
manifestations, 42–43*t*
Charcot-Marie-Tooth (CMT),
211, 479
Chediak-Higashi syndrome, 484
chemodectoma, 545*t*. *See also*
paraganglioma
chemotherapy, 387*t*, 555–556*t*
Chiari I, 57
Chiari II, 57
Chiari III, 57
Chiari IV, 57
chicken pox, 343
childhood psychiatric illnesses, 597
childhood sleep disorders, insomnia, 392

child psychiatry
adult diagnostic criteria, differences
from, 604
attention deficit and disruptive
disorders, 601–602
general concepts of, 595
mental retardation, 597–599
miscellaneous childhood disorders,
603–604
pervasive developmental disorders,
600–601
psychotropics used mostly in
children, 595–597
specific learning disorders, 599–600
tic disorders, 603
choline acetyltransferase, 563
cholinergic agonists, 4*t*
cholinergic antagonists, 4*t*
cholinergic neurons, 391
cholinesterase inhibitors, 173*t*, 175
chorea. *See also* Huntington's disease
dentatorubropallidoluysian
atrophy, 314
etiology, 309–310*t*
Lesch-Nyhan syndrome, 314
neuroacanthocytosis, 313
pantothenate kinase-associated
neurodegeneration, 314
paroxysmal dyskinesias, 315*t*
Sydenham's chorea, 314
choroid plexus carcinoma, 544*t*
chromatolysis, 51
chromosomal aberrations, 31–32*t*, 541*t*
chromosomal abnormalities, 57
chronic alcoholic hallucinosis, 581
chronic inflammatory demyelinating
polyradiculoneuropathy
(CIDP), 215
chronic sensorimotor polyneuropathy,
200–204
chronic traumatic encephalopathy
(CTE), 176
CIDP. *See* chronic inflammatory
demyelinating
polyradiculoneuropathy (CIDP)
ciguatoxin toxin, 381–382
ciliary muscle, 501
cimetidine, 16
circadian rhythm disorders, 392–394
cisplatin, 206
citalopram, 565
claustrum, 90
climbing fibers, 92
clinical dementia rating (CDR) scale, 171
clinical neuroanatomy
basal ganglia and cerebellum, 89–92
brainstem, cranial nerves (CNs), and
special sensory systems, 93–105
cerebral cortex, 64–67
limbic system, 110–112
peripheral nerves, 76–87

clinical neuroanatomy (*cont.*)
   skull, cerebrovascular supply, and
      venous drainage, 61–63
   spinal cord, 68–76
   spinal reflexes and muscle tone, 88–89
   thalamus, hypothalamus, and basal
      ganglia, 105–109
clobazam, 276*t*
clomipramine, 597
clonazepam, 175
clonidine, 596, 597
clozapine, 11, 568
cluster headache
   ICHD-II diagnostic criteria for, 181
   and other trigeminal autonomic
      cephalgias, 179
CN III. *See* oculomotor nerve
CNs. *See* cranial nerves (CNs)
CN VIII. *See* cochlear nerve
coagulopathy, 118
cobblestone lissencephaly (type II), 59
cocaine, 9, 521, 582–583
coccidioidomycosis, 366
coccygeal plexus, 84
cochlea, 525
cochlear ganglion, 99
cochlear nerve, 99
cochlear nuclei, 99
Cogan's syndrome, 530*t*
cognitive impairment, 532
cognitive skill, 600
COL$_4$A$_1$ mutation, 133
colchicine, 206
cold-water caloric testing, 526
collision tumor. *See* gliosarcoma
colloid cyst, 549*t*
Colorado tick fever virus, 348
columns, 68
coma, 162–163
   α coma, 424
   respiratory patterns associated
      with, 163*t*
common carotid arteries, 118–119
comparative genomic hybridization
      (CGH), 28–29
complex repetitive discharges, 408
compound muscle AP (CMAP), 402
concentric sclerosis of balo, 335
concussion, cerebral and sports, 143–144
conduct disorder, 602
conductive hearing loss, 528
cones, 442*t*, 499
confusional arousals, 396
congenital cytomegalovirus (CMV)
      infection, 344
congenital disorders of muscle, 233–235
congenital hydrocephalus, 59
congenital hypomyelinating
      neuropathy, 212
congenital muscular dystrophy, 481
congenital myasthenia, 482

congenital myopathy, 234–235, 505
congenital rubella syndrome, 352
congenital syphilis, 485
conjunctiva, 502
connect dots test, 615
continuous EEG (cEEG) monitoring, 159
contralateral ventral lateral thalamus, 92
contusion, cerebral, 142
conus medullaris syndrome, 68, 76, 197*t*
convergence retraction nystagmus, 512
conversion disorder, 589
coracobrachialis syndrome, 83
cord lesions, 78
corpus callosum, 58, 67
cortical blindness, 610
cortical myoclonus, 316
corticobasal ganglionic degeneration, 308
corticotropin-releasing hormone, 535
coxsackie A, 485
coxsackie B, 485
cramp potentials, 408–409
cranial mononeuropathy, 197
cranial nerves (CNs), 93–105
   CN III, 54, 501
   CN VI, 500
   CN VIII, 526
   paraneoplastic syndromes, 551–552*t*
cranio-cerebral trauma, 139
   concussion in sports, 143–144
   penetrating wounds of the head, 142
   sequelae of head injury, 142–143*t*
craniopharyngioma, 550*t*
creatine, 225
Creutzfeldt-Jakob disease (CJD), 368–369
cristae, 525
critical illness myopathy, 410
critical illness polyneuropathy, 204
crossed-leg palsy, 86
cryoglobulinemia, 203
cryptococcosis, 365
cupula, 525
Cushing's disease, 537–538
cutaneous receptors, 53
cyanide intoxication, 380
cyclosporine, 220
cyclothymia and dysthymia, 604
cyproheptadine, 11
cystic acid, 2
cysticercosis, 371–372
cysts and tumor-like lesions, 549–550*t*
cytogenetic analyses, genetic testing,
      28–29
cytokines, 328
cytomegalovirus, 485. *See also* congenital
      cytomegalovirus (CMV)
      infection
cytoplasmic body myopathy, 235

Dandy-Walker malformation, 58
dapsone, 206
deafness, 100

deblocking techniques, 532
debrancher enzyme deficiency, 240
deep posterior compartment
      syndrome, 87
Dejerine Sottas, 211, 479
delayed cerebral ischemia, 154–157
delayed sleep phase syndrome, 392
delirium
   definition, 167
   tremens, 579–580
delusions, 575
dementia, 32*t*
   alcohol-induced, 581
   Alzheimer's disease and, 171–173
   definitions of, 167
   diagnostic workup, 169–170*t*
   etiologies of, 167–176
   etiology of, 167–169*t*
   frontotemporal, 175
   hydrocephalic, 176
   multi-infarct, 174
   primary progressive aphasia, 176
   prion disorders, 176
   semantic, 175
   of undetermined cause, suggested
      evaluations for, 170–171*t*
dementia-parkinsonism-amyotrophic
      lateral sclerosis complex of
      Guam, 308
dementia with Lewy bodies (DLB). *See*
      diffuse Lewy body disease
De Morsier's syndrome, 522
demyelinating disorders
   acute disseminated
      encephalomyelitis, 335
   acute necrotizing hemorrhagic
      encephalomyelitis, 335–336
   diffuse cerebral sclerosis, 335
   multiple sclerosis in, 328–334
   neuroimmunology, 327–328
   overview, 327
denervation, 407
dentate nucleus lesion, 512
dentatorubropallidoluysian atrophy, 314
deoxyribonucleic acid (DNA), 23
depolarization, 18–19, 20
depression, 604
depressive episode, 572
dermal sinus, 57
dermatomyositis, 481
dermoid cyst, 549*t*
desipramine, 596
desmopressin, 597
desvenlafaxine, 566
developmental disorders, 56–60
Devic's disease, 523
dextroamphetamine, 596
diabetes insipidus (DI), hypothalamic, 539
diabetic amyotrophy, 197–198
diabetic neuropathy, classification of,
      197–198

Diagnostic and Statistical Manual of Mental Disorders, 572
diastematomyelia, 57
diffuse cerebral sclerosis of schilder, 335
diffuse Lewy body disease, 174–175
digital nerve, 87
digital subtraction angiography, 164
dimethyl fumarate, 334
diphtheria, 383
diplopia, 532
direct thrombin inhibitor, 152
disconnection syndromes, 611
dissociated atypical sleep patterns, 456
dissociative fugue, 589
dissociative identity disorder, 589
distal symmetric polyneuropathy, 197
distal ulnar nerve compression syndrome, 82–83
disulfiram, 206, 572
divisions, embryologic, 54*f*
Dix-Hallpike test, 526
DNA transcription, 23–24
DNA variants, nonmutational, 26*t*
dominant frontal lobe, 607
dominant negative mutation, 26
dopamine (DA), 391, 535
    agonists, 304*t*
    catabolism, 561
    diseases associated with, 6*t*
    dopaminergic pathways, 561*t*
    inactivation, 7
    receptors, 7, 561–562
    synthesis, 6–7, 561
dopamine agonist withdrawal syndrome (DAWS), 305
dopaminergic tracts, 6
dopa responsive dystonia, 319
dorsal column lesion, 73
dorsal trigeminothalamic tract, 99
dorsomedial nucleus, 107
downbeat nystagmus, 511
Down syndrome, 598
drug abuse, 118
d-tubocurarine, 4*t*
Duchenne's muscular dystrophy, 480
duloxetine, 566
dysarthria, 532
dysembryoplastic neuroectodermal tumor, 545*t*
dyslexia, 532
dysphagia, 533
dysplastic gangliocytoma, 545*t*
dysplastic ganglioglioma, 545*t*
dysthymia and cyclothymia, 604
dysthymic disorder, 574
dystonia, 34–35*t*, 318–320

eastern EE virus, 346
eating disorders, 590
EBV. *See* Epstein-Barr virus (EBV)
echoviruses, 485

Edinger-Westphal nucleus, 499, 501
EEG. *See* electroencephalography (EEG)
EEG mini-atlas
    absence seizure activity, 297*f*
    alpha coma, 292*f*
    benign epileptiform transients of sleep, 290, 291*f*
    breech, 292*f*
    burst suppression, 293*f*
    diffuse slowing after anoxic brain injury, 291*f*
    electrode pop due to poor impedance and EKG artifact, 299*f*
    focal slowing associated with left central parietal tumor, 293*f*
    frontal intermittent rhythmical delta activity, 294*f*
    frontal lobe ictal seizure, 297*f*
    generalized atonic seizure, 298*f*
    generalized tonic-clonic seizure activity, 298*f*
    muscle artifact, 300*f*
    normal adult awake EEG, 288*f*
    normal deep sleep, 288*f*
    normal light sleep (vertex wave), 289*f*
    normal REM sleep, 290*f*
    periodic lateralized epileptiform discharges in patient with old stroke 6 months prior and no clinical symptoms, 294*f*
    polyspike wave generalized seizure activity, 296*f*
    postictal slowing, 299*f*
    temporal lobe ictal seizure activity and nonconvulsive status epilepticus due to herpes simplex encephalitis, 296*f*
    temporal lobe interctal seizure activity, 296*f*
    triphasic waves in patient with renal failure, 295*f*
efferent fibers, 95–98*t*
electricity, physics and biology of, 415–417
electrocochleogram, 429–430
electroconvulsive therapy (ECT), 566
electrodes, 418
electroencephalography (EEG), 164–165
    abnormal findings of, 423
    amplifiers, 418
    AP generation, 415
    artifact, 419–420
    epileptiform activity, 425, 427
    field potentials and volume conduction, 416
    filters, 418
    generation of EEG rhythms, 416
    generation of epileptiform activity, 417
    important findings, 423–427
    input board, 418
    ion fluxes and membrane potentials, 415

machine, electrodes, and derivations, 418–419
    montage, 419
    normal findings of, 420–422
    periodic lateralized epileptiform discharges, 425
    physics and biology of electricity, 415–417
    procedures, 420
    rhythm and frequency, 419
    status epilepticus, 283
    synaptic transmission, 415–416
    for viral infections of nervous system, 341
electrolyte concentrations, 18*t*
electromyography (EMG)
    basic neurophysiology, 401–403
    clinical applications, 407–409
    equipment, 403–404
    F-response, 412–413
    H-reflex studies, 412
    monitoring, 450
    of neuropathic, neuromuscular, and myopathic processes, 185–186*t*
    of normal muscle, 404–409
    pathologic conditions, 409–410
    of single fiber, 404
electro-oculography (EOG), 450
electroretinograms (ERGs), 445–446
embryologic derivatives, 53*f*
embryologic divisions, 54*f*
embryology, 54–56
    of nervous system and corresponding disorders, 461–463*t*
    normal developmental milestones, 463–464*t*
embryonal tumors, 545–546*t*
Emery-Dreifuss syndrome, 231, 481
emotion/behavior, 536
encephalitis, 250
    periaxialis diffusa, 335
encephalocele, 56
encephalomyelitis, 351
encephalopathy, 465, 555*t*
endemic typhus, 357
endocrine myopathy, 409, 506
endogenous opioids, 586
endolymph, 525
endoplasmic reticulum, disorders involving, 471*t*
enkephalins, 16
enteroviruses, 350
entrapment mononeuropathy, 197
enuresis, treatment, 597
EOG. *See* electro-oculography (EOG)
ependymal cells, 52
ependymal tumors, 543*t*
ependymoma, 543*t*
epidemic typhus, 357
epidermoid cyst, 549*t*
epidural hemorrhage, acute, 141

epilepsy
    animal models of, 249
    associated with sleep, 286t
    causing psychiatric symptoms, 611–612
    definitions, 249
    etiologies, 250–251
    idiopathic, 251t
    incidence and prevalence, 249
    myoclonic. See myoclonic epilepsy
    and sleep, 285–288
    status. See status epilepticus
    surgery, 280
    treatment, 265–281
    women and, 264–265
epileptiform activity
    discharges, 425f
    generation of, 417
epinephrine, 8
episodic memory, 616
epithalamus, 108
EPs. See evoked potentials (EPs)
EPSPs. See excitatory positive-synaptic
        potentials (EPSPs)
Epstein-Barr virus (EBV), 343–344
Epworth sleepiness scale (ESS), 457
Erb-Duchenne palsy, 78, 196
ERGs. See electroretinograms (ERGs)
escitalopram, 565
eslicarbazepine, 277t
esophageal pH, 451
essential tremor, 613
esthesioneuroblastoma. See olfactory
        neuroblastoma
ethanol, neurotoxicity of, 386–387
ethical issues, 531
ethosuximide, 271t
ethyl alcohol (ETOH) withdrawal, 160
ethylene glycol, neurotoxicity of, 378–379
EtOH-related disorders
    epidemiology, 578
    EtOH withdrawal, 579–580
    intoxication, 579
    pharmacology, 578–579
    syndromes, 580–581
    treatment, 579
Eulenburg's disease, 238
evoked potentials (EPs), 429–447
    auditory. See auditory evoked
        potentials
    somatosensory. See somatosensory EPs
    visual. See visual EPs
excessive daytime sleepiness (EDS), 395
excitatory positive-synaptic potentials
        (EPSPs), 20
exons, gene structure, 23
external carotid artery (ECA), 119
external ophthalmoplegia, 522
eye, general examination of, 502–504
eyelids, 499
    disorders of, 504–505
    general examination, 502–504

eye movement. See also nystagmus
    disorders of, 505–510
    extraocular, 503
    horizontal, 499
    pursuit, 500, 503
    torsional, 499

Fabry disease, 133
factitious disorder, 589
factor Xa inhibitors, 152
familial amyloid neuropathy, 210–211
Farber's disease, 468t
far-field recording, 402
fasciculations, 409
fascioscapulohumeral dystrophy, 481
fatal familial insomnia, 369
Fazio-Londe, 480
febrile seizures, 251
femoral mononeuropathy, 188
femoral nerve, 85
fetal alcohol syndrome (FAS), 487,
        580–581
fibers of cerebellum, 91
fibrillary astrocytomas, 542t
fibromuscular dysplasia (FMD), 131
filters, 418
filum terminale, 68, 543t, 553t
fingolimod, 334
first-order neurons, 501
first sleep cycle, 455
fixation, 503
flaviviruses, 346–347
    orbivirus, 348
floppy infant, 466
fluids, 525
flumazenil, 571
fluorescent in situ hybridization
        (FISH), 28
fluoxetine, 565
fluvoxamine, 565
footdrop, 187, 188t
foramina of skull, 61–62t, 66f
Forbes-Cori disease, 480
fosphenytoin, 285
Fragile X syndrome, 598
friedreich's ataxia, 211, 321
frontal eye field, 105
frontal lobes, 65
    attention, 615–616
    executive functioning and reasoning,
        614–615
    specific behavioral signs and
        symptoms of, 607
frontal partial seizure, 261
frontotemporal dementia
        (FTD), 175
fucosidosis, 469t
full outline of unresponsiveness (FOUR)
        score, 162t
functional adaptation, 531
F-waves, 412

GABA (γ-aminobutyric acid), 1, 12–13,
        391, 563
gabapentin, 273t
gain of function mutation, 26
Galactocerebrosidase deficiency. See
        Globoid cell leukodystrophy
gangliocytoma, 544t
ganglioglioma, 544t
ganglion cells, 102
Gases, neurotoxicity of. See Carbon
        monoxide poisoning
gaze-evoked nystagmus, 512
gemistocytic astrocytoma, 543t
generalized convulsive status epilepticus
        (GCSE), 159
generalized seizures, 253–254
general somatic efferent (GSE)
        fibers, 95
general visceral efferent (GVE)
        fibers, 95
genes, 23
    dosage effects of, 25
    mutations, 24–25t
    panels, 30
    patterns of inheritance, 27–28
    transcription, 23–24
    translations, 24
genetics, central dogma of, 23–28
genetic syndromes, associated with brain
        tumors, 41–42t
genetic testing, 28–31
    cytogenetic analyses, 28–29
    genotyping, 29–31
geniculocalcarine tract, 103
genome, definition of, 23
genomic imprinting, 27–28
genotyping, genetic testing, 29–31
germ cell tumors, 550t
germinoma, 550t
Gerstmann-Straüssler-Scheinker
        syndrome, 368–369, 608
GH. See Growth hormone (GH)
ghrelin, 535
giant axonal neuropathy, 210
giant cell arteritis, 130, 515–516
glasgow coma scale, 163t
glatiramer acetate, 333
glial cells, 52
glioblastoma astrocytomas, 542t
gliomatosis cerebri, 543t
gliosarcoma, 543t
globoid cell leukodystrophy, 468t
globuspallidus, 89
glomus body tumor, 530t
glutamate, 1, 11–12, 391
    inactivation, 12
    receptors, 11–12, 563
glycine, 15
glycogen storage diseases, 239–241, 480
GM1 gangliosidosis, 467t
GM2 gangliosidosis, 259t

gold
  neuropathy, 207
  neurotoxicity of, 375
golgi body, disorders involving, 471*t*
golgi tendon organs, 89
gonadotropinomas, 538
gonadotropin-releasing hormone
    (GnRH), 535
granule cells, 91
Graves' disease, 506, 516
group A b-hemolytic streptococci, 362
growth hormone (GH), 539
  releasing hormone, 535
guanfacine, 596
Guillain-Barré syndrome, 212

Haemophilus influenza, 337
hair cells, 99, 102, 525
Hallervorden-Spatz disease, 314
hallucinogens, related disorder, 583
Halstead-Reitan Battery test, 617
Hansen's disease. *See* Leprosy
haploinsufficiency, 25
HDL-2, 313
headaches
  activity-induced, 182–183*t*
  cluster, 181
  frequent episodic tension-type, 181
  medication-overuse, 182
  migraine without aura, 180
  migraine with typical aura, 180
  primary, 179
  secondary, 179–180
  SUNA, 182
  SUNCT, 181
  therapies, 183*t*
head injury. *See also* coma
  minor, 140
  penetrating wounds of, 142
  sequelae of, 142–143*t*
head trauma
  cranio-cerebral trauma, 139
  patient with head injury, 139–143
  related to sports, 143–144
Health Insurance Privacy and Portability
    Act (HIPPA), 592
hearing loss
  conductive, 434–435
  sensorineural, 435
heavy metals, neurotoxicity of, 375–378
hemangioblastoma, 548*t*
hemangiopericytoma, 548*t*
hematopoietic neoplasms, 549*t*
hemicraniectomy watch. *See* malignant
    cerebral edema management
hemimegalencephaly, 58
hemodilution, 157
hemorrhagic transformation
    management, 148
hepatolenticular degeneration, 475*t*
hereditary distal myopathy, 230–231

hereditary hyperekplexia, 262
hereditary motor and sensory
    neuropathies (HMSN), 479
hereditary optic neuropathies, 517–518
hereditary polyneuropathy, 209–212
hereditary sensory and autonomic
    neuropathies (HSAN), 209–210*t*
heredodegenerative disorders, 475–477*t*
herniation syndromes, 161*t*
herpes viruses, 341–342, 485
herpes zoster, 343
heteroplasmy, 28
heterotopias, 59
heterozygosity, loss of, 29
hippocampal sclerosis dementia, 176
histamine, 15, 16, 391, 563
HIV. *See* Human immunodeficiency
    virus (HIV)
HMSN. *See* Hereditary motor and
    sensory neuropathies (HMSN)
HMSN type 1, 479
HMSN type 2a, 479
HMSN type 3, 479
HMSN type 4, 479
holoprosencephaly, 58
homocystic acid, 2
homocystinuria, 473*t*
Hooper Visual Organization Test, 616
Horner's syndrome, 501, 521–522
H-reflex studies, 412
HSV. *See* Herpes viruses
5-HT. *See* 5-hydroxytryptamine (5-HT)
human immunodeficiency virus (HIV),
    352, 355–356, 485
  causing psychiatric symptoms, 613
  neuropathy, 204
human leukocyte antigens (HLA), 328
human T-cell leukemia virus type 1, 356
humeral supracondylar spur syndrome, 82
Huntington's disease, 310–312, 613
hydranencephaly, 60
hydroxyamphetamine, 521
5-hydroxytryptamine (5-HT), 9–11
  agonists, 11
  antagonists, 11
  catabolism, 562
  inactivation, 10
  psychiatric significance, 562
  receptors, 10*t*
  release and storage, 10–11
  synthesis, 10, 562
hyperekplexia, 316
hyperglycemia, 148
hyperhomocysteinemia, 133
hyperkalemic periodic paralysis, 238,
    410, 481–482
hypermagnesemia, 223
hypernychthemeral syndrome (non-24-
    hour sleep-wake syndrome), 393
hyperosmolar therapy, 147
hyperprolactinemia, 537, 537*t*

hypersomnia, 395–396
  medications for, 398
hypertension, 116–117, 157
hyperventilation (HV), 420
hypervolemia, 157
hypnotics, 570–571
hypochondriacal disorder, 589
hypogonadotropic hypogonadism,
    538–539
hypokalemic periodic paralysis, 237–238,
    409, 481
hypomanic episode, 573
hypopituitarism, 538–539
hypothalamic fibers, 502*f*
hypothalamic hamartomas, 550*t*
hypothalamic nuclei and functions,
    108–109*t*
hypothalamus, 105–109, 392, 535–536
hypothyroidism, 538
hypoxic-ischemic encephalopathy
    (HIE), 465

ibuprofen, 180
ICH. *See* Intracerebral hemorrhage (ICH)
ICHD-II diagnostic criteria, 180–182
idiopathic brachial plexopathy, 78
idiopathic epilepsies, 251*t*
idiopathic hypersomnia, 395
igs, 327
illusions, 575
immune response, regulation of, 328
immunomodulators, 333
immunosuppressive medications, other
    side effects of, 388*t*
implicit memory, 616
incontinentia pigmenti, 484
indomethacin, 182
inductive plethysmography, 451
infections
  bacterial, 486
  perinatal, 485
inferior cerebellar peduncle, 91
inferior gluteal nerve, 86
inferior rectus and superior oblique
    muscle, 499
inflammatory myopathies
  DM, 236
  EMG of, 409
  inclusion body myositis, 236
  PM, 235–236
informed consent, 591–592
inhalants, related disorder, 584
inheritance
  modes of, 466
  patterns of, 27
inherited axonal neuropathies, 209–211
inherited demyelinating neuropathies,
    211–212
inner hair cells, 99
insertional activity, 404–405
insomnia, 392, 397–398

intellectual disability. *See* mental retardation
intelligence, 614
interferons, 333
internal carotid artery (ICA), 118–119
internuclear ophthalmoplegia, 509–510
intra-arterial therapy, 157
    neurological monitoring, 149
intracerebral hemorrhage (ICH)
    adjunctive treatments for, 152–153
    etiology, diagnosing, 153–154
    expansion, 151
    supportive treatment of, 151–152
    surgical management of, 153
intracranial vascular malformations, 157–158
intravenous immunoglobulin (IVIg), 214
intraventricular hemorrhage (IVH), 464, 465*t*
introns, gene structure, 23
iodopsin, 442, 499
iris sphincter, 501
iron, neurotoxicity of, 378
irregular sleep–wake cycle, 393
Isaacs' syndrome. *See* Neuromyotonia
ischemic stroke, antiplatelets and anticoagulants for, 128–129*t*
isoniazid, 206

Japanese encephalitis virus, 347
jerk nystagmus, 511
jet lag, 393
jones criteria for acute rheumatic fever, 486
junctional scotoma, 518
juvenile myoclonic epilepsy (JME), 255, 287
juvenile pilocytic astrocytoma (JPA), 542*t*

kainate, 12
Kallmann's syndrome, 539
karyotyping, 28
Kearns-Sayre syndrome, 242, 477*t*
kernicterus, 486–487
ketogenic diet, 264
kinky hair disease, 475*t*
kinocilia, 525
Kleine-Levin syndrome, 395
klumpke's palsy, 78, 196
Klüver-Bucy syndrome, 610
Korsakoff's amnesia, 580
Krabbe's disease. *See* Globoid cell leukodystrophy
Kugelberg-Welander spinal muscular atrophy, 480
kuru, 369

labyrinth, 101–102
lacosamide, 276*t*
La Crosse encephalitis virus, 347–348
lacunar stroke, 124

Lafora's body disease, 256
Lambert-Eaton syndrome, 221–222, 560*t*
laminas, 68–69
lamotrigine, 272–273*t*
Landouzy-Dejerine syndrome, 228
language and speech, neurologic impairments, 532
language function, 617
lateral antebrachial cutaneous nerve, 77
lateral compartment syndrome, 87
lateral cord, 77, 78
lateral corticospinal tract, 56
lateral femoral cutaneous nerve, 85
lateral geniculate body, 103
lateral lemniscus, 99
lateral nuclei, 535
lateral rectus muscle, 499
lateral spinothalamic tract, 74*f*
later sleep cycles, 455
lathyrism, 382–383
latrodectism, 382
Laurence-Moon-Biedl syndrome, 539
lead, 208, 487
    neurotoxicity of, 376–377
learning disorders
    attention deficit disorder, 487
    autism, 487
    diagnosis, 599
    types of, 599–600
Leber's hereditary optic neuropathy (LHON), 477*t*
Leber's optic neuropathy, 517–518
Leigh's disease, 243, 258, 477
Lennox-Gastaut syndrome, 260, 287
lentiviruses, 352
leprosy, 203–204, 360–361
Lesch-Nyhan syndrome, 314, 476*t*, 599
lethal mutations, 26
leukodystrophies, 48–49*t*
    adrenoleukodystrophy, 335
levator palpebrae superioris, 499
levetiracetam, 274*t*
levodopa, 175, 304
levo-α-acetylmethadol, 587
Lhermitte-Duclos disease, 545*t*
Li-Fraumeni cancer susceptibility syndrome, 31–32*t*, 559*t*
light-near dissociation, 520, 522
limb-girdle syndrome, 218, 228, 481
limbic system, 110–112
lipid storage disease, 241
lipogranulomatosis, 468*t*
lipoma, 548*t*
lipomeningocele, 57
lissencephaly, 59
lithium, 8, 206, 567
locus ceruleus, 562
loss of function mutation, 26
Lou Gehrig disease, 224
Louis-Bar syndrome, 483. *See also* ataxia, telangiectasia

lower limb nerves, clinical syndromes of, 85–87
lower trunk lesions, 78
lumbar plexus
    anatomy of, 83
    muscle innervated by, 84–85*t*
lumbar puncture, 338, 340
lumbosacralplexopathy, 196–197
lumbosacral radiculopathy, 193–194*t*
lurasidone, 568
Luria-Nebraska Neuropsychological Battery, 617
luria tests, 615
lyme disease, 200, 363–364
lymphokines, 328
lymphomas, 549*t*
lysergic acid diethylamine (LSD), 11
lysosomal disorders, 467–470*t*
lysosomal storage diseases, 43–45*t*

macroglia, 52
maculae, 525
magnetic resonance imaging (MRI), 341
malignant cerebral edema management, 147
malingering, 589
Malta fever. *See* Brucellosis
mamillotegmental tract, 109
mandibular nerve, 98
manganese, neurotoxicity of, 377–378
manic episode, 13–15, 564, 572–573
MAO. *See* Monoamine oxidase (MAO)
MAO inhibitors (MAOIs), 9
maple syrup urine disease (MSUD), 472*t*
Marburg's variant, 331
Marchiafava-Bignami disease, 385, 581
Marcus Gunn pupil, 103, 519–520
marijuana, related disorder, 582
Martin-Gruber anastomosis, 77, 81
maxillary nerve, 98
McArdle's disease, 480
measles virus, 351–352, 485
Meckel's syndrome, 57
medialantebrachial cutaneous nerve, 77
medial cord, 77, 78
medial forebrain bundle, 109, 111–112*f*
medial geniculate body, 100
medial longitudinal fasciculus (mlf) lesions, 509
medial rectus muscle, 499
median nerve
    anatomy, 81
    brachial plexopathy, 439
    clinical interpretation, 438–439*t*
    clinical syndromes, 81–82
    entrapment, 192–193
    interpeak latencies, 438
    obligate waveforms, 436–438, 437*f*
    radiculopathy, 439–442
medical ethics, 591–592

medication-overuse
  associated with headache, 182
  associated with myopathy, 385
medulloblastoma, 546t
megalencephaly, 58
melanocytoma, 548t
MELAS (mitochondrial encephalopathy, lactic acidosis, and stroke-like episodes), 243, 477t
melatonin, 540
melodic intonation, 532
memantine, 173
membrane channel dysfunction, 20
memory, 532, 616
ménière's syndrome, 529
meninges, tumors of, 547–548t
meningioma, 547–548t
meningitis, 486
meningocele, 56, 57
menkes disease, 475t
menstrual-related hypersomnia, 395
mental retardation, 597–599
meperidine, 586
meralgia paresthetica, 189
mercury, 207–208, 376, 487
MERRF (myoclonic epilepsy with ragged red fibers), 242–243
metabolic disorders, 467–478t
  inherited, 47–48t, 239–243
  glycogen storage diseases, 239–241
  lipid storage disease, 241
  mitochondrial encephalomyopathy, 242–243
  modes of inheritance, 466
metabolic myopathy, 506
metachromatic leukodystrophy, 468t
metastatic tumors, 551t
methadone, 571, 587
methyl alcohol, neurotoxicity of, 378
methylphenidate, 596
1-methyl-4-phenyl-1,2,3,6-tetrahydropyridine (MPTP), 587
methylprednisolone, 332–333
methysergide, 11
metronidazole, 206
MG. See Myasthenia gravis (MG)
MHC (major histocompatibility complex), 328
microarray, genotyping, 29
microcephaly, 58
microglia, 52
micturition, 493–494
middle cerebellar peduncle, 91
middle cerebral artery (MCA), 119–120
middle radicular syndrome, 196
midodrine, 198
migraines, 180
  symptomatic and preventive therapies for, 183t
mild terminal sensorimotor neuropathy, 206

Miller-Dieker syndrome, 59
mirtazapine, 566
mitochondrial disorders, 49–50t, 477–478t
  biotinidase deficiency disease, 258
  epilepsy with ragged red fibers, 257–258
  GM2 gangliosidosis, 259t
  Kearns-Sayre ophthalmoplegia, 242
  Leigh's disease, 243, 258
  MELAS, 243
  MERRF, 242–243
  myopathies, 505
  respiratory chain defects, 243
  Schindler disease, 258
  sialidosis type 1, 258
mitochondrial DNA (mtDNA), 25
  sequencing, 30
mitochondrial encephalopathy, lactic acidosis, and stroke-like episodes (MELAS), 133
mitoxantrone, 333
mixed amphetamine salt, 596
mixed apnea, 394
mixed episode, 573
mixed neuronal-glial tumors, 544–545t
mixed oligoastrocytomas, 544t
mobius syndrome, 510
Moersch-Woltman syndrome. See Stiff-person syndrome
monoamine neurons, 391
monoamine NTs, 1
monoamine oxidase (MAO), 13–15
monoamine oxidase B (MAO-B) inhibitors, 305
monoamines, 1
monoclonalgammopathy, 202
mononeuritis multiplex, 198–200
mononeuropathies
  femoral, 188
  footdrop, 188
  median nerve entrapment, 192–193
  meralgiaparesthetica, 189
  piriformis syndrome, 188
  radial nerve, 191
  sciatic, 187
  tarsal tunnel syndrome, 188–189
  ulnar nerve, 189–190
monosynaptic reflex response, 88
montage, 419
mood disorders, 572–574
mood-stabilizing agents, 567
Morton's neuroma, 87
mossy fibers, 92
motor axonal neuropathies, predominantly, 209
motor end-plate activity, 405
motor impairment, 533
motor neuron diseases, 224–226
motor unit potentials (MUPs), 406–407

movement disorders
  AD ataxias, 36t
  AR ataxias with known gene loci, 36t
  ataxia, 320–323. See also ataxia
  causing psychiatric symptoms, 612–613
  chorea, 309–315. See also chorea
  classification, 301t
  definition of, 301
  dystonia, 34–35t, 318–320
  myoclonus, 315–318
  parkinsonism, 302–309. See parkinsonism
  Parkinson's disease, 32–33t
  tremors, 324t
  trinucleotide-repeat diseases, 34t
moyamoya disease, 132
MRI. See Magnetic resonance imaging (MRI)
mRNA translations, 24
MS. See Multiple sclerosis (MS)
MSLT. See Multiple sleep latency test (MSLT)
mucolipidoses, 469t
mucormycosis, 366–367
Müller's muscle, 499
multifactorial genetic disease, 466
multifocal motor neuropathy, 199
multi-infarct dementia, 174
multiple cranial nerve palsies, 200
multiple endocrine neoplasia type 2b, 212
multiple myeloma, 202, 206
multiple sclerosis (MS)
  acute, 331
  causing psychiatric symptoms, 612
  clinical manifestations, 329–330
  diagnosis, 332
  differential diagnosis, 332
  etiology and epidemiology, 329
  lab findings, 331–332
  pathology, 328
  SSEPs, 436
  treatment, 332–334
  variants, 331
multiple sleep latency test (MSLT), 395, 458–459
multiple system atrophy, 306–307
mumps, 485
  virus, 352
MUPs. See motor unit potentials (MUPs)
muscarinic receptors, 3–4
muscle
  cramps and stiffness, 244–246
  fibers, types of, 185t
  spindles, 88
muscular dystrophy (MD), 227–228, 409, 480–481, 505
musculocutaneous nerve, 77, 83
mushrooms, toxins, 382, 382t
mutational disorders, 20
mutations, 24–26
myasthenia gravis (MG), 217–221

mycobacterium leprae, 360
myelination, 55, 59
myelocystocele, 56
myelomeningocele, 56
myeloschisis, 56
myoclonic epilepsy, 257–260, 477t
myoclonic seizures, 255
myoclonus, 259–260, 315–318
myoclonus-dystonia, 317
myokymia, 246, 408
myopathies, 407, 481–482, 505–506
   channels associated with, 246t
   congenital disorders of the muscle,
      233–235
   degenerative MD, 227
   Emery-Dreifuss syndrome, 231
   EMG of, 409
   endocrine processes, 231–232
   facioscapulohumeral MD, 228
   familial periodic paralysis, 237
   hereditary distal myopathy, 230–231
   infectious forms of, 231
   inflammatory myopathy, 235–236
   inherited metabolic disorders,
      239–243
   limb-girdle MD, 228
   medications associated with
      myopathy, 239
   muscle cramps and stiffness, 243–246
   myotonic dystrophy, 229–230
   oculopharyngeal dystrophy, 230
   X-linked MD, 227–228
myophosphorylase deficiency, 240–241
myosin-losing myopathy, 204
myotonia, 243–244, 408
myotonia congenita, 233
myotonic dystrophy, 229–230, 481, 505
myotubular myopathy, 234, 481
myxopapillary ependymomas, 543t

naloxone, 571, 586, 597
naltrexone, 571, 587, 597
narcolepsy, 40–41t, 395
natalizumab, 333
natural killer cells, 328
necrotizing polymyopathy, 238–239
nefazodone, 566
nemaline myopathy, 234, 481
neocortex, layers of, 64
neonatal myasthenia, 482
neonatal neurology, 464–466
neonatal seizures, 262–263
neonate nervous system, 464
nerve conduction studies (NCS)
   basic neurophysiology, 401–403
   clinical studies, 411
   equipment, 403–404
   F-response, 412–413
   H-reflex studies, 412
   of normal muscle, 404–409
   pathologic conditions, 409–410

nerve conduction velocity (NCV)
   studies, 411
nerve fibers, classification of, 52–53t
nerve sheath cells, tumors of, 547t
nervous system
   chemotherapy, complications of,
      555–556t
   infections of
      bacterial meningitis, 337–339
      fungal infections of, 365–367
      parasitic infections of, 369–372
      prion infections of, 368–369
      spirochete infections of, 363–364
      viral infections, 340–363
   inherited metabolic disease of,
      466–479
neural crest cells, 54
neural tube
   defects, risk factors for, 463
   formation, 55
   segmentation of, 54, 54f
neurapraxia, 186
neurilemmoma, 547t
neurinoma, 547t
neuroacanthocytosis, 313
neurobehavior and neuropsychology
   brain function, comprehensive tests
      of, 617
   frontal lobes, 614–616
   functional-anatomic correlations,
      607–611
   intelligence, 614
   language function, 617
   medical diseases causing psychiatric
      symptoms, 611–614
   memory, 616
   perceptual and motor performance, 616
neuroblastoma, 546t
neurochemistry, 18–20
neuro coding, 162
neuroendocrinology
   hypothalamus, 535–536
   pineal gland, 540
   pituitary, 536–540
neuroepithelial tumors, 541t
   choroid plexus. *See* choroid plexus
      carcinoma
   ependymal. *See* ependymal tumors
   neuronal and mixed neuronal-glial.
      See neuronal mixed neuronal-
      glial tumors
   oligodendroglial. *See* oligodendroglial
      tumors
neurofibroma, 547t
neurofibromatosis type 1 (NF1), 482–483
neurofibromatosis type 2 (NF2), 483
neurogenetics
   central dogma of genetics, 23–28
   channelopathies with neurologic
      manifestations, 42–43t
   dementia, 32t

   genetic syndromes associated with
      brain tumors, 41–42t
   genetic testing, 28–31
   movement disorders, 32–36t
   neuromuscular disorders, 37–40t
   oncogenes and chromosomal
      aberrations in CNS tumors,
      31–32t
   pediatric neurology, 43–50t
   stroke/narcolepsy/seizures, 40–41t
neurogenic arthrogryposis, 480
neurohistology, 51–53
neurohypophysis, 56, 539–540
neuroimaging
   rabies, 349
   viral infections of the nervous
      system, 341
neuroimmunology, 327–328
neuroleptic malignant syndrome, 569
neuroleptics, 8–9
neurological disease, intensive care of
   acute intracerebral hemorrhage,
      150–154
   acute ischemic stroke, 147–149
   brain herniation, 161–162
   coma and brain death, 162–165
   intracranial vascular malformations,
      157–158
   status epilepticus, 159–160
   subarachnoid hemorrhage and delayed
      cerebral ischemia, 154–157
neurologic impairments, management
   of, 532–533
neuromuscular disorders
   acute and chronic inflammatory
      demyelinating
      polyradiculoneuropathy (IDP),
      212–216
   channels associated with, 246t
   general evaluation, 185–186
   history of, 37–40t, 185, 506
   motor neuron diseases, 224–226
   myopathy, 227–246
   neuromuscular junction disorders,
      217–224
   peripheral neuropathic syndromes,
      186–212
neuromuscular junction (NMJ), 19,
      401–402, 482
   disorders
      botulism, toxin-induced, 222–223
      differential diagnosis of, 223–224
      Lambert-Eaton syndrome,
         221–222
      myasthenia gravis (MG), 217–221
      release blockade, 5
neuromyelitis optica (NMO), 331
neuromyotonia, 244, 409
neuronal ceroid lipofuscinosis,
      256–257, 470t
neuronal migrational disorders, 55, 58

neuronal mixed neuronal-glial tumors, 544–545t
neuronal proliferation, 55
neuronal tumors, 544–545t
neurons, 51, 91
neuro-oncology
  central nervous system tumors, 541
  chemotherapy, 555–556t
  common CNS/peripheral nervous system tumors, 542–551t
  common tumor classifications, 552–554t
  paraneoplastic syndromes, 551–552
  radiation side effects, 556
  transplant neurology, 557–558t
neuro-ophthalmology
  anatomy and examination of, 499–501
  clinical assessment, 501–504
  disorders, 504–523
neuro-otology
  anatomy and physiology of, 525–526
  auditory dysfunction, 528–529
  ménière's syndrome, 529
  ototoxic agents, 529
  vestibular and auditory dysfunction examination, 526–527
  vestibular dysfunction, 527–528
neuropathic beriberi, 201
neuropathic disorders, 410t, 507–508
neuropathies, 479
  associated with lymphoma, 206
  EtOH-related syndromes, 581
  heavy metal-induced, 207–209
  medication-induced, 206–207
  motor and sensory. See hereditary motor and sensory neuropathies (HMSN)
neuropeptides, 16, 535
  inactivation, 16
  subtypes, 16
  synthesis, 16
neuro phakomatoses
  ataxia-telangiectasia, 484
  incontinentia pigmenti, 484
  NF1, 482–483
  NF2, 483
  Osler-Weber-Rendu disease, 484
  Sneddon syndrome, 484
  Sturge-Weber syndrome, 483–484
  tuberous sclerosis, 483
  von Hippel-Lindau syndrome, 484
neurophysiology, 18–20
  action potential, 18–19
  neuromuscular junction, 19
  synaptic transmission, 19–20
neurorehabilitation
  aims of, 531–532
  background and general principles, 531
  general prognostic pearls after cerebrovascular accident, 533t

management of specific neurologic impairments, 532–533
mechanisms of functional recovery, 531
specific neurologic impairments management, 532–533
neurotoxicology and nutritional disorders
  animal toxins, 381–382
  bacterial toxins, 383–385
  gases, 379
  heavy metals, 375–378
  miscellaneous, 385–389
  organic solvents, 378–379
  organophosphates, 380
  other industrial toxins, 380
  plant toxins, 382–383
neurotransmitters (NTs), 17t
  ACh, 563
  dopamine, 561–562
  excitatory, 2
  GABA, 563
  glutamate, 563
  histamine, 563
  inhibitory, 2
  major categories of, 1–2
  metabolism, 473t
  norepinephrine, 562–563
  quick reference for, 17
  receptors, 1–18
  serotonin, 562
neurourology
  common neurologic disorders, 496
  evaluation of, 495–496
  management, 496–497
  micturition, 493–494
  neurologic lesion and effect on bladder, 494
  urodynamic findings, 496
  voiding dysfunction classification system, 494
neurulation, disorders of, 56–57
niacin deficiency, 580
nicotine, 4t
  related disorder, 584–585
nicotinic receptors, 3–4
Niemann-Pick disease, infantile, 478t
nightmares, 396
nimodipine, in SAH patient, 157
Nissl substance, 51
nitrofurantoin, 206
nitrous oxide, 389
N-methyl-D-aspartate, 11–12
  receptor antagonist, noncompetitive, 173
NMJ. See neuromuscular junction (NMJ)
nocturnal epilepsies, 397
nocturnal sleep drunkenness. See confusional arousals
non-24-hour sleep-wake syndrome (hypernychthemeral syndrome), 393

nonconvulsive status epilepticus (NCSE), 159
nondominant frontal lobe, 607
nonketotic hyperglycinemia, 473t, 478t
nonnucleoside reverse transcriptase inhibitors, 355
noradrenaline, 391
norepinephrine (NE), 1, 7–8
  catabolism, 562
  inactivation, 8
  psychiatric significance, 562–563
  receptors, 8
  release and vesicle storage, 7–8
  synthesis, 7, 562
NREM sleep, 391, 420–421
  burst during, 456
nystagmus, 503–504, 510–512

obsessive-compulsive disorder (OCD), 577
obstructive sleep apnea (OSA), 394
obturator nerve, 86
occipital eye fields, 105
occipital lobes, 519
  damage, 610–611
occult dysraphic states, 463
ocular bobbing, 513
ocular motor nerves, 499–500
ocular muscles, 499
ocular myoclonus, 513
oculocephalic reflex, 526
oculocraniosomatic myopathy, 223
oculocraniosomatic neuromuscular disease, 242
oculogyric crisis, 513
oculomotor apraxia, 608
oculomotor nerve, 499
  functions of, 500
  medial rectus subnucleus of, 105
  palsy, 507
oculopharyngeal dystrophy, 230, 481
olanzapine, 568
olfactory epithelium, 54
olfactory neuroblastoma, 545t
oligodendrocytes, 52
oligodendroglial tumors, 544t
oligodendroglioma, 544t
olivopontocerebellar atrophy, 307
oncogenes, 31–32t, 541t
oncoviruses, 356
one-and-a-half syndrome, 105, 510
Onuf's nucleus, 493
ophthalmic nerve, 98
opiate overdose, 522
opioids
  receptors, 17t
  related disorder, 585–587
  treatments of abuse, 571–572
oppositional defiant disorder, 602
opsoclonus, 503, 512–513
  myoclonus syndrome, 318, 559t, 560t

optic ataxia, 608
optic chiasm, disorders associated with, 102, 518. *See also* Willebrand's knee
optic disc edema, 513–515
optic nerve, 102
    chiasma, 56
    gliomas, 517
    sheath meningiomas, 516–517
optic Neuritis Treatment Trial, 329, 332–333, 515
optic neuropathies, 515–518
optic tract, 102
optokinetic response, 500
oral contraceptives, 118
orbicularis oculi, 499
orbitofrontal, 607
organic acids, disorders of, 472–473t
organic solvents, neurotoxicity of, 378–379
organophosphates, neurotoxicity of, 224–225, 380
orolingual angioedema, 127
oscillopsia, 532
Osler-Weber-Rendu disease, 484
otoconia, 525
otoliths, 500
ototoxic agents, 529
outer hair cells, 99
oxcarbazepine, 272t
oxytocin, 540

pachygyria, 59
palatal myoclonus, 317
paliperidone, 568
pandysautonomia, 206
panic disorder, 577
pantothenate kinase-associated neurodegeneration (PKAN), 314
papez's circuit, 109
papilledema, 516
paraganglioma
    filum terminale, 543t, 545t, 553t
    glomus jugulare tumor, 545t
parallel fibers, 91
paramyotonia congenita, 233, 238, 480
paramyxovirus. *See* mumps virus
paraneoplastic syndromes, brain and cranial nerves, 551t
parasomnias, 396
parasympathetic pathway, 501
parathyroid disease, 232
parietal lobes, 65–67, 608
Parinaud syndrome, 105, 512
parkinsonism, 569
    acute, 308–309
    corticobasal ganglionic degeneration, 308
    etiologies, 302t, 308–309
    idiopathic. *See* Parkinson's disease
    multiple system atrophy, 306–307

postencephalitic. *See* postencephalitic parkinsonism
progressive supranuclear palsy, 307
Parkinson's disease, 32–33t, 90, 302–303
    causing psychiatric symptoms, 612–613
    pharmacotherapy of, 304–306
paroxetine, 565
paroxysmal autonomic instability with dystonia (PAID), 570
paroxysmal dyskinesias, 315, 315t
paroxysmal events, psychogenic, 262
paroxysmal hemicrania, 182
Parsonage Turner syndrome, 78
partial seizures, 253. *See also* secondary generalized seizures
    frontal, 261
    localization of, 260–261
    parietal and occipital, 261–262
    and sleep, 286–287
    temporal, 260–261, 261f
past pointing, 526
patterns of inheritance, 27–28
PCAb1. *See* anti-purkinje cytoplasmic Ab type 1 (PCAb1)
PCP (phencyclidine) related disorder, 583–584
peabody picture vocabulary test, 617
pediatric epilepsy, 263–264
pediatric neurology
    embryology and development, 461–464
    inborn errors of metabolism, 45–47t
    infections and toxins, 485–487
    learning disorders, 487
    leukodystrophies, 48–49t
    lysosomal storage diseases, 43–45t
    mitochondrial disorders, 49–50t
    neonatal neurology, 464–466
    nervous system, inherited metabolic disease of, 466–479
    neuromuscular disorders, 479–482
    neuro phakomatoses, 482–484
    normal developmental milestones, 463–464
    other metabolic/genetic disorders, 47–48t
    phakomatoses, 43t
pediatric seizures, 263
Pelizaeus-Merzbacher disease, 476t
pellagra, 580
pemoline, 596
pendular nystagmus, 510
penile tumescence, 451
peptides, 1
perilymph, 525
perinatal encephalopathy. *See* cerebral palsy
perinatal infections, 485
periodic leg movements of sleep (PLMS), 457
periodic limb movement disorder (PLMD), 397

periodic paralysis, familial, 237, 237t
periorbital edema, 502, 504
peripheral nerves
    brachial plexus, 76–81
    coccygeal plexus, 84
    disorders
        brachial plexus, 76–80
        classification and degrees of, 186
        clinical syndromes of nerves in lower limb, 85–87
        coccygeal plexus, 84
        lumbar plexus, 83
        median nerve, 81–82
        muscle innervated by the lumbar plexus, 84–85t
        radial nerve, 83
        sacral plexus, 84
        SSEPs, 436
        ulnar nerve, 82–83
    lower limb, clinical syndromes of nerves in, 85–87
    lumbar plexus, 83–84
        muscles innervated by, 84–85t
    median nerve, 81–82
    musculocutaneous nerve, 83
    radial nerve, 83
    ulnar nerve, 82–83
peripheral nervous system (PNS), 493–494
    neurotransmitters of, 1
    tumors, 542–551
periventricular leukomalacia (PVL), 465
periventricular nodular heterotopia, 59
peroneal nerve, 86
peroxisomal disorders, 471t
personality disorders, 590–591
pervasive developmental disorders, 600–601
phakomatoses, 43t
pharmacodynamics, 595
pharmacokinetics, 595
pharmacologic intervention, 531
phenobarbital, 270t
phenylephrine, 522
phenylketonuria, 472t
phenytoin, 206
phobias, 577
phorias, 503
phosphofructokinase deficiency, 241
photic stimulation, 420
photoreceptors, 499
PHT, 265–266t
picornaviruses, 350–351
pineal gland, 540
    tumor, 550–551t
pineoblastoma, 546t, 551t
pineocytoma, 550t
piriformis syndrome, 188
pituitary adenoma, 31t, 550t
pituitary apoplexy, 509

pituitary disorders, 232, 536
    hypopituitarism, 538–539
    neurohypophysis, 539–540
    tumors, 537–538
pituitary gland, 56, 536–540
pituitary hormones, 535
plant toxins, 382*t*, 383
plasma exchange, 334
pleomorphic xanthoastrocytoma
    (PXA), 543*t*
plexopathies, 195–197
PNETs. *See* primitive neuroectodermal
    tumors (PNETs)
poliomyelitis, 486
polioviruses, 350
polymicrogyria, 59
polyneuropathies, 201–203
polysomnography (PSG), 449–457
Pompe's disease, 480
pontine micturition center (PMC), 493
porencephalic development, disorders
    of, 57–58
positional testing (Dix-Hallpike), 526
post-anoxic myoclonus, 317
postencephalitic parkinsonism, 308
posterior cerebral artery (PCA), 121–122
posterior cord, 78
posterior fossa lesions, 554*t*
posterior hypothalamus, 536
posterior interosseous nerve, 83
posterior median sulcus, 68
posterior pituitary hormones, disorder
    of, 539–540
posterolateral sulcus, 68
postganglionic sympathetic fibers, 502*f*
postpolio syndrome, 226
postsynaptic NMJ receptor blockade, 5
posttraumatic stress disorder, 577–578
potassium channel dysfunction, 20
Powassan encephalitis virus, 348
Prader-Willi syndrome, 539, 599
prednisone, 215, 220
preganglionic sympathetic fibers, 501,
    502*f*
presbycusis, 528, 529
presynaptic NMJ release blockade, 5
presynaptic α2-noradrenergic
    agonists, 596
primary amebic meningoencephalitis,
    370–371
primary angiitis of central nervous
    system (PACNS), 130
primary generalized seizures,
    255–257, 287
primary lateral sclerosis, 226
primary melancholia, 574
primary neurulation, disorders of, 56–57
primidone (Mysoline®), 271*t*
primitive neuroectodermal tumors
    (PNETs), 545*t*
procedural memory, 616

progressive multifocal
    leukoencephalopathy (PML),
    349–350
progressive myoclonic ataxias, 317
progressive myoclonic epilepsies, 316
progressive nonfluent aphasia
    (PNFA), 175
progressive supranuclear palsy, 307
proliferation, disorders of, 58
promoters, gene structure, 23
pronator syndrome, 81
pronator teres syndrome, 193
prosopagnosia, 611
protamine sulfate, 152
protease inhibitors, 355
pseudobulbar affect, 607
pseudo-Hurler disease. *See* GM1
    gangliosidosis
pseudoperiodic sharp waves, 427
pseudosymptoms, 589*t*
pseudotumor cerebri, 182
psychiatric disorders, differential
    diagnosis of, 288
psychiatric illnesses, 572–591
psychiatry
    adult. *See* adult psychiatry
    child. *See* child psychiatry
psychochemistry, 561–572
psychosurgery, 572
psychotic disorders, 575–576
psychotropics, 595–597
ptosis, 502, 505
pulvinar, 107
pupillary anatomy, 501
pupillary dilatation pathway, 103–104
pupillary function, disorders of
    adrenergic agents, 519
    afferent pupillary defect, 519–520
    Argyll-Robertson syndrome, 520
    cholinergic agents, 519
    Horner's syndrome, 521–522
    large and poorly reactive pupil, 520
    light-near dissociation, 522
    opiate overdose, 522
pupillary light reflex pathway, 103
pupillary reactivity, 504
Purkinje cells, 91
pursuit eye movement, 500, 503
putamen, 89
pyridostigmine, 220
pyridoxine dependency, 207,
    474*t*, 478*t*

Q fever, 357
quetiapine, 568
quiet sleep, 421
quisqualate-type receptor, 17

rabies, 348–349
radial glia, 55
radial microbrain, 58

radial nerve, 78, 83
    mononeuropathy, 191
radial tunnel syndrome, 191
radiation side effects, 556
radiculopathies, 193–195
    median nerve SSEPs, 439–440
Ramsay-Hunt syndrome, 343. *See also*
    progressive myoclonic ataxias
raphe nuclei, 9
rasagiline, 9, 305
Rasmussen's encephalitis, 263
Rathke cleft cyst, 549*t*
recent memory, 616
recent past memory, 616
receptor organs, 525
receptors, 3–4
red reflex, 504
reduplicative paramnesia, 608
reflex pathway, near, 104–105
Refsum's disease, 479
regeneration, 531
rehabilitation
    AIDP, 214
    aims of, 531–532
relative afferent pupil, 103
REM atonia, isolated, 456
remote memory, 616
REM sleep, 391–392, 421
    without atonia, 456
REM sleep behavior disorder (RBD), 396
REM-spindle sleep, 456
repetitive transcranial magnetic
    stimulation, 566
repolarization, 19
reserpine, 9
respiratory monitoring, 450–451
restless leg syndrome (RLS), 397, 398
restraints, 592
retinal vasculopathy with cerebral
    leukodystrophy (RCVL), 133
retinoblastoma, 31*t*, 546*t*
retrochiasmal visual pathways, 518–519
retroviruses, 353
Rett's syndrome, diagnosis, 601
reversible vasoconstriction syndrome
    (RCVS), 131
rexed laminas, 68
Reye's syndrome, 340, 486
rhabdomyolysis, 238–239
rheumatic fever, 362
rhodopsin, 442, 499
rhomboids, 76
rhythm therapy, 532
riluzole, 225
Rinne's test, 101, 527
risperidone, 568
rivastigmine, 306
Rocky Mountain spotted fever, 357
rods, 442*t*, 499
Romberg's test, 526
Rostral-Edinger-Westphal nucleus, 104

rotigotine, 305
rubella virus, 352, 485
rufinamide (Banzel®), 275t

saccades, 500, 503
sacral plexus, 84
salicylates, 529
Sandhoff disease, 467t
saphenous nerve, 85
sarcoidosis, 199–200
saxitoxin, 382
scarpa's ganglion, 526
Schilder's disease, 335
schizencephaly, 59
schizophrenia, 575–576, 604
schwann cells, 52, 547t
schwannomas, 547t
sciatic mononeuropathy, 187
sciatic nerve, 84, 86, 187
secondary generalized seizures, 262
secondary neurulation, disorders of,
    55, 57
second-order neurons, preganglionic, 501
seesaw nystagmus, 510–511
segmental demyelination, 186
seizures, 40–41t, 252–254
    definitions, 249
    differential diagnosis, 287–288
    incidence and prevalence, 249
    neonatal. See neonatal seizures
    partial. See partial seizures
    pediatric. See pediatric seizures
selective mutism, 604
selective serotonin reuptake inhibitors
    (SSRIs), 175
selegiline, 9, 305
self-injury in developmental disorders,
    medications for, 597
sella tumors, 518
semantic dementia, 175
semantic memory, 616
semicircular canal dehiscence, 527
sensorimotor axonal neuropathies,
    210–211
sensorineural hearing loss, 528
sensory axonal neuropathies,
    predominantly, 209
sensory neuronopathy, 205–206
separation anxiety, 603
septal region, 536
septo-optic dysplasia, 522
serotonin. See 5-hydroxytryptamine
    (5-HT)
serotonin and norepinephrine reuptake
    inhibitors (SNRIs), 565–566
serotonin-specific reuptake inhibitors
    (SSRIs), 564–565
serotonin syndrome, 565
serratus anterior, 76
sertraline, 565
shift-work sleep disorder, 393–394

shingles, 343
sialidosis, 258, 469t
sickle cell disease, 133
simple-partial status epilepticus, 159
simultanagnosia, 608
single gene sequencing, 29–30
skull, foramina of, 61–62t, 66f
sleep
    deprivation, 286, 420
    epilepsy associated with, 285–286
    neurology, 457–459
        polysomnography, 449–457
    and sleep disorders, 391–392
        pharmacology overview, 397–398
    terrors, 396
    wake cycle, 285
sleeping sickness, 371
sleep-onset REM periods, 456
sleep spindles, 107
sleep staging
    basic sleep staging, 451
    leg movement (LM) parameters and
        scoring, 457
    respiratory parameters and scoring, 456
    sleep onset and sleep cycles, 453–456
    sleep parameters and scoring, 452–453t
sleepwalking, 396
slow channel syndrome, 218
smooth pursuit, 503
snake venoms, 381
SNAP. See amplitude of sensory nerve
    AP (SNAP)
SNAP25, 4
SNARE proteins, 4
Sneddon syndrome, 134, 484
Snellen visual acuity test, 502–503
snoring, 394
sodium channel dysfunction, 20
sodium valproate (valproic acid [VA]),
    267–268t
somatic nervous system, 493
somatization disorder, 588–589
somatoform disorders, 588–589
somatosensory evoked potentials, 165
    general clinical interpretation, 436
    generators, 436
    median nerve, 436–440, 437f
    recording, 436
    stimulation parameters, 436
    surgical monitoring, 442
    tibial nerve, 440–441
    ulnar nerve, 440
somatostatin, 535
somatotropin release inhibiting factor, 535
somnambulism. See sleepwalking
spasmus nutans, 510
spasticity, motor impairment, 533
spina bifida, 56
spinal cord, 68, 71f, 73f
    ascending tracts of, 69f, 72t
    descending tracts, 69–70t, 69f

dorsal column lesion, 73
gray matter, 68–69
large central lesion, 72
positional changes in, 56
segments and divisions, 68
small central lesion, 72
white matter, 69
spinalmuscular atrophy (SMA),
    225–226, 479–480
spinal myoclonus, 317
spinal reflexes and muscle tone, 88–89
spinal shock, 75
spiral ganglion, 99
split-brain syndrome, 67
SSEPs. See somatosensory EPs (SSEPs)
Stanford-Binet Test, 614
status epilepticus (SE), 159–160, 283–285
    and sleep, 287
Steele-Richardson-Olszewski
    syndrome, 307
Steinert's disease. See myotonic dystrophy
stem cells, differentiation of, 327f
stereocilia, 525
stiff-person syndrome, 245, 559t, 560t
St. Louis encephalitis virus, 346–347
Strachan's syndrome, 201
strain gauge, 451
stress disorder, posttraumatic, 577–578
stretch reflex, 88–89
striatonigral degeneration, 306
stroke, 40–41t, 115–118
    acute stroke therapy, 125–127
    antiplatelets and anticoagulants,
        128–129t
    brain arteries, infectious and
        inflammatory disease of, 129–130
    cerebral vasculature, diseases
        involving, 131–132
    cerebrovascular disease, genetic
        syndromes in, 132–133
    clinical syndromes, 118–123
    lacunar stroke, 124
    other stroke etiologies, 133–134
    transient ischemic attack (TIA), 124
stroke, risk factors of, 116–118
stroop test, 615–616
struthers, ligament of, 82
strychnine, 15
Sturge-Weber syndrome, 483–484
subacute combined degeneration, 613
subacute necrotizing encephalopathy, 477t
subacute sclerosing panencephalitis,
    351–352, 485
subarachnoid hemorrhage, 154–157
subcortical center, 105
subcortical myoclonus, 316–317
subcutaneous lipomas, 57
subdural hematoma, 140–142
subependymal giant cell astrocytoma
    (SEGA), 542t
subependymoma, 543t

subscapular nerve, 78
substance P, 17
substance-related disorders, 587–588t
   amphetamines, 581–582
   caffeine, 582
   cocaine, 582–583
   EtOH, 578–581
   hallucinogens, 583
   inhalants, 584
   marijuana, 582
   nicotine, 584–585
   opioids, 585–587
   PCP, 583–584
   treatment, 571–572
substantianigra, 89
subthalamic nucleus, 89
sulcus limitans, 54
sumatriptan, 11
SUNA (short-lasting unilateral
      neuralgiform headache with
      cranial autonomic features), 182
SUNCT (short-lasting unilateral
      neuralgiform headache attacks
      with conjunctival injection and
      tearing), 181
superficial radial nerve, 83
superior cerebellar peduncle, 91
superior cervical ganglion, 502f
superior gluteal nerve, 86
superior olivary nucleus, 99
superior rectus and inferior oblique
      muscle, 499
supinator tunnel syndrome. See radial
      tunnel syndrome
supportive care
   AIDP, 214
   botulism, 223
   EBV, 344
   MG, 221
   neuromuscular junction disorders, 224
   VZV, 343
suprachiasmatic nucleus (SCN), 392
suprascapular nerve, 76
surface dyslexia, 67
Susac's syndrome, 134
swallowing and nutrition, visual
      impairment, 533
Sydenham's chorea, 314, 486
sympathetic pathway, 501
synaptic transmission, 19–20

Taenia solium, 371
Takayasu's disease, 130
tanycytes, 52
tardive dyskinesia, 7
tarsal tunnel syndrome, 87, 188–189
Tarui's disease, 480
TCAs. See tricyclic antidepressants (TCAs)
technetium 99
      hexamethylpropyleneamine
      oxime brain scan, 165

telencephalon, 54
temporal lobes
   damage, 609–610
   functions, 67
   sharp waves, 426f
temporal partial seizure, 260–261, 261f
tension-type headache, 179
teriflunomide (Aubagio®), 334
tetanus, 383
tetany, 244–245
tetrabenazine, 9
tetraethyl ammonium chloride, 20
tetrahydrobiopterin, 473t
thalamus, 91, 105–109
thallium, neurotoxicity of, 208, 376, 487
thiamine (B₁) deficiency syndromes, 580
third-order neurons, postganglionic, 501
thoracodorsal nerve, 78
thrombolysis therapy, 125–127
thrombosis of cerebral veins and venous
      sinuses, 133–134
thymectomy, 221
thyroid disorders, causing psychiatric
      symptoms, 614
thyroid myopathy, 231–232
thyroid ophthalmopathy, 506
thyrotropinomas, 538
thyrotropin-releasing hormone, 535
tibial nerve, 87, 440–442
tic disorders, 603
tin, neurotoxicity of, 378
tinnitus, 528–529
tissue plasminogen activator (tPA),
      neurological monitoring
      after, 149
T-lymphocytes, 327
token test, 617
Tolosa-Hunt syndrome, 509
tomaculous neuropathy, 211–212, 479
topiramate (Topamax®), 274–275t
topographic disorientation, 610
torsional nystagmus, 511
Tourette's disorder, 596–597, 603
toxic amblyopia, 517
toxins, 486–487
   animal, 381–382
   auditory, 529
   bacterial, 383–385
   causing neuropathies, 385, 517
   causing seizures, 386
   gases, 379
   heavy metals, 375–378
   industrial, 380
   organic solvents, 378–379
   organophosphates, 380
   plant, 382–383
   specific action of, 386
toxoplasmosis abscess, 358, 370–371, 485
trail-making test, 615
transcranial Doppler (TCD)
      monitoring, 156, 165

transcription, genetic, 23–24
transient ischemic attack (TIA), 115, 124
transient myasthenia, 482
translations, genetic, 24
transverse myelitis, 330
trazodone, 566
treponema pallidum, 75, 485
trichinosis, 231, 372
tricyclic antidepressants (TCAs), 9, 564
trigeminal ganglion, 98
trigeminal reflexes, 99
trigeminothalamic pathways, 98–99
trinucleotide-repeat diseases, 34t,
      310–311t. See also Huntington's
      disease
triphasic waves, 424, 424f
Triple-H therapy, 157
Trisomy 21, 598
trochlear nerve, 500
      palsy, 507–508
tropias, 503
trunk lesions, 78
trypanosomiasis, 371
tryptophan, 385
tuberculoid leprosy, 360
tuberous sclerosis (TS), 483
tumor. See also metastatic tumors
   classifications of, 552–554t
   of meninges, 547–548t
   of nerve sheath cells, 547t
   of sellar region, 550t
   of uncertain histogenesis, 548t
tuning fork tests, 100–101
tyrosine (TYR), 5

ulnar nerve, 77
   anatomy, 82
   clinical syndromes, 82–83
   mononeuropathy, 189–190, 190t
   SSEPs, 440
unethical behavior, 592
unilateral conduction deafness, 101
unilateral partial nerve deafness, 101
unilateral proptosis, 523
unruptured intracranial aneurysms,
      154–155
Unverricht-Lundborg disease, 256
upbeat nystagmus, 511
upper airway resistance syndrome
      (UARS), 394
upper trunk lesion, 78
uremic polyneuropathy, 203
Usher's syndrome, 530t

varicella, 343
varicella zoster virus (VZV), 343
Venezuelan EE virus, 346
venlafaxine, 565
venous anomaly development, 158
venous sinuses, thrombosis of, 133–134
ventral spinal artery occlusion, 75

ventral trigeminothalamic tract, 98–99
ventromedial nuclei, 535
VEPs. *See* Visual EPs (VEPs)
vertebral artery, 122
vestibular dysfunction, examination, 526
vestibular ganglion, 102
vestibular labyrinth, 525
vestibular nuclei, 101*f*, 102
vestibular system, 101–102
vestibulo-ocular reflex, 526
vestibulo-ocular response system, 500
vicarious functions, 531
vigabatrin, 277*t*
vilazodone, 566
vincristine, 207
viral encephalitis, 356. *See also*
    encephalitis
viral infections of nervous system,
    340–341
viral meningitis/encephalitis, 160
vision loss, 532
visual acuity, 502–503
visual agnosia, 532
visual cortex, 103
visual EPs (VEPs), 442–446
visual fields, 503
visual impairment, 532–533
visual system and pathways, disorders of
    AION, 515–516
    Graves' disease, 516
    infectious optic neuropathies, 517
    inflammatory optic neuropathies, 517
    Leber's optic neuropathy, 517–518
    ophthalmoscopic examination,
        517, 518
    optic disc edema, 513–515
    optic nerve gliomas, 517
    optic nerve sheath meningiomas,
        516–517
    optic neuritis, 515
    optic neuropathies, 517–518
    papilledema, 516
vitamin
    deficiencies, 388*t*
    metabolism, disorders of, 474–475*t*
vitamin B$_3$ deficiency, 580
vitamin B$_{12}$ deficiency, 75, 201, 613
vitamin E deficiency, 201
vitamin K antagonist, 152
vocal tic disorder, 603
voiding dysfunction classification
        system, 494
volume conduction, 402
von Hippel-Lindau syndrome, 484,
        548*t*, 559*t*
vortioxetine, 566

wakefulness, 391
    test, maintenance of, 458–459
Waldenström's macroglobulinemia,
        202–203
Walker-Warburg syndrome, 60
Wallenberg lateral medullary
        syndrome, 509
wallerian degeneration, 51, 186
warm-water caloric testing, 526
Weber's test, 100, 527
Wechsler Adult Intelligence Scale, 614
Wechsler Intelligence Scale for
        Children, 614
Werdnig-Hoffman spinal muscular
        atrophy, 479–480
Wernicke's encephalopathy, 580
western equine encephalitis (EE)
        virus, 346
West Nile virus, 226, 347
West's syndrome, 260
Whipple's disease, 362–363
white matter, 69
whole-exome sequencing (WES), 30
whole-genome chromosomal
        microarrays, 29
whole-genome sequencing
        (WGS), 31
Willebrand's knee, 518
Wilson's disease, 319, 613
Wisconsin Card Sorting
        Test, 614–615
witzelsucht, 607, 618
women, and epilepsy, 264–265
working memory, 616
World Health Organization, classification
        for diffuse gliomas, 541*t*

Xa inhibitor, 152
x-linked lissencephaly, 59
x-linked metabolic disease, 466
x-linked recessive patterns of
        inheritance, 27

ziprasidone, 568
zolpidem, 571
zonisamide (Zonegran®), 273–274*t*
zoster ophthalmicus, 343
zygomycosis, 366–367

Printed in the United States
By Bookmasters